ZOONOSES AND COMMUNICABLE DISEASES COMMON TO MAN AND ANIMALS

Third Edition

Volume III

Parasitoses

Scientific and Technical Publication No. 580

PAN AMERICAN HEALTH ORGANIZATION
Pan American Sanitary Bureau, Regional Office of the
WORLD HEALTH ORGANIZATION
525 Twenty-third Street, N.W.
Washington, D.C. 20037 U.S.A.

2003

Also published in Spanish (2003) with the title:
Zoonosis y enfermedades transmisibles comunes al hombre y a los animales:
parasitosis
ISBN 92 75 31991 X (3 volume set)
ISBN 92 75 31992 8 (Vol. 3)

PAHO HQ Library Cataloguing-in-Publication
Pan American Health Organization
   Zoonoses and communicable diseases common to man and animals:
parasitoses
3rd ed. Washington, D.C.: PAHO, © 2003.
3 vol.—(Scientific and Technical Publication No. 580)

ISBN 92 75 11991 0—3 volume set
ISBN 92 75 11993 7—Vol. 3
I. Title II. (Series)
1. ZOONOSES
2. PARASITIC DISEASES
3. DISEASE RESERVOIRS
4. COMMUNICABLE DISEASE CONTROL
5. FOOD CONTAMINATION
6. PUBLIC HEALTH VETERINARY
NLM WC950.P187 2003 v.3 En

This volume was updated by Omar O. Barriga, Professor of Parasitology in the Faculty of Medicine of the University of Chile, and consultant for PAHO's Veterinary Public Health Unit from 1997 to 2001.

CONTENTS

2. Cestodiases

3. Acanthocephaliases and Nematodiases

Section C: ARTHROPODS

LIST OF TABLES

Protozooses

Tables

Helminthiases

Arthropods

PROLOGUE

In recent years, zoonoses and communicable diseases common to man and animals have gained increasing attention worldwide. Human diseases that have their origins in infected animals, such as AIDS or Creutzfeldt-Jakob, have highlighted the need for a better understanding of animal diseases in terms of their epidemiology, mechanism of transmission to man, diagnosis, prevention, and control. Social and demographic changes have also contributed to the importance of gaining and disseminating knowledge about zoonoses. For instance, as people encroach further and further on ecological areas with which they had little contact and whose fauna may not be well known, their exposure to animals—and the infections they transmit—has increased. New knowledge is also being developed in the area of urban ecology. The ease and speed of modern travel also facilitates the spread of diseases once confined to specific geographic areas, as recently occurred with severe acute respiratory syndrome (SARS). Animal migration and trade pose a similar threat, as was shown by the outbreaks in the United States of West Nile fever, and most recently, monkeypox—two diseases not previously known in the Western Hemisphere. Each of these examples highlights the need for improved knowledge and surveillance of and response to zoonoses.

The negative effects of zoonoses are far reaching. High incidence rates continue to cause significant morbidity and mortality in both humans and animals. Their economic impact is seen in lost labor productivity due to illness; reduced travel and tourism to affected areas; reduced livestock and food production; death and destruction of affected animals; and restrictions on and reductions in international trade. Zoonoses can be a serious drain on a country's economy, which in turn can have wide repercussions for a society's health.

To help solve these problems, the Pan American Health Organization (PAHO)—an international public health organization that has devoted itself to improving the health and living conditions of the people of the Americas for over one hundred years—established the Veterinary Public Health Unit. The Unit's overall objective is to collaborate with PAHO's Member Governments in the development, implementation, and evaluation of policies and programs that lead to food safety and protection and to the prevention, control, or eradication of zoonoses, among them foot-and-mouth disease.

To this end, PAHO's Veterinary Public Health Unit has two specialized regional centers: the Pan American Foot-and-Mouth Disease Center (PANAFTOSA), created in 1951 in Rio de Janeiro, Brazil, and the Pan American Institute for Food Protection and Zoonoses (INPPAZ), established on November 15, 1991, in Buenos Aires, Argentina. INPPAZ's precursor was the Pan American Zoonoses Center (CEPANZO), which was created through an agreement with the Government of Argentina to help the countries of the Americas combat zoonoses, and which operated from 1956 until 1990.

Since its creation in 1902, PAHO has participated in various technical cooperation activities with the countries, among them those related to the surveillance, prevention, and control of zoonoses and communicable diseases common to man and animals, which cause high morbidity, disability, and mortality in vulnerable human populations. PAHO has also collaborated in the strengthening of preventive medi-

vii

cine and public health through the promotion of veterinary health education in learning, research, and health care centers. An example of this work is the preparation of several publications, among which the two previous Spanish and English editions of *Zoonoses and Communicable Diseases Common to Man and Animals* stand out.

Scientific knowledge has progressed since the last edition was published in 1986. Also, the countries of the Americas have modified their livestock production strategies in recent years, which has affected the transmission of zoonotic infections and their distribution. The publication of this third edition is an attempt to address these changes. The third edition is presented in three volumes: the first contains bacterioses and mycoses; the second, chlamydioses, rickettsioses, and viroses; and the third, parasitoses.

We believe that this new edition will continue to be useful for professors and students of public health, medicine, veterinary medicine, and rural development; workers in public health and animal health institutions; and veterinarians, researchers, and others interested in the subject. We also hope that this publication is a useful tool in the elaboration of national zoonosis control or eradication policies and programs, as well as in risk evaluation and in the design of epidemiological surveillance systems for the prevention and timely control of emerging and reemerging zoonoses. In summary, we are confident that this book will contribute to the application of the knowledge and resources of the veterinary sciences for the protection and improvement of public health.

MIRTA ROSES PERIAGO
DIRECTOR

PREFACE TO THE FIRST EDITION

This book considers two groups of communicable diseases: those transmitted from vertebrate animals to man, which are—strictly speaking—zoonoses; and those common to man and animals. In the first group, animals play an essential role in maintaining the infection in nature, and man is only an accidental host. In the second group, both animals and man generally contract the infection from the same sources, such as soil, water, invertebrate animals, and plants; as a rule, however, animals do not play an essential role in the life cycle of the etiologic agent, but may contribute in varying degrees to the distribution and actual transmission of infections.

No attempt has been made to include all infections and diseases comprised in these two groups. A selection has been made of some 150 that are of principal interest, for various reasons, in the field of public health. The number of listed zoonoses is increasing as new biomedical knowledge is acquired. Moreover, as human activity extends into unexplored territories containing natural foci of infection, new zoonotic diseases are continually being recognized. In addition, improved health services and better differential diagnostic methods have distinguished zoonoses previously confused with other, more common diseases. A number of diseases described in this book have only recently been recognized, examples of which include the Argentine and Bolivian hemorrhagic fevers, angiostrongyliasis, rotaviral enteritis, Lassa fever, Marburg disease, and babesiosis.

The principal objective in writing this book was to provide the medical professions a source of information on the zoonoses and communicable diseases common to man and animals. Toward that end, both medical and veterinary aspects, which have traditionally been dealt with separately in different texts, have been combined in a single, comprehensive volume. As a result, physicians, veterinarians, epidemiologists, and biologists can all gain an overview of these diseases from one source.

This book, like most scientific works, is the product of many books, texts, monographs, and journal articles. Many sources of literature in medicine, veterinary medicine, virology, bacteriology, mycology, and parasitology were consulted, as were a large number of reports from different biomedical disciplines, in order to provide up-to-date and concise information on each disease. It is expected that any errors or omissions that may have been committed can, with the collaboration of the readers, be corrected in a future edition.

Where possible, explanations were attempted with special emphasis on the Americas, particularly Latin America. An effort was made, one which was not always successful, to collect available information on diseases in this Region. Data on the incidence of many zoonoses are fragmentary and frequently not reliable. It is hoped that the establishment of control programs in various countries will lead to improved epidemiologic surveillance and disease reporting.

More space has been devoted to those zoonoses having greatest impact on public health and on the economy of the countries of the Americas, but information is also included on those regionally less important or exotic diseases.

The movement of persons and animals over great distances adds to the risk of introducing exotic diseases that may become established on the American continent given the appropriate ecologic factors for existence of the etiologic agents. Today, public health and animal health administrators, physicians, and veterinarians must be familiar with the geographic distribution and pathologic manifestations of the various infectious agents so that they can recognize and prevent the introduction of exotic diseases.

We, the authors, would like to give special recognition to Dr. Joe R. Held, Assistant Surgeon-General of the United States Public Health Service and Director of the Division of Research Services of the U.S. National Institutes of Health, who gave impetus to the English translation and reviewed the bacterioses sections.

We would also like to express our utmost appreciation to the experts who reviewed various portions of this book and offered their suggestions for improving the text. These include: Dr. Jeffrey F. Williams, Professor in the Department of Microbiology and Public Health, Michigan State University, who reviewed the chapters dealing with parasitic zoonoses; Dr. James Bond, PAHO/WHO Regional Adviser in Viral Diseases, who read the viroses; Dr. Antonio Pío, formerly PAHO/WHO Regional Adviser in Tuberculosis and presently with WHO in Geneva, and Dr. James H. Rust, PAHO/WHO Regional Adviser in Enteric Diseases, both of whom reviewed the bacterioses; and Dr. F. J. López Antuñano, PAHO/WHO Regional Adviser in Parasitic Diseases, who read the metazooses.

We would like to thank Dr. James Cocozza, PAHO/WHO Veterinary Adviser, for his review of the translation and Dr. Judith Navarro, Editor in the Office of Publications of PAHO, for her valuable collaboration in the editorial revision and composition of the book.

PEDRO N. ACHA
BORIS SZYFRES

PREFACE TO THE SECOND EDITION

The fine reception accorded the Spanish, English, and French versions of this book has motivated us to revise it in order that it still may serve the purpose for which it was written: to provide an up-to-date source of information to the medical profession and allied fields. This book has undoubtedly filled a void, judging by its wide use in schools of public health, medicine, and veterinary medicine, as well as by bureaus of public and animal health.

The present edition has been considerably enlarged. In the seven years since the first edition was published, our knowledge of zoonoses has increased broadly and rapidly, and new zoonotic diseases have emerged. Consequently, most of the discussions have been largely rewritten, and 28 new diseases have been added to the original 148. Some of these new diseases are emerging zoonoses; others are pathologic entities that have been known for a long time, but for which the epidemiologic connection between man and animal has been unclear until recently.

The use this book has had outside the Western Hemisphere has caused us to abandon the previous emphasis on the Americas in favor of a wider scope and geomedical view. Moreover, wars and other conflicts have given rise to the migration of populations from one country or continent to another. A patient with a disease heretofore known only in Asia may now turn up in Amsterdam, London, or New York. The physician must be aware of these diseases in order to diagnose and treat them. "Exotic" animal diseases have been introduced from Africa to Europe, the Caribbean, and South America, causing great damage. The veterinary physician must learn to recognize them to be able to prevent and eradicate them before they become entrenched. It must be remembered that parasites, viruses, bacteria, and other agents of zoonotic infection can take up residence in any territory where they find suitable ecologic conditions. Ignorance, economic or personal interests, and human customs and needs also favor the spread of these diseases.

Research in recent years has demonstrated that some diseases previously considered to be exclusively human have their counterparts in wild animals, which in certain circumstances serve as sources of human infection. On the other hand, these animals may also play a positive role by providing models for research, such as in the case of natural leprosy in nine-banded armadillos or in nonhuman primates in Africa. Of no less interest is the discovery of *Rickettsia prowazekii* in eastern flying squirrels and in their ectoparasites in the United States, and the transmission of the infection to man in a country where epidemic typhus has not been seen since 1922. A possible wild cycle of dengue fever is also discussed in the book. Is Creutzfeldt-Jakob disease a zoonosis? No one can say with certainty, but some researchers believe it may have originated as such. In any case, interest is aroused by the surprising similarity of this disease and of kuru to animal subacute spongiform encephalopathies, especially scrapie, the first known and best studied of this group. Discussion of human and animal slow viruses and encephalopathies is included in the spirit of openness to possibilities and the desire to bring the experience of one field of medicine to another. In view of worldwide concern over acquired immunodeficiency syndrome (AIDS), a brief section on retroviruses has also been added, in which the relationship between the human disease and feline and simian AIDS is noted. Another topic deeply interesting to researchers is the mystery of the radical antigenic changes of type A influenza virus, a cause of explosive pandemics that affect millions of persons around the world. Evidence is mounting that these changes result from recombination with a virus of animal origin (see Influenza). That this should occur is not surprising, given the constant interaction between man and animals. As a rule, zoonoses are transmitted from animal to man, but the reverse may also occur, as is pointed out in the chapters on hepatitis, herpes simplex, and measles. The victims in these cases are nonhuman primates, which may in turn retransmit the infection to man under certain circumstances.

Among emerging zoonoses we cite Lyme disease, which was defined as a clinical entity in 1977; the etiologic agent was found to be a spirochete (isolated in 1982), for which the name *Borrelia burgdorferi* was recently proposed. Emerging viral zoonoses of note in Latin America are Rocio encephalitis and Oropouche fever; the latter has caused multiple epidemics with thousands of victims in northeast Brazil. Outstanding among new viral disease problems in Africa are the emergence of Ebola disease and the spread of Rift Valley fever virus, which has caused tens of thousands of human cases along with great havoc in the cattle industry of Egypt and has evoked alarm around the world. Similarly, the protozoan *Cryptosporidium* is emerging as one of the numerous agents of diarrheal diseases among man and animals, and probably has a worldwide distribution.

As the English edition was being prepared, reports came to light of two animal diseases not previously confirmed in humans. Three cases of human pseudorabies virus infection were recognized between 1983 and 1986 in two men and one woman who had all had close contact with cats and other domestic animals. In 1986, serologic testing confirmed infection by *Ehrlichia canis* in a 51-year-old man who had been suspected of having Rocky Mountain spotted fever. This is the first known occurrence of *E. canis* infection in a human. These two diseases bear watching as possible emerging zoonoses.

The space given to each zoonosis is in proportion to its importance. Some diseases that deserve their own monographs were given more detailed treatment, but no attempt was made to cover the topic exhaustively.

We, the authors, would like to give special recognition to Dr. Donald C. Blenden, Professor in the Department of Medicine and Infectious Diseases, School of Medicine, and Head of the Department of Veterinary Microbiology, College of Veterinary Medicine, University of Missouri; and to Dr. Manuel J. Torres, Professor of Epidemiology and Public Health, Department of Veterinary Microbiology, College of Veterinary Medicine, University of Missouri, for their thorough review of and valuable contributions to the English translation of this book.

We would also like to recognize the support received from the Pan American Health Organization (PAHO/WHO), the Pan American Health and Education Foundation (PAHEF), and the Pan American Zoonoses Center in Buenos Aires, Argentina, which enabled us to update this book.

We are most grateful to Dr. F. L. Bryan for his generous permission to adapt his monograph "Diseases Transmitted by Foods" as an Appendix to this book.

Mr. Carlos Larranaga, Chief of the Audiovisual Unit at the Pan American Zoonosis Center, deserves our special thanks for the book's artwork, as do Ms. Iris Elliot and Mr. William A. Stapp for providing the translation into English. We would like to express our most sincere gratitude and recognition to Ms. Donna J. Reynolds, editor in the PAHO Editorial Service, for her valuable collaboration in the scientific editorial revision of the book.

PEDRO N. ACHA
BORIS SZYFRES

INTRODUCTION

This new edition of *Zoonoses and Communicable Diseases Common to Man and Animals* is published in three volumes: I. Bacterioses and mycoses; II. Chlamydioses and rickettsioses, and viroses; and III. Parasitoses. Each of the five parts corresponds to the location of the etiologic agents in the biological classification; for practical purposes, chlamydias and rickettsias are grouped together.

In each part, the diseases are listed in alphabetical order to facilitate reader searches. There is also an alphabetical index, which includes synonyms of the diseases and the etiologic agents' names.

In this edition, the numbers and names of the diseases according to the *International Statistical Classification of Diseases and Related Health Problems*, Tenth Revision (ICD-10), are listed below the disease title. However, some zoonoses are not included in ICD-10 and are difficult to classify within the current scheme.

In addition, for each disease or infection, elements such as synonyms; etiology; geographical distribution; occurrence in man and animals; the disease in man and animals; source of infection and mode of transmission; role of animals in the epidemiology; diagnosis; and control are addressed. Patient treatment (for man or other species) is beyond the scope of this work; however, recommended medicines are indicated for many diseases, especially where they are applicable to prophylaxis. Special attention is paid to the epidemiological and ecological aspects so that the reader can begin to understand the determining factors of the infection or disease. Some topics include simple illustrations of the etiologic agent's mode of transmission, showing the animals that maintain the cycle of infection in nature. Similarly, other graphics and tables are included to provide additional information on the geographical distribution or prevalence of certain zoonoses.

The data on the occurrence of the infection in man and animals, along with data on the geographical distribution, may help the reader judge the relative impact that each disease has on public health and the livestock economy in the different regions of the world, given that the importance of different zoonoses varies greatly. For example, foot-and-mouth disease is extremely important from an economic standpoint, but of little importance in terms of public health, if animal protein losses are not considered. In contrast, Argentine and Machupo hemorrhagic fevers are important human diseases, but their economic impact is minimal, if treatment costs and loss of man-hours are not taken into account. Many other diseases, such as brucellosis, leptospirosis, salmonellosis, and equine encephalitis, are important from both a public health and an economic standpoint.

Finally, each disease entry includes an alphabetical bibliography, which includes both the works cited and other relevant works that the reader may consult for more information about the disease.

Section A

PROTOZOOSES

AFRICAN TRYPANOSOMIASIS

ICD-10 B56 African trypanosomiasis; B56.0 Gambiense trypanosomiasis;
B56.1 Rhodesiense trypanosomiasis;
B56.9 African trypanosomiasis, unspecified

Synonyms: Sleeping sickness, trypanosomiasis; *gambiense* trypanosomiasis: infection due to *Trypanosoma brucei gambiense*, West African sleeping sickness; *rhodesiense* trypanosomiasis: infection due to *Trypanosoma brucei rhodesiense*, East African sleeping sickness.

Etiology: African trypanosomiasis in man is caused by two subspecies of *Trypanosoma (Trypanozoon) brucei*: *T. brucei gambiense* and *T. brucei rhodesiense*, both of which are transmitted by the bite of tsetse flies (genus *Glossina*) (Bales, 1991; Dumas and Bouteille, 1996; Chimelli and Scaravilli, 1997). These trypanosomes are considered to belong to the salivarian group because of the way in which they are transmitted through the vector's bite. Infection caused directly by a bite is considered inoculative, or via the anterior station, as opposed to contaminative, or via the posterior station, when the infection is transmitted by means of the fly's excrement (see the chapter on Chagas' Disease).

The two subspecies that affect man, *T. b. gambiense* and *T. b. rhodesiense*, as well as *T. b. brucei*, are morphologically indistinguishable. The latter species, while it does not affect man, is pathogenic for domestic animals in Africa, such as donkeys, horses, goats, camels, mules, sheep, dogs, and cattle. The forms that are present in blood, cerebrospinal fluid, and lymph are pleomorphic trypomastigotes (see Chagas' Disease). The forms range from long, thin parasites (measuring 30 μm by 1.5 μm on average, with a subterminal kinetoplast, a long flagellum extending from the anterior tip of the body, and an undulating membrane between the flagellum and the body) to short, fat parasites (averaging 15 μm by 3.5 μm, with a near-terminal kinetoplast and no external flagellum). The long forms multiply in the fluids of the definitive host by binary longitudinal division. The short forms are the infective elements for the vector and do not divide in the human host.

For a long time, the three subspecies *T. b. brucei*, *T. b. gambiense*, and *T. b. rhodesiense* were distinguished on the basis of their infectivity and pathogenicity for rats, their sensitivity to the drug tryparsamide, and their pathogenicity for man. To make a definitive distinction between *T. b. brucei* and the human trypanosomes, human volunteers were employed, with the consequent risks. In practice, differentiation between the two human pathogens is still fundamentally based on the course and geographic distribution of the infection. Now more precise techniques are available for identifying the parasites. The blood incubation infectivity test (BIIT) consists of incubating the trypanosomes in human serum or plasma and then inoculating them in rats. In this procedure, *T. b. brucei* loses its infectivity for rats whereas the subspecies that affect humans maintain it. Nevertheless, studies have revealed wide variation in the susceptibility of these trypanosomes to the effects of human serum, and some evidence exists that *T. b. brucei* can become resistant to the action of the serum. This would mean that *T. b. brucei* could become infective for man when flies infected by animals feed on human blood (Minter, 1982). Another important and increasingly used method is characterization of the trypanosomes according to the electrophoretic movement of their isozymes, which makes it possible to distinguish the different zymodemes (see definition under Chagas' Disease). Truc and Tybayrenc (1993) have described 23 zymodemes in Central Africa, which can be divided into two groups, one corresponding to *T. b. gambiense* and the other to *T. b. brucei*. Recent findings suggest that the different zymodemes are related not only to the species but also to the geographic distribution and clinical characteristics of the infection (Smith and Bailey, 1997). Also, the use of polymerase chain reaction has made it possible to identify *T. b. gambiense* (Schares and Mehlitz, 1996).

In man, the trypanosomes of African trypanosomiasis multiply in the blood, lymph, cerebrospinal fluid, and intercellular spaces, but they do not penetrate cells. In the vector, the short, fat trypanosomes consumed in the process of ingesting a blood meal multiply in the lumen of the mid and hindgut for about 10 days, after which they turn into thin forms and migrate toward the proventriculus, where they multiply for another 10 days; from there they travel to the salivary glands, where they attach themselves to the epithelial cells and turn into epimastigotes (see Chagas' Disease). The epimastigotes continue to multiply and are rapidly transformed into short, fat, metacyclic trypomastigotes, sometimes without a flagellum, which are the forms that are infective for man. Although the complete cycle of the trypanosome inside the tsetse fly can range from 15 to 35 days (average 21 days), the infection cycle up to the formation of metacyclic trypomastigotes is completed in only about 10% of the flies that ingest the parasite. The infected flies remain so for the rest of their lives and inoculate trypanosomes every time they take a blood meal.

Geographic Distribution: African trypanosomiasis in man occurs between 15° N and 20° S Latitude in Africa, which is the vector's area of distribution. *T. b. rhodesiense* is found in multiple foci in eastern Africa over an area stretching from Ethiopia to Botswana, while *T. b. gambiense* is found in central and western Africa, from northwestern Senegal to northeastern Sudan in the north to Angola in the south. Outside the endemic area, there are occasional cases in tourists and immigrants from endemic countries.

Occurrence in Man: In the past, there were devastating epidemics of *gambiense* trypanosomiasis, brought on by the migration of settlers during colonization. At the beginning of the twentieth century, 500,000 people died within a decade in the Congo basin alone, and there were about 200,000 fatalities (two-thirds of the population) in the province of Busoga, Uganda (Goodwin, 1970). Following the implementation of control measures, by 1950 and 1960 prevalence of the disease had dropped to very low levels in some areas (0.1% to 2%) and annual incidence was estimated at less than 10,000 cases. In 1972, there were 4,126 new cases in the Democratic Republic of Congo (formerly Zaire) and 3,000 in the rest of Africa (De Raadt, 1976). However, starting in the 1970s, the disease flared up again alarmingly in some of its old foci (Kusoe, 1993; Cattand, 1994; Jusot *et al.*, 1995). This increase was a reflection of the massive new movements of people both within and outside the endemic areas as a result of wars and social and political instability in many African countries. The situation was aggravated by shortages of human and material resources for surveillance and medical care programs in the affected countries (Mhlanga, 1996). In 1982, the World Health Organization (WHO) reported that *gambiense* trypanosomiasis was endemic in 23 African countries, 45 million inhabitants were at risk, and that every year there were nearly 10,000 new infections (*Bull World Health Organ*, 1982). Currently, African trypanosomiasis in man is endemic in 36 African countries south of the Sahara; the two forms of the disease together pose a risk for approximately 50 million people; and about 25,000 new cases are being reported annually, with the likelihood that not all cases were being notified (Bales, 1991; Kusoe, 1993).

Gambiense trypanosomiasis, which is chronic, tends to occur in epidemics, whereas *rhodesiense* trypanosomiasis, which has a more acute course, occurs sporadically, and gives rise to far fewer epidemics. The latter infection is endemic among livestock-raising tribes in eastern Africa and frequently affects hunters, fishermen, and travelers. Overall incidence is rather low because the people avoid areas infested by the vector.

The Disease in Man: The human disease usually has three phases: the primary lesion, parasitemia, and invasion of the central nervous system. Two or three days after the bite of an infected fly, a painful inflammation (chancre) appears at the inoculation site, and it disappears after two to three weeks (McGovern *et al.*, 1995). The primary lesion is observed more frequently in infections caused by *T. b. rhodesiense* than in those produced by *T. b. gambiense*. From the chancre site, the trypanosomes invade the bloodstream, and the patient suffers from irregular and intermittent fever, mirroring the waves of parasitemia. Other signs during this acute period are painless adenopathies, especially in the posterior cervical lymph nodes, as well as edema of the eyelids and joints. The most common symptoms of the acute phase are cephalalgia, insomnia, arthralgia, weight loss, and generalized erythema and pruritus, particularly in the sternal region. In later stages of the disease, the symptomatology is related to the affected organ. Invasion of the central nervous system is common, and a large variety of psychological, motor, and sensory perturbations may be seen. Following the meningitis that develops early in the course of the infection, a rupture occurs in the choroid plexus which allows the parasites to invade sites in the brain. The result is encephalitis, consisting of generalized inflammation with perivascular infiltrations of B and T lymphocytes, plasmocytes, and macrophages. The blood-brain barrier becomes permeable, and this condition may give rise to vasogenic cerebral edema. Astrocytes and microglia are activated, and, together with immune cells, they begin to produce cytokines, which also contribute to progression of the disease (Pentreath *et al.*, 1994). There is irritability, paresthesia, and insomnia, and later on, cerebral edema can cause severe headaches and edema of the optic papillae. There can also be neurologic manifestations such as epileptic seizures, chorea, psychotic episodes, euphoria, somnolence, lethargy, and coma.

As it was noted earlier, *gambiense* trypanosomiasis usually follows a slow and chronic course. Weeks or months may elapse between the first and second phase, and months or years may elapse between the second and third phase. *Rhodesiense* trypanosomiasis has a more acute course and its phases are less marked; death may come within a few months, in contrast to patients with *T. b. gambiense* infection, who can live for many years. Cardiac complications are more common in *rhodesiense* trypanosomiasis, and some patients die before reaching the neurologic phase (Greenwood and Whittle, 1980; WHO, 1979).

Both forms of African trypanosomiasis severely alter the patient's immune system. The main characteristics are synthesis of large amounts of gamma globulin, autoantibody formation, and immunodeficiency (Vincendeau *et al.*, 1996). The parasites in the bloodstream are covered with variable glycoprotein surface antigen (VGSA), which generates powerful immune responses that rapidly suppress parasitemia. These responses include antibody production and activation of macrophages that produce tumor necrosis factor alpha (TNF-α) and nitric acid (NO). Some parasites, however, manage to express another of the more than 1,000 genes coded for this antigen and are covered with a different glycoprotein, thereby initiating a new wave of parasitemia. These waves recur every 7 to 15 days until the patient, if left untreated, dies. The succession of new antigens is a powerful stimulus for the immune response, which participates in both the defense and the pathology of the disease. Although there is epidemiologic evidence of protective immunity in *gambiense* trypanosomiasis (Khonde *et al.*, 1995), individual antigenic variation is effective protection for the parasite against the immunity of the host. In terms of immunopathology, there is no evidence that high gamma globulin levels or an abundance of immune complexes play an important role in pathology of the human disease. Nevertheless, there is experimental evidence suggesting that autoantibodies to components of the central nervous system, such as anti-galactocerebrosides and tryptophan anti-analogous antibodies, may play a part in the development of encephalitis (Hunter *et al.*, 1992). Although T lymphocytes diminish the parasite's capacity to proliferate, they continue to produce gamma interferon (IFN-γ). The macrophages and astrocytes, for their part, produce TNF-α. Although IFN-γ and TNF-α, together with their specific antibodies and the NO of the macrophages, have powerful properties to fight the trypanosomes, it has been demonstrated that TNF-α levels are directly related to the severity of the disease (Okomo-Assoumou *et al.*, 1995).

The Disease in Animals: Infections caused by African trypanosomes in animals have a variety of local names, but they are most often referred to as *nagana*. *T. b. gambiense* has been inoculated in or isolated occasionally from animals, including laboratory animals, antelopes, swine, chickens, dogs, and cows, but there is no evidence that it causes disease or sustained parasitemia. However, *T. b. rhodesiense* can cause an infection, which is usually asymptomatic, in domestic animals such as cattle and sheep; wild animals, including antelopes, hyenas, and lions; and also laboratory animals. *T. b. brucei*, on the other hand, infects a wide variety of animals, including carnivores, swine, equines, ruminants, and laboratory animals. It causes an important disease in camels, equines, cats, dogs, and small ruminants. The disease is chronic and occasionally fatal in cattle; it is rarely fatal in swine. Man is resistant to the infection. There are other African trypanosomes of great importance for domestic animals, but none of them infects man (Levine, 1985): *T. congolense* affects carnivores, swine, equines, and ruminants; *T. vivax* affects equines and ruminants; and *T. simiae* affects camels and swine. The primary symptoms in animals are lymphadenopathy, intermittent fever, anemia, and progressive emaciation (Urquhart, 1980). Depending on the species, the age of the host, and the parasite load, the disease may be acute or chronic.

Trypanosomiasis in animals has played a role in configuring African societies: awareness of the parasite's fatal effect on horses protected the original inhabitants from foreign invasions, while its effect on cattle has prevented ranchers from taking advantage of 7 million km² of pastureland to raise high-yield European cattle. Another form of trypanosomiasis that occurs both in Africa and outside the continent is caused by *T. evansi*. It is transmitted by tabanid flies and is especially pathogenic for camels, equines, and dogs.

Source of Infection and Mode of Transmission: Man is the main reservoir of *T. b. gambiense* and the source of infection for the vector. Because the infection is prolonged and includes intervals between febrile attacks during which the patient feels relatively well, affected individuals may move about and propagate the infection in new areas where the vectors exist. There is no evidence that lower animals play a role in human *T. b. gambiense* infection, even though animal-to-animal transmission has been demonstrated in the laboratory (Molyneux, 1983) and parasites from swine, sheep, and dogs have been shown to be identical to human parasites in their sensitivity to human sera or their isoenzymatic profile (Scott *et al.*, 1983; Schares and Mehlitz, 1996). The success of control programs aimed exclusively at eliminating the human parasite would indicate that animal reservoirs are not important in *gambiense* trypanosomiasis. Nevertheless, the presence of animal reservoirs could account for maintenance of the *T. b. gambiense* infection in areas where isolated human cases have occurred with long intervals between them.

The main vectors of *T. b. gambiense* infection are the tsetse flies *Glossina fuscipes, G. palpalis*, and *G. tachinoide*. These species belong to the *palpalis*, or riverine, group of flies, which inhabit dense vegetation along the shores of rivers and lakes. Human infection occurs almost always in the vicinity of watercourses or places where water pools in rural settings; tourists are rarely affected. The male and female tsetse flies are biological vectors, but they can transmit the infection mechanically during epidemics, when there are many patients with parasitemia. In general, the infection rate in the vectors is low. In addition, according to some reports, congenital transmission can occur in man.

By contrast, in the case of *rhodesiense* trypanosomiasis, lower animals, especially cattle, play an important role as reservoirs. *T. b. rhodesiense* has been isolated from a number of wild and domestic animals; but only antelopes, hyenas, lions, sheep, and cattle develop sufficiently high and prolonged parasitemia to serve as effective reservoirs. These animals are responsible for persistence of the parasite in areas that have not been inhabited by humans for years.

The main vectors in eastern Africa are *Glossina morsitans, G. pallidipes*, and *G. swynnertoni*. These species belong to the *morsitans* group of flies, which inhabit savannahs and forested areas and prefer to feed on cattle and wild animals. The more acute nature of the human infection, coupled with the fact that the habitat of the vectors is not near homes, makes *rhodesiense* trypanosomiasis more sporadic than the *gambiense* form and less capable of causing epidemics. The main victims of the *rhodesiense* form are hunters, tourists, and persons who have contact with wild animal habitats where the infection is enzootic.

Diagnosis: The disease may be suspected when its main symptoms and signs are present, in particular intermittent fever, enlarged posterior cervical lymph glands, and cutaneous erythema. Biochemical tests do not reveal any remarkable alterations except higher cell counts and increased IgM in cerebrospinal fluid, which are considered pathognomonic of invasion of the central nervous system (Bisser *et al.*, 1997). The infection is confirmed by demonstrating the presence of the parasite in aspirate from the chancre or the lymph glands, in bone marrow, or in blood taken during the acute phase, or cerebrospinal fluid during the chronic phase. The sample to be observed may be either fresh or fixed and stained. In acute-phase patients, aspiration of the lymph glands is more effective for detecting *T. b. gambiense* than *T. b. rhodesiense*. On the other hand, peripheral parasitemia is higher in *rhodesiense* than in *gambiense* trypanosomiasis, and it is therefore easier to demonstrate the presence of *T. b. rhodesiense* by examining thick blood films. In both cases, however, the levels of parasitemia fluctuate and are higher during febrile attacks. It is easier to find parasites in blood by centrifugation in hematocrit tubes and examination of the leukocyte layer, or by minifiltration in DEAE-cellulose, centrifugation, and examination of the exudate (Bailey and Smith, 1994). To demonstrate the presence of *T. b. rhodesiense,* samples of blood or cerebrospinal fluid can be inoculated intraperitoneally in mice, which develop detectable parasitemia within the second week. It is difficult to infect rodents with *T. b. gambiense.* When the foregoing methods have been unsuccessful, an attempt may be made to examine bone marrow or culture it in special media such as glucose, lacto-albumin, serum, hemoglobin, or GLSH. Sediment from cerebrospinal fluid should be examined immediately after it is collected. Serologic reactions such as the card agglutination test, indirect hemagglutination, enzyme-linked immunosorbent assay (ELISA), and indirect immunofluorescence are useful for epidemiologic studies, but they are of limited value for individual diagnosis: healthy individuals may have developed antibodies to animal trypanosomes inoculated by tsetse flies which did not produce infection, and these antibodies can cross-react with the antigens of *T. b. gambiense* and *T. b. rhodesiense.*

Control: The two main approaches to controlling the African trypanosomiases are to reduce the principal reservoirs of infection and the presence of the vectors. In diminishing the reservoirs of *gambiense* trypanosomiasis, detecting and treating the human infection should be emphasized to reduce the source of infection for the vectors. The challenge is greater with *rhodesiense* trypanosomiasis, because measures must also be taken to control the livestock population, both wild (e.g., antelopes) and domestic (e.g., cattle). The latter can be reduced by converting the savannahs where livestock graze into cropland, which is not propitious for the proliferation of tsetse flies. Reduction of the vector population, which is much more efficient in controlling *rhodesiense* trypanosomiasis, can be achieved either through the targeted destruction of the flies' habitats or the use of insecticides. Both approaches, however, can cause major ecologic changes. Moreover, the mass use of insecticides is costly and not very efficient, because the flies are protected by vegetation in their habitats. Tsetse fly traps have been developed that are very effective, especially when they are impregnated with insecticides (Langley, 1994). Another approach would be to saturate the natural environment with male flies sterilized in the laboratory, which was successful in eradicating the fly *Cochliomyia hominivorax* in Libya in 1991. Empirical observations and mathematical models suggest that reducing the vector population is most efficient during epidemics, while reducing the human reservoir is more effective in endemic situations (Gouteux and Artzrouni, 1996). Other appropriate measures include preventing host-vector contact by the use of protective clothing, netting that keeps out flies, repellants, or simply not going into areas where there are high densities of tsetse flies. In highly endemic areas, the indiscriminate donation of blood should be prohibited. Chemoprophylaxis for visitors to endemic areas is not recommended because pentamidine and suramin are only effective against *T. b. gambiense*, they are somewhat toxic, their use can mask symptoms of the disease until it invades the central nervous system, and generalized application promotes parasite resistance to the drugs. Moreover, most tourists are more exposed to *T. b. rhodesiense* than to *T. b. gambiense*. Wery (1990) considers that the most important advances in the control of *gambiense* trypanosomiasis have been the improvements in serologic diagnosis, the demonstration of parasitemia, and the introduction of low-cost, efficient traps for tsetse flies.

The problem of antigenic variation in the African trypanosomes has impeded the production of a vaccine, but there is epidemiologic evidence that the disease generates protective immunity: while 30% of the uninfected population in the Democratic Republic of Congo is at risk of contracting the infection, only 15% of those previously infected run a similar risk (Khonde *et al.*, 1995). These facts suggest that a vaccination is possible.

Bibliography

Bailey, J.W., D.H. Smith. The quantitative buffy coat for the diagnosis of trypanosomes. *Trop Doct* 24:54–56, 1994.

Bales, J.D. African trypanosomiasis. *In*: Strickland, G.T., ed. *Hunter's Tropical Medicine*, 7th ed. Philadelphia: Saunders; 1991:617–628.

Bisser, S., B. Bouteille, J. Sarda, *et al.* Apport des examens biochimiques dans le diagnostic de la phase nerveuse de la trypanosomose humaine africaine. *Bull Soc Pathol Exot* 90:321–326, 1997.

Cattand, P.P. Trypanosomiase humaine africaine. Situation epidemiologique actuelle, une recrudescence alarmante de la maladie. *Bull Soc Pathol Exot* 87:307–310, 1994.

Chimelli, L., S. Scaravilli. Trypanosomiasis. *Brain Pathol* 7:599–611, 1997.

Control of sleeping sickness due to *Trypanosoma brucei gambiense*. *Bull World Health Organ* 60:821–825, 1982.

De Raadt, P. African sleeping sickness today. *Trans R Soc Trop Med Hyg* 70:114–116, 1976.

Dumas, M., B. Bouteille. Trypanosomose humaine africaine. *C R Seances Soc Biol Fil* 190:395–408, 1996.

Goodwin, L.G. The pathology of African trypanosomiases. *Trans R Soc Trop Med Hyg* 64:797–817, 1970.

Gouteux, P.J., M. Artzrouni. Aut-il ou non un controle des vecteurs dans la lutte contre la maladie du sommeil? Une approche bio-mathématique du problème. *Bull Soc Pathol Exot* 89:299–305, 1996.

Greenwood, B.M., H.C. Whittle. The pathogenesis of sleeping sickness. *Trans R Soc Trop Med Hyg* 74:716–725, 1980.

Hunter, C.A., F.W. Jennings, J.F. Tierney, M. Murray, P.G. Kennedy. Correlation of autoantibody titres with central nervous system pathology in experimental African trypanosomiasis. *J Neuroimmunol* 41:143–148, 1992.

Jusot, J.F., S.J. de Vlas, G.J. van Oortmarssen, A. De Muynck. Apport d'un modèle mathématique dans le controle d'une parasitose: cas de la trypanosomiase humaine africaine à *Trypanosoma brucei gambiense. Ann Soc Belg Med Trop* 75:257–272, 1995.

Khonde, N., J. Pepin, T. Niyonsenga, F. Milord, P. De Wals. Epidemiological evidence for immunity following *Trypanosoma brucei gambiense* sleeping sickness. *Trans R Soc Trop Med Hyg* 89:607–611, 1995.

Kuzoe, F.A. Current situation of African trypanosomiasis. *Acta Trop* 54:153–162, 1993.

Langley, P.A. Understanding tsetse flies. *Onderstepoort J Vet Res* 61:361–367, 1994.

Levine, N.D. *Veterinary Protozoology.* Ames: Iowa State University Press; 1985.

McGovern, T.W., W. Williams, J.E. Fitzpatrick, M.S. Cetron, B.C. Hepburn, R.H. Gentry. Cutaneous manifestations of African trypanosomiasis. *Arch Dermatol* 131:1178–1182, 1995.

Mhlanga, J.D. Sleeping sickness: Perspectives in African trypanosomiasis. *Sci Prog* 79 (Pt 3):183–214, 1996.

Minter, D.M. Trypanosomes. *In:* Manson, P., F.I.C. Apted. *Manson's Tropical Diseases,* 18th ed. London: Ballière Tindall; 1982.

Molyneux, D.M. Selective primary health care: Strategies for control of disease in developing world. VIII African trypanosomiasis. *Rev Infect Dis* 5:945–956, 1983.

Okomo-Assoumou, M.C., S. Daulouede, J.L. Lemesre, A. N'Zila-Mouanda, P. Vincendeau. Correlation of high serum levels of tumor necrosis factor-alpha with disease severity in human African trypanosomiasis. *Am J Trop Med Hyg* 53:539–543, 1995.

Pentreath, V.W., P.J. Baugh, D.R. Lavin. Sleeping sickness and the central nervous system. *Onderstepoort J Vet Res* 61:369–377, 1994.

Schares, G., D. Mehlitz. Sleeping sickness in Zaire: A nested polymerase chain reaction improves the identification of *Trypanosoma (Trypanozoon) brucei gambiense* by specific kinetoplast DNA probes. *Trop Med Int Health* 1:59–70, 1996.

Scott, C.M., J.L. Frezil, A. Toudic, D.G. Godfrey. The sheep as a potential reservoir of human trypanosomiasis in the Republic of the Congo. *Trans R Soc Trop Med Hyg* 77:397–401, 1983.

Smith, D.H., J.W. Bailey. Human African trypanosomiasis in south-eastern Uganda: Clinical diversity and isoenzyme profiles. *Ann Trop Med Parasitol* 91:851–856, 1997.

Truc, P., M. Tibayrenc. Population genetics of *Trypanosoma brucei* in central Africa: Taxonomic and epidemiological significance. *Parasitology* 106(Pt 2):137–149, 1993.

Urquhart, G.M. The pathogenesis and immunology of African trypanosomiasis in domestic animals. *Trans R Soc Trop Med Hyg* 74:726–729, 1980.

Vincendeau, P., M.C. Okomo-Assoumou, S. Semballa, C. Fouquet, S. Daulouede. Immunologie et immunopathologie de la trypanosomose Africaine. *Med Trop* (Mars) 56:73–78, 1996.

Wery, M. Les lents progrès du controle de la maladie du sommeil. *Ann Parasitol Hum Comp* 65(Suppl 1):89–93, 1990.

World Health Organization (WHO). *Parasitic Zoonoses. Report of a WHO Expert Committee, with the Participation of FAO.* Geneva: WHO; 1979. (Technical Report Series 637).

AMEBIASIS

ICD-10 A06

Synonyms: Amebiosis, amebic dysentery, entamebiasis.

Etiology: Of the numerous species of the genus *Entamoeba* found in mammals, only *E. histolytica* and *E. polecki* are of zoonotic interest. *E. dispar* was recently identified as a separate species, but knowledge about it is still quite limited. *E. histolytica* is essentially a human parasite which is also capable of infecting a number of non-human primates. In addition, it has been occasionally isolated from dogs, cats, swine, and rats, and it has produced experimental infection in rabbits and other rodents (Tsutsumi, 1994). *E. polecki* was isolated from swine and goats in 1912 and has also been identified in humans (Giboda *et al.*, 1988), although Levine (1985) contends that the original description was inadequate to distinguish it from *E. histolytica*. Another human species, *E. dispar*, was thought for many years to be a "small race" of *E. histolytica* because it is very similar in appearance but does not have the same pathogenic power; it has now been identified as a separate species (Jackson, 1998).

Amebas have two developmental stages: the trophic (or vegetative), during which the trophozoite is formed, and the cystic (or resistant) stage, when the cyst appears. The trophozoites live in the large intestine of the host, moving around by means of pseudopodia and multiplying by binary fission. As they progress through the host intestine toward the outside, they divide into smaller forms, cease taking in nourishment, and develop a thin, resistant wall around themselves in preparation for turning into cysts. At first the cysts are mononuclear; they then subdivide by two consecutive mitoses, producing two and ultimately four nuclei. At that point the cysts are eliminated in the feces of the host. If they are ingested by another host via contaminated food or water, upon reaching the small intestine they break up into four new trophozoites which then migrate to the large intestine, where the multiplication process resumes.

Geographic Distribution: Worldwide.

Occurrence in Man: *E. histolytica* infection is especially prevalent in tropical and subtropical areas, and it is more frequent in developing countries than industrialized ones. An estimated 400 to 500 million people in the world are infected, and between 5% and 10% of them present symptoms (García and Bruckner, 1997). In recent decades, prevalence of the infection has declined notably in the industrialized countries. In the US, for example, the rate in the general population fell from 7% in 1961 to approximately 2% at the end of the 1990s. On the other hand, in the developing world the disease continues to be an important cause of morbidity and mortality. According to reports published in 1996–1997, the infection was found in 0.3% of 1,917 apparently healthy children in Spain, 7.8% of 862 children with diarrhea in Kenya, 19.4% of 33,253 hospital fecal samples in Beirut and 1.2% of 11,611 similar samples in Tripoli, between 20% and 29% of 980 normal adults in Egypt, 18.6% of 1,267 individuals in Nicaragua, and 8.7% of a group of 342 persons in Venezuela.

The prevalence of *E. dispar* is unknown because laboratories only rarely distinguish it from *E. histolytica*. Its frequency may be high, however, since symptoms are present in only 5% to 10% of the infections attributed to *E. histolytica*.

E. polecki infection is rare in humans, and most reports refer to individual cases. However, the prevalence of this species may be greater than has been reported so far because of the difficulty of distinguishing it from *E. histolytica* (Levine, 1985). It would appear to be more frequent in southeastern parts of Asia: the parasite was found in 19% of 184 children in Papua New Guinea (Desowitz and Barnish, 1986); 4.6% of 1,478 refugees from Cambodia, the Lao People's Democratic Republic, and Viet Nam arriving in the US (DeGirolami and Kimber, 1983); and 3.2% of 435 refugees from Cambodia and Viet Nam arriving in France (Chaker *et al.,* 1982).

Occurrence in Animals: Infection with *E. histolytica* is relatively common in nonhuman primates. The parasite has been isolated from dogs and rats, and on occasion from naturally infected cats and swine; it has also been reported in cattle (Levine, 1985). Experimental infections have been produced in numerous rodents (mice, rats, guinea pigs, hamsters, and jerboas) and also in rabbits (Tsutsumi, 1994).

Infection with *E. polecki* appears to be common in swine. Pakandl (1994) reported high prevalence of this parasite among newly weaned swine in the former Czechoslovakia. It is rarely identified in diagnostic laboratories.

The Disease in Man: Most *E. histolytica* infections are asymptomatic, but they should be regarded as potentially pathogenic because there is always the danger that they could develop into a progressive and invasive disease (WHO, 1981). Amebiasis is particularly common in young adults and may be manifested by an invasion of the small intestine, liver, or, more rarely, other tissues. In the intestinal disease, the parasite invades the tissues and produces small ulcers in the intestinal mucosa which spread underneath in the submucosal tissue by means of lysis. On rare occasions it can cause perforation of the intestine or produce granulomas in the wall of the large intestine. The symptoms range from mild abdominal discomfort with bloody mucous diarrhea, alternating with periods of constipation or remission, to acute or fatal dysentery with fever, chills, and bloody or mucous diarrhea (amebic dysentery) (Benenson, 1995). Hematogenic dissemination may carry the parasites to the liver, where they produce a focal necrosis which is often incorrectly referred to as an amebic liver abscess. The symptoms of intestinal amebiasis correspond to febrile and painful hepatosplenomegaly. However, unlike hepatic fascioliasis, there is no peripheral eosinophilia. Occasionally, the parasite may invade the lungs, skin, genital organs, spleen, brain, or pericardium.

Human infection with *E. polecki* is usually asymptomatic. In the few cases of intestinal disease that have been described, the symptoms were considerably milder than those produced by *E. histolytica* and there was no invasion of extraintestinal tissues.

The Disease in Animals: Like human infections, animal infections with *E. histolytica* are usually asymptomatic. Both the clinical intestinal form and the hepatic form occur in lower primates, and spider monkeys are particularly susceptible (Amyx *et al.,* 1978). It is not known whether the disease occurs in swine. In dogs, there have been reports of occasional cases of intestinal disease and, more rarely, invasion of the liver and other tissues. Shimada *et al.* (1992) described a case of *E. histolytica* disease in a cat. Among laboratory rodents, the hamster and the jerboa are susceptible to hepatic invasion, but the guinea pig and the rat are resistant. Although combined immunodeficient mice are fully susceptible to hepatic amebiasis, normal mice are highly resistant.

E. polecki does not appear to be pathogenic for swine (Dunlap, 1975).

Source of Infection and Mode of Transmission: Humans are the reservoir of *E. histolytica*. There is no evidence of animal-to-human transmission. The infection is acquired by the ingestion of products contaminated with the fecal matter from infected persons. Although contaminated water (Marshall *et al.*, 1997) and raw vegetables (Monge and Arias, 1996) are sources of infection, well-documented risk factors include persons who handle contaminated food and those with poor hygienic habits who may contaminate the household food supply. In addition, flies are efficient vectors of the cysts. The trophozoites, which are virtually the only forms present in diarrheic stools, are of little importance as transmitters of the infection because they are not very resistant to desiccation or the action of gastric juices. The cysts, which are found in abundance in pasty or formed feces, are the principal elements of transmission, since they survive in the soil for eight days at temperatures between 28°C and 34°C and for 40 days at 2°C to 6°C. For this reason, the chronic patient and the healthy carrier are more effective sources of infection than the acute patient. In the last two decades it has also been documented that sexual practices which include anal-oral or anal-genital-oral contact are an important risk factor for infection.

Except in the case of monkeys, it is believed that animals acquire the infection from human reservoirs. Apparently *E. histolytica* can be propagated among lower primates: of 29 chimpanzees admitted to a particular colony, only 2 had *E. histolytica* on the day of their arrival, whereas 4 years later 10 of the 29 were infected (Miller and Bray, 1966).

The reservoir of *E. polecki* is swine, and the human infection is contracted either by the ingestion of protozoan cysts in contaminated water or food or via the hands of a person who has been in contact with fecal matter from this reservoir. Human-to-human transmission is also suspected: of three patients diagnosed in Venezuela, two had not had any contact with animals (Chacin-Bonilla, 1983).

Diagnosis: Clinical manifestations alone are not sufficient to differentiate dysentery caused by amebiasis from other causes of dysentery. Laboratory diagnosis is based on three fecal examinations, each taken half a day apart, and serologic tests in special cases. Direct examination of diarrheic feces almost always reveals trophozoites, whereas cysts and occasional trophozoites are found in formed and pasty feces. Samples of diarrheic fecal matter should be examined as soon as possible after collection unless steps are taken to preserve the trophozoites, for which purpose trichromic or iron hematoxylin stain is recommended (García and Bruckner, 1997). Samples from formed or pasty feces may be examined using stool concentration methods and direct microscopic observation of cysts. The diagnosis of *E. histolytica* requires carefully performed procedures and personnel well trained in distinguishing between the macrophages, leukocytes, trophozoites, and cysts of this and other parasites.

The clinical manifestations of extraintestinal amebiasis are not sufficient for a definitive diagnosis. Tests such as the enzyme-linked immunosorbent assay make it possible to identify 90% of all cases, although this technique only detects 10% of intestinal cases (Restrepo *et al.*, 1996). Tests designed to identify foreign bodies, such as radioisotopic imaging, ultrasound, and computerized tomography, may help to locate the lesion, but they are not diagnostic of the disease.

Differential diagnosis between *E. histolytica* and *E. polecki* is difficult and can only be accomplished by studying the cysts. Although the distinction between the pathogenic species *E. histolytica* and the nonpathogenic *E. dispar* cannot be made on the basis of morphological criteria alone, there are immunologic and isoenzymatic differences which have recently made it possible to identify the species in specialized laboratories (Jackson, 1998). The *E. polecki* cysts have a single nucleus, unevenly distributed chromatin in the nuclear periphery, rare glycogen vacuoles in the cytoplasm, usually an opaque cytoplasmic inclusion body which is much larger than the nucleus, and up to 30 chromatoidal bars. On the other hand, mature *E. histolytica* cysts have four nuclei, uniformly distributed chromatin, frequent glycogen vacuoles in the cytoplasm, no cytoplasmic inclusion body, and fewer than 10 chromatoidal bars (Levin and Armstrong, 1970). Giboda *et al.* (1988) have established additional criteria.

Control: Basically, amebiasis is controlled by avoiding contamination of the environment with human feces and educating the general public—children in particular, in order to reach the people in the household who handle food—and commercial food handlers about proper hygiene to prevent transmission of the infection. The following measures are essential in order to avoid contamination: proper disposal of human excreta, protection of water sources from fecal contamination, treatment of chronic patients and healthy carriers who are spreading cysts, and supervision of food preparation in public places where raw food is eaten. Food should be covered when there are flies or dust in the air. Health education should stress the danger of drinking water or eating raw vegetables that might be contaminated, as well as the importance of washing one's hands after defecating and before preparing food. Education programs should be targeted toward high-risk groups such as homosexuals and swineherds in order to prevent infections caused by *E. polecki*. In endemic areas, water and food should be either boiled or treated with nine drops of 2% tincture of iodine per liter of water for 30 minutes. Travelers visiting endemic areas should consume only bottled water (including ice made from bottled water) and cooked food.

Bibliography

Amyx, H.L., D.M. Asher, T.E. Nash, C.J. Gibbs, Jr., D.C. Gajdusek. Hepatic amebiasis in spider monkeys. *Am J Trop Med Hyg* 27:888–891, 1978.

Benenson, A.S., ed. *Control of Communicable Diseases in Man*, 16th ed. An official report of the American Public Health Association. Washington, D.C.: APHA; 1995.

Chaker, E., M. Kremer, T.T. Kien. Quatorze cas d'*Entamoeba* polecki chez des refugies du Sud-Est asiatique: remarques sur l'aspect morphologique du parasite. *Bull Soc Pathol Exot Filiales* 75:484–490, 1982.

Chacin-Bonilla, L. *Entamoeba polecki* infection in Venezuela. Report of a new case. *Trans R Soc Trop Med Hyg* 77:137, 1983.

DeGirolami, P.C., J. Kimber. Intestinal parasites among Southeastern Asian refugees in Massachusetts. *Am J Clin Pathol* 79:502–504, 1983.

Desowitz, R.S., G. Barnish. *Entamoeba polecki* and other intestinal protozoa in Papua New Guinea Highland children. *Ann Trop Med Parasitol* 80:399–402, 1986.

Dunlap, J.S. Protozoa. *In*: Dunne, H.W., A.D. Leman, eds. *Diseases of Swine,* 4th ed. Ames: Iowa State University Press; 1975.

García, L.S., D.A. Bruckner. *Diagnostic Medical Parasitology,* 3rd ed. Washington, D.C.: ASM Press; 1997.

Giboda, M., N. Vokurkova, P. Kopacek, O. Ditrich, J. Gutvirth. *Entamoeba polecki*: Morphology, immunology, antigen study and clinic of the first infections in Czechoslovakia. *Folia Parasitol* (Praha) 35:11–16, 1988.

Jackson, T.P. *Entamoeba histolytica* and *Entamoeba dispar* are distinct species: Clinical, epidemiological and serological evidence. *Int J Parasitol* 28:181–186, 1998.

Levin, R.L., D.E. Armstrong. Human infection with *Entamoeba polecki. Am J Clin Pathol* 54:611–614, 1970.

Levine, N.D. *Veterinary Protozoology.* Ames: Iowa State University Press; 1985.

Marshall, M.M., D. Naumowitz, Y. Ortega, C.R. Sterling. Waterborne protozoan pathogens. *Clin Microbiol Rev* 10:67–85, 1997.

Miller, M.J., R.S. Bray. *Entamoeba histolytica* infections in the chimpanzee *(Pan satyrus). J Parasit* 52:386–388, 1966.

Monge, R., M.L. Arias. Presencia de microorganismos patógenos en hortalizas de consumo crudo en Costa Rica. *Arch Latinoam Nutr* 46:292–294, 1996.

Pakandl, M. The prevalence of intestinal protozoa in wild and domestic pigs. *Vet Med* (Praha) 39:377–380, 1994.

Restrepo, M.I., Z. Restrepo, C.L. Elsa Villareal, A. Aguirre, M. Restrepo. Diagnostic tests for amoebic liver abscess: Comparison of enzyme-linked immunosorbent assay (ELISA) and counterimmunoelectrophoresis (CIE). *Rev Soc Bras Med Trop* 29:27–32, 1996.

Shimada, A., Y. Muraki, T. Awakura, *et al.* Necrotic colitis associated with *Entamoeba histolytica* in a cat. *J Comp Pathol* 106:195–199, 1992.

Tsutsumi, V. Los modelos experimentales *in vivo* en la amebiasis. *Gac Med Mex* 130:450–453, 1994.

World Health Organization (WHO). *Intestinal Protozoan and Helminthis Infections. Report of a WHO Scientific Group.* Geneva: WHO; 1981. (Technical Report No. 666).

BABESIOSIS

ICD-10 B60.0

Synonyms: Piroplasmosis, babesiasis.

Etiology: Of the 73 species of *Babesia* that have been described as parasites of mammals, only slightly more than a dozen are important for domestic animals and only five occasionally infect man: 1) *B. microti,* a parasite of rodents; 2) *B. divergens,* a parasite of cattle in Europe; 3) a species related to the dog parasite *B. gibsoni,* isolated in Africa and Asia (but undistinguishable from *B. microti*) and also in the state of Washington, US, where it was given the preliminary designation WA1; 4) a species related to *B. divergens* isolated in Missouri, US, and assigned the preliminary designation MO1; and 5) a species related to *B. microti* isolated in Taiwan and identified preliminarily as TW1 (Barriga, 1997; Herwaldt *et al.,* 1996; Shih *et al.,* 1997). Since the diagnosis of *Babesia* is still based mainly on the morphology of the parasites, it is possible that man may be infected by other species which have not yet been identified with certainty.

Babesias parasitize the red blood cells of vertebrate hosts and are transmitted in nature by ticks. When an infected tick bites a mammal, pyriform parasites (sporozoites measuring 1.5–3 µm long) are introduced through the tick's saliva and rapidly penetrate the host's erythrocytes. The majority of the parasites grow inside the red blood cells as pyriform trophozoites or merozoites, the rest as gametocytes. The trophozoites or merozoites often divide asexually into two organisms, forming a "V." *B. microti* sometimes divides into four parasites that form a tetrad or Maltese cross. When they achieve full growth and measure between 1 µm and 5 µm in length, the parasites break free of the erythrocytes, often destroying them in the process, and invade new ones. This cycle is repeated until either the infection is brought under control or the host dies. The gametocytes, on the other hand, develop inside the host's erythrocytes until they become an oval or round parasite, at which point they stop growing. These gametocytes are the precursors of the parasite's sexual stage, which continue to multiply inside the tick.

Babesiosis is typically a chronic infection. Even after the infection is controlled, the parasite usually maintains a low-level presence in the host erythrocytes for a very long time. In domestic animals, this period often lasts for the rest of their life.

When a tick vector—*Ixodes scapularis* (formerly *I. dammini*) in the case of *B. microti*, or *I. ricinus* in the case of *B. divergens*—sucks blood containing the parasites, the merozoites are destroyed in the digestive tract, but the gametocytes mature and become male and female gametes, which fuse and form mobile zygotes. The latter in turn become kinetes, which migrate to the hemocele and from there invade numerous organs of the tick, where they divide asexually and invade even more organs. Some of the kinetes invade oocytes; once inside the egg, they can be passed on to the next generation of ticks via transovarial transmission. Other kinetes invade the salivary glands, where they are transformed into sporozoites after the gland has undergone certain developmental changes that take place while the arthropod ingests its blood meal. Because of the time required for this process to occur, sporozoites are not inoculated until a few days after the infected tick begins to feed (Mehlhorn and Schein, 1985).

Geographic Distribution: Animal babesias occurs almost everywhere in the world where ticks exist, including both the tropical zones and many temperate areas as well. In the US, human infections have been identified and attributed to the following: *B. microti* (especially in New England), WA1 (in Washington State and northern California), and MO1 (in Missouri). In Europe, cases of babesiosis caused by *B. divergens* have been reported in Belgium, France, Ireland, Russia, Scotland, Spain, Sweden, and the former Yugoslavia. In Taiwan, cases due to TW1 were identified. Osorno *et al.* (1976) found antibodies to an undetermined species of *Babesia* in 38 of 101 samples taken from residents in a rural area of Mexico, and they successfully isolated the parasite from three of the samples by inoculation in hamsters.

Occurrence in Man: Clinical human babesiosis is infrequent. The first case was confirmed in the former Yugoslavia in 1957 and attributed to *B. divergens*. Since 1990, there have been reports in the US of 100 cases in the states of Massachusetts and New York; 2 in the midwest in the states of Wisconsin and Minnesota; 10 in the states of Washington and California; and 1 in the state of Missouri. In addition, some 22 cases have been identified in Europe and there has been 1 case in Taiwan. The total number of cases described in the world is estimated to be fewer than 200. Although most of the cases in Europe and the first cases in the US occurred in splenectomized individuals, in the last decade numerous cases have been described, especially in the US, in patients who were immunodeficient for other reasons or previously healthy. However, there is evidence that the infection is much more frequent than the disease. For example, 6.3% of 1,285 residents of Connecticut were found to be seropositive for *B. microti* (Krause *et al.*, 1991), 9% of 574 residents of Rhode Island were also seropositive for *B. microti* (Krause *et al.*, 1992), and 17.8% of 230 semirural residents of northern California were seropositive for WA1 (Fritz *et al.*, 1997).

Occurrence in Animals: Animal babesiosis is widespread throughout the world, with the highest prevalence in the tropics. It is one of the most important diseases of cattle in Africa, the Middle East and other parts of Asia, Australia, Central America, and the northern half of South America. The disease poses a risk for 50% to 70% of the cattle in the world and causes heavy economic losses, and has been compared to malaria in man. *B. divergens* occurs only in Europe and some parts of the former USSR. It is distinguished from the other major babesias of cattle (*B. bigemina, B. bovis*, and *B. major*) by its relatively smaller size, measuring only 1.5 µm x 1.0 µm, compared with at least 2.0 µm in length in the case of all the others (Barriga, 1997). *B. microti* is found on numerous wild rodents in the US and Europe, and it is a common laboratory research model. In the US, blood examinations of the white-footed mouse (*Peromyscus leucopus*) on Nantucket Island, Massachusetts, revealed *B. microti* in 35.4% of the blood smears examined and 67% of the specimens inoculated in hamsters (Spielman *et al.,* 1981). In Germany, it was found in 38% of 255 field voles (*Microtus agrestis*) (Krampitz, 1979). Nevertheless, the only known cases of human infection due to this species have been found on the eastern coast of the US.

The Disease in Man: The cases in Europe of *B. divergens* infection usually occur in splenectomized individuals (80%). They are characterized by severe illness, often with pyrexia, chills, anemia, muscular pain, prostration, hemoglobinuria, and jaundice. The case fatality rate is about 50%. The spleen plays a very important role in resistance to the parasite, and splenectomy is undoubtedly a predisposing factor. By the same token, the disease may be more severe in immunodeficient individuals. In the Americas, the nonsplenectomized patients infected with *B. microti* had a disease that developed gradually, with anorexia, fatigue, fever, sweating, and generalized muscle pain. Some patients may have mild splenomegaly and hepatomegaly, and mild to severe hemolytic anemia is common as well. Parasitemia may affect fewer than 1% or up to 10% or more of the erythrocytes. In blood smears, it is difficult to distinguish the predominant form of *B. microti* from the small ring forms of *Plasmodium*, which they closely resemble. Recovery is slow, with malaise and fatigue persisting for several months (Ruebush, 1984). *B. microti* rarely causes death, even in splenectomized or immunodeficient patients. The incubation period between the tick bite and the appearance of symptoms can range from 7 to 28 days.

Because of epidemiologic similarities with infections caused by *Borrelia burgdorferi* and *Ehrlichia* spp., human babesiosis in the US can coexist with infections caused by these other agents (Mitchell *et al.*, 1996).

The Disease in Animals: In the affected domestic species the symptomatology of babesiosis is similar, characterized by the triad of fever, anemia, and jaundice.

Anemia occurs when the parasites emerge from the erythrocytes and cause the immunologic destruction of these cells. The increased amount of free hemoglobin in plasma often produces hemoglobinuria. *B. bovis* tends to attach itself to the capillary endothelium in much the same way that *Plasmodium falciparum* does in man, thereby blocking circulation. The sensitivity of nervous tissue to anoxia often results in symptoms of agitation and convulsions. Babesiosis in cattle can range from mild to fatal, and those animals that recover usually harbor a subclinical infection and act as healthy carriers. Calves and young equines 6 to 9 months of age are relatively resistant to the infection and disease. In endemic areas, most animals acquire an asymptomatic infection when they are young that confers premunition (i.e., resistance to subsequent infections). By contrast, animals arriving from parasite-free areas usually develop a severe form of the disease.

B. microti in rodents appears to be asymptomatic, but no extensive studies have been done on the subject.

Source of Infection and Mode of Transmission: The reservoirs for domestic animals and rodents are other infected animals, which are often healthy carriers. The reservoirs for man are wild rodents, especially the white-footed mouse *P. leucopus* and meadow vole *Microtus pennsylvanicus*, both of which have been demonstrated to be infected with *B. microti* in the US, and cattle infected with *B. divergens* in Europe. The *B. microti* infection is transmitted in nature by the tick *I. scapularis* and the *B. divergens* infection, by *I. ricinus*.

In the case of *B. microti*, the larva of *I. scapularis* acquires the infection from wild rodents and the nymph, which acquires the infection via transstadial transmission from the larva, passes the infection along when it bites a human host. In a study on Nantucket Island, Massachusetts, US, 5% of the *I. scapularis* nymphs collected were infected. However, the protozoan is not passed from the nymph to the adult tick. Since the adult tick feeds on deer that are not susceptible to *B. microti*, it does not have the opportunity to become infected and therefore does not transmit the infection (Lane and Crosskey, 1993). The *B. microti* enzootic areas are characterized by an abundance of rodents, which serve as hosts for the larvae and nymphs of the vector, while deer serve as the host for adult ticks. Most of the human infections in the US occur in July and August, when nymphs are most abundant (Ruebush *et al.*, 1981).

In the case of *B. divergens*, only the adult *I. ricinus* tick feeds on cattle and is capable of acquiring the infection. However, *B. divergens* is transmitted to the next generation of ticks both through the egg (transovarial transmission) and subsequently during the different developmental stages of the tick (transstadial transmission). Thus, *I. ricinus* can transmit *B. divergens* at any stage in its life cycle.

There have been about eight reports of human *Babesia* infection due to blood transfusion (Mintz *et al.*, 1991). Asymptomatic donors carry the infection for up to 12 months after they initially acquire the infection themselves.

Diagnosis: A diagnosis of babesiosis should be suspected when the clinical symptoms coincide with an epidemiological history of tick bites or visits to enzootic areas. It is confirmed in febrile or acute cases when parasites are seen inside erythrocytes on Giemsa-stained thin or thick blood smears. Differentiation from *Plasmodium*, especially *P. falciparum*, may require the help of experts. Unlike *Plasmodium*, *Babesia* does not produce pigment (hemozoin) in the parasitized red blood cells. In more chronic cases with low parasitemia, a diagnosis can be made using serologic examinations such as the indirect immunofluorescence test or the inoculation of blood into susceptible animals. In chronic cases, or before babesias appear in the blood in detectable numbers, the polymerase chain reaction can be used to detect the specific nucleic acids of the parasite (Krause *et al.*, 1996).

Control: For domestic animals in endemic areas, the most effective control measure is to prevent intense infestation by the tick vectors. There is now a vaccine that invokes an immunologic response against *Boophilus microplus* infestation in cattle; as this tick is the main vector of babesiosis in cattle, the reduction of tick infestation also reduces the transmission of the disease (de la Fuente *et al.*, 1998). Cattle introduced into endemic areas may be protected by the administration of commercially available live vaccines or by artificial premunition, i.e., inoculating them with blood from healthy carrier cattle to induce a mild infection and then treating them subcuratively. Since the human infection is usually sporadic and occurs only after visits to endemic areas, it is recommended that on such occasions people use protective clothing or tick repellents, and following the visit, that they examine themselves closely for nymphs, which are very small. Those living in endemic areas should control rodents inside the home and cut down shrubbery surrounding the dwelling to control the presence of nymphs.

Bibliography

Barriga, O.O. *Veterinary Parasitology for Practitioners*, 2nd ed. Edina: Burgess International Group; 1997.

De la Fuente, J., M. Rodríguez, M. Redondo, C. Montero, J.C. García-García, L. Méndez, *et al.* Field studies and cost-effectiveness analysis of vaccination with Gavac™ against the cattle tick, *Boophilus microplus*. *Vaccine* 16(4):366–373, 1998.

Fritz, C.L., A.M. Kjemtrup, P.A. Conrad, *et al.* Seroepidemiology of emerging tickborne infectious diseases in a Northern California community. *J Infect Dis* 175:1432–1439, 1997.

Herwaldt, B., D.H. Persing, E.A. Precigout, *et al.* A fatal case of babesiosis in Missouri: Identification of another piroplasm that infects humans. *Ann Intern Med* 124:643–650, 1996.

Krampitz, H.E. *Babesia microti*: Morphology, distribution and host relationship in Germany. *Zentralbl Bakteriol* [Orig A] 244:411–415, 1979.

Krause, P.J., S.R. Telford, R. Ryan, *et al.* Geographic and temporal distribution of babesial infection in Connecticut. *J Clin Microbiol* 29:1–4, 1991.

Krause, P.J., S.R. Telford, R.J. Pollack, *et al.* Babesiosis: An underdiagnosed disease of children. *Pediatrics* 89 (6 Pt 1):1045–1048, 1992.

Krause, P.J., S.R. Telford, A. Spielman, *et al.* Comparison of PCR with blood smear and inoculation of small animals for diagnosis of *Babesia microti* parasitemia. *J Clin Microbiol* 34:2791–2794, 1996.

Lane, R.P., R.W. Crosskey, eds. *Medical Insects and Arachnids*. London: Chapman & Hall; 1993.

Mehlhorn, H., E. Schein. The piroplasms: Life cycle and sexual stages. *Adv Parasitol* 23:37–103, 1984.

Mintz, E.D., J.F. Anderson, R.G. Cable, J.L Hadler. Transfusion-transmitted babesiosis: A case report from a new endemic area. *Transfusion* 31:365–368, 1991.

Mitchell, P.D., K.D. Reed, J.M. Hofkes. Immunoserologic evidence of coinfection with *Borrelia burgdorferi*, *Babesia microti*, and human granulocytic *Ehrlichia* species in residents of Wisconsin and Minnesota. *J Clin Microbiol* 34:724–727, 1996.

Osorno, M., C. Vega, M. Ristic, C. Robles, S. Ibarra. Isolation of *Babesia* spp. from asymptomatic human beings. *Vet Parasitol* 2:111–120, 1976.

Ruebush, T.K. Babesiosis. *In*: Warren, K.S., A.A.F. Mahmoud, eds. *Tropical and Geographical Medicine*. New York: McGraw-Hill; 1984.

Ruebush, T.K., D.D. Juranek, A. Spielman, J. Piesman, G.R. Healy. Epidemiology of human babesiosis on Nantucket Island. *Am J Trop Med Hyg* 30:937–941, 1981.

Shih, C.M., L.P. Liu, W.C. Chung, S.J. Ong, C.C. Wang. Human babesiosis in Taiwan: Asymptomatic infection with a *Babesia microti*-like organism in a Taiwanese woman. *J Clin Microbiol* 35:450–454, 1997.

Spielman, A., P. Etkind, J. Piesman, T.K. Ruebush, D.D. Juranek, M.S. Jacobs. Reservoir hosts of human babesiosis on Nantucket Island. *Am J Trop Med Hyg* 30:560–565, 1981.

BALANTIDIASIS

ICD-10 A07.0

Synonyms: Balantidiosis, balantidial dysentery.

Etiology: *Balantidium coli* is a ciliated protozoan that affects swine, primates (including humans) and, rarely, guinea pigs, dogs, and rats. It has been isolated from 27 species of vertebrates (Wenyon, 1926), but its identification is dubious in many cases. The vegetative form (or trophozoite) measures 30–150 μm in length and 25–120 μm in width; it is ovoid, with a slightly elongated end in which there is a triangular cell mouth, or cytostome, and it is covered with short cilia in a spiral pattern. Osmoregulatory and food vacuoles are frequently found in its cytoplasm. The infective form (the cyst) measures 45–65 μm in diameter, is round, and contains the ciliated organism, sometimes mobile and often with vacuoles, within a thick but transparent double wall (Neva and Brown, 1994). As is characteristic of ciliates, both forms have a large kidney-shaped nucleus, or macronucleus, which is responsible for vegetative functions, and a smaller spherical nucleus, or micronucleus, which is not always visible and is responsible for sexual reproduction, when it occurs. Unlike other protozoa, the parasite does not multiply inside the cyst. Hence, the *Balantidium* cyst possesses the same number of nuclei as the trophozoite (García and Bruckner, 1997).

The trophozoites live in the lumen of the large intestine and, occasionally, invade the mucosa and other tissues. They replicate by transverse binary fission and, sometimes, by budding or conjugation. As they move towards the outside of the body, many become encysted. The cysts form in the fecal matter as it passes through the intestine or in the soft feces that are excreted.

Geographic Distribution: *B. coli* is found throughout the world, but it is more prevalent in tropical and temperate regions. In man, it is most often found in individuals who are in contact with swine and those exposed to poor environmental hygiene conditions.

Occurrence in Man: Balantidiasis is an uncommon disease in humans. Worldwide, only 772 cases of balantidial dysentery had been reported up to 1960. Asymptomatic infection is less rare, but it is not frequent, either. Four surveys carried out between 1988 and 1996 in apparently healthy populations found prevalences of 0.05% in Mexico, 0.3% in Venezuela, 0.5% in children in Argentina, and 1.8% in children in Bolivia. Of 18,512 people examined in Benin, only 0.26% were infected. Wittner and Tanowitz (1992) report that the infection is extremely uncommon in travelers returning to the US from developing countries. Occasionally, however, circumstances arise that facilitate the infection of a sizable segment of population. A study conducted in Ecuador during a gastroenteritis epidemic found that 19.3% of the children examined were infected. In studies in indigenous communities of Bolivia and Peru and in isolated rural populations in Chile, presumably with poor sanitary conditions, the infection was detected in 8%, 6%, and 4.5%, respectively, of those surveyed.

Occurrence in Animals: The infection is very frequent in swine. Prevalences of 60% to 90% have been reported in animals in a single herd and in 60% or more of the herds examined. Based on the form of the parasite and its macronucleus, a separate species, *B. suis*, has been described in swine, but most authorities do not accept this species as different from *B. coli*. Natural infection in dogs and rodents seems to be exceptional.

The Disease in Man: Disease from *B. coli* in man usually affects the mucosa of the large intestine, but it can also invade the liver and the lung, though this rarely happens (Vidan *et al.*, 1985; Ladas *et al.*, 1989). In symptomatic infections, the parasite first causes congestion and hyperemia of the mucosa and then small ulcers, which may spread and ultimately destroy large areas of epithelium. The organisms generally invade the intestinal crypts and cause inflammation due to lymphocytes and eosinophils, as well as microabscesses and necrosis. They may spread into the muscularis mucosae and, on rare occasions, perforation of the intestinal wall has occurred. Secondary bacterial infection is common. In acute cases, the patient presents with severe diarrhea, often with mucus, blood, and pus in the stools. In chronic cases, the patient may alternate between diarrhea and constipation and suffer from abdominal pain, anemia, and cachexia. The pathology and symptomatology for *B. coli* are similar to those associated with *Entamoeba histolytica*.

The Disease in Animals: The parasite is apparently not pathogenic in swine. It invades the intestinal mucosa only when prior damage enables its entry and, even in these cases, it does not appear to cause any reaction in the tissues. Infection of dogs and rats is rare, and invasion of the tissues in these species is even less frequent. Primates may possess some natural resistance to *B. coli* infection and disease. Yang *et al.* (1995) reported that two monkeys treated with hydrocortisone and infected with cysts of human origin developed diarrhea, while two untreated monkeys developed only the asymptomatic infection.

Source of Infection and Mode of Transmission: In many cases, the infection in man has been conclusively linked to contamination of water and food by feces of infected pigs or to close contact with pigs. However, the infection exists in Muslim countries where pigs are not raised (Geddes, 1952), and epidemics have occurred in mental hospitals where no pigs were present (Faust *et al.*, 1970). Hence, it appears that person-to-person transmission is possible where environmental sanitation conditions are poor.

The *B. coli* trophozoite cannot survive for very long in a dry environment, so it is unlikely that infection would be acquired through ingestion of viable trophozoites. The cyst is a much more efficient means of transmission than the trophozoite, since it can survive outside the body for two weeks or more at ambient temperatures. Ingested cysts excyst in the intestine and begin to multiply as trophozoites.

Diagnosis: The symptomatology of balantidiasis is such that it cannot be differentiated clinically from other causes of dysentery. Similarly, it is not possible to distinguish it from amebiasis through endoscopic observation of intestinal lesions. Diagnosis is based on detection of trophozoites, which are most commonly found in watery diarrheal stools, or cysts, which are particularly abundant in formed stools. The trophozoite, obtained from stool specimens or endoscopic samples, can be seen by microscopic examination of wet mounts at low magnification (100X). Permanent stained preparations are not recommended because the parasite, owing to its size and thickness, stains deeply and its internal structures then cannot be observed. The cysts can be visualized by means of fecal parasite concentration methods.

Control: The most efficient control method is probably to educate the public about basic personal hygiene practices in areas in which contact between humans and swine is common. On pig farms, care should be taken to prevent animal waste from contaminating water used for drinking or irrigation, and manure should not be used as fertilizer on crops of vegetables that are eaten raw. Suspicious water or food should be boiled because normal chlorination will not kill the cysts. Where there is a potential for person-to-person transmission, the usual personal hygiene practices for preventing infections of fecal origin, combined with effective treatment of infected individuals, should reduce the risk of transmission.

Bibliography

Faust, E.C., P.F. Russell, C.R. Jung. *Craig and Faust's Clinical Parasitology.* Philadelphia: Lea & Febiger; 1970.

García, L.S., D.A. Bruckner. *Diagnostic Medical Parasitology,* 3rd ed. Washington, D.C.: ASM Press; 1997.

Geddes, McC.A. Balantidiasis in South Persia. *Br Med J* 1:629–631, 1952.

Ladas, S.D., S. Savva, A. Frydas, A. Kaloviduris, J. Hatzioannou, S. Raptis. Invasive balantidiasis presented as chronic colitis and lung involvement. *Dig Dis Sci* 34:1621–1623, 1989.

Neva, F.A., H.W. Brown. *Basic Clinical Parasitology,* 6th ed. Norwalk, Connecticut: Appleton & Lange; 1994.

Vidan, J.R., A. Frauca, B. Martínez, F. Borda. Parasitosis hepática por *Balantidium coli. Med Clin* (Barc) 85:299–300, 1985.

Wenyon, C.M. *Protozoology: A Manual for Medical Men, Veterinarians and Zoologists.* London: Baillière, Tindall and Cox; 1926.

Wittner, M., H.B. Tanowitz. Intestinal parasites in returned travelers. *Med Clin North Am* 76:6, 1433–1448, 1992.

Yang Y., L. Zeng, M. Li, J. Zhou. Diarrhoea in piglets and monkeys experimentally infected with *Balantidium coli* isolated from human faeces. *J Trop Med Hyg* 98(1):69–72, 1995.

CHAGAS' DISEASE

ICD-10 B57

Synonyms: American trypanosomiasis, Chagas-Mazza disease, infection due to *Trypanosoma cruzi.*

Etiology: Chagas' disease is produced by the flagellate protozoan *Trypanosoma (Schizotrypanum) cruzi.* This protozoan has a complex developmental cycle that involves mammals and an arthropod vector. In mammals, *T. cruzi* is found in two forms: extracellular trypomastigotes (formerly "trypanosomal forms") in the bloodstream, and intracellular amastigotes (formerly "leishmanial forms") in tissue. In the vector, it also exists in two forms, both of them extracellular: epimastigotes (formerly "crithidial forms") in the intestine and *in vitro* cultures, and trypomastigotes or metacyclic trypanosomes in the insect's rectum. Thin blood smears prepared with Giemsa's stain show that the trypomastigotes are fusiform, doubled over in the shape of a "U" or "C"; some of them are narrow and about 20 μm long, while others are wider and shorter, measuring about 15 μm long. Near the tip of the parasite there is a large bulging kinetoplast with an attached flagellum that protrudes from the rear end of the body. Between the flagellum and the body is a thin, wavy membrane with two or three undulations. The nucleus, located near the center of the body, is large and bulky. The amastigotes are oval, measuring about 2 μm by 3 μm, and have a nucleus, a kinetoplast, and a short intracellular flagellum which can be seen only at high levels of magnification. The epimastigotes are fusiform and about 20 μm long; the kinetoplast is in front of the nucleus, and the membrane and flagellum are shorter. The metacyclic trypanosomes are longer, thinner, and straighter than the trypomastigotes seen in the bloodstream.

Electrophoresis of isozymes of various *T. cruzi* isolates has made it possible to group the strains of the parasite according to their predominant isozymes, known as zymodemes. Miles (1983) introduced this technique for the study of *T. cruzi* and identified 3 zymodemes in Brazil, each of them with different epidemiological characteristics. Subsequent studies have identified 7 zymodemes in Brazil, 11 more in Bolivia, Chile, Colombia, and Paraguay (Bogliolo *et al.*, 1986), and 12 in Argentina (Blanco and Montamat, 1998). Some authors have suggested that there is a correlation between zymodemes and the epidemiological or clinical characteristics of the parasites, but others have not been able to confirm this hypothesis (Lauria-Pires and Teixeira, 1996). The species *Trypanosoma (Herpetosoma) rangeli* is found in some parts of Central America and northern South America; like *T. cruzi,* it is transmitted to man and a variety of mammals by the bite of certain reduviid bugs. Although this species does not cause disease in man or animals, it produces prolonged parasitemia and can be mistaken for *T. cruzi.* The bloodstream trypomastigotes of *T. rangeli* are narrower and longer than those of *T. cruzi,* measuring about 30 μm, with a smaller nucleus and a much smaller kinetoplast, which is located farther from the posterior tip of the parasite.

Some 150 mammal species are susceptible to *T. cruzi,* ranging from marsupials such as the opossum (*Didelphis marsupialis*) to primates. Prevalence can be high in cats, dogs, rodents, and both domestic and wild lagomorphs, which taken together constitute an important reservoir for human infection. Birds and cold-blooded vertebrates are refractory to *T. cruzi* infection, but domestic birds are important food sources for the vector.

The vectors are reduviid bugs of the family Triatomidae. It has been confirmed that about a hundred species are susceptible to the infection, but the most important vectors are *Triatoma infestans* in southern Peru; *Panstrongylus megistus* in northern Argentina, southern Brazil, and Paraguay; and *Rhodnius prolixus* in northern South America, parts of Central America, and Mexico. The vector becomes infected when it feeds on the blood of an infected mammal and ingests trypomastigotes. These forms reach the midgut of the insect, turn into epimastigotes, and divide abundantly by binary fission. After the bug has been infected for 15 to 30 days, the infective metacyclic trypanosomes begin to appear in its rectum. The bug usually remains infected for several months or the rest of its life.

Unlike the African trypanosomes (see the chapter on African Trypanosomiasis), which produce infection through the bite of a vector, *T. cruzi* infects its definitive host through the vector's excrement. This modality is referred to as contaminative infection, or transmission from the "posterior station," as opposed to inoculative infection, or transmission from the "anterior station." Animals may also become infected by ingesting infected vectors. The metacyclic trypanosomes penetrate the organism either through normal healthy mucosa or broken skin, often caused by scratching; they then invade the macrophages of the dermis or subcutaneous tissue, transform into amastigotes, and multiply by binary fission. Between four and five days after infecting the host cell, the amastigotes then turn into trypomastigotes, which destroy the original cell and invade neighboring cells or spread through the bloodstream to the cells of other organs, especially macrophages, cardiac and striated muscle fibers, and the neuroglia. The trypomastigotes do not multiply in the bloodstream; instead, they turn into amastigotes once again inside the cells and repeat the cycle of intracellular multiplication and destruction of the cell. Some authors have described intermediate forms between trypomastigotes and amastigotes (promastigotes, epimastigotes) when the parasite abandons the cells, but if such forms exist, they are rarely seen in a mammal host. At the beginning of the infection, there are large numbers of trypomastigotes in the bloodstream, but over time, the frequency of the blood-cell cycles tapers off, and as a result, after a few weeks the level of parasitemia drops considerably and the parasite remains restricted to tissue.

Geographic Distribution: *T. cruzi* infection exists only in the Americas, within an area extending from 42° N latitude in the US (from California to Maryland) to approximately 34° S in Chile and 42° S in Argentina. Vectors and wild reservoirs have also been found throughout much of the Caribbean, which was previously considered free of the infection (PAHO, 1984). Autochthonous Chagas' disease has not been confirmed outside the Americas (Marsden, 1997).

Occurrence in Man: Chagas' disease is essentially a problem affecting southern Mexico and Central and South America. According to estimates based on seroepidemiologic studies, at the beginning of the 1980s, 10 to 20 million people in Latin America were infected and 65 million were at risk for the infection; in addition, 10% of those infected in South America could be expected to develop symptoms and clinical signs of chronic Chagas' disease (PAHO, 1984). By the mid-1990s, it was estimated that the disease had affected between 16 and 18 million people, that 50 million were at risk, and that up to 30% of those infected would develop the chronic disease, with a fatal outcome (Moncayo, 1992; Wanderley and Correa, 1995).

The highest prevalence of vector-borne infection is found in rural and periurban areas, but the distribution is uneven and depends on the presence of the vector, whether it lives in dwellings, and whether conditions in the home facilitate contact between the vector and man. In three rural villages in northwestern Argentina, the level of serologic prevalence was 34% (Gurtler et al., 1998). In a rural community of São Paulo State, Brazil, cross-sectional studies found a seroprevalence rate of 16.6% (ranging from 2.9% to 61.9%) in 1971–1972, but after a long campaign to control the vector, by 1989–1991, the level had dropped to 10.1% (with a range from 0.4% to 44.8%). In both studies, the lowest prevalence was found in children, and the highest, in the elderly (Passos et al., 1997). Jaramillo et al. (1997) found a prevalence of 7.1% in Belize; 8.2% in El Salvador; 5.1% in Guatemala; and 6.2% in Honduras. In the southern US, where the infection exists but there are no domiciliary vectors and conditions do not exist for vectors to invade human homes, five acute vector-borne infections have been reported (Benenson, 1995).

Although to a lesser extent, transmission by transfusion also contributes to maintaining the infection. In endemic areas, the importance of this mechanism depends on the prevalence of the infection in the population: in Mexico, it was found that 17% of blood donors had antibodies to T. cruzi (Rangel et al., 1998), while in the US, there have been 3 cases of T. cruzi infection by transfusion, and in some areas of Los Angeles and Miami, where there are large numbers of immigrants from Latin America, 34 of 49,565 blood donors were serologically positive for the infection (Leiby et al., 1997).

Congenital transmission has been documented in several studies: in Paraguay, 3% of 172 mothers who were serologically positive for T. cruzi transmitted the infection to their babies (Russomando et al., 1998); in Argentina, 5.3% of 62 mothers (Arcavi et al., 1993), 4% of 149 (Zaidenberg and Segovia, 1993), and 2.6% of 341 (Streiger et al., 1995) did so; and in Bolivia, 9.5% of 910 mothers also passed the infection on (Azoge, 1993). In the US, Di Pentima et al. (1999) found that 0.3% of 3,765 pregnant women in the city of Houston had antibodies to T. cruzi and speculated that congenital infection could occur in this area. Leiby et al. (1999) found two blood donors with antibodies to T. cruzi who had been born in the US and had never traveled to endemic areas. Since these donors had a family history of heart disease and complications, the authors suggested that the infections might have been congenital.

Attention has often been called to the public health importance of Chagas' disease, particularly because of the high rate of cardiopathy in chronic patients. In central Brazil, visceromegalies such as megacolon and megaesophagus are also a consequence of the chronic disease. In some areas, Chagas' disease is the most frequent cause of myocardiopathy and even the leading cause of death. Deaths from Chagas cardiopathy were confirmed in 7 of 10 Latin American cities studied in an investigation of mortality (Puffer and Griffith, 1967). The mortality rate was exceptionally high in the city of Ribeirão Prêto, Brazil: Chagas' disease was the cause of 13% of all deaths in the population aged 15 to 74 years—29% of 25-to 44-year-old men and 22% of the women in the same age group. Chagas' disease is primarily a rural affliction, but its sequelae in chronic patients are also seen in cities. Vector transmission occurs in cities as well, as migrants from the countryside bring the disease and even the vector along with them.

Occurrence in Animals: The natural infection has been found in 150 species of mammals, both domestic and wild. However, because of the difficulty in identifying the agent, it is not certain that all the strains that have been isolated correspond to *T. cruzi*. Several animal species serve as reservoirs in different ecologic settings. In Paraguay, the direct agglutination test was positive for *T. cruzi* in 3 of 37 cattle (8.1%), 2 of 20 swine (10%), 16 of 44 dogs (36.4%), and 3 of 8 cats (37.5%), while 3 equines, an opossum, and 3 armadillos were negative (Fujita *et al.*, 1994). Among domestic animals, dogs and cats are common and important hosts of the parasite. In a group of towns in northwestern Argentina, 41.2% of 68 dogs and 39.3% of 28 cats were positive on xenodiagnosis (Gurtler *et al.*, 1993). In Texas, US, 11 symptomatic cases of Chagas' disease in dogs were reported between 1987 and 1996 (Meurs *et al.*, 1998). Several studies have confirmed that in endemic areas the prevalence of infection is higher in these species than it is in man. In the Yaracuy Valley in Venezuela, 70 of 140 dogs (50%) tested were positive on xenodiagnosis. In Chile, 9.1% of 3,321 dogs and 11.9% of 1,805 cats were positive. Xenodiagnosis also revealed that 8.4% of the human population was positive. Other domestic animals can also serve as reservoirs (Miles, 1983). In a serologic survey of 34 rural localities in Region IV of Chile, the hemagglutination test showed antibodies for *T. cruzi* in 7.8% of 232 goats, 11.7% of 145 rabbits, and 4.8% of 42 sheep, and high rates of infection were also confirmed in dogs and cats (Correa *et al.*, 1982). The guinea pig *Cavia porcellus,* a common domestic animal in the high Andean plateau, plays a very important epidemiologic role in the transmission of Chagas' disease in that region, with infection rates ranging from 10.5% to 61% in different localities in Bolivia.

Natural infection has also been confirmed in a large number of wild animal species. Although any mammal in contact with infected vectors can acquire the infection, not all species are equally preponderant in maintaining the Chagas enzootic in the wild. Studies conducted in Brazil and Venezuela have shown that opossums of the genus *Didelphis (D. albiventris* and *D. marsupialis)* play a very important role. Xenodiagnosis of 750 mammals representing 31 species from the dry tropical forests in the highland plains of Venezuela was positive in 10 species; in all, 143 infections were found, and 83% of them were in *D. marsupialis,* even though the infected animals represented only 30% of the mammals in the sample. Seasonal fluctuations were observed, with the infection rate rising at the end of the rainy season and affecting more than 80% of the opossum population (Telford *et al.,* 1981). These marsupials have prolonged parasitemia, which can last for more than 12 months (Mello, 1982). Opossums are important because of their tendency to approach human homes, thus serving as a link between the wild and domestic cycles of the infection. Armadillos, which are common in Latin America, have been found to be parasitized in a number of countries. In Georgia, US, parasitemia was found in 13 of 30 (43%) raccoons tested. The cardiac muscle was examined histopathologically in 10 of the cases; in each case a mild, multifocal interstitial inflammation was observed, and a parasitic cyst was found in one of them. Apparently the infection does not cause pathology in this species (Pietrzak and Pung, 1998).

The Disease in Man: In cases of vector transmission, the incubation period lasts 7 to 14 days and sometimes longer. When the infection is transmitted by infected blood, incubation takes between 30 and 40 days. Three phases of infection are distinguished: acute, indeterminate, and chronic. The acute phase can range from an asymptomatic course, which is most common, to a severe or fatal disease. In 59 acute-phase patients treated in Venezuela between 1988 and 1996, the disease presented 19 different forms. In its most frequent manifestation, the symptomatology included fever, myalgia, cephalalgia, and Romaña's sign (unilateral eyelid swelling which seems to be mainly an allergic reaction to the bite), observed in 20% of the patients (particularly children). Fifteen percent of the cases were asymptomatic, and 11.9% manifested fever only. Nearly 50% of the children had an inoculation chagoma (swelling with involvement of a satellite lymph node, apparently caused by local multiplication of the parasite), but in about 25% of the patients no signs of a portal of entry were observed. The case fatality rate for the acute form is about 8%, and the deaths occur mainly in children with cardiac or central nervous system complications (Anez *et al.*, 1999).

The indeterminate phase consists of a period of latent infection with low parasitemia and no clinical symptoms, which can last indefinitely or progress to the chronic disease. This period is characterized by positive serology or xenodiagnosis without any clinical cardiac, digestive, or central nervous system manifestations and no electrocardiographic or radiologic alterations. In endemic areas, this form is seen especially in the first three decades of life (Dorea, 1981). Autopsies of persons dying from an accident who were in this phase have revealed foci of myocarditis and a reduced number of neurons in the parasympathetic plexus.

The chronic form is seen in 10% to 30% of infected individuals, usually appearing 10 to 15 years after the acute phase. Chagas cardiopathy is the most important chronic form. After the first manifestations, which almost always consist of extrasystoles and precordialgia, an electrocardiogram will show complete or partial blockage of the right branch of the bundle of His. Signs of heart failure are seen during this phase, and autopsies show a weakened ventricular wall with aneurysms. Often the chronic phase is manifested only by abnormalities in the electrocardiogram, with no clinical symptomatology. Histopathologic examination reveals areas of fibrosis and infiltration of mononuclear cells but not the presence of parasites, conditions not usually found in the chronic form of the disease (see hypotheses presented below). The heart lesion corresponds to a microfocal, diffuse, fibrosing myocarditis. At the same time, there is a significant reduction in the number of parasympathetic ganglia (González Cappa and Segura, 1982). In Argentina, it is estimated that about 20% of all Chagas patients suffer from myocarditis. In several endemic areas of Latin America, there is a digestive form of Chagas' disease that produces visceromegalies such as megacolon and megaesophagus, and less frequently, neurologic, myxedematous, and glandular forms. Patients with acquired immunodeficiency syndrome may experience reactivation of the disease, with nervous (75%) or cardiac (44%) involvement, or myositis of the esophagus and stomach (Ferreira *et al.*, 1997).

The pathogenesis of the chronic phase is not yet understood. The lack of correlation between the lesions in the myocardium or digestive apparatus and the presence of parasites has given rise to three main hypotheses to account for the pathogenesis of these manifestations: 1) when the pseudocysts rupture, *T. cruzi* "toxin" is released and destroys the muscle cells or the neurons; 2) antigen from the *T. cruzi* pseudocysts is absorbed by the adjacent cells, inducing an immune response that destroys these cells; or 3) the parasite and the muscle cells or neurons share antigens in common; therefore, immune reactions to the parasite also destroy the host cells. Since no toxin has been found that might account for the damage, the autoimmune hypotheses have been gaining ground in recent years, even though the supporting evidence is only circumstantial (Kierszembaum, 1999). Some investigators have proposed that the lesions may be due to inflammatory reactions to parasites that remain inside the tissues (Brener and Gazzinelli, 1997).

When immunocompetent individuals acquire the infection from a blood transfusion, there are usually no symptoms of the disease, but these people may develop prolonged fever, adenopathies, and later, splenomegaly. In immunodeficient patients, however, the infection can cause a high fever and progressively compromise their general state of health.

In the congenital disease, the most frequent signs are hepatosplenomegaly, premature birth (weight under 2.5 kg), changes in the retina, meningoencephalitis, and cardiac insufficiency with alterations in the electroencephalogram. Fever is unusual.

The Disease in Animals: It is generally believed that *T. cruzi* infection is asymptomatic in wild animals, but this impression may be largely due to the lack of detailed clinical examination. Electrocardiographic studies and ventricular angiograms of rats (*Rattus rattus*) naturally infected with *T. cruzi* have revealed auricular and ventricular arrhythmias, second degree AV block, blockage of the right outflow tract, and dilation of the right chambers. The same alterations are seen in dogs with chronic *T. cruzi* infections (Blandon *et al.*, 1995). The acute phase, which begins after an incubation period of 5 to 42 days, is characterized by moderate fever, palpebral edema in some cases, pronounced hepatomegaly, multiple adenopathies, cardiac perturbations, and alterations in the nervous system. The acute phase lasts from 10 to 30 days and sometimes longer, following which the disease passes to the indeterminate phase, which can extend for years without clinical manifestations. Dogs with acute experimental infections have exhibited alterations in the neurons of the Auerbach plexus and myositis in the lower third of the esophagus (Caliari *et al.*, 1996), but they did not have any visceromegalies. As in man, the chronic form is characterized by myocarditis. Of 26 dogs experimentally infected with blood trypomastigotes, 13 died spontaneously during the acute phase, while 12 of 38 dogs infected with metacyclic trypanosomes survived to the chronic phase and lived for 1 or 2 years. These animals had the same cardiac alterations that are seen in man during the acute and chronic phase (Lana *et al.*, 1992). Clinical, electrocardiographic, and echocardiographic manifestations in dogs with chronic Chagas' disease were compatible with right heart disease. Six dogs survived less than 6 months, while 5 of them lived more than 30 months, the outcome varying according to the age of the animal at the time of initial examination (Meurs *et al.*, 1998). There have also been occasional reports of alterations in the brain and the peripheral nerves during the acute and chronic phases. The infection was found in a female dog and seven of her eight pups in Virginia, US, suggesting that in dogs the infection can be transmitted either via the placenta or through the mother's milk.

Source of Infection and Mode of Transmission: The source of Chagas' infection is always the infected mammal. In the case of vector transmission, the reservoir may be any peridomestic animal that infects the vector, which in turn, infects other animals, including man. In nature, Chagas' disease appears to exist preferably in the wild, invading the domestic environment only when there are domiciliary vectors and ecological conditions that enable them to live in human homes. Since these conditions do not exist in the US, the infection has remained in the wild in that country. However, in many poor rural areas of Latin America, there are vectors that live exclusively or preferably inside houses, or at least have the potential to do so, and the dwellings have the kind of cracks that the insect needs in order to reproduce and hide during the day. The infection is particularly prevalent in these areas. Migrants who move from the countryside to the outskirts of cities can carry the vectors in their personal effects and infest new residential areas. Often, migrants or *T. cruzi*-infected vectors settle in periurban areas where Chagas' disease is already endemic. Several studies have shown that one of the major risk factors for human infection is the presence and number of dogs in the home, and some studies have implicated cats as well, especially when these animals are infected. This observation would indicate that dogs are a primary source of food and infection for the vectors (Gurtler *et al.*, 1998). Chickens in the household are also a risk factor because, even though these animals are not susceptible to *T. cruzi*, the vector feeds on them. *T. cruzi* can also be introduced in the human environment through peridomestic wild animals such as armadillos, guinea pigs, opossums, and others. Rats have visible and prolonged infections, and they can also be a source of infection (Blandon *et al.*, 1995). Moreover, even in the chronic phase of the disease, a human can be a potential source of infection, as revealed in a 13-year follow-up study of 202 chronic-phase patients: xenodiagnosis showed that the levels of parasitemia were consistently maintained in 146 of the patients and actually rose in 14 of them, while in 42 of the cases did these levels decline (Castro *et al.*, 1999). These results notwithstanding, there are statistical studies indicating that the presence of infected dogs is much more important in the infection of vectors than is the presence of infected humans (Gurtler *et al.*, 1991).

A number of the vectors are fully adapted to cohabiting with humans—for example, *Triatoma infestans*, which has a wide area of distribution that encompasses Argentina, Bolivia, Brazil, Chile, Paraguay, Peru, and Uruguay. Such species play a key role in human infection because of their facility of contact with people. Then there are species, found both in homes and in the wild, that are important because they introduce *T. cruzi* into the domestic environment; an example is *Rhodnius prolixus*, which is widely active in Colombia, Ecuador, Venezuela, much of Central America, and Mexico. Still other species are in the process of domiciliary adaptation—for example, *Triatoma sordida* in Argentina, Bolivia, and Brazil; *Panstrongylus megistus* in the eastern part of Brazil; *T. brasiliensis* in the Brazilian northeast; and *T. maculata* in Venezuela. Finally, there are species that are fundamentally wild and rarely invade the peridomestic environment; examples are *T. spinolai* in Chile, *T. protracta* in North America, and *T. sanguisuga* in the US. Although these species do not play a significant role in human infection, they maintain the endemicity of Chagas' disease in the wild. Some of the vectors, such as *T. infestans*, defecate while they feed, thus easily contaminating the skin or mucosae of the host and facilitating transmission of the infective agent. These species are most important in transmission to man. Other species, such as *T. protracta,* defecate later and are therefore less significant for human infection, but they can play a role in the case of animals that chew and eat them in an effort to get rid of them.

The ecology of Chagas' disease is closely linked to underdevelopment and poverty in rural and marginal urban areas of Latin America. Precariously built dwellings made of adobe and mud, as well as roofs of palm thatch or straw, afford ideal conditions for triatomine colonization. The bugs also take up residence in chicken houses, rabbit hutches, corrals, pigsties, aviaries, sheds, and wood piles in areas surrounding the homes.

Although less prevalent than vector transmission, congenital transmission and transmission via blood transfusion are also important sources of human infection (see The Disease in Man), especially because they introduce the agent in areas where the vectors do not exist. Unlike toxoplasmosis, Chagas' disease can be passed on congenitally when the mother is in the chronic phase of the infection. Although transmission can also occur from the ingestion of food contaminated with the excrement of infected triatomines, the importance of this route in the epidemiology of the disease remains to be assessed. There have also been accidental infections in laboratories and from organ transplants from infected donors.

Diagnosis: The specific diagnostic methods for Chagas' disease are direct identification of the parasite and testing for immunologic reactions. Recent efforts have focused on detection of the parasite's DNA using the polymerase chain reaction (PCR) technique. Since *T. cruzi* remains in the blood for only a short time, direct demonstration is used mainly in the acute phase, whereas the immunologic tests are used in the indeterminate and chronic phases.

In direct observation, fresh blood is examined either between slide and coverslip or in thin or thick films stained using Giemsa's method. However, the effectiveness of these diagnostic procedures is limited except in very acute cases and with congenital infection in children under 6 months old. Microscopic examination of tissues often fails to yield any parasites. A technique that is more efficient is the Strout method (Flores *et al.*, 1966), in which the blood sample is allowed to coagulate, the serum is centrifuged at a low speed (200 G) to eliminate the rest of the blood cells and then at a high speed (600 G) to concentrate the trypanosomes, and finally, the sediment is observed. All the procedures mentioned become less effective as the level of parasitemia declines. For borderline cases, the most effective direct methods are xenodiagnosis, hemoculture (Anez *et al.*, 1999), and inoculation in animals, in all of which the few parasites present in the patient's blood are multiplied. In xenodiagnosis, the patient is bitten by uninfected vectors that have been produced in the laboratory and fed on chickens (to prevent accidental *T. cruzi* infections), and the insects' feces are examined 30 and 60 days later to detect the presence of the parasite. This method is 100% effective in acute-phase patients, but less than 50% effective with those in the indeterminate and chronic phases. Culture of blood or tissue samples is done preferably using Novy-MacNeal-Nicolle medium, and incubation takes 30 days. Finally, another method of diagnosis consists of inoculating samples in uninfested mice or rats and subsequently observing these animals for parasitemia.

As the patient progresses to the indeterminate or chronic phase, the presence of parasites in the bloodstream is too low to apply direct methods and indirect immunologic methods must be used. The complement fixation test (or Guerreiro Machado reaction) was common in the past, but it is now considered that the most sensitive and specific tests are direct agglutination, indirect immunofluorescence, and the enzyme-linked immunosorbent assay (Anez *et al.*, 1999). Specificity, and to some extent sensitivity, depends on the antigens used, and recombinant antigens are being studied for this purpose (Umezawa *et al.*, 1999). Also being investigated is PCR, which detects parasite DNA and should obtain reactions that are both highly specific and sufficiently sensitive (Gomes *et al.*, 1999).

Cases of congenital infection in infants up to 6 months of age can be considered acute cases; thereafter, they should be considered indeterminate or chronic cases. When serology is used in congenital cases, the focus should be on finding IgM or IgA antibodies, because the mother's IgG antibodies cross the placenta and can simulate an infection in healthy children.

Although *T. rangeli* can be mistaken for *T. cruzi*, the two can be differentiated by morphology, immunologic techniques based on selected antigens (Acosto *et al.*, 1991), or PCR.

Control: The drugs available for the treatment of acute-phase Chagas' disease are toxic and unreliable in terms of eradicating the infection, and there is no curative treatment for chronic infection (Levi *et al.*, 1996); therefore, it is highly important to control transmission. A number of countries, Brazil in particular, have independently undertaken control campaigns (da Rocha e Silva *et al.*, 1998). In 1991, six Southern Cone countries (Argentina, Bolivia, Brazil, Chile, Paraguay, and Uruguay) launched a regional control initiative with the support of the World Health Organization (Schofield and Dias, 1999). By 1999, vector transmission had been interrupted in Uruguay and significantly reduced in Argentina, Chile, and Brazil, but it had not yet been curtailed in Bolivia or Paraguay.

To ultimately control vector transmission, homes must be improved by eliminating the cracks and crevices in which the vectors establish their colonies. However, since this is a costly, long-term undertaking, a more immediate alternative is to treat the surfaces of infested dwellings with residual insecticides. Synthetic pyrethroids are most often used, and the employment of synthetic insect hormones is under study. It is desirable to remove dogs and cats from the human environment because they are not only an important food source for the vector but also a major reservoir for *T. cruzi* (Gurtler *et al.*, 1998). The areas to be treated are identified through reports received, observation of the vector's presence in homes (often found after the spraying of repellents), and detection of persons with positive serology for *T. cruzi*. Although the last approach is the most efficient and reliable, its drawback is that it only identifies a Chagas endemic area after the people have become infected. The verification of *T. cruzi*-positive serology in domestic dogs appears to give similar results (Castanera *et al.*, 1998). One possible approach to identifying endemic areas prior to the appearance of *T. cruzi* infection might be by detecting antibodies to the vector (instead of the protozoan) in humans or domestic animals (Barriga, 2000). It is necessary to maintain surveillance following initial eradication of the domiciliary vectors; it has been shown that they can establish foci outside the home after the application of insecticides and return to their original densities in one to six years. Moreover, wild species can occupy the habitats abandoned by the domestic vectors.

Transmission by blood transfusion is prevented through the presumptive identification of blood donors using questionnaires to find out if they come from Chagasic areas, through blood tests, or by treating the donated blood with gentian violet (250 mg/L) for 24 hours or longer, with or without the addition of ascorbic acid and exposure to light (Morães-Souza and Bordin, 1996).

Congenital infection is combated through timely treatment of infected mothers, but there are no reliable reports on the effectiveness of this method.

Although numerous studies have been conducted with a view to producing a vaccine against Chagas' disease, success has been impeded by the difficulty of distinguishing between protective antigens and those that might generate pathology in the long term.

Bibliography

Acosta, L., A.J. Romanha, H. Cosenza, A. Krettli. Trypanosomatid isolates from Honduras: Differentiation between *Trypanosoma cruzi* and *Trypanosoma rangeli*. *Am J Trop Med Hyg* 44:676–683, 1991.

Anez, N., H. Carrasco, H. Parada, *et al.* Acute Chagas' disease in western Venezuela: A clinical, seroparasitologic, and epidemiologic study. *Am J Trop Med Hyg* 60:215–222, 1999.

Arcavi, M., G. Orfus, G. Griemberg. Incidencia de la infección chagásica en embarazadas y en recién nacidos en área no endémica. *Medicina (B Aires)* 53:217–222, 1993.

Azogue, E. Women and congenital Chagas' disease in Santa Cruz, Bolivia: Epidemiological and sociocultural aspects. *Soc Sci Med* 37:503–511, 1993.

Barriga, O.O. Los hospederos generan anticuerpos circulantes y cutáneos contra las picadas de *Triatoma infestans* e inhiben su alimentación. *In*: VII Jornada Anual SOCHIPA, Libro de resúmenes, p. 22. Temuco: Sociedad Chilena de Producción Animal; 2000.

Benenson, A.S., ed. *Control of Communicable Diseases in Man*, 16th ed. An Official Report of the American Public Health Association. Washington, D.C.: APHA; 1995.

Blanco, A., E.E. Montamat. Genetic variation among *Trypanosoma cruzi* populations. *J Exp Zool* 282:62–70, 1998.

Blandon, R., I.M. Leandro, C.M. Johnson. Evaluación clínica, electrocardiográfica y angiográfica de los reservorios naturales de la enfermedad de Chagas en la República de Panama. *Rev Med Panama* 20:108–115, 1995.

Bogliolo, A.R., E. Chiari, R.O. Silva-Pereira, A.A. Silva-Pereira. A comparative study of *Trypanosoma cruzi* enzyme polymorphism in South America. *Braz J Med Biol Res* 19:673–683, 1986.

Brener, Z., R.T. Gazzinelli. Immunological control of *Trypanosoma cruzi* infection and pathogenesis of Chagas' disease. *Int Arch Allergy Immunol* 114:103–110, 1997.

Caliari, E.R., M.V. Caliari, M. de Lana, W.L. Tafuri. Estudo quantitativo e qualitativo dos plexos de Auerbach e Meissner do esôfago de cãos inoculados com o *Trypanosoma cruzi*. *Rev Soc Bras Med Trop* 29:17–20, 1996.

Castanera, M.B., M.A. Lauricella, R. Chuit, R.E. Gurtler. Evaluation of dogs as sentinels of the transmission of *Trypanosoma cruzi* in a rural area of north-western Argentina. *Ann Trop Med Parasitol* 92(6):671–683, 1998.

Castro, C., V. Macêddo, A. Prata. Comportamento da parasitemia pelo *Trypanosoma cruzi* em chagásicos crônicos durante 13 anos. *Rev Soc Bras Med Trop* 32:157–165, 1999.

Correa, V., J. Briceño, J. Zuñiga, *et al.* Infección por *Trypanosoma cruzi* en animales domésticos de sectores rurales de la IV Región, Chile. *Bol Chil Parasitol* 37:27–78, 1982.

da Rocha e Silva, E.O., D.M. Wanderley, V.L. Rodrigues. *Triatoma infestans*: importancia, controle e eliminação da espécie no Estado de São Paulo, Brasil. *Rev Soc Bras Med Trop* 31:73–88, 1998.

Di Pentima, M.C., L.Y. Hwang, C.M. Skeeter, M.S. Edwards. Prevalence of antibody to *Trypanosoma cruzi* in pregnant Hispanic women in Houston. *Clin Infect Dis* 28:1281–1285, 1999.

Dorea, R.C.C. Doença de Chagas na Amazônia: aspectos epidemiológicos regionais e considerações a propósito de um caso pediátrico. *Hileia Méd* 3:81–109, 1981.

Ferreira, M.S., S. de Nishioka, M.T. Silvestre, A.S. Borges, F.R. Nunes-Araujo, A. Rocha. Reactivation of Chagas' disease in patients with AIDS: Report of three new cases and review of the literature. *Clin Infect Dis* 25:1397–1400, 1997.

Flores, M.A., A. Trejos, A. R. Paredes, A.Y. Ramos. El método de concentración de Strout en el diagnóstico de la fase aguda de la enfermedad de Chagas. *Bol Chil Parasitol* 21:38–39, 1966.

Fujita, O., L. Sanabria, A. Inchaustti, A.R. De Arias, Y. Tomizawa, Y. Oku. Animal reservoirs for *Trypanosoma cruzi* infection in an endemic area in Paraguay. *J Vet Med Sci* 56:305–308, 1994.

Gomes, M.L., L.M. Galvão, A.M. Macedo, S.D. Pena, E. Chiari. Chagas' disease diagnosis: Comparative analysis of parasitologic, molecular, and serologic methods. *Am J Trop Med Hyg* 60:205–210, 1999.

González Cappa, S.M., E.L. Segura. Enfermedad de Chagas. *Adel Microbiol Enf Infec* (B Aires) 1:51–102, 1982.

Gurtler, R.E., M.C. Cecere, D.N. Rubel, *et al.* Chagas disease in north-west Argentina: Infected dogs as a risk factor for the domestic transmission of *Trypanosoma cruzi*. *Trans R Soc Trop Med Hyg* 85:741–745, 1991.

Gurtler, R.E., M.C. Cecere, R.M. Petersen, D.N. Rubel, N.J. Schweigmann. Chagas disease in north-west Argentina: Association between *Trypanosoma cruzi* parasitaemia in dogs and cats and infection rates in domestic *Triatoma infestans*. *Trans R Soc Trop Med Hyg* 87:12–15, 1993.

Gurtler, R.E., R. Chuit, M.C. Cecere, M.B. Castanera, J.E. Cohen, E.L. Segura. Household prevalence of seropositivity for *Trypanosoma cruzi* in three rural villages in northwest Argentina: Environmental, demographic, and entomologic associations. *Am J Trop Med Hyg* 59:741–749, 1998.

Jaramillo, R., J.P. Bryan, J. Schur, A.A. Pan. Prevalence of antibody to *Trypanosoma cruzi* in three populations in Belize. *Am J Trop Med Hyg* 57:298–301, 1997.

Kierszenbaum, F. Chagas' disease and the autoimmunity hypothesis. *Clin Microbiol Rev* 12:210–223, 1999.

Lana, M. de, E. Chiari, W.L. Tafuri. Experimental Chagas' disease in dogs. *Mem Inst Oswaldo Cruz* 87:59–71, 1992.

Lauria-Pires, L., A.R. Teixeira. Virulence and pathogenicity associated with diversity of *Trypanosoma cruzi* stocks and clones derived from Chagas' disease patients. *Am J Trop Med Hyg* 55:304–310, 1996.

Leiby, D.A., E.J. Read, B.A. Lenes, *et al.* Seroepidemiology of *Trypanosoma cruzi*, etiologic agent of Chagas' disease, in US blood donors. *J Infect Dis* 176:1047–1052, 1997.

Leiby, D.A., M.H. Fucci, R.J. Stumpf. *Trypanosoma cruzi* in a low- to moderate-risk blood donor population: Seroprevalence and possible congenital transmission. *Transfusion* 39:310–315, 1999.

Levi, G.C., I.M. Lobo, E.G. Kallas, V. Amato Neto. Etiological drug treatment of human infection by *Trypanosoma cruzi*. *Rev Inst Med Trop Sao Paulo* 38:35–38, 1996.

Marsden, P.D. The control of Latin American Chagas' disease. *Rev Soc Bras Med Trop* 30:521–527, 1997.

Mello, D.A. Aspectos do ciclo silvestre do *Trypanosoma cruzi* em regiões de cerrado (Município de Formosa, Estado de Goias). *Mem Inst Oswaldo Cruz* 76:227–246, 1981.

Meurs, K.M., M.A. Anthony, M. Slater, M.W. Miller. Chronic *Trypanosoma cruzi* infection in dogs: 11 cases (1987–1996). *J Am Vet Med Assoc* 213:497–500, 1998.

Miles, M.A. The epidemiology of South American trypanosomiasis—Biochemical and immunological approaches and their relevance to control. *Trans R Soc Trop Med Hyg* 77:5–23, 1983.

Moncayo, A. Chagas' disease: Epidemiology and prospects for interruption in the Americas. *World Health Stat Q* 45:276–279, 1992.

Morães-Souza, H., J.O. Bordin. Strategies for prevention of transfusion-associated Chagas' disease. *Transfus Med Rev* 10:161–170, 1996.

Pan American Health Organization (PAHO). Situación de la enfermedad de Chagas en las Américas. *Bol Oficina Sanit Panam* 97:159–165, 1984.

Passos, A.D., J.L. Nogueira, J.F. de Castro Figueiredo, U.A. Gomes, A.L. Dal-Fabbro. Evolução da positividade sorológica para a doença de Chagas numa comunidade rural brasileira. *Rev Panam Salud Publica* 2:247–252, 1997.

Pietrzak, S.M., O.J. Pung. Trypanosomiasis in raccoons from Georgia. *J Wildl Dis* 34:132–136, 1998.

Puffer, R.R., G. Wynne Griffith. *Patterns of Urban Mortality.* Washington, D.C.: Pan American Health Organization; 1967. (Scientific Publication No. 151.)

Rangel, H., R. Gatica, C. Ramos. Detection of antibodies against *Trypanosoma cruzi* in donors from a blood bank in Cuernavaca, Morelos, Mexico. *Arch Med Res* 29:79–82, 1998.

Russomando, G., M.M. de Tomassone, I. de Guillen, *et al.* Treatment of congenital Chagas' disease diagnosed and followed up by the polymerase chain reaction. *Am J Trop Med Hyg* 59:487–491, 1998.

Schmunis, G.A., F. Zicker, F. Pinheiro, D. Brandling-Bennett. Risk for transfusion-transmitted infectious diseases in Central and South America. *Emerg Infect Dis* 4:5–11, 1998.

Schofield, C.J., J.C. Dias. The Southern Cone Initiative against Chagas' disease. *Adv Parasitol* 42:1–27, 1999.

Streiger, M., D. Fabbro, M. del Barco, R. Beltramino, N. Bovero. Chagas congénito en la ciudad de Santa Fe. Diagnóstico y tratamiento. *Medicina (B Aires)* 55:125–132, 1995.

Telford, S.R., Jr., R.J. Tonn, J. González, P. Betancourt. Dinámica de las infecciones tripanosómicas entre la comunidad de los bosques tropicales secos en los llanos altos de Venezuela. *Bol Dirección Malariol Saneam Ambient* 21:196–209, 1981.

Umezawa, E.S., S.F. Bastos, M.E. Camargo, *et al.* Evaluation of recombinant antigens for serodiagnosis of Chagas' disease in South and Central America. *J Clin Microbiol* 37:1554–1560, 1999.

Wanderley, D.M., F.M. Correa. Epidemiology of Chagas' heart disease. *Rev Paul Med* 113:742–749, 1995.

Zaidenberg, M., A. Segovia. Enfermedad de Chagas congénita en la ciudad de Salta, Argentina. *Rev Inst Med Trop Sao Paulo* 35:35–43, 1993.

CRYPTOSPORIDIOSIS

ICD-10 A07.2

Synonym: *Cryptosporidium* infection.

Etiology: The genus *Cryptosporidium*, together with *Isospora, Cyclospora, Sarcocystis,* and *Toxoplasma*, contains protozoa of the coccidia group in the phylum Apicomplexa (formerly Sporozoa). Since the genus was recognized in 1907 by Tyzzer, more than 20 species of *Cryptosporidium* have been described, but at present only 6 are accepted as valid. The only species that affects both humans and other mammals is *C. parvum* (Barriga, 1997). However, it appears that some varieties of this parasite infect only humans and other varieties infect humans, cattle, and mice. *C. parvum* normally lives in the small intestine, where it forms oocysts that are excreted in the host's feces. Each oocyst contains four small banana-shaped sporozoites, which are the infective stage of the parasite. When a susceptible host ingests the oocysts, the sporozoites shed their protective cover and penetrate the epithelial cells of the new host's intestine. Each sporozoite differentiates into a spherical parasite, the trophozoite, which in turn multiplies asexually to form two types of meronts (formerly called schizonts), each about 5 μm in diameter. Type I meronts produce six to eight new banana-shaped parasites (merozoites). Type II meronts form four oval-shaped merozoites, the gametocytes. Once mature, the merozoites leave the host cell and invade new epithelial cells, where they produce more merozoites (type I) or gametocytes (type II). The gametocytes also invade new intestinal cells, where they differentiate into male cells (microgametocytes) and female cells (macrogametocytes).

The microgametocytes produce numerous filamentous microgametes 1–2 μm in length, which leave the host cell and fertilize the macrogametocytes, forming a zygote. The zygote matures in the host cell and produces four naked sporozoites— i.e., not inside sporocysts—which are already infective. Most of the mature zygotes (around 80%) develop a tough outer cover measuring 2.5–5 μm in diameter and become infective oocysts. These oocysts are excreted by the host in feces and contaminate the environment. The rest of the mature zygotes have only a thin outer membrane. Because these thin-walled oocysts are easily ruptured, their sporozoites remain in the intestine, reinfecting the same host (Fayer and Ungar, 1986).

Geographic Distribution: Worldwide. Cases of human cryptosporidiosis have been reported from more than 50 countries on 6 continents (Benenson, 1997).

Occurrence in Man: The first two clinical cases of human cryptosporidiosis were identified in 1976 in two immunodeficient patients. Since then, many cases and numerous epidemics have been recognized. Various surveys have indicated that the oocyst prevalence in feces ranges from 1% to 2% in Europe, 0.6% to 4.3% in North America, and 10% to 20% in the developing countries. However, serologic evidence of past infections has shown positivity rates of 25% to 35% in industrialized countries and up to 65% in developing countries. The most well-known epidemic occurred in 1993 in Milwaukee, Wisconsin, US, where a total of 1.6 million people were exposed, 403,000 wcre infected, and 7 died (Lisle and Rose, 1995). Infection is much more common than the clinical disease and most frequently occurs in children under 2 years of age, contacts of infected individuals, livestock handlers, travelers to developing countries, homosexuals, and, especially, immunodeficient individuals. In Australia, *Cryptosporidium* was found in 4.1% of stool samples from 884 patients with gastroenteritis, but not in samples from 320 patients without gastroenteritis (Tzipori *et al.*, 1983). In the US, however, while *Cryptosporidium* was similarly found in the stool samples of around 4% of patients with gastroenteritis, it was also found in 13% of samples from healthy individuals.

Occurrence in Animals: Several species of *Cryptosporidium* infect both warm- and cold-blooded animals. *C. parvum* infects numerous mammals in addition to humans, in particular other primates, cattle and other ruminants, horses, carnivores, and rodents. In all the affected domestic species, very young unweaned animals are more susceptible to the infection and the disease than adults, and calves appear to be most susceptible. The first clinical case of cryptosporidiosis in animals was identified in a calf in 1971. Subsequently, the infection has been found in up to 80% of calves under 1 month of age and up to 62% of apparently healthy adult cattle. In horses, the infection has been found in 15%–31% of suckling foals, but only 0.6% of adult horses. Of calves with diarrhea studied in the US, 25% were found to be infected.

The Disease in Man: In individuals with healthy immune systems, cryptosporidiosis may be asymptomatic or may occur as a self-limiting disease. The illness is characterized by profuse watery diarrhea that begins explosively one or two weeks after infection and generally lasts 8–20 days, often accompanied by abdominal pain, nausea, vomiting, low-grade fever (under 39°C), and weight loss. In immunodeficient individuals, the symptoms are more severe and may include as many as 71 evacuations per day, with fluid loss of up to 25 liters (Ryan, 1994). Rather than being self-limiting, the disease may persist until the individual's death. In such patients, the parasite has sometimes been found to invade the respiratory and biliary tracts (Clavel *et al.*, 1996).

The Disease in Animals: Cryptosporidiosis is fairly common in young calves. The infection generally appears during the first three weeks of life and affects animals between 3 and 35 days of age. The clinical manifestations are diarrhea, tenesmus, anorexia, and weight loss. It is difficult to distinguish diarrhea caused by *Cryptosporidium* from diarrhea caused by other agents. Anderson (1982) reported that in calves aged 1–15 days from 47 herds, only 17 out of 51 were found to be excreting *Cryptosporidium* oocysts, although all had diarrhea. In horses, swine, and domestic carnivores, the disease has occasionally been reported in very young or immunodeficient animals (Barriga, 1997). Infected rodents do not appear to develop signs of disease. Birds are rarely affected by the species of the parasite that infect mammals.

Source of Infection and Mode of Transmission: The sources of infection for humans are other infected people and infected cattle. There is no solid evidence that other animals are an important source of human infection. Although *Cryptosporidium*-infected cats have been found in association with AIDS patients, it is not clear who infected whom. However, recent studies indicate that *C. parvum* exhibits genetic polymorphism, with one genotype infecting only humans and another infecting humans, cattle, and mice (Peng *et al.*, 1997). These genotypes might represent different species, but unequivocal identification of *Cryptosporidium* species is difficult.

The source of infection for domestic animals is other domestic animals. Cross-transmission studies have demonstrated that parasites isolated from humans, goat kids, deer, lambs, and calves can infect and cause diarrhea in pigs, lambs, and calves, while they produce an asymptomatic infection in chickens, colts, and laboratory animals (Tzipori, 1983). Isolates from humans and calves have also been transmitted to kids, puppies, cats, mice, and calves (Current, 1983). *Cryptosporidium* species that infect birds do not infect mammals, and species that infect mammals rarely infect birds.

The infection is transmitted through ingestion of foods and water contaminated with fecal matter from an infected individual, direct contact with infected feces, or ingestion of water from sources contaminated by effluents from sewerage systems or cattle farms. Children, childcare workers who change diapers, bed-ridden patients and their caregivers, people who work with cattle, and individuals who engage in anal sex have a high risk of being infected through direct contact with fecal matter.

Diagnosis: Diarrhea from *Cryptosporidium* is hard to distinguish clinically from diarrheal illnesses due to other causes. Diagnosis of cryptosporidiosis is suspected on the basis of both clinical symptoms and epidemiological history and is confirmed by demonstrating the presence of oocysts in the patient's feces. However, because oocysts are small (2.5–5 μm in diameter), they are difficult to see with direct microscopic examination of fecal samples. They are therefore more easily detected by means of techniques involving concentration in sugar solutions, such as Sheather's solution, and by phase contrast microscopy. Giemsa or methylene blue staining makes the oocysts more visible but also turns yeast contaminants the same color, making it impossible to distinguish them from the parasite. Ziehl-Neelsen stain, on the other hand, turns oocysts red but does not stain yeast. Auramine-rhodamine and safranine-methylene blue are also useful for distinguishing oocysts. A recently developed technique uses fluorescent monoclonal antibodies specific to *Cryptosporidium* to visualize the parasites in fecal or environmental specimens. The specificity of serologic diagnosis by means of immunofluorescence assay or enzyme-linked immunosorbent assay was initially dubious, but the tests have been refined and now show satisfactory levels of sensitivity and specificity. Although serologic diagnosis is useful for epidemiological studies, the antibodies may appear too late for clinical purposes in immunocompetent patients or may not appear in sufficient quantities in immunodeficient patients.

Procedures for recovering and identifying *Cryptosporidium* in environmental waters are highly variable, inefficient, and time-consuming. The currently recommended practice involves passing large volumes of water through special filters, centrifuging the material trapped by the filters to concentrate it, purifying the concentrate in a Percoll-sucrose gradient, staining with fluorescent antibodies, and, finally, examining the material microscopically.

Control: For an individual, prevention of cryptosporidiosis consists of avoiding the ingestion of raw foods or water that may be contaminated with human or animal feces and avoiding contact with feces (Juraneck, 1995). Cooking high-risk foods and washing hands carefully before eating should also reduce the danger of infection. People should avoid immersion in water containing effluents from sewerage systems or cattle farms. *Cryptosporidium* oocysts are highly resistant to all disinfectants. For example, the CT value (concentration of disinfectant in milligrams per liter multiplied by contact time in minutes) for killing 99% to 99.9% of the *Cryptosporidium* oocysts present in water is 6 to 10 for ozone and 9,600 for chlorine. In contrast, the corresponding values for *Giardia intestinalis* are 0.17 and 15. Exposure to water temperatures of 25°C and 8°C for 4 weeks kills only 50% and 25% of oocysts, respectively (Barriga, 1997). Under favorable conditions, they are probably capable of surviving for several months in nature.

Treatment of drinking water in well-run plants with good filters removes around 99.9% of oocysts.

Bibliography

Anderson, B.C. Cryptosporidiosis: A review. *J Am Med Assoc* 180:1455–1457, 1982.

Barriga, O.O. *Veterinary Parasitology for Practitioners*, 2nd ed. Edina: Burgess International Group; 1997.

Benenson, A.S., ed. *Control of Communicable Diseases Manual*, 16th ed. An official report of the American Public Health Association. Washington, D.C: APHA; 1995.

Clavel, A., A.C. Arnal, E.C. Sanchez, *et al.* Respiratory cryptosporidiosis: Case series and review of the literature. *Infection* 24:341–346, 1996.

Current, W. L., N.C. Reese, J.V. Ernst, *et al.* Human cryptosporidiosis in immunocompetent and immunodeficient persons. Studies of an outbreak and experimental transmission. *New Engl J Med* 308(21):1252–1257, 1983.

Fayer, R., B.L. Ungar. *Cryptosporidium* spp. and cryptosporidiosis. *Microbiol Rev* 50:458–483, 1986.

Juraneck, D.D. Cryptosporidiosis: Sources of infection and guidelines for prevention. *Clin Infect Dis* Suppl 1:S57–61, 1995.

Lisle, J.T., J.B. Rose. *Cryptosporidium* contamination of water in the US and the UK: A mini-review. *J Water SRT-Aqua* 44:103–117, 1995.

Peng, M.M., L. Xiao, A.R. Freeman, *et al.* Genetic polymorphism among *Cryptosporidium parvum* isolates: Evidence of two distinct human transmission cycles. *Emerg Infect Dis* 3:567–573, 1997.

Ryan, K.J., ed. *Sherris Medical Microbiology: An Introduction to Infectious Diseases*, 3rd ed. Norwalk, Connecticut: Appleton & Lange; 1994.

Tzipori, S. Cryptosporidiosis in animals and humans. *Microbiol Rev* 47:84–96, 1983.

Tzipori, S., M. Smith, C. Birch, G. Bames, R. Bishop. Cryptosporidiosis in hospital patients with gastroenteritis. *Am J Trop Med Hyg* 32:931–934, 1983.

CUTANEOUS LEISHMANIASIS

ICD-10 B55.1

Synonyms: Chiclero ulcer, espundia, pian-bois, uta, and buba (in the Americas); oriental sore, Aleppo boil, Baghdad sore, Delhi sore, and other local names (in the Old World).

Etiology: Leishmaniasis is caused by flagellate protozoa of the family Trypanosomatidae, genus *Leishmania*. The life cycle of leishmanias is relatively simple. The flagellate forms of the parasite—oval amastigotes measuring 2 to 5 μm in diameter (see the chapter on Chagas' Disease)—exist within macrophages of a definitive vertebrate host, including humans. Small flies of the family Phlebotomidae (genus *Phlebotomus* in the Old World and *Lutzomyia* in the Americas) ingest the parasites when they feed on the host's blood. Once in the fly's intestine, the amastigotes become promastigotes—extracellular forms with a flagellum emerging from the anterior end, which are fusiform and measure 14 to 20 μm long and 2 to 4 μm wide. The promastigotes then multiply in the intestine of the vector. In the insect, two promastigote forms can be observed: a wider, relatively immotile form that attaches to the wall of the intestine, and another, thinner, motile form that moves freely in the insect's intestinal lumen and proboscis. The first form incubates easily in human serum; the second does not. Presumably, the latter are metacyclic infective forms for the vertebrate which, by regurgitation from the intestine, are inoculated by the fly through the proboscis at its next blood meal (Kettle,

1995). Once inside the vertebrate, the promastigotes become amastigotes, invade the cutaneous macrophages, and multiply in a parasitophorous vacuole. These parasites are equipped with several adaptation mechanisms that enable them to overcome the lethal effects of macrophages and lysosomes on microorganisms (Antoine, 1995). Their multiplication eventually causes the host cell to rupture, and the released amastigotes then invade new macrophages.

Though there have been reports of morphological differentiation of *Leishmania* by computerized image analysis (Youssef *et al.*, 1997), it is virtually impossible to distinguish between species by means of conventional microscopy. Moreover, leishmanias seem to be undergoing an active process of evolution: isolates from parasites that cause identical diseases have shown different biochemical characteristics, while isolates from parasites that cause different diseases have similar biochemical features (Barral *et al.*, 1991). Some authors have proposed dividing the genus into two subgenera: *Leishmania*, encompassing forms that multiply in the foregut of their vectors (suprapylaria reproduction), and *Vianna*, comprising leishmania that develop in the midgut and hindgut (peripylaria reproduction). It is widely accepted that very similar groups of leishmanias exist. Those groups have been classified as species or complexes, which in turn comprise various lesser categories or subspecies. The complexes associated with cutaneous or visceral leishmaniasis in the Americas have been identified by polymerase chain reaction (Harris *et al.*, 1998). The species or subspecies of each complex are distinguished mainly by their geographic distribution, the clinical manifestations of the disease they cause, and epidemiologic characteristics.

Current efforts are endeavoring to classify leishmanias by means of serologic methods (agglutination, specificity of excretory antigens, and fluorescence with monoclonal antibodies), biochemical methods (enzymatic profile, nuclear and kinetoplast DNA (kDNA) density, and metabolic characteristics), and molecular biology techniques (genomic DNA sequencing and karyotype analysis), as a result of which new species are being proposed (Kreutzer *et al.*, 1991). Investigators now speak of serodemes (populations that are differentiated by their reactivity, using antibody batteries), zymodemes (populations distinguished by the composition of their isozymes), and schizodemes (populations that can be distinguished by the size of their DNA fragments when they are treated with batteries of restriction enzymes). For example, Chouicha *et al.* (1997) studied 10 enzymatic systems from 137 isolates of *L. braziliensis* obtained in Bolivia, Brazil, and Colombia, and were able to identify 44 closely related zymodemes. Kapoor *et al.* (1998) distinguished *L. tropica* from *L. donovani,* the agent of visceral leishmaniasis in Africa and Asia, and identified different isolates of *L. donovani* using cDNA probes and kDNA fragments.

The complexes that produce cutaneous leishmaniasis in the Americas are *L. mexicana* (which encompasses the species *L. mexicana, L. amazonensis,* and *L. venezuelensis*); *L. braziliensis* (*L. braziliensis, L. panamensis, L. guyanensis*); and *L. peruviana*. In the Old World, the agents of the disease belong to the *L. tropica* complex (*L. tropica, L. major,* and *L. aethiopica*) (Chulay, 1991). The complexes that cause American cutaneous leishmaniasis can be distinguished by such characteristics as vector, parasite localization in the insect's intestine, the pathogenicity of the agent on hamster skin, and the growth in culture media (Lainson and Shaw, 1974). The vectors of the *L. mexicana* complex leishmanias are phlebotomines of the group *Nyssomyia*. These parasites undergo suprapylaria development. When inoculated in hamster skin, they reproduce quickly, forming histiocytomas in which amastigotes are abundant and metastasis is common. They grow profusely in Novy, MacNeal, and Nicolle (NNN) culture medium. In contrast, leishmanias of the *L. braziliensis* complex, for which the vectors are phlebotomines of the groups *Psychodopygus* and *Nyssomyia*, undergo peripylaria development and multiply very slowly in hamster skin, producing small nodules or ulcers with few amastigotes that do not metastasize and whose growth in NNN culture media is slow or moderate (Bonfante-Garrido, 1983).

Geographic Distribution (Table 1): Some leishmanias appear to be indigenous to the Americas, while others were most likely imported from the Old World. Momen *et al.* (1993) found similarities between the isozymes of *L. chagasi* in Central and South America and those of *L. infantum* in the Mediterranean and Asia. They also found zymodemes characteristic of *L. major* from Africa and Asia in parasites isolated in the Americas.

Human cutaneous leishmaniasis in the Americas occurs from southern Mexico to northern Argentina, with sporadic cases in permanent residents and travelers who visit northern Mexico (Melby *et al.*, 1992). In the Caribbean islands, indigenous leishmaniasis exists only in the Dominican Republic (Zeledón, 1992). In South America, on the other hand, only Chile and Uruguay are free of the parasite. Detailed information on the distribution of leishmanias in the Americas can be found in Grimaldi *et al.* (1989). In the Old World, there are known endemic areas along the Mediterranean coast and in the Middle East, several countries of Asia (Azerbaijan, Kazakhstan, Tajikistan, Turkmenistan, and Uzbekistan), northern China, and northwestern India. In Africa, in addition to the foci on the Mediterranean coast, others exist in the western-central, eastern-central, and southern parts of the continent.

Within the *L. mexicana* complex, the subspecies *L. mexicana* is distributed in Belize, Brazil (Vale do Ribeira in the state of São Paulo) (Machado *et al.*, 1983), Guatemala, Mexico (Yucatan Peninsula and foci in Veracruz and Oaxaca), and the US (Texas, Oklahoma, Ohio, and possibly Michigan) (Sellon *et al.*, 1993). *L. amazonensis* is distributed in Mato Grosso in the Amazon Basin of Brazil, and *L. venezuelensis* was described in 1980 and isolated in Venezuela on the banks of the Turbio River in the state of Lara (Bonfante-Garrido, 1984).

Within the *L. braziliensis* complex, the distribution area of *L. braziliensis* encompasses eastern Bolivia, jungle areas of Brazil, Colombia, Ecuador, Paraguay, Peru, and Venezuela (Bonfante-Garrido, 1983). *L. guyanensis* is distributed north of the Amazon in Brazil and in French Guiana, Guyana, and Suriname. *L. panamensis* is present in Costa Rica, Honduras, Panama, and possibly in other Central American countries. *L. peruviana* is limited to the Peruvian Andes and is found only at altitudes of 900 to 3,000 m. In several regions of the Americas, *L. braziliensis* coexists with *L. mexicana*.

As for the complex *L. tropica* in the Old World, the subspecies *L. tropica* is found in some Mediterranean countries (Greece, Tunisia, and Turkey) and in Afghanistan, Iran, Iraq, Israel, Kuwait, and Uganda. In many other countries, such as the former Soviet Union, its identification is dubious owing to lack of information over the last 15 years or because it was eradicated (WHO, 1984). *L. major* exists in the Arabian peninsula, Afghanistan, Algeria, Burkina Faso, Egypt, India, Iran, Iraq, Israel, Jordan, Libya, Mali, Morocco, Mauritania, Pakistan, Senegal, Sudan, Syria, and Turkey. *L. aethiopica* is found in Ethiopia and Kenya (WHO, 1984).

TABLE 1. Features of *Leishmania* infections.

Species	Syndrome	Geographic distribution	Principal reservoir	Principal vector
Leishmania mexicana complex				
L. mexicana	Cutaneous, rarely diffuse	Belize, Brazilian Amazon, Guatemala, Mexico, Venezuela	Rodents	*Lutzomyia olmeca*
L. amazonensis	Cutaneous and diffuse	Brazilian Amazon	Rodents and marsupials	*Lutzomyia flaviscutellata*
L. venezuelensis	Cutaneous	Venezuela	Unknown	*Lutzomyia olmeca*
L. braziliensis complex				
L. braziliensis	Cutaneous and mucocutaneous	Bolivia, Brazil, Colombia, Paraguay, Peru, Venezuela	Rodents, dogs	*Lutzomyia wellcomei*
L. panamensis	Cutaneous, rarely mucocutaneous	Colombia, Costa Rica, Panama	Sloths	*Lutzomyia trapidoi*
L. guyanensis	Cutaneous	French Guiana, Guyana, Suriname	Sloths, anteaters	*Lutzomyia umbratilis*
L. peruviana	Cutaneous	Argentina, Peru	Dogs	*Lutzomyia peruensis*
				Lutzomyia verrucarum
L. tropica complex				
L. tropica	Cutaneous	Middle East, Mediterranean coast, Southeast Asia	Man, dogs	*Phlebotomus sergenti*
				Phlebotomus papatasi
L. major	Cutaneous	Middle East, Southeast Asia, Sub-Saharan Africa	Gerbils	*Phlebotomus papatasi*
				Phlebotomus caucasicus
L. aethiopica	Cutaneous and diffuse	Ethiopia, Kenya	Hyraxes	*Phlebotomus longipes*
				Phlebotomus pedifer
L. donovani complex				
L. donovani	Visceral	India, Nepal, Pakistan, Sub-Saharan Africa, Western Africa	Man, dogs, rodents	*Phlebotomus argentipes*
				Phlebotomus orientalis
				Phlebotomus martini
L. infantum	Visceral	Mediterranean coast, Central Asia, China, Middle East	Domestic and wild canids	*Phlebotomus perniciosus*
				Phlebotomus major
				Phlebotomus caucasicus
				Phlebotomus chinensis
				Phlebotomus sergenti
L. chagasi	Visceral	Central and South America	Canids	*Lutzomyia longipalpis*

Occurrence: Leishmaniasis is believed to be endemic in 88 countries—72 of them developing countries—on four continents. It is estimated that every year between 1.5 and 2 million new cases occur, of which only 600,000 are officially reported. An estimated 320–350 million people are at risk of acquiring the infection and 12 million are already infected (Desjeux, 1992; WHO, 2003). Ninety percent of all cases of cutaneous leishmaniasis occur in Afghanistan, Brazil, Peru, Saudi Arabia, and Syria (WHO, 2003). Despite some local successes in controlling the infection, it seems to be expanding in range and increasing in prevalence. Cutaneous leishmaniasis prevalence rates vary considerably, but most endemic countries are reporting an increase in cases or an expansion in the disease's distribution. For example, in 1972, a total of 22,368 human cases of leishmaniasis (cutaneous and visceral) were reported in the Americas, 20,348 of them from Mesoamerica, especially Guatemala (29.6 per 100,000 population), and 2,020 from South America (2.9 per 100,000 population) (PAHO, 1975). Since 1987, Brazil has been reporting between 23,000 and 26,000 cases of cutaneous leishmaniasis annually, with 2,511 cases of visceral leishmaniasis in 1985 alone (Lacerda, 1994). Although part of this increase may be due to improved reporting, Jorquera *et al.* (1998) found a prevalence of 16.7% in three communities in Venezuela, and prevalences of 47% were recorded in Ecuador (Armijos *et al.*, 1997), 34% in Brazil (Pignatti *et al.*, 1995), 10.7–20% among 11,517 children in Iran (Sharifi *et al.*, 1998), and 64.8% in 4 communities in Iran (Yaghoobi-Ershadi and Javadian, 1995).

The Disease in Man: Cutaneous leishmaniasis is a polymorphous disease that may affect only the skin or both the skin and the mucous membranes. It manifests initially as itchy erythematous lesions, which later form papules and then painless ulcers. The incubation period is between one week and several months. There may be one or many lesions, and they may sometimes be nonulcerative and diffuse. Though the lesions generally heal spontaneously within weeks or months, they may persist for as long as a year, or more. Spontaneous healing of leishmaniasis in man has been shown to depend on cell-mediated immunity and production of gamma interferon (Carvalho *et al.*, 1995). In AIDS patients, the manifestations are atypical and relapses are frequent (Agostoni *et al.*, 1998). In the Americas, the disease occurs in several clinical forms, depending mainly, but not solely, on the species of the etiologic agent involved.

a) Leishmaniasis due to *L. mexicana mexicana* predominates in Central America and southeastern Mexico. It causes a benign infection with only one or a few skin ulcers, known as chiclero ulcer, chiclero ear, or bay sore. The lesion is usually located on the earflap or, less often, on the face or extremities. It begins with an erythematous papule that then ulcerates and, when the scab comes off, bleeds easily. The lesions on the earflap are deforming, tend to be chronic, and may last many years, while those on other parts of the body heal spontaneously in about six months. A distinctive feature of this form of cutaneous leishmaniasis is that it may spread to the lymph nodes, though this very rarely occurs. In Mexico, no cases of mucocutaneous leishmaniasis have been detected, but two or three cases of cutaneous lesions that invaded the contiguous mucosa have been reported. The vectors are not especially attracted to man, and the main victims tend to be people who spend a lot of time in the forest, the vector's habitat, such as the gum tappers (*chicleros*) who work there during the rainy season when phlebotomine flies are plentiful.

b) *L. mexicana amazonensis* leishmaniasis occurs in the Amazon basin of Brazil and neighboring countries. Human cases due to this agent are rare because the vectors are nocturnal and not normally anthropophilic, and they inhabit marshy areas where man does not ordinarily live. The infection causes single or multiple lesions that rarely heal spontaneously. Around 30% of patients have diffuse cutaneous lesions characterized by thickening of the skin in the form of scattered plaques, papules, or nodules, found mainly on the face and legs.

c) *L. mexicana pifanoi* causes a diffuse cutaneous leishmaniasis similar to lepromatous leprosy, with which it is often confused. This diffuse form of leishmaniasis has been described in Venezuela, but it also occurs in other areas. Outside the Americas, cases have been reported from Ethiopia and Kenya. This form appears in individuals with immune system deficiencies. Patients with diffuse cutaneous leishmaniasis are anergic and do not react to the Montenegro skin test. The lesions harbor a large number of parasites. Healthy volunteers inoculated with parasites from patients with diffuse cutaneous leishmaniasis developed a localized lesion at the inoculation site which healed without sequelae. For that reason, the occurrence of this form is believed to be due more to deficient immune response in the host than to some special property of the parasite. Human cases of diffuse cutaneous leishmaniasis are infrequent.

d) *L. mexicana venezuelensis* leishmaniasis causes ulcerous lesions and, less frequently, nodules or ulceronodular lesions.

e) *L. braziliensis braziliensis* causes the mucocutaneous form of leishmaniasis known as espundia. The disease begins with a papular lesion on the face or extremities that may develop into a painless ulcer that seldom heals spontaneously. A characteristic feature of this form is metastasis to the mucocutaneous parts of the body. A sizable proportion of untreated patients develop lesions on the nasal septum, mouth, nasopharynx, and, sometimes, even the anorectal region, penis, scrotum, and vulva. These metastases may occur simultaneously with the primary lesion or, more often, much later, and may cause severe destruction of the affected tissue, disfiguring the patient. The secondary lesions are ulcerous or indurated.

f) Leishmaniasis due to *L. braziliensis guyanensis* occurs in Guyana, French Guiana, Suriname, and northern Brazil; it causes characteristic lesions on the skin, which frequently spread via the lymph vessels and produce ulcers known as pian bois all over the body.

g) *L. braziliensis peruviana* leishmaniasis exists in villages in Andean valleys of Peru and causes a form of cutaneous leishmaniasis called uta, characterized by a single lesion that tends not to metastasize and heals spontaneously. The disease mainly affects children.

h) *L. braziliensis panamensis* causes ulcerous skin lesions and, occasionally, affects the mucosa.

Despite these descriptions, most clinical physicians indicate that it is very difficult to differentiate between subspecies of leishmanias based only on the lesions they cause.

In the Old World, cutaneous leishmaniasis occurs in three main forms:

a) *L. major* causes the rural or wet form of leishmaniasis that occurs in semi-desert and desert regions. The lesion begins as a papule on the exposed parts of the body (face and extremities), which develops into a wet ulcer. The lesions may spread, either directly or via the lymph system. The disease lasts two to eight months, and fibrosis during spontaneous healing leaves a permanent scar.

b) *L. tropica* causes the dry form of leishmaniasis, which occurs in urban and peri-urban areas primarily in the Middle East. The initial papule develops slowly, and ulceration, when it occurs, is also slow to develop. The disease has a long course—a year or more—and leaves a permanent scar. In contrast to the wet form, the lesions contain large numbers of parasites.

c) *L. aethiopica* causes three types of lesions: the oriental button or furuncle, the mucocutaneous form, and diffuse cutaneous leishmaniasis. The lesions develop slowly and may or may not ulcerate later. Spontaneous healing occurs after one to three years, or sometimes longer (WHO, 1984).

The Disease in Animals: In the Americas, until recently only *L. braziliensis peruviana*, the agent of human cutaneous leishmaniasis, and *L. donovani chagasi*, the agent of human visceral leishmaniasis, had been identified in dogs. However, *L. braziliensis* has since been found in dogs in São Paulo, Brazil. Owing to the difficulty of identifying the parasite species, the etiologic agent of leishmaniasis in dogs is sometimes called simply *L. canis* (Santos *et al.*, 1998). The prevalence in dogs may be high. In 270 dogs from endemic areas of Rio de Janeiro, Brazil, Santos *et al.* (1998) found that 31.5% had acute or chronic lesions, results of indirect immunofluorescence were positive in 25.1%, and the skin test yielded positive results in 40.5%.

In the Old World, dogs are affected by *L. tropica*, which causes a cutaneous disease in man, and by subspecies of *L. donovani*—except for those isolated in India—which causes a visceral disease in humans. Regardless of which species causes the infection, dogs often exhibit both cutaneous and visceral manifestations. In endemic areas, leishmaniasis may also occur in equines, which develop nodular lesions and sometimes scabs or ulcers, but only on or around the earflap.

In Venezuela, of 116 donkeys examined, 28 had one or more ulcerous lesions and 17 (15%) had positive microscopy. Based on its behavior in hamsters and culture media, the authors classified the agent as *L. braziliensis* (Bonfante-Garrido *et al.*, 1981). In general, infections in wild animals are inapparent. In rodents and other wild animals, apparent infections by the agents of the *L. mexicana* complex produce skin alterations, mainly at the base of the tail and, occasionally, on the ears and toes. Lesions consist of swellings with hair loss and, sometimes, ulcers, in which the presence of amastigotes can be demonstrated. Infection in these hosts is prolonged. *L. mexicana amazonensis* infection has also been found in the rodent *Proechimys guyannensis* and other animals in the Amazon Basin. In these cases, the skin remains normal in appearance but the parasites are dispersed in the dermis. The parasites of the *L. braziliensis* complex produce a systemic infection in wild animals, but skin lesions are rarely seen. The parasites can be cultured from blood, viscera (spleen, liver), and apparently normal skin.

Source of Infection and Mode of Transmission: In the Americas, the reservoirs of cutaneous leishmaniasis are generally rodents or edentate animals (Table 1). The infection is transmitted from one wild animal to another by means of phlebotomine flies of the genus *Lutzomyia*. Humans are infected accidentally by the bite of these phlebotomines when they enter enzootic areas in the jungle. Recent studies have shown that a large number of wild mammal species are infected, but not all of these animals can be considered primary hosts, either because they are not very abundant or their infection rate is too low for them to play that role. The exception is dogs, the only known nonhuman hosts of *L. b. peruviana*. However, Lainson (1983) suspected that dogs are actually a secondary host of this infection (uta) and that the primary host is a wild animal. Infected domestic rats (*Rattus rattus*) have been found in Brazil. In Manaus, Brazil, opossums of the species *Didelphis marsupialis* may also serve as a link between the wild enzootic and the peridomestic cycles (WHO, 1984). It is possible that the infections produced by the *L. mexicana* complex are maintained in nature not by a single specific host, but by a wide variety of species associated with a particular type of habitat (WHO, 1984). In some areas of the Americas, the relative roles of the various infected animal species have not been clearly defined.

In the Old World, the vectors belong to the genus *Phlebotomus*. The main reservoir of *L. major* in the former Soviet Union is the great gerbil *Rhombomys opimus*. Infected colonies of this desert or semidesert rodent have been found in Iran, the southern part of the former Soviet Union, and from northern Afghanistan to Mongolia. In northwestern India and in Israel and Morocco, the reservoirs are *Meriones* spp. The infection in these rodents is quite prolonged. In Algeria, northwestern Libya, and Israel, *Psammomys obesus* serves as the reservoir, while in Ethiopia and Senegal, the reservoirs are species of *Mastomys*, *Tatera*, and *Arvicanthis*.

The agent *L. tropica* has been isolated from dogs and from *Rattus rattus*, but most investigators believe that the maintenance host is man. Lainson (1982) does not share that opinion, however, pointing out that person-to-person transmission is unlikely, since this agent causes few skin lesions in humans and those lesions contain only scant numbers of amastigotes.

In Ethiopia and Kenya, *L. aethiopica* infection is maintained by hyraxes, such as *Procavia capensis*, *Heterohyrax brucei*, and *Dendrohyrax arboreus*.

Cutaneous leishmaniasis is a zoonosis. Humans are accidental hosts who acquire the infection when they enter enzootic forest areas for occupational purposes (e.g., lumberjacks, gum tappers, oilfield workers, cattlemen, and farmers). Cutaneous leishmaniasis may be a serious problem in rural settlements within the jungle. Permanent human settlements in enzootic areas generate significant ecological changes, especially deforestation, replacement of wildlife with domestic animals, and replacement or modification in the prevalence of some insects as species better adapted to the new environment become dominant. These ecological changes also modify the epidemiology of cutaneous leishmaniasis: in Vale do Ribeira, São Paulo, Brazil, 80% of cutaneous leishmaniasis patients worked near their homes and had no contact with the jungle. The devastation of the natural environment altered the species composition of the phlebotomine population in that region and *Psychodopygus intermedius*—a species that prefers secondary growth, enters human dwellings, and is anthropophilic—became dominant (Tolezano *et al.*, 1980).

In the western-central region of Venezuela, the disease used to occur exclusively among the inhabitants of villages located near mountainous areas with dense vegetation. However, cases have been diagnosed in several neighborhoods on the outskirts of the city of Barquisimeto (Bonfante-Garrido *et al.*, 1984). It is not yet known whether this was due to some ecological change, but the appearance of the disease in an urban environment shows that cutaneous leishmaniasis is not always sylvatic or rural and that its epidemiology is changing. Among the American cutaneous leishmaniases, uta in Peru is exceptional because no wild reservoirs of the parasite are known. In the Old World, *L. major* infection is a rural zoonosis, whereas *L. tropica* infections appear to be transmitted between humans in an urban environment.

Diagnosis: The simplest specific diagnostic method consists of confirming the presence of amastigotes in lesions. For that purpose, the lesion is cleaned with 70% alcohol to remove any necrotic matter. Then, a sample is taken from the edge or base of the lesion (nodule or ulcer of the skin or mucosa) by aspiration, scraping, or biopsy. The sample is mounted on a slide and stained using the Giemsa or Wright technique. Numerous amastigotes may be seen in the case of lesions that are recent or active, but in lesions that are chronic or healing, it can be difficult or impossible to demonstrate the presence of parasites by direct smear microscopy or biopsy. Parasitologic diagnosis is especially difficult in the mucocutaneous form (Cuba Cuba *et al.*, 1981).

Isolation of the agent can be accomplished by culturing the sample in an appropriate medium, such as NNN or Schneider's Drosophila, with a supplement of 30% fetal bovine serum. The promastigotes grow in these media and can be observed within a week. Another procedure is intracutaneous or intranasal inoculation of the suspicious material into hamsters, but it may take two months or more to obtain a positive result. The best results are obtained by culturing and inoculating hamsters simultaneously. Parasites of the *L. mexicana* complex grow abundantly in laboratory media. When inoculated into the nose of a hamster, a histiocytoma containing many amastigotes forms within a few weeks, and the infection spreads by metastasis. In contrast, parasites of the *L. braziliensis* complex grow poorly in artificial culture media, and when inoculated in hamsters produce a small nodule or ulcer that takes six months or more to form. These lesions contain few amastigotes and do not metastasize.

Numerous immunologic tests have been used to diagnose cutaneous leishmaniasis, including the Montenegro skin test, immunofluorescence, direct agglutination, latex agglutination, gel immunodiffusion, and enzyme-linked immunosorbent assay (ELISA). The Montenegro skin test is a delayed hypersensitivity reaction, which is read 48–72 hours after intradermal injection of a suspension of promastigotes. It is group-specific but not species-specific, and it is useful in epidemiologic surveys. Though frequently positive in the cutaneous and mucocutaneous forms, the Montenegro test is ordinarily negative in the visceral and diffuse cutaneous forms. It does not produce cross-reactions with the agents of American or African trypanosomiasis, and its application will not affect the titer for any subsequent serologic reactions (Amato Neto *et al.*, 1996). The indirect immunofluorescence test, perhaps the most widely used of the serologic reactions, yields better results with an amastigote antigen than with a promastigote antigen; however, there is no correlation between the titer required to produce a reaction and clinical manifestations, duration, or number of lesions (Cuba Cuba *et al.*, 1981). An IgA conjugate proved superior to IgG when used to diagnose the mucocutaneous form (Lainson, 1983).

Serology for the cutaneous leishmaniases of the Old World is generally negative (WHO, 1984). In general, serology is positive in only 70% to 80% of cases, at low titers—except in the mucosal forms—and only after two to three months following initial infection. Polymerase chain reaction had a sensitivity of 86% when used alone and 93% when used in combination with Southern blotting. In contrast, microscopy of histological sections and impression smears exhibited a sensitivity of only 76% and 48%, respectively (Andresen *et al.*, 1996).

Control: Cutaneous leishmaniases in the Americas are mainly diseases of forest areas, with sylvatic reservoirs and vectors. Hence, it is impossible to control them by eliminating reservoirs and vectors. The only effective method of prevention is to avoid endemic areas or use repellents and protective clothing to avoid being bitten by the insect vectors. In special circumstances, the environment may be modified by means of deforestation to eliminate vector habitats. In camps or in domestic and peridomestic areas where *L. peruviana* and *L. tropica* exist, the walls of rooms can be sprayed with insecticide and windows can be covered with fine mesh to control the vectors. Use of insecticides in antimalaria campaigns in Southeast Asia led to virtual disappearance of visceral and cutaneous leishmaniasis from the region. Patients infected with *L. b. braziliensis* should be treated as soon as possible to prevent development of the mucocutaneous form, as should those infected with *L. mexicana amazonensis* to prevent the occurrence of diffuse cutaneous leishmaniasis. It is believed that uta could be prevented by eliminating infected dogs in the endemic areas of Peru. However, the elimination of reservoirs has not generally been effective against the urban cutaneous leishmaniasis in the Old World.

In Iran, Israel, and the former Soviet Union, immunization with virulent strains of *L. major* has been practiced to prevent infection with that agent and with *L. tropica*. The inoculation is intended to prevent later infections that cause deforming lesions on the face, and it is applied on a part of the body where the scar will not be visible or unattractive. Inoculated individuals are advised to remain outside endemic areas until immunity is established. This type of immunization is not recommended, though it may be useful for people who must enter high-risk areas. Armijos *et al.* (1998) achieved 72.9% protection in Ecuadorian children by administering a killed promastigote vaccine with BCG adjuvant.

Bibliography

Agostoni, C., N. Dorigoni, A. Malfitano, *et al.* Mediterranean leishmaniasis in HIV-infected patients: Epidemiological, clinical, and diagnostic features of 22 cases. *Infection* 26:93–99, 1998.

Amato Neto, V., C.R. De Marchi, M.C. Guimarães, A. Salebian, L.C. Cuce, L. Matsubara. Avaliação de eventual influência da intradermorreação de Montenegro sobre prova sorologica para o diagnóstico da Leishmaniose tegumentar americana. *Rev Hosp Clin Fac Med Univ Sao Paulo* 51:217–219, 1996.

Andresen, K., A. Gaafar, A.M. El-Hassan, *et al.* Evaluation of the polymerase chain reaction in the diagnosis of cutaneous leishmaniasis due to *Leishmania major*: A comparison with direct microscopy of smears and sections from lesions. *Trans R Soc Trop Med Hyg* 90:133–135, 1996.

Antoine, J.C. Biologie des interactions macrophages *Leishmania*. *Pathol Biol* (Paris) 43: 215–223, 1995.

Armijos, R.X., M.M. Weigel, R. Izurieta, *et al.* The epidemiology of cutaneous leishmaniasis in subtropical Ecuador. *Trop Med Int Health* 2:140–152, 1997.

Armijos, R.X., M.M. Weigel, H. Aviles, R. Maldonado, J. Racines. Field trial of a vaccine against New World cutaneous leishmaniasis in an at-risk child population: Safety, immunogenicity, and efficacy during the first 12 months of follow-up. *J Infect Dis* 177:1352–1357, 1998.

Barral, A., D. Pedral-Sampaio, G. Grimaldi, Jr., *et al.* Leishmaniasis in Bahia, Brazil: Evidence that *Leishmania amazonensis* produces a wide spectrum of clinical disease. *Am J Trop Med Hyg* 44:536–546, 1991.

Blackwell, J.M. Parasite genome analysis. Progress in the *Leishmania* genome project. *Trans R Soc Trop Med Hyg* 91:107–110, 1997.

Bonfante-Garrido, R. Leishmanias y leishmaniasis tegumentaria en América Latina. *Bol Of Sanit Panam* 95:418–426, 1983.

Bonfante-Garrido, R., E. Melendez, R. Torres, N. Murillo, C. Arredondo, I. Urdaneta. Enzootic equine cutaneous leishmaniasis in Venezuela. *Trans R Soc Trop Med Hyg* 75:471, 1981.

Bonfante-Garrido, R., S. Barroeta, M. A. Mejía de Alejos, *et al.* Leishmaniasis tegumentaria urbana en Barquisimeto, Venezuela. *Bol Of Sanit Panam* 97:105–110, 1984.

Carvalho, E.M., D. Correia Filho, O. Bacellar, R.P. Almeida, H. Lessa, H. Rocha. Characterization of the immune response in subjects with self-healing cutaneous leishmaniasis. *Am J Trop Med Hyg* 53:273–277, 1995.

Chouicha, N., G. Lanotte, F. Pratlong, C.A. Cuba Cuba, I.D. Velez, J.P. Dedet. Phylogenetic taxonomy of *Leishmania (Viannia) braziliensis* based on isoenzymatic study of 137 isolates. *Parasitology* 115:343–348, 1997.

Chulay, J.D. Leishmaniasis, cutaneous leishmaniasis of the Old World, and cutaneous leishmaniasis of the New World. *In*: Strickland, G.T., ed. *Hunter's Tropical Medicine*, 7th ed. Philadelphia: Saunders; 1991.

Cuba Cuba, C.A., P.D. Marsden, A.C. Barreto, R. Rocha, R.R. Sampaio, L. Patzlaff. Parasitologic and immunologic diagnosis of American (mucocutaneous) leishmaniasis. *Bull Pan Am Health Organ* 15:249–259, 1981.

Desjeux P. Human leishmaniases: Epidemiology and public health aspects. *World Health Stat Q* 45:267–275, 1992.

Grimaldi, G., R.B. Tesh, D. McMahon-Pratt. A review of the geographic distribution and epidemiology of leishmaniasis in the New World. *Am J Trop Med Hyg* 41:687–725, 1989.

Harris, E., G. Kropp, A. Belli, B. Rodríguez, N. Agabian. Single-step multiplex PCR assay for characterization of New World *Leishmania* complexes. *J Clin Microbiol* 36:1989–1995, 1998.

Jorquera, A., E. Ledezma, L. De Sousa, *et al.* Epidemiologic characterization of American cutaneous leishmaniasis in an endemic region of eastern Venezuela. *Am J Trop Med Hyg* 58: 589–593, 1998.

Kapoor, G.S, S.K. Arora, S. Sehgal. Genetic polymorphism of *Leishmania* species using kinetoplast DNA restriction fragment length polymorphism and cDNA probe of *Leishmania donovani*. *Med Microbiol Immunol (Berl)* 186:209–214, 1998.

Kettle, D.S. *Medical and Veterinary Entomology*, 2nd ed. Wallingford: CAB International; 1995.

Kreutzer, R.D., A. Corredor, G. Grimaldi, *et al.* Characterization of *Leishmania colombiensis* sp. n (Kinetoplastida: Trypanosomatidae), a new parasite infecting humans, animals, and phlebotomine sand flies in Colombia and Panama. *Am J Trop Med Hyg* 44:662–675, 1991.

Lacerda, M.M. The Brazilian leishmaniasis control program. *Mem Inst Oswaldo Cruz* 89:489–495, 1994.

Lainson, R. Epidemiología e ecología de leishmaniose tegumentar na Amazonia. *Hileia Med* (Belem) 3:35–40, 1981.

Lainson, R. Leishmaniasis. *In*: Jacobs, L., P. Arámbulo, section eds. Vol. 1: *CRC Handbook Series in Zoonoses*. Boca Raton: CRC Press; 1982.

Lainson, R. The American leishmaniases: some observations on their ecology and epidemiology. *Trans R Soc Trop Med Hyg* 77:569–596, 1983.

Lainson, R., J.J. Shaw. Las leishmanias y la leishmaniasis del Nuevo Mundo, con particular referencia al Brasil. *Bol Oficina Sanit Panam* 76:93–114, 1974.

Machado, M. I., R.V. Milder, G. Grimaldi, H. Momen. Identification *of Leishmania mexicana mexicana* in the state of Sao Paulo, Brazil. *Rev Inst Med Trop S Paulo* 25:97, 1983.

Melby, P.C., R.D. Kreutzer, D. McMahon-Pratt, A.A. Gam, F.A. Neva. Cutaneous leishmaniasis: Review of 59 cases seen at the National Institutes of Health. *Clin Infect Dis* 15:924–937, 1992.

Momen, H., R.S. Pacheco, E. Cupolillo, G. Grimaldi, Jr. Molecular evidence for the importation of Old World *Leishmania* into the Americas. *Biol Res* 26:249–255, 1993.

Pan American Health Organization (PAHO). *Reported Cases of Notifiable Diseases in the Americas, 1970–1972.* Washington, D.C.: PAHO; 1975. (Scientific Publication 308).

Pignatti, MG., R.C. Mayo, M.J. Alves, S.S. Souza, F. Macedo, R.M. Pereira. Leishmaniose tegumentar americana na região nordeste do estado de São Paulo-Brasil. *Rev Soc Bras Med Trop* 28:243–247, 1995.

Santos, E.G., M.C. Marzochi, N.F. Conceição, C.M. Brito, R.S. Pacheco. Epidemiological survey on canine population with the use of immunoleish skin test in endemic areas of human American cutaneous leishmaniasis in the state of Rio de Janeiro, Brazil. *Rev Inst Med Trop Sao Paulo* 40:41–47, 1998.

Sellon, R.K., M.M. Menard, D.J. Meuten, E.J. Lengerich, F.J. Steurer, E.B. Breitschwerdt. Endemic visceral leishmaniasis in a dog from Texas. *J Vet Internal Med* 7:16–19, 1993.

Sharifi, I., A.R. Fekri, M.R. Aflatonian, A. Nadim, Y. Nikian, A. Kamesipour. Cutaneous leishmaniasis in primary school children in the south-eastern Iranian city of Bam, 1994–95. *Bull World Health Organ* 76:289–293, 1998.

Tolezano, J.E., S.A. Macoris, J.M.P. Diniz. Modificação na epidemiologia da leishmaniose tegumentar no Vale do Ribeira, Estado de São Paulo, Brasil. *Rev Inst A Lutz* 40:49–54, 1980.

World Health Organization (WHO). *The Leishmaniases.* Report of a WHO Expert Committee. Geneva: WHO; 1984. (Technical Report Series 701).

World Health Organization (WHO). *Control of the Leishmaniases. Report of a WHO Expert Committee.* Geneva: WHO; 1990:155. (Technical Report Series 793).

World Health Organization (WHO). The Leishmaniases and *Leishmania*/HIV Co-infections. May 2000 [web page]. Available at www.who.int/inf-fs/en/fact116.html. Accessed January 2003.

Yaghoobi-Ershadi, M.R., E. Javadian. Leishmaniose cutanée zoonotique au nord d'Ispahan. Le point sur l'infection humaine en 1991. *Bull Soc Pathol Exot* 88:42–45, 1995.

Youssef, M.Y., M.M. Eissa, S.T. el Mansoury. Confirmation of clinical differentiation of three Leishmania strains by computerized image analyser system. *J Egypt Soc Parasitol* 27:553–561, 1997.

Zeledon, R. Leishmaniasis in the Caribbean Islands. A review. *Ann N Y Acad Sci* 653:154–160, 1992.

CYCLOSPORIASIS

Etiology: Cyclosporiasis is caused by *Cyclospora cayetanensis*, a coccidium related taxonomically to the genus *Eimeria* and clinically to the genera *Cryptosporidium* and *Isospora*. The earliest reports of the disease—from Peru in 1986—referred to cyanobacteria-like bodies found in human feces. Subsequent studies revealed their coccidial nature. Apparently, similar organisms had been observed in New Guinea in 1977 and had been confused with *Isospora* (Sterling and Ortega, 1999).

The life cycle of *Cyclospora* is not yet fully known, but various observations, as well as the organism's similarities to other coccidia, suggest that parasites ingested in mature oocysts lodge in the epithelial cells of the duodenum and jejunum, where they multiply asexually to form merozoites. It is not known whether these forms must leave the host cell and invade new cells to begin the next phase of sexual multiplication, which concludes with the formation of oocysts. The oocysts, which must sporulate in the external environment to become infective, are passed from the body in feces. The mature oocyst contains two sporocysts, each of which contains two sporozoites (Ortega *et al.*, 1998).

Geographic Distribution: Probably worldwide. The first cases were seen in Nepal, New Guinea, and Peru, but since then the infection has been confirmed in the Americas, North Africa, Southeast Asia, Australia, Bangladesh, Western Europe, Indonesia, Pakistan, Papua New Guinea, the UK, and the Middle East (Drenaggi *et al.*, 1998).

Occurrence in Man: The distribution of *Cyclospora* is similar to that of *Cryptosporidium*, although it is only a third to a half as prevalent (various surveys have found prevalence rates of 1% to 20%). It infects mainly children between 2 and 4 years of age, and the prevalence diminishes rapidly with age. Approximately one-third of infected individuals are symptomatic. Although the infection does affect travelers and immunocompromised patients, it does not appear to be predominantly associated with these groups.

Occurrence in Animals: Animals do not appear to be susceptible to cyclosporiasis. Eberhard *et al.* (2000) attempted to infect nine strains of mice (including some immunodeficient animals), rats, chickens, ducks, rabbits, hamsters, ferrets, pigs, dogs, and various monkeys with oocysts obtained from Guatemala, Haiti, Nepal, Peru, and the US. None of the animals manifested clinical signs of infection or disease.

The Disease in Man: The disease in humans is characterized by watery diarrhea, which begins abruptly after an incubation period of 12 hours to 11 days. In immunocompetent individuals, it lasts from six to eight weeks, while in immunodeficient patients it may persist for up to three months (Looney, 1998). In a study in Egypt, the diarrhea lasted 28 ± 8 days in children and 37 ± 12 days in adults, with more than 5 evacuations per day (Nassef *et al.*, 1998). Of 63 infected individuals in Peru, 68% were asymptomatic and the highest prevalence occurred among children aged 2 to 4 years. The prevalence decreases in winter and with age (Madico *et al.*, 1997). Patients usually experience anorexia and weight loss. Examinations have shown malabsorption, atrophy of villi, and crypt hyperplasia (Connor, 1997). Not all infected individuals develop the disease. In Haiti, 15%–20% of the population examined were found to be carriers of *Cyclospora* oocysts, but few had diarrhea (Eberhard *et al.*, 1999).

The Disease in Animals: *Cyclospora* does not appear to infect animals (see Occurrence in Animals).

Source of Infection and Mode of Transmission: Cyclosporiasis is acquired through ingestion of raw fruits and vegetables and contaminated water. The second outbreak of cyclosporiasis in the US affected 1,400 people and was attributed to consumption of raspberries from Guatemala (Katz *et al.*, 1996). A later study, in which 5,552 stool samples were collected from workers on raspberry farms in Guatemala, found infection rates of between 2.3% and 6.7%, with children showing the highest rates (Bern *et al.*, 1999). The highest prevalence occurred during the warm months. In Peru, Ortega *et al.* (1997) found that 14.5% of vegetables obtained from markets were contaminated with *Cryptosporidium* and 1.8% with *Cyclospora*. In two outbreaks in the US, basil seems to have been the vehicle (López *et al.*, 1999), while in Spain, cases have been attributed to consumption of raspberries, buffalo milk, and raw fish (Gascon *et al.*, 2001). The study by Bern *et al.* (1999) in Guatemala revealed that the principal risk for infection among those affected was consumption of untreated water. A study of the water in domestic containers in Egypt showed that 56% was contaminated with *Giardia*, 50% with *Cryptosporidium*, 12% with *Blastocystis*, 9% with *Cyclospora*, and 3% with microsporidia (Khalifa *et al.*, 2001). Using microscopy and molecular biology techniques, Sturbaum (1998) identified *Cyclospora* oocysts in wastewater.

Diagnosis: *Cyclospora* infection is suggested by the patient's symptoms and by epidemiological circumstances, especially in travelers who have visited endemic areas. The diagnosis is confirmed by detection of the double-walled oocysts measuring 8–10 microns in diameter in stool samples. The oocysts are concentrated by formol-ether sedimentation and flotation in Sheather's sucrose solution. They can be detected by staining, autofluorescence under ultraviolet light, phase contrast microscopy, or polymerase chain reaction (Ortega *et al.*, 1998). The stains used most frequently (to make it easier to visualize the organisms and to differentiate them from yeasts) are trichrome stains, Ziehl-Neelsen, Giemsa, safranin with methylene blue, calcofluor white, and auramine phenol. Safranin has been found to be the most effective and appropriate stain for use in diagnostic laboratories (Negm, 1998).

Control: Cyclosporiasis can be prevented by applying the classic measures for control of parasitoses transmitted via the fecal-oral route: washing foods that are eaten raw, boiling suspicious water, and washing hands before eating. Treatment of water contaminated with *Giardia*, *Cryptosporidium*, *Blastocystis*, *Cyclospora*, or microsporidia with chlorine at 4 or 8 parts per million (ppm) or with ozone at 1 ppm showed that ozone was more effective in destroying the parasites, but that it did not totally inactivate *Cyclospora* or *Blastocystis* (Khalifa *et al.*, 2001).

Bibliography

Bern, C., B. Hernandez, M.B. Lopez, *et al.* Epidemiologic studies of *Cyclospora cayetanensis* in Guatemala. *Emerg Infect Dis* 5:766–774, 1999.

Drenaggi, D., O. Cirioni, A. Giacometti, *et al.* Cyclosporiasis in a traveler returning from South America. *J Travel Med* 5:153–155, 1998.

Connor, B.A. *Cyclospora* infection: A review. *Ann Acad Med Singapore* 26(5):632–636, 1997.

Eberhard, M.L., E.K. Nace, A.R. Freeman, *et al.* *Cyclospora cayetanensis* infections in Haiti: A common occurrence in the absence of watery diarrhea. *Am J Trop Med Hyg* 60(4):584–586, 1999.

Eberhard, M.L., Y.R. Ortega, D.E. Hanes, *et al.* Attempts to establish experimental *Cyclospora cayetanensis* infection in laboratory animals. *J Parasitol* 86(3):577–582, 2000.

Gascon, J., M. Alvarez, E.M. Valls, *et al.* Ciclosporiasis: estudio clinicoepidemiológico en viajeros con *Cyclospora cayetanensis* importada. *Med Clin* (Spain) 116(12):461–464, 2001.

Khalifa, A.M., M.M. El Temsahy, I.F. Abou El Naga. Effect of ozone on the viability of some protozoa in drinking water. *J Egypt Soc Parasitol* 31(2):603–616, 2001.

Katz, D., S. Kumar, J. Malecki, *et al.* Cyclosporiasis associated with imported raspberries, Florida, 1996. *Public Health Rep* 114(5):427–438, 1999.

Looney, W.J. *Cyclospora* species as a cause of diarrhoea in humans. *Br J Biomed Sc* 55:157–161, 1998.

Lopez, A.S., D.R. Dodson, M.J. Arrowood, *et al.* Outbreak of cyclosporiasis associated with basil in Missouri in 1999. *Clin Infect Dis* 32(7):1010–1017, 2001.

Madico, G., J. McDonald, R.H. Gilman, *et al.* Epidemiology and treatment of *Cyclospora cayetanensis* infection in Peruvian children. *Clin Infect Dis* 24(5):977–981, 1997.

Nassef, N.E., S.A. el-Ahl, O.K. el-Shafee, *et al.* Cyclospora: A newly identified protozoan pathogen of man. *J Egypt Soc Parasitol* 28(1):213–219, 1998.

Negm, A.Y. Identification of *Cyclospora cayetanensis* in stool using different stains. *J Egypt Soc Parasitol* 28(2):429–436, 1998.

Ortega,Y.R., C.R. Sterling, R.H. Gilman. *Cyclospora cayetanensis. Adv Parasitol* 40: 399–418, 1998.

Ortega, Y.R., C.R. Roxas, R.H. Gilman, *et al.* Isolation of *Cryptosporidium parvum* and *Cyclospora cayetanensis* from vegetables collected in markets of an endemic region in Peru. *Am J Trop Med Hyg* 57(6):683–686, 1997.

Sterling, C.R., Y.R. Ortega. *Cyclospora*: An enigma worth unraveling. *Emerg Infect Dis* 5(1):48–53, 1999.

Sturbaum, G.D., Y.R. Ortega, R.H. Gilman, *et al.* Detection of *Cyclospora cayetanensis* in wastewater. *Appl Environ Microbiol* 64(6):2284–2286, 1998.

GIARDIASIS

ICD-10 A07.1

Synonyms: Lambliasis, *Giardia* enteritis.

Etiology: The taxonomy of the species of the genus *Giardia* is still controversial. Three morphological forms are currently accepted: *G. intestinalis,* which affects man, domestic animals, and other mammals; *G. muris,* which affects birds, rodents, and reptiles; and *G. agilis,* which affects amphibians (Barriga, 1997; Meyer, 1990). Although in the past many species were described and named according to the host in which they were found—for example, *G. canis, G. bovis,* and *G. caviae*—there are no clearly defined criteria for differentiating them. Giardia infection in man is caused by *G. intestinalis,* also called *G. duodenalis, G. lamblia,* and, sometimes, *Lamblia intestinalis.* Although *Lamblia* was the original name given to the genus by Lambl when he first described it in 1859, Stiles changed it to *Giardia* in 1915. It is possible, however, that *G. intestinalis* is a complex of several species or subspecies (Adam, 1991).

G. intestinalis is a flagellate protozoan whose life cycle includes trophozoites in the vegetative stage and cysts in the transmission stage. The trophozoites are pyriform and measure 10 μm to 19 μm long, 5 μm to 12 μm wide, and 2 μm to 4 μm thick. They have four pairs of flagella which extend towards the rear part of the organism, two nuclei, two claw-shaped median bodies in the middle of the body, and a convex ventral disk in the front half of the body, with which they cling to the intestinal mucosa. Those forms live in the anterior portion of the host's small intestine, particularly in the duodenum, where they multiply by binary fission. Many of the trophozoites are carried to the ileum, where they secrete a resistant wall and become ovoid cysts measuring 7 µm to 10 µm by 8 µm to 13 µm. After encysting, the parasite's organs divide again. The mature cyst thus has four nuclei, four median bodies, and eight flagella. Division of the cytoplasm does not occur until the parasite excysts. The cysts leave the host in feces. They can survive for more than two months in water at 8°C and around one month at 21°C; however, they are sensitive to desiccation, freezing, and sunlight. They are also relatively sensitive to ordinary disinfectants. Solutions of quaternary ammonium recommended for disinfecting the environment will kill them in one minute at 20°C, but normal concentrations of chlorine in drinking water do not affect them. The mature cyst is the infective element for a new host. Once ingested, the parasite excysts in the duodenum, divides, and begins to multiply normally.

Geographic Distribution: Worldwide.

Occurrence in Man: Giardiasis is endemic throughout the world. Its prevalence generally ranges from 2% to 4% in industrialized countries, but it may be over 15% among children in developing countries. Both the infection and the disease are more common in children than in adults. Giardiasis may also occur in epidemic form. Of 25 and 22 disease epidemics spread through ingestion of drinking or recreational waters, which affected 2,366 and 2,567 people in the US in 1993–1994 and 1995–1996, respectively, *G. intestinalis* was the most common pathogen. In the first epidemic, together with *Cryptosporidium*, it caused 40% of the cases, while in the second epidemic, together with *Shigella sonnei*, it was responsible for 9% of the cases (Kramer *et al.,* 1996; Levy *et al.,* 1998). In 1974, in a population of 46,000 inhabitants in the state of New York, US, 4,800 people (10.4%) contracted clinical giardiasis as a result of contamination of drinking water supplies. In epidemic situations, all age groups are affected equally. In previously uninfected populations, morbidity rates may be as high as 20% or more of the total population (Knight, 1980). Outbreaks are relatively common in institutions for children, such as orphanages and daycare centers. *G. intestinalis* is also frequently a cause of "travelers' diarrhea." In a group of 21 people whose feces tested negative for *Giardia*, the protozoan's cysts were later found in those of 15 out of 17 who became ill after visiting Leningrad (Kulda and Nohynková, 1978). The infection is less frequent in AIDS patients, perhaps because the virus interferes with the parasite's activity in the intestinal mucosa (Lindo *et al.,* 1998).

Occurrence in Animals: The infection has been confirmed in a wide variety of domestic and wild mammal species. Surveys from all over the world have found prevalences of 20% to 35% in young dogs; 10% to 15% in young cats; 5% to 90% in calves; 6% to 80% in lambs; 17% to 32% in foals; and 7% to 44% in young pigs (Xiao, 1994). As with man, the infection is less frequent in adult animals. In a study in which feces of 494 dogs were examined for parasites, the infection was detected in 3.4% of adult males, 7% of adult females, and 53.2% of puppies. A study in Colorado, US, found cysts of the parasite in 10% of the cattle, 18% of the beavers, and 6% of the coyotes examined. A giardiasis outbreak among nonhuman primates and zoo personnel was recorded in Kansas City, Missouri, US. High rates of infection have also been found in rats and other rodents, both synanthropic and wild, but whether the agent was *G. intestinalis* or *G. muris* has not been determined (Meyer and Jarroll, 1982).

The Disease in Man: The majority of infections are subclinical (Flanagan, 1992; Farthing, 1996). Rajeshwari *et al.* (1996) found that impairment of the humoral immune response was the deciding factor in whether or not the infection was symptomatic in children. In symptomatic individuals, the incubation period is generally 3–25 days (Benenson, 1997). The symptomatology consists mainly of diarrhea and bloating, frequently accompanied by abdominal pain. Nausea and vomiting occur less frequently. The acute phase of the disease lasts 3–4 days. In some persons, giardiasis may be a prolonged illness, with episodes of recurring diarrhea and flatulence, urticaria, and intolerance of certain foods. These and other allergic manifestations associated with giardiasis disappear after treatment and cure. Meloni *et al.* (1995) examined 97 isolates of *G. intestinalis* from humans and various animals and differentiated 47 zymodemes. In another study, Cevallos *et al.* (1995) found a correlation between certain zymodemes and the pathology caused by the parasite in rats. However, Rajeshwari *et al.* (1996) demonstrated that neither the zymodeme of the parasite nor the presence of associated bacterial infections influenced the occurrence or the pathogenicity of the infection in children.

The Disease in Animals: As in man, the infection is usually asymptomatic. The manifestations of the disease in dogs and cats are also similar to those in man. However, experimental infections in ruminants produced only mild diarrhea in calves and weight loss in lambs (Zajac, 1992; Olson *et al.*, 1995). The disease is more frequent in young animals.

Source of Infection and Mode of Transmission: Man is the principal reservoir of human giardiasis. The source of infection is feces containing the parasite's cysts, which often contaminate water. Although the infection in individuals is often self-limited and disappears within a few months, continuous transmission to other hosts in endemic areas ensures the agent's persistence. The existence of asymptomatic infected individuals and chronic patients, coupled with the cysts' resistance to environmental factors, are important factors in the epidemiology. The median infective dose (ID_{50}) of giardiasis for man is only 10 cysts, but infected individuals may later excrete up to 900 million cysts per day in their feces. Elimination of cysts can be intermittent and the quantity can vary greatly (Knight, 1980).

The most frequent mode of transmission appears to be ingestion of water contaminated with cysts (Hill, 1993). Direct hand-to-hand or hand-to-mouth transmission of cysts from an infected person to a susceptible person is also common, especially among children, personnel in institutions that care for children or adults, and food-handlers. Rezende *et al.* (1997) studied 264 food-handlers in 57 schools in Minas Gerais (Brazil) at various times of the year and found 8%, 2%, and 3% to be infected. Indirect transmission from fecal contamination of food is less frequent than direct transmission from infected food-handlers, but it may occur as a result of irrigating or washing foods with contaminated water or by means of mechanical vectors. However, as the cysts are susceptible to environmental factors such as desiccation, high or low temperatures, and sunlight, they cannot survive for long on foods. All the epidemics that have occurred in various cities have been due to contamination of drinking water or water in pools, lagoons, and ponds. An association has been described between giardiasis, hypochlorhydria, and pancreatic disease among children suffering from protein-calorie malnutrition, which is very frequent in developing countries. Giardiasis and hypochlorhydria are more common in people of blood type A than in people of other types (Knight, 1980).

Some animals probably also serve as reservoirs for human infection. The giardias that infect man and domestic and wild animals are morphologically identical, and several experiments have demonstrated that cross-species infections can occur. *G. intestinalis* cysts of human origin have produced infection in several animal species, including dogs, raccoons (*Procyon lotor*), rats (*Rattus norvegicus*), gerbils (*Gerbillus gerbillus*), guinea pigs, mouflon sheep (*Ovis musimon*), bighorn sheep (*Ovis canadensis*), and pronghorn antelope (*Antilocapra americana*). In another experiment, two of three human volunteers and four of four dogs were infected with *Giardia* cysts from beavers, but hamsters, guinea pigs, mice, and rats did not become infected. A human volunteer who ingested cysts from a blacktail deer was infected, but dogs similarly exposed were not (WHO, 1981). However, neither positive nor negative results are completely reliable: the former may be due to resurgence of a previous infection and the latter to resistance acquired through earlier infections (Meyer and Radulescu, 1979). The most extensive outbreak of human giardiasis attributed to an animal source occurred in 1976 in Camas, a city of 6,000 inhabitants in the state of Washington, US, where 128 cases of giardiasis were confirmed. Part of the Camas water supply came from two remote mountain streams, and though epidemiologic investigation revealed no human source of contamination, several infected beavers were found in the area of the streams. Specific-pathogen-free puppies have also been infected with *Giardia* cysts from beavers. Another apparent example of cross-transmission occurred in 1978 in a zoo in the US, where six primates and three female employees contracted the infection from an infected gibbon that had been placed in a special care unit (Armstrong *et al.*, 1979). Meloni *et al.* (1995) found certain similarities between isolates from humans and those from other animals, as well as extensive genetic variation in human *Giardia* isolates. The authors interpreted this discovery as evidence of zoonotic transmission of the parasite.

Diagnosis: Diagnosis is generally made by identifying parasites in the patient's feces. Cysts prevail in formed feces, while trophozoites are more commonly found in diarrheal stools. Different methods should be used in each case to preserve and process samples. Concentration methods are useful for the detection of cysts. As cysts are eliminated intermittently, at least three samples, taken every other day, should be examined to rule out the infection. Excretion of trophozoites is also irregular. The recommended procedures for detecting them are simultaneous examination of fresh stool samples, in which the parasite can be identified by its characteristic flagellar movement, and examination of fixed and stained samples, in which the parasite can be identified by its characteristic morphology. Some experts recommend taking up to six samples and looking for trophozoites in fixed and stained preparations, even in formed feces (García and Bruckner, 1997). Aspiration of duodenal fluid or duodenal biopsy can also be performed to reveal the presence of trophozoites. Specific fluorescent antibodies have been used as a diagnostic method for detecting cysts, as these techniques facilitate visualization under the microscope with a sensitivity 2.3 times greater than observation without fluorescence (Winiecka-Krusnell, 1995). The enzyme-linked immunosorbent assay (ELISA) has also been used to demonstrate the presence of *G. intestinalis* antigens in feces (Hill, 1993). Although the presence of antibodies and cell-mediated immune responses have been reported in patients, immunobiological procedures are not very specific (Isaac-Renton *et al.*, 1994) and do not indicate whether an infection is current or residual. The possibility of using polymerase chain reaction to detect specific DNA sequences in patients' feces or blood is currently being studied. In any event, it should be borne in mind that there is not always a causal relationship between symptoms and the discovery of giardias in an ill person, and it is therefore necessary to rule out infections due to other intestinal microorganisms or other pathologies.

Control: As the cysts of *G. intestinalis* can live for long periods in water, public water supplies should be protected against contamination by human and animal fecal matter. Adequate systems of sedimentation, flocculation, and filtration can remove *Giardia* from water, allowing the use of surface water supply systems (CDC, 1977). Sanitary elimination of feces is another important measure. In developing countries, prevailing socioeconomic conditions make it difficult to prevent infection in children. Instruction in personal hygiene is essential in institutions for children. Individual prevention measures include boiling or filtering suspicious water. Tourists should drink only bottled water in places where the purity of tap water cannot be guaranteed. Although there is no evidence that domestic animals are a significant source of infection for man, dogs and cats with giardiasis should be treated because they may frequently come into contact with children (Meyer and Jarroll, 1982).

Whereas treatment of infected individuals, coupled with prophylactic measures, has reduced the prevalence of parasitic infections caused by other organisms, it has not been successful in the case of giardiasis (Dorea *et al.*, 1996). Studies have shown that vaccinated dogs develop some resistance to the disease (Olson *et al.*, 1996). These results may be promising for humans as it has been shown that people with natural infections also develop a certain degree of resistance, which lasts at least five years (Isaac-Renton *et al.*, 1994). Most methods for testing suspicious water are tedious, complicated, and not very efficient; however, some highly effective and sensitive techniques have been developed (Bielec *et al.*, 1996; Kaucner and Stinear, 1998).

Bibliography

Adam, R.D. The biology of *Giardia* spp. *Microbiol Rev* 55(4):706–732, 1991.

Armstrong, J., R.E. Hertzog, R.T. Hall, G.L. Hoff. Giardiasis in apes and zoo attendants, Kansas City, Missouri. *CDC Vet Public Health Notes*, January(7-8), 1979.

Barriga, O.O. *Veterinary Parasitology for Practitioners*, 2nd ed. Edina: Burgess International Group; 1997.

Benenson, A.S., ed. *Control of Communicable Diseases Manual,* 17th edition. Washington, D.C.: American Public Health Association; 1997.

Bielec, L., T.C. Boisvert, S.G. Jackson. Modified procedure for recovery of *Giardia* cysts from diverse water sources. *Lett Appl Microbiol* 22(1):21–25, 1996.

Cevallos, A., S. Carnaby, M. James, J.G. Farthing. Small intestinal injury in a neonatal rat model of giardiasis is strain dependent. *Gastroenterology* 109(3):766–773, 1995.

Dorea, R.C., E. Salata, C.R. Padovani, G.L. dos Anjos. Control of parasitic infections among school children in the peri-urban area of Botucatu, Sao Paulo, Brazil. *Rev Soc Bras Med Trop* 29(5):425–430, 1996.

Farthing, M.J. Giardiasis. *Gastroenterol Clin North Am* 25(3):493–515, 1996.

Flanagan, P.A. *Giardia*—diagnosis, clinical course and epidemiology. A review. *Epidemiol Infect* 109(1):1–22, 1992.

García, L.S., D.A. Bruckner. *Diagnostic Medical Parasitology*, 3rd ed. Washington, D.C.: ASM Press; 1997.

Hill, D.R. Giardiasis: Issues in diagnosis and management. *Infect Dis Clin North Am* 7(3):503–525, 1993.

Isaac-Renton, J.L., L.F. Lewis, C.S. Ong, M.F. Nulsen. A second community outbreak of waterborne giardiasis in Canada and serological investigation of patients. *Trans R Soc Trop Med Hyg* 88(4):395–399, 1994.

Kaucner, C., T. Stinear. Sensitive and rapid detection of viable *Giardia* cysts and *Cryptosporidium parvum* oocysts in large-volume water samples with wound fiberglass cartridge filters and reverse transcription-PCR. *Appl Environ Microbiol* 64(5):1743–1749, 1998.

Knight, R. Epidemiology and transmission of giardiasis. *Trans R Soc Trop Med Hyg* 74: 433–436, 1980.

Kramer, M.H., B.L. Herwaldt, G.F. Craun, R.L. Calderón, D.D. Juranek. Surveillance for waterborne-disease outbreaks—United States, 1993–1994. *MMWR Morb Mortal Wkly Rep CDC Surveill Summ* 45(1):1–33, 1996.

Kulda, J., E. Nohynková. Flagellates of the human intestine and of intestines of other species. *In*: Kreier, J.P., ed. Vol. 2: *Parasitic Protozoa*. New York: Academic Press; 1978.

Levy, D.A., M.S. Bens, G.F. Craun, R.L. Calderón, B.L. Herwaldt. Surveillance for waterborne-disease outbreaks—United States, 1995–1996. *MMWR Morb Mortal Wkly Rep CDC Surveill Summ* 47(1):1–34, 1998.

Lindo, J.F., J.M. Dubon, A.L. Ager, *et al*. Intestinal parasitic infections in human immunodeficiency virus (HIV)-positive and HIV-negative individuals in San Pedro Sula, Honduras. *Am J Trop Med Hyg* 58(4):431–435, 1998.

Meloni, B.P., A.J. Lymbery, R.C. Thompson. Genetic characterization of isolates of *Giardia duodenalis* by enzyme electrophoresis: Implications for reproductive biology, population structure, taxonomy, and epidemiology. *J Parasitol* 81(3):368–383, 1995.

Meyer, E.A., ed. *Giardiasis*. Amsterdam: Elsevier; 1990.

Meyer, E.A., S. Radulescu. *Giardia* and giardiasis. *Adv Parasit* 17:1–47, 1979.

Meyer, E.A., E.L. Jarroll. Giardiasis. *In*: Jacobs, L., P. Arámbulo. Vol. 1: *CRC Handbook Series in Zoonoses*. Boca Raton: CRC Press; 1982.

Olson, M.E., T.A. McAllister, L. Deselliers, *et al*. Effect of giardiasis on production in a domestic ruminant (lamb) model. *Am J Vet Res* 56(11):1470–1474, 1995.

Olson, M.E., D.W. Morck, H. Ceri. The efficacy of a *Giardia lamblia* vaccine in kittens. *Can J Vet Res* 60(4):249–256, 1996.

Rajeshwari, K., N. Jaggi, V. Aggarwal, K.K. Kalra, S.K. Mittal, U. Baveja. Determinants of symptomatic giardiasis in childhood. *Trop Gastroenterol* 17(2):70–76, 1996.

Rezende, C.H. de, J.M. Costa-Cruz, M.L. Gennari-Cardoso. Enteroparasitoses em manipuladores de alimentos de escolas públicas em Uberlândia (Minas Gerais), Brasil. *Rev Panam Salud Publican* 2(6):392–397, 1997.

United States of America, Department of Health and Human Services, Centers for Disease Control and Prevention (CDC). Water-borne giardiasis outbreaks. Washington, New Hampshire. *Morb Mortal Wkly Rep* 26:169–170, 1977.

Winiecka-Krusnell, J., E. Linder. Detection of *Giardia lamblia* cysts in stool samples by immunofluorescence using monoclonal antibody. *Eur J Clin Microbiol Infect Dis* 14(3): 218–222, 1995.

World Health Organization (WHO). *Infecciones intestinales por protozoos y helmintos. Informe de un Grupo Científico de la OMS*. Geneva: WHO; 1981. (Technical Report Series 666).

Xiao, L. *Giardia* infections in farm animals. *Parasitol Today* 10:436–438, 1994.

Zajac, A.M. Giardiasis. *Comp Cont Educ Vet Pract* 14:604–611, 1992.

INFECTIONS CAUSED BY FREE-LIVING AMEBAE

ICD-10 B60.1 Acanthamebiasis; B60.2 Naegleriasis

Synonyms: Naegleriasis, primary amebic meningoencephalitis, acanthamebiasis, granulomatous amebic encephalitis, amebic conjunctivitis, and amebic keratoconjunctivitis.

Etiology: Three genera of free-living amebae are capable of infecting man and other mammals: *Naegleria* (*N. fowleri*), *Acanthamoeba* (*A. astronyxis, A. castellanii, A. culbertsoni,* and *A. polyphaga*), and *Balamuthia* (*B. mandrillaris*). *Balamuthia* was included under the order Leptomyxida (the leptomyxid amebae) until Visvesvara *et al.* (1993) created this new genus and species in 1993. All three genera have both trophozoites and cystic forms in their respective life cycles (Martínez and Visvesvara, 1997). Although free-living amebae belonging to the genera *Hartmanella* and *Vahlkampfia* have been isolated from human nasal passages, they apparently do not cause pathology.

The trophozoites of *N. fowleri* can exist in either ameboid or flagellate form. The ameboid form is elongated (more rounded on the anterior end and more pointed on the posterior) and measures between 7 μm and 20 μm. The cytoplasm is granular, contains vacuoles, and forms blunt lobular pseudopodia at its widest point. The nucleus has one large nucleolus at the center and does not have peripheral chromatin. The flagellate form occurs when ameboid forms in tissue or culture are transferred to fresh water, especially at temperatures between 27°C and 37°C. It is pear-shaped and slightly smaller than the ameboid form, with two flagellae at its broader end. The cytoplasm and nucleus are similar to those of the ameboid form, but it does not reproduce. The cysts are round, measuring between 7 μm and 10 μm, with a nucleus similar to that of the trophozoites, and they are surrounded by a smooth thick double wall. Both the trophozoites and the cysts are present in water and soil; only the ameboid forms and the cysts grow in cultures; and only the ameboid forms are found in host tissue and cerebrospinal fluid.

The trophozoites of *Acanthamoeba* spp. occur only in the ameboid form, which is elongated and can vary widely in size, from 15 μm to 25 μm or longer. The nucleus is very similar to that of *Naegleria*, but the pseudopodia are long and narrow, and they are often distally bifurcated. The cysts are similar to those of *Naegleria*, but they are slightly larger and have an undulated wall. Both trophozoites and cysts are observed in host tissue, and both forms live in water and soil as well.

The trophozoites of *B. mandrillaris* have branches extending in all directions and they can measure between 15 μm and 60 μm. Sometimes they have two nuclei, and they have a central nucleolus. They do not have flagellate forms. The pseudopodia have secondary branchings. The cysts, which can measure from 15 μm to 30 μm, also have a single nucleus, and the outer wall is undulated. Both trophozoites and cysts can be found in host tissue. Little is known about the natural reservoir of *Balamuthia*.

Geographic Distribution: Free-living amebae appear to exist throughout the world. Clinical cases have been recorded in widely distant locations, including Australia, Brazil, US, Europe, India, and Zambia (Strickland, 1991).

Occurrence in Man: Infections with free-living amebae have only been known since the 1960s. As of 1996, there had been 179 reported cases of primary amebic meningoencephalitis caused by *N. fowleri*, 103 cases of granulomatous amebic encephalitis caused by *Acanthamoeba* spp., and 63 cases of granulomatous amebic encephalitis caused by *B. mandrillaris* (Martínez and Visvesvara, 1997). In addition, as of 1993, there have been 570 known cases of keratitis caused by *Acanthamoeba* spp. (Benenson, 1995).

Occurrence in Animals: *Naegleria* is capable of infecting experimentally inoculated mice and sheep. *Acanthamoeba* can infect sheep (Van der Lugt and Van der Merve, 1990) and dogs (Pearce *et al.*, 1985) in nature, and in the laboratory, it can infect the cornea of swine, rabbits, and mice. The invasive capacity of this protozoan appears to vary. Other researchers have found that it does not attack the cornea of horses, guinea pigs, rabbits, chicken, mice, rats, or cows, but that it can produce severe damage in the cornea of man, swine, and Chinese hamsters (Niederkorn *et al.*, 1992). *Balamuthia* has been isolated from fatal infections in horses, gorillas, mandrills, and sheep (García and Bruckner, 1997). The range of susceptible animals is probably greater, but there have been few reports of infection because of the difficulty of diagnosing this genus and because the disease in animals receives less attention than its human counterpart.

The Disease in Man: *Naegleria* mainly affects young, immunocompetent, healthy individuals. The ameba penetrates the host via the nasal cavity, where it causes local inflammation and ulceration, and goes on to invade the olfactory nerves and ultimately the meninges, where it multiplies and produces an acute inflammation with abundant neutrophils and monocytes along with hemorrhagic necroses (primary amebic meningoencephalitis). The disease is fatal. After an incubation period of three to seven days, the initial symptoms include sore throat, blocked nasal passages, and intense cephalalgia, subsequently followed by fever, vomiting, and stiff neck. Mental confusion and coma develop three to four days after the first symptoms, and death occurs between three and four days later.

Acanthamoeba spp. preferentially attack individuals who are immunodeficient, undernourished, or weakened by other conditions. This ameba usually invades the host through the skin, the respiratory tract, or the genitourinary tract, spreading through the bloodstream until it reaches the brain and the meninges. The exact length of incubation is unknown, but central nervous system symptoms apparently do not develop until weeks or even months after the primary infection. Often there is a slow-growing cutaneous or pulmonary granulomatous lesion which tends to follow a subacute or chronic course (granulomatous amebic encephalitis). The predominant lesions are foci of granulomatous inflammation, necroses, thromboses, and hemorrhages. The most prevalent symptoms include cutaneous papules, nodules, ulcers or abscesses, congestion, secretion from or ulcers in the nasal passages, sinusitis, cephalalgia, mental or motor disturbances, meningeal signs, or sensory deficiencies. Occasionally the parasite is recovered from other organs such as the skin, kidneys, liver, or pancreas. *Acanthamoeba* often infects the ocular cornea, causing keratitis, uveitis, and chronic corneal ulcers, which can lead to blindness, especially in persons who wear contact lenses. Both *Acanthamoeba* and *Naegleria* are capable of ingesting microorganisms in their environment such as *Legionella* and acting as vectors of the respective infections (Tyndall and Domingue, 1982).

Less information is available about *Balamuthia*, which was not identified until 1993. It can attack both previously healthy and weakened individuals. Although its mechanism of penetrating the host is still unknown, it can produce a subacute or chronic illness similar to that associated with *Acanthamoeba* (Denney *et al.*, 1997) and it can also cause granulomatous amebic encephalitis.

The Disease in Animals: Very little information is available about the disease in animals, but the cases reported so far have resembled the disease in humans (Simpson *et al.*, 1982; Pearce *et al.*, 1985; Niederkorn *et al.*, 1992; Visvesvara *et al.*, 1993).

Source of Infection and Mode of Transmission: The source of *Naegleria* and *Acanthamoeba* infections appears to be contaminated water and soil. Muñoz *et al.* (1993) examined 100 freshwater samples collected from different sources and found *Naegleria* present in 7.6% and *Acanthamoeba* in 31.5%. The main source of *Naegleria* infection is poorly maintained swimming pools, lakes, etc. The ameba enters the nasal passages of swimmers, especially in summer or when the water has been artificially heated. This ameba is destroyed when pools are adequately chlorinated. The flagellate trophozoite forms probably play the most important role in infection, since they are more mobile and appear to predominate in warm water. The cysts are capable of overwintering, and it is believed that the arrival of warm summer weather causes them to break open and assume the form of flagellate trophozoites. Contaminated water is also the source of infection caused by *Acanthamoeba*, and probably by *Balamuthia* as well. However, the fact that some patients have had no history of contact with suspicious water would indicate that the infection can also be acquired from contaminated soil through breaks in the skin, by the inhalation of dust containing parasite cysts, or by the inhalation of aerosols containing cysts or trophozoites. An important source of the ocular infection is the use of contact lenses that have been poorly disinfected or kept in contaminated cases. *Acanthamoeba* is more resistant to environmental agents than *Naegleria*, as evidenced by the fact that it can tolerate conventional chlorination. It has been determined that 82% of all samples of cysts survive 24 years in water at 4°C, and in vitro cultures have been known to retain their virulence for mice as long as eight years. The reservoir and mode of transmission of *Balamuthia* are unknown.

Diagnosis: Diseases caused by free-living amebae cannot be differentiated from other etiologies on the basis of clinical manifestations alone. Under the microscope it is difficult, though possible, to identify the parasites in tissue on the basis of their morphology; however, at low levels of magnification they can be easily mistaken for macrophages, leukocytes, or *Entamoeba histolytica*. *E. histolytica* has a thin nuclear membrane and a small nucleolus that stains only faintly, unlike the free-living amebae, which have a very distinct nuclear membrane and a larger nucleolus that stains brightly. In lesions caused by *Naegleria*, the only forms present are ameboid trophozoites, which are often perivascular, and polymorphonuclear cells are abundant in the reaction. On the other hand, in lesions produced by *Acanthamoeba* and *Balamuthia* there are both trophozoites and cysts, vasculitis is present, and the reaction is characterized by an abundance of mononuclear cells, either with or without multinucleate cells (Anzil *et al.*, 1991). The wall of *Acanthamoeba* cysts found in tissue turns red with periodic acid-Schiff stain and black when methenamine silver is used. The morphology of the amebae in cerebrospinal fluid can be observed by conventional or phase-contrast microscopy in fresh preparations or those to which Giemsa or Wright's stain has been applied. *Naegleria* grows on non-nutrient agar cultures in the presence of *Escherichia coli* and in sodium chloride at less than 0.4% solution, while *Acanthamoeba* grows in the absence of bacteria and in sodium chloride at less than 0.85% solution. Because *Naegleria* trophozoites are destroyed at cold temperatures, the samples should never be refrigerated. The diagnosis of *Balamuthia* is not yet well defined. Although the trophozoite is characterized by its branching, the cysts are very similar to those of *Acanthamoeba*; only the occasional presence of binucleate *Balamuthia* cysts makes it possible to use conventional microscopy to differentiate *Balamuthia* from *Acanthamoeba*. *Balamuthia* does not grow well on agar in the presence of bacteria, but it does proliferate in mammal tissue cultures. Immunologic reactions with patient sera have not been successful. However, it has been possible to identify exact genera and species using immunofluorescence with monoclonal or polyclonal antibodies at reference centers such as the US Centers for Disease Control and Prevention. Recently, there have been encouraging results with the use of molecular biology techniques to identify and separate species.

Control: Infections caused by free-living amebae are not sufficiently common to justify general control measures. Education of the public regarding appropriate swimming-pool maintenance and the importance of not swimming in suspicious water should reduce the risk of infection. To prevent the parasites from invading the nasal passages, those practicing aquatic sports should avoid submersing the head in water or else use nose clips. In addition, persons who are immunodeficient or have debilitating diseases should be careful not to let broken skin come in contact with natural water or damp soil and avoid breathing dust or aerosols. Contact-lens wearers should not swim with their lenses on to avoid contamination, and lenses should be disinfected either by heating them to a temperature of at least 70°C or by using hydrogen peroxide solutions, which are more effective against *Acanthamoeba* than conventional sodium chloride solutions. Control to protect against animal cases does not appear to be necessary. There is no evidence of human-to-human transmission or transmission from animals to humans. These infections mainly occur in humans and in animals that transmit them from one to another.

Bibliography

Anzil, A.P., C. Rao, M.A. Wrzolek, G.S. Visvesvara, J.H. Sher, P.B. Kozlowski. Amebic meningoencephalitis in a patient with AIDS caused by a newly recognized opportunistic pathogen, *Leptomyxid ameba. Arch Pathol Lab Med* 115:21–25, 1991.

Benenson, A.S., ed. *Control of Communicable Diseases in Man*, 16th ed. An official report of the American Public Health Association. Washington, D.C.: APHA; 1995.

Denney, C.F., V.J. Iragui, L.D. Uber-Zak, *et al.* Amebic meningoencephalitis caused by *Balamuthia mandrillaris*: Case report and review. *Clin Infect Dis* 25:1354–1358, 1997.

García, L.S., Bruckner, D.A. *Diagnostic Medical Parasitology,* 3rd ed. Washington, D.C.: ASM Press; 1997.

Martínez, A.J., G.S. Visvesvara. Free-living, amphizoic and opportunistic amebas. *Brain Pathol* 7:583–598, 1997.

Muñoz, V., H. Reyes, B. Astorga L., E. Rugiero P., S. Del Río, P. Toche. Amebas de vida libre en hábitats de aguas dulces de Chile. *Parasitol Día* 17:147–152, 1993.

Niederkorn, J.Y., J.E. Ubelaker, J.P. McCulley, *et al.* Susceptibility of corneas from various animal species to *in vitro* binding and invasion by *Acanthamoeba castellanii. Invest Ophthalmol Vis Sci* 33:104–112, 1992.

Pearce, J.R., H.S. Powell, F.W. Chandler, G.S. Visvesvara. Amebic meningoencephalitis caused by *Acanthamoeba castellani* in a dog. *J Am Vet Assoc* 187:951–952, 1985.

Simpson, C.P., E. Willaert, F.C. Neal, A.R. Stevens, M.D. Young. Experimental *Naegleria fowleri* meningoencephalitis in sheep: Light and electron microscopic studies. *Am J Vet Res* 43:154–157, 1982.

Strickland, G.T., ed. *Hunter's Tropical Medicine,* 7th ed. Philadelphia: Saunders; 1991.

Tyndall, R.L., E.L. Domingue. Cocultivacion of *Legionella pneumophila* and free-living amoebae. *Appl Environ Microbiol* 44:954–959, 1982.

Van der Lugt, J.J., H.E. Van der Merwe. Amoebic meningoencephalitis in a sheep. *J S Afr Vet Assoc* 61:33–36, 1990.

Visvesvara, G.S., F.L. Schuster, A.J. Martínez. *Balamuthia mandrillaris*, N. G., N. Sp., agent of amebic meningoencephalitis in humans and other animals. *J Eukaryot Microbiol* 40:504–514, 1993.

MALARIA IN NONHUMAN PRIMATES

ICD-10 B53.1 Malaria due to simian plasmodia

Synonyms: Monkey malaria, monkey paludism.

Etiology: Malaria is a disease caused by protozoa of the phylum Apicomplexa, genus *Plasmodium.* The four species that infect man are *P. falciparum, P. malariae, P. ovale,* and *P. vivax.* Some 20 species are presumed to infect nonhuman primates: the large simians are affected by 4 species of the family Pongidae, gibbons by 4 species of the family Hylobatidae, Old World monkeys by 8 species of the family Cercopithecidae, New World monkeys by 2 species of the family Cebidae, and lemurs by 2 species of the family Lemuridae (Collins and Aikawa, 1977). However, the taxonomy of some species is uncertain. Table 2 shows some characteristics of the most common species.

Seven of the species that affect nonhuman primates have been transmitted experimentally to humans: *P. brasilianum, P. cynomolgi, P. eylesi, P. inui, P. knowlesi, P. schwetzi,* and *P. simium.* In addition, some species, such as *P. cynomolgi, P. knowlesi, P. simium,* and, possibly, *P. eylesi,* have been found in natural or accidental infections, though this rarely occurs. Nonhuman primates can also be infected

TABLE 2. *Plasmodium* **species that infect primates.**

Species	Host	Geographic range	Periodicity	Relapses
P. brasilianum	New World monkeys	Central and South America	Quartan	Uncertain
P. coatneyi	Old World monkeys	Malaysia	Tertian	No
P. cynomolgi	Old World monkeys	Southeast Asia	Tertian	Yes
P. eylesi	Gibbons	Malaysia	Tertian	Uncertain
P. falciparum	Humans	Tropics	Tertian	No
P. fieldi	Old World monkeys	Malaysia	Tertian	Yes
P. gonderi	Old World monkeys	Central Africa	Tertian	No
P. hylobati	Gibbons	Malaysia	Tertian	No
P. inui	Old World monkeys	India and Southeast Asia	Quartan	No
P. knowlesi	Old World monkeys	Malaysia	Quotidian	No
P. malariae	Humans	Tropics and subtropics	Quartan	No
P. ovale	Humans	Asia and Africa	Tertian	Yes
P. reichenowi	Chimpanzees	Central Africa	Tertian	No
P. schwetzi	Gorillas and chimpanzees	Tropical Africa	Tertian	Yes
P. simiovale	Old World monkeys	Sri Lanka	Tertian	Yes
P. simium	New World monkeys	Brazil	Tertian	Uncertain
P. vivax	Humans	Tropics and subtropics	Tertian	Yes

with natural or adapted strains of the plasmodia that normally affect humans: *Aotus* and *Saimiri* monkeys with *P. falciparum* or *P. vivax*, and chimpanzees with *P. ovale*.

For many years, it was believed that the plasmodia of man did not have a common origin (monophyletic) but rather were descended from different ancestral species (polyphyletic), and the relationship of some species that infect man to some species that infect simians was frequently the subject of speculation. Escalante *et al.* (1998) compared cytochrome *b* gene sequences from 4 species of human parasites, 10 species of simian parasites, 1 species of rodent parasite, and 2 species of avian parasites. They concluded that the plasmodia of man are indeed polyphyletic. *P. falciparum* and *P. reichenowi* are closely related to one another and share a common ancestor with avian malaria parasites. *P. vivax* forms a different but closely related group with the plasmodia of Old World monkeys, especially *P. simium*. *P. ovale* and *P. malariae* form a separate group, although there is very little relationship between them. An interesting finding is that, contrary to widely held opinion, no inverse relationship exists between virulence of the parasite and length of the plasmodium-host association. Neither is there any relationship between phylogenetic proximity of the parasites and certain characteristics of malarial disease, such as virulence, periodicity, and occurrence of relapses. Notwithstanding the foregoing, biologic and pathogenic similarities have led to the use of certain nonhuman primate *Plasmodium* species as the preferred models for *Plasmodium* species that infect man: *P. cynomolgi* for *P. vivax, P. brasilianum* for *P. malariae, P. fieldi* and *P. simiovale* for *P. ovale*, and *P. coatneyi* for *P. falciparum*. In addition, Lal *et al.* (1988) demonstrated that the immunodominant repeat domain was the same for *P. brasilianum* and *P. malariae* and for *P. reichenowi* and *P. falciparum*.

The life cycle of plasmodia of nonhuman primates, like that of the plasmodia that infect man, includes host mammals and insect vectors. An infected mosquito of the genus *Anopheles* injects sporozoites of the parasite into a susceptible host when it takes a blood meal. In less than an hour, the sporozoites disappear from the blood and enter the cells of the hepatic parenchyma. There, they begin to multiply by multiple fission to form thousands of filamentous parasites, the merozoites, which leave the host cell after five days or more. In some species, there is a single generation of hepatic merozoites, but in others, dormant forms, hypnozoites, are produced. The hypnozoites may become active again months or years later and cause reinfection (Cogswell, 1992) (Table 2). This stage of replication in the liver is known as the exo-erythrocytic cycle. The growth and asexual division of the sporozoites to form merozoites is termed merogony (formerly called schizogony).

Once released, the merozoites invade the erythrocytes to form a trophozoite within a vacuole. The trophozoite is originally ovoid, but then it forms a ring structure with a vacuole in the center. At this stage, the trophozoite begins to feed on the cytoplasm of the erythrocyte, and a dark pigment, hemozoin, is deposited into its food vacuoles. As the trophozoite matures, the central vacuole disappears and the nucleus begins to divide by successive mitosis, forming a multinucleate cell, the meront (formerly called the schizont). Later, the cytoplasm of the erythrocyte divides into portions that envelop each nucleus to form numerous merozoites. The mature merozoites rupture the blood cell and enter the bloodstream, where they invade other erythrocytes, and the same cycle is repeated. This multiplication in the erythrocytes is known as the erythrocytic cycle. Like the process that occurs in the liver, the growth and asexual division of the original parasites to form merozoites is known as merogony. The cycle of merozoite formation in the red blood cells takes 24 hours in some species (e.g., *P. knowlesi*) and 48 or 72 hours in others. As the recurrent fevers of malaria coincide with the mass release of merozoites from the red cells, they occur daily or every third or fourth day. Malaria is classified as quotidian, tertian, or quartan, respectively, according to the periodicity of these febrile attacks (Table 2).

After several rounds of asexual reproduction in the erythrocytes, some merozoites become female cells, or macrogametocytes, and male cells, or microgametocytes, which are the infective forms for the vector. The process of gamete formation is known as gametogony. When an *Anopheles* mosquito ingests the gametocytes during a blood meal, they mature in the insect's alimentary tract and become macrogametes (ova) and microgametes (sperm). A sperm fertilizes each ovum, forming a motile zygote, the ookinete, which penetrates the epithelium of the insect's midgut, is engulfed by a membrane, and forms an oocyst in the intestinal wall. Inside the oocyst, the zygote multiplies by successive mitosis to produce an enormous number of filamentous parasites, the sporozoites, which ultimately break out of the oocyst and are distributed in the hemocele of the insect. The process of sporozoite formation is known as sporogony. The sporozoites invade all of the mosquito's tissues, and those that reach the salivary glands may be passed to a vertebrate host with the saliva of the insect at its next blood meal.

Geographic Distribution: Although the prevailing opinion is that the plasmodia of simians originated in Southeast Asia, Escalante *et al.* (1998) suggest that the origin of primate malaria parasites is African and posit that from there they spread to Southeast Asia with their host mammals and vectors. Their current geographic distribution coincides with that of their preferred hosts (Table 2). In the Americas, *P. brasilianum* is widely distributed among the neotropical monkeys of Brazil,

Colombia, Panama, Peru, and Venezuela, while *P. simium* is found in the southern and eastern regions of Brazil.

Occurrence in Man: Infection of man with plasmodia of nonhuman primates is considered very rare. The literature records only two confirmed human cases acquired under natural conditions: one caused by *P. knowlesi* in Malaysia and another by *P. simium* in Brazil. Two other cases have been reported but not confirmed: one by *P. knowlesi* and the other by *P. eylesi*, both in Malaysia. All these cases occurred prior to 1970. However, it was subsequently discovered that more than 90% of the adults in four tribes in northern Brazil had antibodies against *P. brasilianum* or *P. malariae* (these species cannot be differentiated using conventional serology), although the incidence of malaria was very low and parasitemia was below 0.02% (de Arruda *et al.,* 1989). The presence of *P. brasilianum* was confirmed in numerous monkeys and in *Anopheles darlingi* mosquitoes in the area. This finding suggests that *P. brasilianum* infection is occurring in the indigenous population.

P. knowlesi was transmitted experimentally to human volunteers through the inoculation of blood or the bite of infected mosquitoes. After 170 serial passages, however, the infection became so virulent that the passages were stopped (Collins and Aikawa, 1977). *P. cynomolgi* was inoculated accidentally into humans and was then transmitted to man and monkeys by infected mosquitos. Although the level of parasitemia in humans was low, the disease was moderately serious. Infection by *P. brasilianum*, *P. inui*, or *P. schwetzi* in volunteers produced low levels of parasitemia and mild symptoms (Collins and Aikawa, 1977). *P. schwetzi* was also transmitted experimentally to man and produced a mild disease. Transmission of *P. reichenowi* to man was attempted, but without success (Flynn, 1973). Deane (1992) reported an accidental human infection with *P. simium* in southeastern Brazil.

Occurrence in Animals: *P. brasilianum* has been found in numerous monkey species of the family Cebidae in neotropical regions. The infection rate is close to 15% in howler monkeys of the genus *Alouatta*, spider monkeys of the genus *Ateles*, and capuchin or white monkeys of the genus *Cebus*. Natural infection by *P. simium* has been found in brown howler monkeys (*Alouatta fusca*) and in woolly spider monkeys (*Brachyteles arachnoides*). The prevalence of malaria has been reported to be 10% among simians in the Amazon region and 35% and 18% in the southeastern and southern regions of Brazil, respectively. Although *P. brasilianum* is present in all those areas, *P. simium* is found only along the southeastern and southern coast. Virtually all the parasites were detected in monkeys of the family Cebidae (Deane, 1992). Among nonhuman primates in Asia and Africa, the prevalence of the infection seems to be high in areas with large numbers of monkeys and appropriate anopheline vectors. Conversely, there are areas with sparse monkey populations in both the New World and the Old World where the infection does not occur.

The Disease in Man: Human malaria caused by plasmodia of simian origin resembles a mild and benign infection caused by human plasmodia (see Occurrence in Man). In general, the disease is of short duration, parasitemias are low, and relapses are rare. Recuperation is spontaneous, and very few patients require treatment. The periodicity of malarial attacks depends on the parasite species (Table 2).

The Disease in Animals: In general, malaria in simians is a mild disease that resolves spontaneously in the parasite's natural hosts. However, *P. knowlesi* infection is serious in rhesus monkeys and in baboons. *P. brasilianum* can cause acute disease in American monkeys and, occasionally, may even be fatal for spider, howler, and capuchin monkeys. *P. eylesi* causes high parasitemia in mandrills. *P. gonderi* has a chronic course, *P. georgesi* produces a relapsing malaria, and *P. petersi* causes a brief infection in *Cercocebus* monkeys, which are the natural hosts for these species (Poirriez *et al.*, 1995). In rhesus monkeys (*Macaca mulatta*), *P. coatneyi* and *P. fragile* cause neurological signs similar to those that occur in humans infected with *P. falciparum* (Aikawa *et al.*, 1992; Fujioka *et al.*, 1994). *P. cynomolgi* causes placentitis in rhesus monkeys (Saxena *et al.*, 1993). After infection with *P. ovale*, monkeys of the genus *Saimiri* develop parasites in the liver but do not progress to erythrocytic stages (Millet *et al.*, 1994).

Source of Infection and Mode of Transmission: Malaria of both humans and nonhuman primates is transmitted by the bite of infected anopheline mosquitoes. Which species of mosquitoes transmit malaria of nonhuman primates in the forests of Africa, the Americas, and a large part of Asia is still not well known. In northwestern Malaysia, the vector of *P. cynomolgi* has been shown to be *Anopheles balabacensis balabacensis,* which also transmits human malaria in that region. However, the cycles of disease transmission in humans and nonhuman primates are generally independent of one another because the vectors of human plasmodia feed at ground level, while those of simian plasmodia feed in the treetrops. In northern Brazil, *P. brasilianum* has been found in *Anopheles darlingi* mosquitoes. It has been demonstrated that the distribution of *P. simium* and *P. brasilianum* in that country is governed by the presence of the mosquitoes *A. cruzi* and *A. neivai*, which feed in the forest canopy. This explains the rarity of human infection by plasmodia of simian origin. Nevertheless, in some regions of Brazil, such as the mountainous and wooded coastal areas of the state of Santa Catarina, *A. cruzi* is the vector of human malaria and possibly also of simian malaria, while in other regions it is exclusively a vector of the simian disease. In Santa Catarina, however, it was found that *A. cruzi* feeds both at ground level and in the treetops. In such conditions, human infection caused by simian plasmodia may occur naturally. In western Malaysia, a similar situation exists: the vector is the same for the human and nonhuman cycles, and zoonotic infections may thus occur. However, the risk appears to be limited to those who live in or enter jungle areas, and it is unlikely that the infection could spread to other human communities. In tropical Africa, where chimpanzees are infected by *P. malariae, P. rodhaini,* and *P. schwetzi,* humans might become infected when they enter the habitat of these primates. However, malariologists point out that the plasmodia of nonhuman primates pose little risk for the human population, since *P. malariae* from chimpanzees cannot infect *Anopheles gambiae,* the vector of human malaria, and *P. schwetzi* does not develop fully in that mosquito.

Diagnosis: Routine diagnosis in man and in monkeys is done by examining the parasite in thick blood films stained with Giemsa stain. Differentiation of the species of *Plasmodium* that infect nonhuman primates is based mainly on morphologic features of the parasite's various stages of development. Another criterion is host specificity. Specific diagnosis is very difficult, for example in the case of *P. brasilianum* and *P. simium,* which are similar to the human plasmodia *P. malariae* and *P. vivax,* respectively. Because the routine diagnostic techniques for differentiating *Plasmodium* species are imprecise, it is possible that some human malaria cases of simian origin have been diagnosed erroneously as being caused by human malarial agents. Another difficulty in diagnosis by microscopic examination of blood preparations is the low parasitemia that occurs in nonhuman primates. To get around this difficulty, inoculation of blood into susceptible monkeys is recommended. Although serologic reactions are useful as a means of confirming malarial infection, they are rarely specific enough to identify the *Plasmodium* species involved.

Control: Malaria experts agree that malaria of nonhuman primates does not constitute an obstacle for programs to control and eradicate human malaria. The human infection has been eradicated from some parts of Brazil, although high rates of infection in monkeys persist. Given the small number of confirmed cases of human infection by plasmodia of simian origin and the benign nature of the clinical manifestations, special control measures are not justified.

To prevent the disease, nonimmune persons who must go into the jungle should use insect repellents on exposed body parts and on clothing. Regular use of chemoprophylaxis would be justified only if the nonimmune person had to live in an area where human malaria is endemic.

Bibliography

Aikawa, M., A. Brown, C.D. Smith, *et al.* A primate model for human cerebral malaria: *Plasmodium coatneyi*-infected rhesus monkeys. *Am J Trop Med Hyg* 46:391–397, 1992.

Bruce-Chwatt, L.J. Malaria zoonosis in relation to malaria eradication. *Trop Geogr Med* 20:50–87, 1968.

Coatney, G.R. Simian malarias in man: Facts, implications, and predictions. *Am J Trop Med Hyg* 17:147–155, 1968.

Coatney, G.R. The simian malarias: Zoonoses, anthroponoses, or both? *Am J Trop Med Hyg* 20:795–803, 1971.

Cogswell, F.B. The hypnozoite and relapse in primate malaria. *Clin Microbiol Rev* 5:26–35, 1992.

Collins, W.E., M. Aikawa. Plasmodia of nonhuman primates. *In:* Kreier, J.P., ed. Vol. 3: *Parasitic Protozoa.* New York: Academic Press; 1977.

Deane, L.M. Epidemiology of simian malaria in the American continent. *In: First Inter-American Conference on Conservation and Utilization of American Nonhuman Primates in Biomedical Research.* Washington, D.C.: Pan American Health Organization; 1977. (Scientific Publication 317).

Deane, L.M. Simian malaria in Brazil. *Mem Inst Oswaldo Cruz* 87(Suppl 3):1–20, 1992.

Deane, L.M., M.P. Deane, J. Ferreira Neto. Studies on transmission of simian malaria and on a natural infection of man with *Plasmodium simium* in Brazil. *Bull World Health Organ* 35:805–808, 1966.

de Arruda, M., E.H. Nardin, R.S. Nussenzweig, A.H. Cochrane. Sero-epidemiological studies of malaria in Indian tribes of the Amazon Basin of Brazil. *Am J Trop Med Hyg* 41:379–385, 1989.

Escalante, A.A., D.E. Freeland, W.E. Collins, A.A. Lal. The evolution of primate malaria parasites based on the gene encoding cytochrome *b* from the linear mitochondial genome. *Proc Natl Acad Sci USA* 95:8124–8129, 1998.

Flynn, R.J. *Parasites of Laboratory Animals.* Ames: Iowa State University Press; 1973.

Fujioka, H., P. Millet, Y. Maeno, *et al.* A nonhuman primate model for human cerebral malaria: Rhesus monkeys experimentally infected with *Plasmodium fragile. Exp Parasitol* 78:371–376, 1994.

Garnham, P.C. Recent research on malaria in mammals excluding man. *Adv Parasit* 11:603–630, 1973.

Lal, A.A., V.F. de la Cruz, W.E. Collins, G.H. Campbell, P.M. Procell, T.F. McCutchan. Circumsporozoite protein gene from *Plasmodium brasilianum*. Animal reservoirs for human malaria parasites? *J Biol Chem* 263:5495–5498, 1988.

Millet, P., C. Nelson, G.G. Galland, *et al. Plasmodium ovale*: Observations on the parasite development in *Saimiri* monkey hepatocytes in vivo and in vitro in contrast with its inability to induce parasitemia. *Exp Parasitol* 78:394–399, 1994.

Poirriez, J., E. Dei-Cas, L. Dujardin, I. Landau. The blood-stages of *Plasmodium georgesi, P. gonderi* and *P. petersi*: Course of untreated infection in their natural hosts and additional morphological distinctive features. *Parasitology* 111:547–554, 1995.

Ruch, T.C. *Diseases of Laboratory Primates.* Philadelphia: Saunders; 1959.

Saxena, N., V.C. Pandey, P.N. Saxena, S. Upadhyay. Hydrolytic enzymes of rhesus placenta during *Plasmodium cynomolgi* infection: Ultrastructural and biochemical studies. *Indian J Exp Biol* 31:54–56, 1993.

Warren, M. Simian and anthropoid malarias—their role in human disease. *Lab Anim Care* 20:368–376, 1970.

World Health Organization (WHO). *Parasitology of Malaria. Report of a WHO Scientific Group.* Geneva: WHO; 1969. (Technical Report Series 433).

World Health Organization (WHO). *Parasitic Zoonoses. Report of a WHO Expert Committee with the Participation of FAO.* Geneva: WHO; 1979. (Technical Report Series 637).

MICROSPORIDIOSIS

ICD-10 B60.8 Other specified protozoal diseases

Etiology: Microsporidiosis is an emerging human infection caused by protozoa of the family Microspora. Although there are some 700 species that infect vertebrates and invertebrates, the species identified to date as parasites of man are *Enterocytozoon bieneusi, Encephalitozoon intestinalis* (formerly *Septata intestinalis*), *Encephalitozoon hellem, Encephalitozoon cuniculi*, and some species of the genera *Nosema, Pleistophora, Trachipleistophora*, and *Vittaforma* (Scaglia *et al.,* 1994). *Enterocytozoon* causes intestinal infections almost exclusively, while *Encephalitozoon* may cause intestinal or systemic infections which may spread to various organs. Parasites of the genera *Nosema, Pleistophora, Trachipleistophora*, and *Vittaforma* are uncommon in man and do not affect the intestine (Field *et al.,* 1996). The first known human infection was by *E. bieneusi* in 1985. Differentiation of genera and species requires experience and is generally based on ultrastructural morphology, antigenic composition, or DNA sequencing. Proof of the existence of isolates with genetic differences exists, at least within *E. bieneusi,* but it is not yet known if those differences are associated with differences in clinical or epidemiological conditions (Rinder *et al.,* 1997). The genera *Cryptosporidium, Isospora*, and *Cyclospora* belong to a completely different phylum: Apicomplexa (formerly Esporozoa). However, because they are also transmitted by elements commonly called "spores" and because they cause intestinal pathology, they are frequently grouped with the microsporidia under the name "intestinal spore-forming protozoa" (Goodgame, 1996).

Microsporidia are small intracellular protozoa that undergo a phase of asexual multiplication—merogony—followed by a phase of sexual multiplication—sporogony—during which they produce spores, or oocysts, inside the infected cell. The spores are released from the host cell and are eliminated into the external environment, where they may infect other individuals. They are small, double-walled bodies measuring 1 μm to 3 μm which contain a parasitic cell, or sporoplasm, with one or two nuclei. At their anterior end, they have an extrusion apparatus, the polaroplast, which everts the polar tube or filament that is coiled around the polaroplast and sporoplasm within the spore. Infection takes place when the polar tube is extruded and penetrates the host cell, allowing the sporoplasm to pass through it and enter the host.

Geographic Distribution: Apparently worldwide. Cases have been reported in Argentina, Australia, Botswana, Brazil, Canada, Czech Republic, Germany, France, India, Italy, Japan, New Zealand, Netherlands, Spain, Sri Lanka, Sweden, Switzerland, Thailand, Uganda, UK, USA, and Zambia (CDC, 2003).

Occurrence in Man: Microsporidiosis is one of the most frequent complications occurring in immunodeficient patients, but it is rare in immunocompetent individuals. It has also been reported in transplant patients (Rabodonirina *et al.*, 1996). As of 1994, more than 400 cases had been recognized, most in immunodeficient patients. The most frequent microsporidium is *E. bieneusi,* followed by *E. intestinalis,* which is about 10 times less prevalent. Other species are even less frequent. In North America, Australia, and Europe, prevalences of 12% to 50% have been reported in AIDS patients (Voglino *et al.*, 1996). The infection generally causes chronic diarrhea in immunodeficient patients. Coyle *et al.* (1996) found the infection in 44% of AIDS patients with diarrhea but in only 2.3% of AIDS patients without diarrhea. In Germany, microsporidia were identified in 36% of 50 AIDS patients with diarrhea and in 4.3% of 47 AIDS patients without diarrhea. The parasites were detected in 60% of patients with chronic diarrhea but in only 5.9% of patients with acute diarrhea. In 18 of the patients, the agent was *E. bieneusi* and in 2, it was *E. intestinalis* (Sobottka *et al.*, 1998). In Spain, Del Aguila *et al.* (1997) found the infection in only 1.2% of HIV-positive children, whereas the percentage among HIV-positive adults was 13.9%. In Niger, Bretagne *et al.* (1993) found the infection in 7% of 60 HIV-positive children and in 0.8% of 990 asymptomatic HIV-negative children. In Zimbabwe, van Gool *et al.* (1995) found the infection in 10% of 129 adults with AIDS, but in none of 106 children with AIDS and none of 13 adults and 12 children without AIDS.

Occurrence in Animals: Microsporidiosis occurs in a great number of vertebrate and invertebrate species, but as it is not generally pathogenic for vertebrates, its discovery is accidental, and there are thus no reliable statistics on its frequency. Only *E. cuniculi* has been proven to be zoonotic (Deplazes *et al.*, 1996). However, *E. bieneusi* has been found in macaques (Chalifoux *et al.*, 1998) and *E. intestinalis* in donkeys, cows, goats, pigs, and dogs (Bornay-Llinares *et al.*, 1998), and it is therefore believed that these species could also be zoonotic. In addition, *E. bieneusi* has been transmitted to macaques with AIDS and to immunodeficient pigs (Kondova *et al.*, 1998), and *E. hellem* has been transmitted to mice (Snowden, 1998).

The Disease in Man: *E. bieneusi* infects the small intestine and, sometimes, the hepatobiliary tract in immunodeficient individuals. The clinical manifestations include chronic diarrhea with passage of watery or semi-watery stools numerous times (2–8) a day, but without evidence of intestinal hemorrhage; malabsorption with atrophy of the microvilli, which is aggravated by the ingestion of food; and subsequent progressive and irreversible weight loss. Spontaneous remissions are sometimes seen, but they are short-lived. The diarrhea can ultimately lead to dehydration and malnutrition. Although the causes of the intestinal disease are not well understood, it is presumed that it is due to loss of microvilli and enterocytes. *E. intestinalis* also causes chronic diarrhea and malabsorption, and it may spread to the nasal sinuses and the kidneys (Dore *et al.*, 1996; Moss *et al.*, 1997). *E. hellem* has been isolated from the corneal epithelium and the conjunctiva and has been found in generalized infections. As in the lower animals, the few human cases of *E. cuniculi* have been systemic and have affected mainly the brain and the kidneys. *Trachipleistophora hominis* may affect the skeletal musculature, the cornea, and the upper respiratory tract (Field *et al.*, 1996); *Vittaforma* may infect the cornea.

The Disease in Animals: Most infections in vertebrates seem to be asymptomatic, except for *E. cuniculi* infection, which occasionally causes disease with foci of micronecrosis and formation of granulomas in the brain, kidneys, endothelia, and other organs of rabbits, rats, mice, and dogs.

Source of Infection and Mode of Transmission: The presence of microsporidia spores in the host stools and urine suggests that the infection could be transmitted by fecal or urinary contamination of the environment, especially water. Recent studies have demonstrated the presence of *E. bieneusi*, *E. intestinalis*, and *Vittaforma corneae* in surface and underground waters and in effluents from sewerage systems (Dowd *et al.*, 1998), which supports that presumption. *E. cuniculi* can be transmitted by parenteral inoculation in rabbits and rodents, and it is believed that it is transmitted congenitally in mice.

Diagnosis: Diagnosis of microsporidiosis is difficult owing to the small size of the spores. Specimens are obtained, inter alia, from body fluids, feces, duodenal aspirates, urinary sediment, and corneal scrapings, and they are then stained using methods that facilitate microscopic examination. Fluorescence with calcofluor white is the most sensitive method but, as it also stains yeast cells, it may give false positive results. Weber's modified trichrome stain is almost as sensitive as calcofluor white, but it is more specific because it does not stain yeasts; however, it is slower. The slowest and least sensitive test is indirect immunofluorescence using polyclonal antibodies (Didier *et al.*, 1995). In biopsies, the parasites can be detected by means of Gram or Giemsa stains or fluorescent antibodies; however, these procedures must be performed by experienced personnel. Microsporidia have been grown in cell cultures to which stains are applied to reveal the parasitized cells (Croppo *et al.*, 1998). Systemic immunologic reactions are of little use from a clinical standpoint because they do not indicate whether the infection is recent or active. Polymerase chain reaction has also been used successfully to identify microsporidia in feces and biopsies (Gainzarain *et al.*, 1998). This method may also replace electron microscopy as the only reliable procedure for differentiating species (Croppo *et al.*, 1998).

Control: Because it is not fully understood how microsporidia are transmitted, there is not yet an effective control protocol. However, the discovery of microsporidia spores in surface and underground waters and sewage by Dowd *et al.* (1998) suggests that immunodeficient individuals should avoid oral exposure to water from suspicious sources such as pools, streams, and lakes, and that questionable drinking water should be boiled.

Bibliography

Bornay-Llinares, F.J., A.J. da Silva, H. Moura, *et al.* Immunologic, microscopic, and molecular evidence of *Encephalitozoon intestinalis* (*Septata intestinalis*) infection in mammals other than humans. *J Infect Dis* 178:820–826, 1998.

Bretagne, S., F. Foulet, W. Alkassoum, J. Fleury-Feith, M. Develoux. Prévalence des spores d'*Enterocytozoon bieneusi* dans les selles de patients sidéens et d'enfants africains non infectés par le VIH. *Bull Soc Pathol Exot* 86:351–357, 1993.

Chalifoux, L.V., J. MacKey, A. Carville, *et al.* Ultrastructural morphology of *Enterocytozoon bieneusi* in biliary epithelium of rhesus macaques (*Macaca mulatta*). *Vet Pathol* 35:292–296, 1998.

Coyle, C.M., M. Wittner, D.P. Kotler, *et al.* Prevalence of microsporidiosis due to *Enterocytozoon bieneusi* and *Encephalitozoon (Septata) intestinalis* among patients with AIDS-related diarrhea: Determination by polymerase chain reaction to the microsporidian small-subunit rRNA gene. *Clin Infect Dis* 23:1002–1006, 1996.

Croppo, G.P., G.P Croppo, H. Moura, *et al.* Ultrastructure, immunofluorescence, Western blot, and PCR analysis of eight isolates of *Encephalitozoon (Septata) intestinalis* established in culture from sputum and urine samples and duodenal aspirates of five patients with AIDS. *J Clin Microbiol* 36:1201–1208, 1998.

Del Aguila, C., R. Navajas, D. Gurbindo, *et al.* Microsporidiosis in HIV-positive children in Madrid (Spain). *J Eukaryot Microbiol* 44:84S–85S, 1997.

Deplazes, P., A. Mathis, R. Baumgartner, I. Tanner, R. Weber. Immunologic and molecular characteristics of *Encephalitozoon*-like microsporidia isolated from humans and rabbits indicate that *Encephalitozoon cuniculi* is a zoonotic parasite. *Clin Infect Dis* 22:557–559, 1996.

Didier, E.S., J.M. Orenstein, A. Aldras, D. Bertucci, L.B. Rogers, F.A. Janney. Comparison of three staining methods for detecting microsporidia in fluids. *J Clin Microbiol* 33:3138–3145, 1995.

Dore, G.J., D.J. Marriott, M.C. Hing, J.L. Harkness, A.S. Field. Disseminated microsporidiosis due to *Septata intestinalis* in nine patients infected with the human immunodeficiency virus: Response to therapy with albendazole. *Clin Infect Dis* 21:70–76, 1995.

Dowd, S.E., C.P. Gerba, I.L. Pepper. Confirmation of the human-pathogenic microsporidia *Enterocytozoon bieneusi, Encephalitozoon intestinalis,* and *Vittaforma corneae* in water. *Appl Environ Microbiol* 64:3332–3335, 1998.

Gainzarain, J.C., A. Canut, M. Lozano, *et al.* Detection of *Enterocytozoon bieneusi* in two human immunodeficiency virus-negative patients with chronic diarrhea by polymerase chain reaction in duodenal biopsy specimens and review. *Clin Infect Dis* 27:394–398, 1998.

Goodgame, R.W. Understanding intestinal spore-forming protozoa: *Cryptosporidia, Microsporidia, Isospora,* and *Cyclospora. Ann Internal Med* 124:429–441, 1996.

Field, A.S., D.J. Marriott, S.T. Milliken, *et al.* Myositis associated with a newly described microsporidian, *Trachipleistophora hominis,* in a patient with AIDS. *J Clin Microbiol* 34:2803–2811, 1996.

Kondova, I., K. Mansfield, M.A. Buckholt, *et al.* Transmission and serial propagation of *Enterocytozoon bieneusi* from humans and Rhesus macaques in gnotobiotic piglets. *Infect Immun* 66:5515–5519, 1998.

Levine, N.D. *Veterinary Protozoology.* Ames: Iowa State University Press; 1985.

Moss, R.B., L.M. Beaudet, B.M. Wenig, *et al. Microsporidium*-associated sinusitis. *Ear Nose Throat J* 76:95–101, 1997.

Rabodonirina, M., M. Bertocchi, I. Desportes-Livage, *et al. Enterocytozoon bieneusi* as a cause of chronic diarrhea in a heart-lung transplant recipient who was seronegative for human immunodeficiency virus. *Clin Infect Dis* 23:114–117, 1996.

Rinder, H., S. Katzwinkel-Wladarsch, T. Loscher. Evidence for the existence of genetically distinct strains of *Enterocytozoon bieneusi. Parasitol Res* 83:670–672, 1997.

Scaglia, M., L. Sacchi, S. Gatti, *et al.* Isolation and identification of *Encephalitozoon hellem* from an Italian AIDS patient with disseminated microsporidiosis. *APMIS* 102:817–827, 1994.

Snowden, K.F., E.S. Didier, J.M. Orenstein, J.A. Shadduck. Animal models of human microsporidial infections. *Lab Anim Sci* 48:589–592, 1998.

Sobottka, I., D.A. Schwartz, J. Schottelius, *et al.* Prevalence and clinical significance of intestinal microsporidiosis in human immunodeficiency virus-infected patients with and without diarrhea in Germany: A prospective coprodiagnostic study. *Clin Infect Dis* 26:475–480, 1998.

United States of America, Department of Health and Human Services, Centers for Disease Control and Prevention (CDC). Parasites and Health: Microsporidiosis. [web page] Available at www.dpd.cdc.gov/dpdx/HTML/Microsporidiosis.htm. Accessed 31 January 2003.

van Gool, T., E. Luderhoff, K.J. Nathoo, C.F. Kiire, J. Dankert, P.R. Mason. High prevalence of *Enterocytozoon bieneusi* infections among HIV-positive individuals with persistent diarrhoea in Harare, Zimbabwe. *Trans R Soc Trop Med Hyg* 89:478–480, 1995.

Voglino, M.C., G. Donelli, P. Rossi, *et al.* Intestinal microsporidiosis in Italian individuals with AIDS. *Ital J Gastroenterol* 28:381–386, 1996.

SARCOCYSTOSIS

ICD-10 A07.8 Other specified protozoal intestinal diseases

Synonym: Sarcosporidiosis.

Etiology: Of more than a hundred species of *Sarcocystis* that infect mammals, only two are known to parasitize the human intestine: *S. suihominis* and *S. hominis* (also known as *S. bovihominis*). For many years the oocysts of these species were mistakenly assigned to the genus *Isospora* and referred to as *Isospora hominis.* A third species appears to have been found in the intestines of five immunodeficient patients in Egypt (el Naga *et al.,* 1998). A presumed sarcocyst, *S. lindemanni,* was observed for the first time in human muscle in 1968; the ecologic relationship between this species and man is uncertain.

Sarcocysts are coccidia belonging to the phylum Apicomplexa. Although these coccidia are related to *Isospora, Cryptosporidium, Cyclospora,* and *Toxoplasma,* they require both an intermediate and a definitive host. The definitive host of *S. hominis* and *S. suihominis* is man, and the intermediate hosts are cattle and swine, respectively (Markus, 1978).

The life cycle of sarcocysts appears to be similar in all the species. The definitive host acquires them upon ingesting meat infected with the parasite. The infected striated muscle contains mature, whitish-colored cysts (sarcocysts), which are usually oval and range in size from microscopic to clearly visible by direct observation. The sarcocyst has a wall around it with internal septa that divide the cyst into compartments filled with hundreds or thousands of slowly dividing fusiform parasites, called bradyzoites. Once the cyst is ingested, the bradyzoites are released into the intestine and invade the cells of the lamina propia, where they are immediately transformed by gametogony into sexuated parasites, which in turn fuse and form oocysts by sporogony. There is no asexual multiplication phase in the intestine of the definitive host. The oocysts mature in the intestine, destroy the host cell, and then exit the body in the feces. When they are eliminated they already contain two sporocysts, each with four sporozoites.

The intermediate host acquires the infection upon consuming oocysts or mature sporocysts. The sporozoites are released into the intestine, penetrate the intestinal mucosa, invade the bloodstream, and multiply asexually by merogony in the endothelial cells of the small blood vessels for one or two generations. These forms, called tachyzoites, do not form cysts; instead, they multiply rapidly, invade the fibers of striated muscle, form the sarcocyst wall, and multiply asexually by merogony for several generations into intermediate forms known as merozoites, the forms that generate the infective bradyzoites (Rommel, 1989).

Geographic Distribution: Human intestinal sarcocystosis appears to occur worldwide. Muscular sarcocystosis has been reported only in Egypt, India, Malaysia, and Thailand.

Occurrence in Man: The human intestinal infection is found in most parts of the world, with an incidence of 6% to 10% (WHO, 1981). However, these figures are affected by the custom of eating raw meat. For example, in the Lao People's Democratic Republic the prevalence of *S. hominis* was higher than 10% in adults, and in Tibet the rate for *S. hominis* was 21.8%, while that for *S. suihominis* ranged from 0.06% to 7%. About 30 cases of human muscular sarcocystosis have been reported, most of them in Malaysia, where the prevalence of sarcocystosis in general was 21% in routine autopsies (Wong and Pathmanathan, 1992).

Occurrence in Animals: The prevalence of muscular infection caused by *Sarcocystis* spp. in cattle and swine is very high, sometimes reaching more than 90%. Cattle also harbor the species *S. cruzi* (alternatively referred to as *S. bovicanis*) and *S. hirsuta* (or *S. bovifelis*), whose definitive hosts are dogs and cats, respectively, while swine are associated with *S. miescheriana* (or *S. suicanis*) and *S. porcifelis*, the definitive hosts of which are dogs and cats, respectively. Since it is difficult to differentiate species in the intermediate host, it is not known what percentage of prevalence corresponds to the parasites that are infective for man. The World Health Organization (1981) estimates that nearly half the muscular cysts in cattle and swine correspond to *S. hominis* or *S. suihominis*. Indeed, in India it was found that the prevalence of *S. suihominis* in swine was 47% and that of *S. miescheriana* was 43% (Saleque and Bhatia, 1991). Other studies have shown that rhesus monkeys can be infected with *S. hominis* and maintain an intestinal infection for at least a week.

The Disease in Man: Intestinal sarcocystosis is usually asymptomatic. Experimentally infected volunteers experienced nausea, abdominal pain, and diarrhea 3 to 6 hours after eating raw or undercooked beef containing *S. hominis*. Abdominal pain and diarrhea recurred 14 to 18 days after ingestion of the beef, coinciding with the maximum elimination of sporocysts in feces. Clinical symptoms were more pronounced after the subjects ate pork containing cysts of *S. suihominis*. Symptomatic infection is generally observed when the meat consumed contains a large number of merozoites. In Thailand, several cases of sarcocystosis involved acute intestinal obstruction, requiring resection of the affected segment of the small intestine. Histopathological examination of the resected segments revealed eosinophilic or necrotizing enteritis. It is possible that a bacterial superinfection also may have been involved in the necrotizing enteritis (Bunyaratvej *et al.*, 1982).

Human muscular sarcocystosis is usually discovered fortuitously during examination of muscle tissue for other reasons. Although the infection is nearly always asymptomatic, in some cases muscular weakness, muscular pain, myositis, periarteritis, and subcutaneous tumefaction have been observed. However, in none of these cases was there conclusive proof that the muscular cysts were the definite cause of the clinical symptoms.

The Disease in Animals: There are several species of sarcocysts in nonhuman mammals, which can occasionally cause intestinal or systemic disease. However, *S. hominis* does not cause disease in cattle, and *S. suihominis* only rarely causes severe disease in swine (Barriga, 1997). When 29 suckling pigs were given 50,000 to 500,000 sporocysts of *S. suihominis*, severe pathologic manifestations were observed 12 days after inoculation, and about half the animals died.

Source of Infection and Mode of Transmission: The source of infection for human intestinal sarcocystosis is beef or pork containing mature sarcocysts. Only the bradyzoites, which appear about two and a half months after infection of the intermediate host, are infective for the definitive host. The mode of transmission is through the ingestion of raw or undercooked infected meat. The sources of infection for cattle and swine are the oocysts or sporocysts of *S. hominis* and *S. suihominis*, respectively, shed in the feces of infected individuals. The mode of transmission is through contamination of pastures or feedlots with feces and the eventual ingestion thereof by cattle or swine. The sarcocysts have strict host specificity, so it is clear that other vertebrate species are not directly involved in transmission.

The epidemiology of human muscular sarcocystosis has not yet been clarified. It may be that *S. lindemanni* is a parasite of man, albeit an infrequent one, with an unknown carnivorous or omnivorous definitive host that has the opportunity to consume human cadavers. Some authors have suggested that the reports of human cases of sarcosporidia are based on erroneous diagnoses. Taking into account the morphology of the sarcocysts, Beaver (1979) and Kan and Pathmanathan (1991) have suggested that man might be an aberrant host of sarcocysts that normally infect the musculature of monkeys. The relative frequency of the infection in areas where there are large numbers of monkeys gives some credence to this hypothesis.

Diagnosis: Human intestinal sarcocystosis can be diagnosed by confirming the presence of oocysts or mature sporocysts in feces starting on day 9 or 10 following the ingestion of infected meat. The outer wall of the oocysts is very thin and often ruptures, which accounts for the presence of sporocysts in feces. The most efficient way to recover them from feces is by zinc sulfate flotation. *S. hominis* sporocysts measure 13 to 17 μm by 10.8 μm, and those of *S. suihominis*, 11.6 to 13.9 μm by 10 to 10.8 μm (Frenkel *et al.*, 1979). Both exhibit interior residue, but neither of them has a Stieda body.

Muscular cysts in cattle and swine are found along the length of the muscle fiber and are whitish in color, often microscopic in size, and have the shape of a long cylinder. The cyst wall forms internal septa that separate the bradyzoites into banana-shaped compartments measuring 6 to 20 μm by 4 to 9 μm (Gorman, 1984). The cysts are found most often in the cardiac muscle, esophagus, and diaphragm of adult cattle and swine. They can be observed by trichinoscopy and, more effectively, by microscopy following tryptic digestion of the infected meat. The sarcocysts are similar to those in man, but they can sometimes be as long as 5 cm and are visible to the naked eye.

Serologic tests (indirect immunofluorescence and ELISA) are not considered useful in diagnosing the intestinal infection (WHO, 1981), but studies are being done to assess their effectiveness in the diagnosis of muscular infection (Habeeb *et al.*, 1996).

Control: Cattle or swine should be prevented from ingesting infected human feces, and humans should avoid eating raw or undercooked meat. In the first case, measures should be taken to properly dispose of human waste in rural settings where there are large numbers of cattle and swine. Except in areas where there are high rates of human infection, it is probably not necessary to treat infected individuals in order to reduce contamination of the environment. The population should be educated about the risk of infection when raw meat is consumed, and veterinary inspection of slaughterhouses should be improved. Freezing of meat reduces the number of viable cysts.

Bibliography

Barriga, O.O. *Veterinary Parasitology for Practitioners*, 2nd ed. Edina: Burgess International Group; 1997.

Beaver, P.C., K. Gadgil, P. Morera. *Sarcocystis* in man: A review and report of five cases. *Am J Trop Med Hyg* 28:819–844, 1979.

Bunyaratvej, S., P. Bunyawongwiroj, P. Nitiyanant. Human intestinal sarcosporidiosis: Report of six cases. *Am J Trop Med Hyg* 31:36–41, 1982.

el Naga, I.F., A.Y. Negm, H.N. Awadalla. Preliminary identification of an intestinal coccidian parasite in man. *J Egypt Soc Parasitol* 28:807–814, 1998.

Frenkel, J.K., A.O. Heydorn, H. Mehlhorn, M. Rommel. Sarcocystinae: *Nomina dubia* and available names. *Z Parasitenkd* 58:115–139, 1979.

Gorman, T. Nuevos conceptos sobre sarcosporidiosis animal. *Monogr Med Vet* 6:5–23, 1984.

Habeeb, Y.S., M.A. Selim, M.S. Ali, L.A. Mahmoud, A.M. Abdel Hadi, A. Shafei. Serological diagnosis of extraintestinal sarcocystosis. *J Egypt Soc Parasitol* 26:393–400, 1996.

Kan, S.P., R. Pathmanathan. Review of sarcocystosis in Malaysia. *Southeast Asian J Trop Med Public Health* 22 Suppl:129–134, 1991.

Markus, M.B. Sarcocystis and sarcocystosis in domestic animals and man. *Adv Vet Sci Comp Med* 22:159–193, 1978.

Rommel, M. Recent advances in the knowledge of the biology of cyst-forming coccidia. *Angew Parasitol* 30:173–183, 1989.

Saleque, A., B.B. Bhatia. Prevalence of *Sarcocystis* in domestic pigs in India. *Vet Parasitol* 40:151–153, 1991.

Wong, K.T., R. Pathmanathan. High prevalence of human skeletal muscle sarcocystosis in south-east Asia. *Trans R Soc Trop Med Hyg* 86:631–632, 1992.

World Health Organization (WHO). *Intestinal Protozoan and Helminthic Infections. Report of a WHO Scientific Group*. Geneva: WHO; 1981. (Technical Report Series 666.)

TOXOPLASMOSIS

ICD-10 B58 Toxoplasmosis; P37.1 Congenital toxoplasmosis

Etiology: The agent of these infections is *Toxoplasma gondii*, a coccidium belonging to the phylum Apicomplexa and related to *Sarcocystis. T. gondii* can complete its evolutionary cycle in the intestine of the cat and other felines, which are the definitive hosts. In addition, it can, and usually does, take advantage of an intermediate host, which may be any of some 200 species of vertebrates. The fact that man is an intermediate host makes it medically important.

When the parasites are ingested by a cat (see Source of Infection and Mode of Transmission), they invade the feline's intestinal cells and multiply asexually by merogony for several generations. They then multiply sexually by gametogony and produce immature oocysts that cause the host cells to rupture, after which they are eventually evacuated in the feces. The oocysts measure 10 μm by 12 μm and have a single zygote inside. The cat sheds the oocytes for a period of 1 or 2 weeks, and then the cat develops immunity. Outside the host, the oocysts mature in 1 to 5 days, depending on the temperature and humidity of the environment, at which point they form sporulated oocysts (11 μm by 13 μm), each containing two sporozoites (6 μm by 8 μm) without a Stieda body and each of the latter containing four more sporozoites (2 μm by 6–8 μm) inside it (Dubey and Beattie, 1988).

In the intermediate host, which can include man and the cat, parasites are released in the small intestine and invade the epithelial cells, where they multiply until they rupture the cells. They are then disseminated by the lymphatic system or the bloodstream, either as free forms or inside macrophages or leukocytes. Although most of the parasites are captured by the lymph nodes, they can also be found inside macrophages or monocytes, and in some cases they bypass the lymph nodes and spread throughout the rest of the organism. These parasites, or tachyzoites, are banana-shaped and measure 6 μm by 2 μm. They are very active, and their cycles of invasion, multiplication, and cell rupture continue for one to two weeks, until the host develops a degree of immunity. At that point they begin to be replaced in the tissues by bradyzoites (7 μm by 1.5 μm, also banana-shaped), which are more slow-moving. The bradyzoites accumulate in the cytoplasm of the parasitized cells and encase themselves in a membrane, forming a cyst. Tachyzoites, also referred to as proliferative forms or trophozoites, are typical of the acute, or active, phase of the infection, while bradyzoites, also known as cystic forms or cystozoites, are typical of the latent, or chronic, infection and can persist in tissue throughout the life of the host. These forms can parasitize any nucleated cell, but tachyzoites show a preference for macrophages and monocytes, while bradyzoites are seen more often in muscle and nerve tissue.

Geographic Distribution: Worldwide. This is one of the most widespread of all the zoonoses.

Occurrence in Man: The infection is very common, but the clinical disease is relatively rare. Studies have shown that between 16% and 40% of the population in the US and Great Britain and from 50% to 80% of the people in continental Europe and Latin America have antibodies to the parasite, indicating that they have been infected at some time (Barriga, 1997). Most of those with bradyzoite cysts, given that they often persist for the life of the host, have a latent infection. The prevalence rate is usually higher in warm, humid climates than in cold, dry ones, and it is also higher at lower elevations and in older persons. The seropositivity rate in human populations, for whom the cause of infection is mainly the consumption of infected meat (see Source of Infection and Mode of Transmission), is low in children up to 5 years of age, but then it begins to increase and reaches its highest levels in the population 20 to 50 years old. In areas where the main cause of infection is the ingestion of contaminated soil, the infection rate is also high in children because of their inclination to get dirt on their hands.

The clinical disease usually occurs sporadically and has low levels of incidence. However, occasionally there are small epidemics attributed to the consumption of infected meat (Choi *et al.*, 1997) or contaminated water (Mullens, 1996). The epidemic reported by Mullens (1996) affected more than 110 persons and it may be the largest one on record. In 1979, an outbreak of acute toxoplasmosis affected 39 of 98 soldiers in a company that had been practicing maneuvers in the jungles of Panama. The source of infection was deemed to be the consumption of water from a stream that may have been contaminated with the feces of wild felines (Benenson *et al.*, 1982).

The infection or disease also occurs in recipients of organ transplants. Gallino *et al.* (1996) studied 121 heart transplant patients in Switzerland and found that 16 had recent *T. gondii* infections, 5 of them with clinical manifestations; 61% of the cases were infections that had been transmitted along with the transplanted organ and 7% were reactivations of a latent infection that the recipient had had before.

The congenital infection is particularly important because of the severity of the sequelae in both the fetus and the newborn. In the US, some 3,000 babies are born every year with congenital toxoplasmosis and the annual cost of treating this disease is between US$ 31 and US$ 40 million. The frequency of toxoplasmosis has been calculated at 1 per 4,000 births in the US, and in France the rate is 1 per 1,500. In Norway, Jenum *et al.* (1998) found that 10.9% of 35,940 pregnant women had been infected before pregnancy and that 0.17% became infected during pregnancy, most notably in the first trimester. Twenty-three percent of those who were infected gave birth to infected babies: 13% of the fetuses became infected during the first trimester, 29% in the second trimester, and 50% in the third. In Great Britain, a study found the infection in 6.8% to 17.8% of pregnant women, and 0.4% of these infections were recent. It is estimated that the rate of congenital infection is about 10 newborns for every 10,000 deliveries. In Spain, the infection affects 56.7% of the general population, but primary infection in pregnant women is only 0.056% (Rodríguez et al., 1996). In a region of Colombia, the rate of congenital infection has been estimated at between 30 and 120 for every 8,000 pregnancies (Gómez-Marín et al., 1997).

Toxoplasmosis is more severe in immunodeficient individuals, whose condition appears to facilitate the infection. Bossi et al. (1998) found that 399 (24.5%) of 1,628 AIDS patients had encephalitis caused by Toxoplasma, which is rare in immunocompetent persons; 97% of the patients had antibodies to the parasite, 13% had relapses, and 84% died during the course of the study. A study in Thailand revealed an infection rate of 13.1% in pregnant women who were HIV-negative and 21.1% in women who were HIV-positive (Chintana et al., 1998).

Occurrence in Animals: The infection has been confirmed in some 200 species of vertebrates, including primates, ruminants, swine, equines, carnivores, rodents, marsupials, insectivores, and numerous avian species. Wild, as well as domestic, felines have been infected with Toxoplasma. In Córdoba, Argentina, when 23 specimens of wild cats (Oncifelis geoffroyi, Felis colocolo, or Felis eira) were studied using both serologic and parasitologic tests, oocysts were found in 37% of the animals and positive serologic reactions in 59% (Pizzi et al., 1978). Among domestic animals, high reactor rates have been found in cats, sheep, goats, and swine; lower levels in horses and dogs; and low levels in cattle. In some places, 25% to 45% of the cats are seropositive. For example, studies conducted in Costa Rica using either serologic tests or isolation of the parasite showed that 60 of 237 cats (25.3%) were infected. In 55 of the animals (23%) the parasite was identified by isolation from feces and inoculation in mice, and 82% of the isolations corresponded to cats under 6 months of age. It is of interest to point out that 60% of the cats found to have oocysts in their feces were negative in the serologic tests, which indicates that they were suffering from a primary infection (Ruiz and Frenkel, 1980). In the US, two studies of cats demonstrated the presence of the parasite in the brain of 24.3% and 11% of the felines, respectively (Dubey, 1973). In animals, as in man, the seropositivity rate increases with age.

Confirmation of the parasite's presence in the meat of food animals is of special interest for public health, since undercooked meat is one of the principal sources of infection for man. In Europe, parasitism rates in excess of 50% have been found in the meat of sheep and swine slaughtered in abattoirs. In Canada, the infection was found in 3.5% to 13.2% of pigs that underwent federal inspection, while in Japan the rates are much lower. Cattle, on the other hand, are more resistant to the infection: they have low, brief serologic titers, and parasites are isolated from them only rarely (Dubey and Streitel, 1976). Although there have been sporadic reports in the past of abundant T. gondii isolations from cattle, it is now believed that the organism was actually Neospora caninum, a tissue coccidium discovered in 1988, which has been found in ruminants, equines, and dogs (Barriga, 1997).

Most infections in animals are clinically inapparent. The clinical forms are similar to those seen in man. The cases occur sporadically, with the following exceptions: in sheep and goats the congenital infection is common, and in swine there have been infrequent epizootic outbreaks in several parts of the world. Dogs can develop manifestations that are mistaken for distemper, but such cases are rare. The greatest damage caused by toxoplasmosis in sheep and goats, and sometimes swine, is abortion and the birth of infected offspring, in which perinatal fatality can be as high as 50%.

The Disease in Man: Toxoplasmosis acquired postnatally is usually a mild disease. Most of the infections are inapparent, and of the symptomatic infections, about 90% produce mild fever, persistent lymphadenopathy in one or more lymph nodes, and asthenia. Toxoplasmosis can easily be mistaken for influenza or infectious mononucleosis. As a rule, the patient recovers spontaneously in a few weeks or months. About 4% of symptomatic patients have neurological manifestations ranging from cephalalgia, lethargy, and facial paralysis to hemiplegia, severe reflex alterations, and coma. A small proportion of symptomatic patients may exhibit muscular signs with myositis and weakness. There are also reports of myocarditis and pneumonitis caused by *Toxoplasma*, but such cases do not appear to be common. Unlike the foregoing manifestations of acute toxoplasmosis, an ocular form with subsequent uveitis may be seen in adolescents, either as a reactivation of congenital toxoplasmosis or as a delayed manifestation of postnatally acquired toxoplasmosis. Encephalitis caused by *T. gondii* is common in immunodeficient patients but rare in immunocompetent individuals. Ferrer *et al.* (1996) reviewed 63 cases and found that the most frequent clinical manifestations were focal neurological signs (80.9%), cephalalgia (53.3%), and fever (42.4%). Only 6% of the patients had new infections; 87.3% of the cases were reactivations of an earlier infection. The average survival was 11.5 months. Retinitis and pneumonitis caused by *Toxoplasma* are also common in AIDS patients.

Although congenital toxoplasmosis is not very frequent, it can cause severe disease and sequelae. Fetal infection occurs only when the pregnant mother acquires an acute or primary infection, either symptomatic or not, that generates parasitemia and permits transplacental transmission. Since the infection confers lifelong immunity, intrauterine transmission of the parasite does not occur in subsequent pregnancies except when the mother is severely immunocompromised. Observations indicate that the seriousness of the congenital infection depends on the duration of the fetal infection and that the most severe cases stem from infection in the first trimester of pregnancy (WHO, 1979). Early transmission causes few cases of fetal infection, but the risk of severe fetal illnesses is great. Only about 13% of children with toxoplasmosis acquired the infection during the first trimester *in utero* (Jenum *et al.*, 1998), but an estimated 80% of them can be expected to suffer severe disease. Of the approximately 29% who become infected in the second trimester, 30% will have serious disease. Of the 50% who become infected in the third trimester, 70% to 90% are born with an inapparent infection, but they may develop ocular or neurological sequelae after several weeks or months. The symptoms of congenital toxoplasmosis are highly varied. Early infection can cause pre- or postnatal death or severe damage to the fetus. Later infection can cause generalized disease *in utero*, subsequent invasion of the nervous system, and the birth of children with sequelae such as hydrocephaly, chorioretinitis, or cerebral calcifications. Even later infection may result in the birth of a child already in the active stage of chorioretinitis or encephalitis. When the infection occurs shortly before delivery, the child may be born with an inapparent infection; or with fever, eruptions, hepatomegaly, splenomegaly, or pneumonia; or with a generalized infection that compromises the hematopoietic, reticuloendothelial, or pulmonary systems.

Ocular toxoplasmosis deserves special mention. The most common manifestation of this form is retinochoroiditis (more than 80% of the cases), but there can be other lesions and alterations, such as strabismus, nystagmus, and microphthalmia. Ocular lesions are common in newborn infants with toxoplasmosis, and they are almost always bilateral. Later manifestations of the lesion tend to be unilateral.

Most of the pathology of toxoplasmosis appears to involve the destruction of host cells during the multiplication of tachyzoites. It has also been shown that the production of cytokines during the immune response to the parasite can influence the pathology.

The Disease in Animals: As in man, the infection is very common but the clinical disease is relatively infrequent. Its effects are particularly important in sheep and goats because it causes abortions and disease in newborns, resulting in serious economic losses, especially in Australia, Great Britain, and New Zealand. In Tasmania, Australia, *T. gondii* was believed to have been the etiology in 46% of the outbreaks of abortion and neonatal mortality in sheep between 1962 and 1968 (Munday, 1975). Congenitally infected lambs lack muscular coordination, they are physically weak, and they are unable to feed themselves. Congenital toxoplasmosis occurs in lambs only when the ewe is infected during pregnancy. When the fetus is infected between days 45 and 55 of gestation, it usually dies; if the infection is acquired in the third month of pregnancy, the lambs are born but they are sick; if it occurs after 4 months, the lambs may be born with the infection but they are asymptomatic. Disease in adult sheep is rare. Some authors have defended the use of sheep rather than mice as animal models for the human infection, because the clinical characteristics of ovine congenital toxoplasmosis are similar to those seen in man. In swine, there have been reports of outbreaks with manifestations such as pneumonia, encephalitis, and abortion (Dubey, 1977).

Dogs have a high infection rate, and the clinical picture can resemble distemper. Cats also have a high infection rate. Both the intestinal and the systemic infections tend to be asymptomatic in cats, but cases have been reported with generalized, intestinal, encephalic, and ocular manifestations, particularly in young animals. Artificially infected young cats have developed diarrhea, hepatitis, myocarditis, myositis, pneumonia, and encephalitis. Toxoplasmosis has also been observed in rabbits, guinea pigs, and other laboratory animals, sometimes with fatal outcome. Because toxoplasmosis is a strong trigger for helper lymphocyte type 2 immune reactions (cell-mediated immunity), the infection may interfere with experimental results.

Toxoplasmosis in birds can be very common, but it is rarely symptomatic. In Costa Rica *T. gondii* was isolated from 54% of 50 chickens even though no antibodies were found. In acute cases, necrotic foci have been observed in the liver, spleen, lungs, and lymph nodes.

Source of Infection and Mode of Transmission: The human infection can be acquired *in utero* or postnatally. In the US, it is estimated that fewer than 0.1% of infected adults have acquired the infection congenitally. After birth, the intermediate hosts, including man, can be infected by eating raw or undercooked meat, especially pork or lamb, or by ingesting mature oocysts from earth, water, or food contaminated with the feces of infected cats. In Thailand, a study of 1,200 pregnant women showed that 13% were infected. The rate was 19.5% in women who ate undercooked meat and only 9.6% in those who did not. When this factor was excluded, the rate was 31.8% for women who had cats in their home and 19.3% for those who did not (Chintana *et al.*, 1998). In Ireland, Taylor *et al.* (1997) found an infection rate of 12.8% in 1,276 children between 4 and 18 years of age. Presumably, infection acquired from infected earth or food played an important role, because the rate was higher in rural areas (16.6%) than in cities (10.2%); these results correlated with titers for *Toxocara canis*, which is acquired from ingesting contaminated earth. As in other studies, no correlation was found with the presence of domestic cats. This result may be due to the fact that the populations studied were mainly infected through the consumption of contaminated meat, or else because cats shed oocysts for only 1 or 2 weeks; hence, the infection correlates more with the existence of a contaminated environment that with the presence of these animals.

Cats and other felines are very important links in the epidemiology of toxoplasmosis. Unlike man, other omnivores and carnivores can become infected by ingesting food, especially meat, contaminated with oocysts. Sheep, which are one of the main sources of human infection, become infected only by ingesting oocysts. It appears that cats are a significant factor in the contamination of pastures, because a single infected cat produces millions of oocysts, which survive in the ground for almost a year as long as they are protected from the sun and from drying out. The results of studies conducted on islands near Australia lend credence to this idea: only 2% of the sheep raised on the islands without cats had antibodies to *T. gondii*, whereas antibodies were found in 32% of the sheep on the islands with cats. Apparently, the main sources of infection for cats are rodents or birds infected with bradyzoite cysts: some experiments have shown that oocysts infect a smaller proportion of cats than do cysts and that most cats develop antibodies against the parasite at around the age when they begin to hunt. Although there have been reports of cats infected with tachyzoites, these forms cannot be very efficient because they are destroyed by gastric acid. At some point between 3 and 21 days after the initial infection, the cat begins to shed oocysts in its feces for a period of 1 or 2 weeks, thus contaminating the environment. The infection generates sufficient immunity to stave off any future clinical infections for the rest of the cat's life. However, the oocysts can remain viable for about a year in environments that are cool, humid, and shady. Even though it is difficult to diagnose clinical infection in a cat, positive serology indicates that the animal has already had an infection, and in that case it poses no risk of contamination because it will no longer shed any oocysts.

It has been pointed out that there is a correlation between meat handling and the prevalence of seropositivity. In a serologic survey of 144 employees and workers at a slaughterhouse in Belo Horizonte, Brazil, the prevalence of positive reactors was 72%, with the highest rate among meat inspectors (92%) and the lowest rate among workers in the corrals (60%) (Riemann *et al.*, 1975). Higher reactor rates have also been found in housewives who handle meat in the kitchen compared with the general population. Presumably, their hands become contaminated by infected meat and transmission occurs via the oral route. Recent studies have suggested that coprophilic flies and cockroaches may act as transport hosts carrying cat fecal oocysts to human food, which would account for infections in vegetarians. Contamination of the soil with oocysts from wild felines would account for infections contracted by indigenous peoples living along the banks of the upper Xingú River in Brazil, who do not keep domestic cats and do not eat raw meat.

The literature also cites a few cases of transmission to man through raw milk (Riemann *et al.*, 1975; Chiari and Neves, 1984), eggs, transfusions, and accidental inoculations in the laboratory, but these cases are not significant from the epidemiologic standpoint. Congenital transmission in humans, despite its clinical significance, is also unimportant epidemiologically, both because it is relatively rare and also because the infected person is a source of infection only for the fetus during the acute phase. Congenital transmission is infrequent in all animals except sheep and goats. Because the latter are a source of infection for man, they are the only species that are epidemiologically significant.

Diagnosis: Specific diagnosis can be made in acute-phase patients by directly visualizing the parasite in fluid or tissue, but this is a difficult and low-yield process. The parasite can also be isolated from organic fluid or tissue by intraperitoneal inoculation in mice. In chronic cases, samples of muscle or brain tissue may be subjected to peptic digestion before inoculation (this procedure is not recommended in acute cases because the tachyzoites are destroyed by gastric acid). During the first week after inoculation, tachyzoites may appear in the peritoneal exudate of the mice. At 6 weeks, serologic diagnosis is performed on the surviving animals, and, if the result is positive, the mice are sacrificed to confirm the presence of cysts in the brain.

A diagnosis may also be obtained with serologic tests. The following procedures are generally used: Sabin-Feldman (S-F) dye test, indirect immunofluorescence (IIF), indirect hemagglutination (IHA), complement fixation (CF), direct agglutination (DA), and enzyme-linked immunosorbent assay (ELISA). The S-F dye test is based on the fact that live tachyzoites do not ordinarily stain with methylene blue but they do stain if they have been subjected to the lethal action of antibodies and complement; if the patient is infected, the serum to be studied provides the anti-*Toxoplasma* antibodies. With membrane antigen, the S-F test, IIF, and ELISA are sensitive, specific, and often preferred over clinical tests because they give earlier results and make it possible to diagnose active infection. However, the S-F test is being replaced by IIF, even though the results are equivalent, because the former entails manipulating live parasites and breeding mice. Positive results from IHA can be obtained later and over a longer period, but it is of little use during the acute phase of the infection. CF is a more difficult test to perform and does not offer any advantages over the ones already mentioned; consequently, its use is in decline. DA with membrane antigen is a simple, low-cost technique that diagnoses acute infections. It was recently introduced to test for infections in patients with AIDS. Some of these serologic tests, particularly ELISA, have been modified for use in diagnosing infection in food animals. Polymerase chain reaction has been used to confirm the presence of parasite DNA in adult or fetal fluids.

Clinicians are especially interested in developing a test that can distinguish between the acute and chronic forms of the infection, given the importance of the former in congenital transmission. IIF and ELISA are particularly appropriate for this purpose because they make it possible to determine the presence of IgM antibodies, which appear and disappear before the IgG antibodies. In acute acquired toxoplasmosis, IgM antibodies peak during the first month of the disease and persist for an average of eight months, although in some patients they may be present for years. In the case of acute infection, it is believed that the study of IgG antibody avidity (the total combined power of an antibody molecule and its antigen, which depends on the number of binding sites and the affinity of each) and the presence of IgA antibodies give better results than merely verifying the presence of IgM antibodies (Rodríguez *et al.*, 1996).

Because IgM does not cross the placenta, the presence of these antibodies in the serum of newborns is reliable evidence that the fetus developed them *in utero* and that the infant was born with the infection. In the US, the Food and Drug Administration recently studied six commercial kits to ascertain the presence of IgM antibodies for toxoplasmosis and found that they all had greater than 93% sensitivity; however, the specificity of three of them was lower than 90% (Wilson *et al.*, 1997). For diagnosing toxoplasmosis in the fetus, the most useful tests are ultrasound, demonstration of specific IgM antibodies in the umbilical cord, and verification of parasite DNA in amniotic fluid (Beazley and Egerman, 1998).

It has also been proposed to investigate the presence of IgE antibodies for *Toxoplasma* as an indicator of acute infection, even though they appear after the infection and persist for only three to five months. Unfortunately, the specificity of the antibodies is high (98%), but their sensitivity is low (76%); hence, the absence of IgE antibodies does not rule out acute infection (Gross *et al.*, 1997). Another procedure used for determining the presence of acute infection is the evolution of IgG antibody titers, for which purpose a quantitative serologic test is used and is repeated after two to four weeks. If the titers increase after more than three dilutions, it may be speculated that the patient's immune system is responding actively to the parasite and therefore he or she must be in the active phase of the infection.

The toxoplasmin skin test reveals past infections and is mainly useful in epidemiologic studies. The reaction demonstrates type IV delayed hypersensitivity. The positive response appears several months after the initial infection and may last for life.

The intestinal infection in cats is diagnosed by feces flotation procedures, which permit observation of the small immature oocysts that are characteristic of the parasite. However, it is difficult to find positive cats with this test because they shed oocysts for only 1 to 2 weeks starting 3 to 21 days after primary infection. In the US, it has been estimated that, even though the infection affects 15% to 40% of the feline population, fewer than 1% of the cats are shedding oocysts at any given moment. Nevertheless, the infection in cats can be diagnosed remotely by serology. If a cat is serologically positive, it has already had the infection. Since feline toxoplasmosis leaves strong immunity against reinfection, the animal will not contaminate the environment by shedding oocysts in the future.

Control: Two circumstances facilitate human postnatal *Toxoplasma* infection: the ingestion of bradyzoites in infected undercooked meat, and the ingestion of oocysts via hands or food contaminated with the feces of infected cats. Hence, the control of human toxoplasmosis consists of avoiding these circumstances. Although the measures apply to everyone, pregnant women and immunodeficient individuals merit special attention, the former because of the possibility of congenital infection and the latter because of the risk of developing a severe case. Sanitary education should be directed particularly toward high-risk populations, and it should focus on teaching people to avoid eating raw or undercooked meat and, in the case of food handlers, to prevent their hands from becoming contaminated. Meat, particularly pork and lamb, should be cooked until there is no reddish color left. Just as it is not recommended to use microwave ovens to kill *Trichinella*, the same is true for *Toxoplasma*, because these ovens do not cook meat evenly. Alternatively, freezing the meat for more than three days at −15°C or for more than two days at −20°C has been shown to kill most of the bradyzoite cysts. Food handlers should avoid tasting raw meat, and they should wash their hands carefully after touching it because water destroys the tachyzoites.

Populations at risk should also be taught to prevent infection from oocysts. People who keep cats in their homes, especially young animals that are just beginning to hunt, should dispose of the cat's fecal matter daily and rinse out the receptacles for the feces with boiling water, thus eliminating the oocysts before they have a chance to sporulate and become infective. These cats should be kept indoors and fed canned, cooked, or previously frozen food to keep them from hunting and catching infected rodents and birds and thus becoming infected. A serologically negative cat in the home of a pregnant woman should be removed from the household because it could acquire a primary infection and contaminate the environment with oocysts. It has been shown in the laboratory that the addition of monensin (a carboxylic ionophore produced by *Streptomyces cinnamonensis*) to dry cat food can suppress the excretion of oocysts in feces (Frenkel and Smith, 1982). Pregnant women and immunodeficient individuals should not perform tasks that expose them to potentially contaminated soil (for example, gardening) unless they use waterproof gloves and wash their hands carefully afterward. Fruit and vegetables that grow near the ground should be washed or cooked, since they might be contaminated. Flies and cockroaches should be controlled to prevent them from serving as transport hosts for the fecal oocysts of cats.

It would appear that an effective means of controlling infection in newborns is to identify pregnant women with acute infection and treat them. In Switzerland, 10 of 17 mothers treated during pregnancy had babies with antibodies to *T. gondii* and only 1 of them was infected, while 4 of 7 untreated mothers had infected babies (Berger *et al.*, 1995).

Preventing infection in sheep and swine requires eliminating cats and wild felines from stables and pastures, which would be a major challenge. Veterinary inspection of slaughterhouses, which has been effective in controlling trichinosis and teniasis, is not being done for toxoplasmosis.

For some years, work has been under way to develop vaccines against toxoplasmosis for cats (Freyre *et al.*, 1993), sheep (Wastling *et al.*, 1995), and swine (Dubey *et al.*, 1998). So far, the only successful effort has been a modified live parasite vaccine for sheep, which is administered before impregnation to prevent congenital infections.

Bibliography

Allain, J.P., C.R. Palmer, G. Pearson. Epidemiological study of latent and recent infection by *Toxoplasma gondii* in pregnant women from a regional population in the U.K. *J Infect Dis* 36:189–196, 1998.

Barriga, O.O. *Veterinary Parasitology for Practitioners*, 2nd ed. Edina: Burgess International Group; 1997.

Beazley, D.M., R.S. Egerman. Toxoplasmosis. *Semin Perinatol* 22:332–338, 1998.

Benenson, M.W., E.T. Takafuji, S.M. Lemon, R.L. Greenup, A.J. Sulzer. Oocyst-transmitted toxoplasmosis associated with ingestion of contaminated water. *N Engl J Med* 307:666–669, 1982.

Berger, R., S. Merkel, C. Rudin. Toxoplasmose und Schwangerschaft—Erkenntnisse aus einem Nabelschnurblut-Screening von 30,000 Neugeborenen. *Schweiz Med Wochenschr* 125:1168–1173, 1995.

Bossi, P., E. Caumes, P. Astagneau, *et al.* Caracteristiques epidemiologiques des toxoplasmoses cérébrales chez 399 patients infectés par le VIH suivis entre 1983 et 1994. *Rev Med Interne* 19:313–317, 1998.

Chiari, C. de A., D.P. Neves. Toxoplasmose adquirida através da ingestão de leite de cabra. *Mem Inst Osw Cruz* 79:337–340, 1984.

Chintana, T., Y. Sukthana, B. Bunyakai, A. Lekkla. *Toxoplasma gondii* antibody in pregnant women with and without HIV infection. *Southeast Asian J Trop Med Public Health* 29:383–386, 1998.

Choi, W.Y., H.W. Nam, N.H. Kwak, *et al.* Foodborne outbreaks of human toxoplasmosis. *J Infect Dis* 175:1280–1282, 1997.

Dubey, J.P. Feline toxoplasmosis and coccidiosis: A survey of domiciled and stray cats. *J Am Vet Med Assoc* 162:873–877, 1973.

Dubey, J.P., R.H. Streitel. Prevalence of *Toxoplasma* infection in cattle slaughtered at an Ohio abattoir. *J Am Vet Med Assoc* 169:1197–1199, 1976.

Dubey, J.P. *Toxoplasma, Hammondia, Besnoitia,* sarcocystis and other tissue cyst-forming coccidia of man and animals. *In*: Kreier, J.P., ed. Vol. 3: *Parasitic Protozoa.* New York: Academic Press; 1977.

Dubey, J.P., C.P. Beattie. *Toxoplasmosis of Animals and Man.* Boca Raton: CRC Press; 1988.

Dubey, J.P., J.K. Lunney, S.K. Shen, O.C. Kwoc. Immunity to toxoplasmosis in pigs fed irradiated *Toxoplasma gondii* oocysts. *J Parasitol* 84:749–752, 1998.

Ferrer, S., I. Fuentes, P. Domingo, *et al.* Toxoplasmosis encefálica en pacientes con infección por el virus de la inmunodeficiencia humana (VIH). Características clínico-radiológicas y terapeúticas en 63 pacientes. *Ann Med Interna* 13:4–8, 1996.

Frenkel, J.K., K.M. Hassanein, R.S. Hassanein, E. Brown, P. Thulliez, R. Quintero-Núñez. Transmission of *Toxoplasma gondii* in Panama City, Panama: A five-year prospective cohort study of children, cats, rodents, birds, and soil. *Am J Trop Med Hyg* 53:458–468, 1995.

Frenkel, J.K., D.D. Smith. Inhibitory effects of monesin on shedding of *Toxoplasma* oocysts by cats. *J Parasitol* 68:851–855, 1982.

Freyre, A., L. Choromanski, J.L. Fishback, I. Popiel. Immunization of cats with tissue cysts, bradyzoites, and tachyzoites of the T-263 strain of *Toxoplasma gondii. J Parasitol* 79:716–719, 1993.

Gallino, A., M. Maggiorini, W. Kiowski, *et al.* Toxoplasmosis in heart transplant recipients. *Eur J Clin Microbiol Infect Dis* 15:389–393, 1996.

Gómez-Marín, J.E., M.T. Montoya-de-Londoño, J.C. Castaño-Osorio. A maternal screening program for congenital toxoplasmosis in Quindio, Colombia and application of mathematical models to estimate incidences using age-stratified data. *Am J Trop Med Hyg* 57:180–186, 1997.

Gross, U., O. Keksel, M.L. Darde. Value of detecting immunoglobulin E antibodies for the serological diagnosis of *Toxoplasma gondii* infection. *Clin Diagn Lab Immunol* 4:247–251, 1997.

Jenum, P.A., B. Stray-Pedersen, K.K. Melby, *et al.* Incidence of *Toxoplasma gondii* infection in 35,940 pregnant women in Norway and pregnancy outcome for infected women. *J Clin Microbiol* 36:2900–2906, 1998.

Mullens, A. "I think we have a problem in Victoria": MDs respond quickly to toxoplasmosis outbreak in BC. *CMAJ* 154:1721–1724, 1996.

Munday, B.L. Prevalence of toxoplasmosis in Tasmanian meat animals. *Aust Vet J* 51:315–316, 1975.

Pizzi, H.L., C.M. Rico, O.A.M. Pessat. Hallazgo del ciclo ontogénico selvático del *Toxoplasma gondii* en félidos salvajes (*Oncifelis geofroyi, Felis colocolo y Felis eira*) de la Provincia de Córdoba. *Rev Milit Vet* (B Aires) 25:293–300, 1978.

Riemann, H.P., A.T. Smith, C. Stormont, *et al*. Equine toxoplasmosis: A survey for antibodies to *Toxoplasma gondii* in horses. *Am J Vet Res* 36:1797–1800, 1975.

Rodriguez, J.C., M.J. Alcantara, G. Royo. Toxoplasmosis en el embarazo: nuevas técnicas diagnósticas. *Enferm Infecc Microbiol Clin* 14:145–149, 1996.

Ruiz, A., J.K. Frenkel. *Toxoplasma gondii* in Costa Rican cats. *Am J Trop Med Hyg* 29:1150–1160, 1980.

Taylor, M.R., B. Lennon, C.V. Holland, M. Cafferkey. Community study of *Toxoplasma* antibodies in urban and rural schoolchildren aged 4 to 18 years. *Arch Dis Child* 77:406–410, 1997.

Wastling, J.M., D. Harkins, S. Maley, *et al*. Kinetics of the local and systemic antibody response to primary and secondary infection with S48 *Toxoplasma gondii* in sheep. *J Comp Pathol* 112:53–62, 1995.

Wilson, M., J.S. Remington, C. Clavet, G. Varney, C. Press, D. Ware. Evaluation of six commercial kits for detection of human immunoglobulin M antibodies to *Toxoplasma gondii*. The FDA Toxoplasmosis Ad Hoc Working Group. *J Clin Microbiol* 35:3112–3115, 1997.

World Health Organization (WHO). *Parasitic Zoonoses: Report of a WHO Expert Committee, with the Participation of FAO*. Geneva: WHO; 1979. (Technical Report Series 637.)

VISCERAL LEISHMANIASIS

ICD-10 B55.0

Synonyms: Kala-azar, black fever, Dum-dum fever, Sikari disease, Burdwan fever, Shahib's disease, infantile splenic fever, febrile tropical splenomegaly, post-kala-azar dermal leishmaniasis.

Etiology: Although visceral leishmaniasis is generally caused by *Leishmania chagasi* in the Americas and by *L. donovani* or *L. infantum* in the Old World (Wilson and Streit, 1996), cases of visceral leishmaniasis due to *L. amazonensis* have been reported (Barral *et al.*, 1991), as have cases of cutaneous leishmaniasis due to *L. infantum* (Giudice *et al.*, 1998). Moreover, *L. donovani* often causes cutaneous lesions in man, and some subspecies of *L. braziliensis* and *L. major* are viscerotropic in lower animals. Parasites characterized as *L. tropica* have also been isolated from patients with visceral leishmaniasis in India and Israel (Lainson, 1982).

Leishmania chagasi, L. donovani, and *L. infantum* are considered subspecies or members of a principal species or species complex called *L. donovani sensu lato.* The leishmanias that cause the visceral form of the disease are indistinguishable morphologically from those that cause the cutaneous and mucocutaneous forms (see classification and taxonomy of leishmanias in the chapter on Cutaneous Leishmaniasis).

The subspecies of *L. donovani sensu lato* were distinguished initially by differing ecological, clinical, and epidemiological characteristics. Later, serologic, enzymatic, and molecular biology methods began to be used to differentiate them (Minodier *et al.*, 1997). Among the serologic techniques, the most well-known is the Adler, or Noguchi-Adler, test, which relies on the fact that leishmanias clump together and become immobilized when cultured in the serum of patients who have suffered homologous infection. By means of this test, *L. d. donovani* can be distinguished from *L. d. infantum* and from the species that cause cutaneous leishmaniasis in the Americas and in the Old World. However, *L. d. infantum* cannot be differentiated from *L. d. chagasi*.

In humans and other mammal reservoirs, the parasite takes the form of intracellular amastigotes within the macrophages. In the phlebotomine vectors and in culture, it occurs as a flagellate form, or the free promastigote, which is found in the intestinal lumen and in the proboscis of the vector. Its life cycle is similar to that described for cutaneous leishmaniasis, with the difference that the parasites do not concentrate in the subcutaneous or submucosal macrophages but rather are distributed throughout the body with the circulating macrophages, and they multiply preferentially in the spleen, the bone marrow, and the liver.

Geographic Distribution: Ninety percent of new annual cases of visceral leishmaniasis come from five countries: Bangladesh, Brazil, India, Nepal, and Sudan (WHO, 2003). However, there are endemic areas and foci of kala-azar in several places in the world. *L. d. donovani* occurs in Bangladesh and India and possibly in China and Nepal. *L. d. infantum* is distributed across eastern, western, and central Africa; the former Soviet republics of Central Asia; the Mediterranean coast of Europe and Africa; Afghanistan; Saudi Arabia; north and northwest China; Egypt; Iran; Iraq; Israel; and Yemen. *L. d. chagasi* is found in the northeastern region and parts of the eastern region of Brazil, although small foci have also been confirmed in the northern and center-west regions. Sporadic cases of the disease have been diagnosed in northern Argentina, Bolivia, Colombia, Ecuador, El Salvador, Guatemala, Honduras, Mexico, Paraguay, Suriname, Venezuela, and on the islands of Guadeloupe and Martinique. Some reports indicate that the infection could be spreading to new areas in some countries, such as Brazil, Israel (Baneth *et al.*, 1998), and Sudan, and that the number of cases and the geographic distribution of both visceral and cutaneous leishmaniasis is expanding in several countries that border the Mediterranean (Gradoni *et al.*, 1996; Harrat *et al.*, 1996; Lagardere *et al.*, 1992).

Occurrence in Man: In most countries, visceral leishmaniasis occurs sporadically; however, it may sometimes reach epidemic proportions. In 1978, in northern Bihar, India, some 50,000 cases occurred, and the infection spread to western Bengal, with 7,500 cases reported in the first eight months of 1982. The largest number of cases occurred in a village in the same area in 1984 and 1985, but, with treatment, the number then declined steadily until 1988, when no more cases were reported (Dhiman and Sen, 1991). In China, the number of cases has declined, thanks to rigorous control efforts. Prior to 1960, as many as 600,000 cases were reported in the northeastern and northwestern parts of the country, whereas in 1979, only 48 cases were reported, most of them in the northeast. As of 1990, the figures remained at the same level (Guan, 1991). In Iraq, 1,969 clinical cases were reported in 1974, but in the following years, the number decreased to about 500 cases a year. In Sudan, between 3,000 and 5,000 cases a year were reported, although the prevalence was estimated to be much higher. However, between 1984 and 1994 an epidemic of visceral leishmaniasis broke out in a region of southern Sudan where the disease had not previously occurred, causing 100,000 deaths in a population of 280,000 inhabitants, with average mortality ranging from 38%–57% (Seaman et al., 1996). In Brazil, endemicity is highest in the states of Ceará and Bahia; 3,078 cases were reported in that country between 1971 and 1980, 44.6% of them occurring in Ceará (WHO, 1984). Between 1989 and 1991, a survey of 243 people in a village of Bahia confirmed a new leishmaniasis focus: cutaneous tests were positive in close to 30% of those surveyed and serologic tests indicated recent infection in 14%. Of 460 dogs examined, serologic tests were positive in 6% (Cunha et al., 1995). Information for the country as a whole indicates that visceral leishmaniasis in Brazil peaked in 1985, when 2,511 cases were reported, and that it had decreased significantly by 1991.

Although the exact incidence of visceral leishmaniasis is not known, the number of cases occurring each year around the world is estimated in the tens of thousands. In the Americas, the western Mediterranean, and northern Africa, those most affected are children under 1 year of age (infantile kala-azar), while in other areas, children over the age of 5 and young adults are most affected (Marinkele, 1981).

Occurrence in Animals: Studies of the prevalence of leishmaniasis in animals generally focus on dogs because they constitute the main source of infection for humans in many areas and because they are the most frequent victims of the infection in southern Europe. However, both wild canids and rodents can also be reservoirs in specific areas.

In the state of Ceará, Brazil, a survey conducted between 1953 and 1962 found the infection in 1.9% of 35,272 dogs with clinical symptomatology and in 1.5% of 285,592 apparently healthy dogs (Deane and Deane, 1962). In the state of Bahia, 10,132 dogs were examined between 1962 and 1969 and 1.7% were positive; in the known foci of human kala-azar, prevalence rates were as high as 25% (Sherlock and Almeida, 1970). In another study of 1,681 dogs in the state of Bahia, 23.5% were found to have antibodies against Leishmania and L. chagasi parasites were isolated from eight dogs (Paranhos-Silva et al., 1996). Infection rates of 4% and 12% were also found in Lycalopex vetulus foxes in Brazil. In northern Iran, 4 of 161 jackals and 3 of 100 dogs whose viscera and skin were examined for parasites tested positive, and for 6 of 48 jackals and 6 of 34 dogs results of immunofluorescence tests were seropositive (Hamidi et al., 1982). In a leishmaniasis focus in Tuscany, Italy, 2.9% of 103 dogs were seropositive and 1% showed clinical symptoms. In another focus, 23.9% of 250 dogs examined were seropositive, 10% had lesions, and 7% had positive microscopy (Gradoni et al., 1980).

The Disease in Man: The incubation period is generally two to six months, but it may range from 10 days to several years. The promastigotes inoculated by a phlebotomine into human skin are engulfed by macrophages, where they become amastigotes. In some patients, especially in Africa, a primary granuloma of the skin, called a leishmanioma, forms several months before systemic symptoms appear. Leishmanias multiply slowly by binary fission in the macrophages. Some parasitized macrophages spread to the local lymph nodes. From there they enter the bloodstream and reach the viscera, particularly the spleen, the liver, and the bone marrow, where the leishmanias then multiply rapidly in the fixed macrophages, producing reticuloendotheliosis, which ultimately destroys the macrophages.

In inhabitants of endemic areas, the disease's onset is insidious and its course is chronic. However, in persons from areas free from the disease, onset may be abrupt. Fever is prolonged and undulating, often with two daily peaks. Some patients experience cough, diarrhea, and symptoms of intercurrent infections. The disease is characterized by splenomegaly and, later, by hepatomegaly. Lymphadenopathy is common in some regions, such as Africa and the Mediterranean. Other symptoms may include anemia with leukopenia, edema, darkening of the skin, and emaciation. The abdomen sometimes becomes distended from the splenomegaly and the hepatomegaly. Petechiae and hemorrhage of the mucous membranes are frequent and are indicative of clotting problems. Secondary infections are also common. Mortality is very high in untreated patients. *L. donovani* infection is not always accompanied by serious symptoms; it may occur asymptomatically or produce only mild symptoms, depending on the host's degree of resistance. The immune system of some patients is able to control the infection, but the proportion of people who recover spontaneously is not known.

In the infection foci studied in Ceará, Brazil, 67% of the patients were 0 to 4 years old. In the Mediterranean basin, the prevalence of infections caused by *L. d. infantum* by age group is similar. In India, in contrast, the infection is more prevalent in young adults.

In the Americas, cutaneous kala-azar lesions are very rarely seen, but the parasites have been found in macroscopically normal skin. In India, in contrast, the skin of patients often takes on a gray hue (the name kala-azar means "black fever"), especially on feet, hands, and abdomen. In Kenya and Sudan in Africa, and in the Mediterranean and China, patients may develop nodular lesions. Another type of lesion that frequently appears about a year after treatment with antimony is post–kala-azar dermal leishmaniasis. These sequelae are common in the Old World, occurring in up to 56% of cases (Zijlstra *et al.*, 1995); however, they are rare in the Americas.

There is solid evidence from both experimental animals and man that the immune response of the T helper 1 lymphocytes (cell-mediated immunity)—especially the production of gamma interferon and tumor necrosis factor alpha—protects against leishmaniasis, and the infection may resolve spontaneously or remain asymptomatic. There is also some evidence that these reactions might contribute to tissue damage in cutaneous leishmaniasis (Ribeiro de Jesus *et al.*, 1998).

Visceral leishmaniasis in AIDS patients is similar to the disease in immunocompetent individuals, but it is more severe and far more prevalent, recurs more frequently, and is more often resistant to antimonials (Altes *et al.*, 1991; López-Vélez *et al.*, 1998). In several organ transplant recipients, the disease recurred after treatment, resulting in the death of some patients (Berenguer *et al.*, 1998).

The Disease in Animals: Visceral leishmaniasis in domestic dogs also occurs in geographic foci. Frequently, but not always, the prevalence in man and dogs in the same area is similar, although there may be areas of canine infection where no human infection exists. The disease causes cutaneous and systemic lesions, but the former are more evident. The incubation period is three to seven months. The severity of the disease varies. The cutaneous lesions are non-pruritic and include areas of alopecia, desquamation, and inflammation. They occur mostly around the eyes, ears, face, and feet. Although the lesions may evolve and become nodules, ulcerations, and scabs, it is uncommon for pustules to form. The most frequent systemic manifestations are intermittent fever, anemia, hypergammaglobulinemia, hypoalbuminemia, lymphadenopathy, splenomegaly, lethargy, and weight loss. Episodes of diarrhea, glomerulonephritis, and polyarthritis sometimes also occur. Antimonial treatment is not very effective and recurrences are frequent (Barriga, 1997). Severity of clinical symptoms does not appear to be related to parasite load, as very heavily parasitized dogs may have mild symptomatology. In Brazil, more than 30% of infected dogs had no apparent clinical symptoms (Hipólito et al., 1965). Infection in the fox Lycalopex vetulus in northeast Brazil is similar to that of dogs. Some animals may have clinically inapparent infections, while others manifest different forms of the disease, including very serious and even fatal cases.

Source of Infection and Mode of Transmission: The epidemiology of the disease varies from region to region and from one area to another. In the Americas, the reservoirs of visceral leishmaniasis are dogs and the wild canids. The infection is spread among canids and from these animals to man by the bite of the phlebotomine fly Lutzomyia longipalpis. The epidemic significance of the man-dog link seems to vary from area to area; while some authors have found no correlation between the prevalence in humans and in dogs (Paranhos-Silva et al., 1996) or no change in the human prevalence after removal of infected dogs (Dietze et al., 1997), other authors believe that elimination of infected dogs does reduce the prevalence of the infection in humans (Ashford et al., 1998).

The most important endemic area in the Americas is in northeastern Brazil; the main foci are distributed across a semiarid region that is subject to prolonged droughts. The disease is basically rural, with a few cases occurring in populations or places on the outskirts of cities. The distribution of kala-azar is focal. The largest concentration of cases occurs in foothill areas or in mountain valleys, where the disease is endemic with periodic epidemic outbreaks. In the flatlands, on the other hand, cases are sporadic and occur primarily in the most humid areas, near rivers.

In Brazil, the geographic distribution of the disease coincides with that of the vector. The main, and possibly the only, vector in the endemic area of northeastern Brazil is the phlebotomine L. longipalpis, an abundant insect that reaches its highest density about two months after the heaviest rains and is resistant to drought. The vector is found both outdoors and indoors. It feeds on dogs, wild animals, and, less often, man.

Dogs are an especially suitable reservoir because they offer the vector direct access to the parasitized macrophages of their cutaneous lesions. In studies conducted in Ceará, Brazil, parasites were detected in the skin of 77.6% of 49 dogs with visceral leishmaniasis but only in 16.3% of 43 human patients examined. In addition, humans have been found to have a lesser number of parasites in their skin than dogs. Amastigotes are scarce in human skin and only rarely serve as a source of infection for the vector.

A wild host of visceral leishmaniasis in northeastern Brazil is the fox Lycalopex vetulus, which often comes near houses to hunt chickens. Amastigotes are abundant in the fox's skin, and it is a great source of infection for the vector (Garnham, 1971). In the tropical rain forest region of the lower Amazon, such as the state of Pará, where the number of cases in humans and domestic dogs is low, the reservoir of the parasite is suspected to be a wild canid. In this region, L. donovani has been isolated from the fox *Cerdocyon thous* (Lainson *et al.*, 1969; Silveira *et al.*, 1982).

In the Mediterranean basin, dogs are also the principal reservoir, while several species of the genus *Phlebotomus* serve as vectors. In the Middle East, jackals and dogs are the hosts and the main sources of infection for phlebotomines. In India, by contrast, no dogs or other animals have been found to be infected, and man is the main reservoir (Bhattacharya and Ghosh, 1983). Prevalence of the disease was very high in the country's large cities, but it was reduced significantly as a result of an antimalaria campaign that eliminated both mosquitoes and phlebotomines. When the campaign was discontinued, Bihar experienced an epidemic resurgence of kala-azar (see Geographic Distribution and Occurrence in Man). In the absence of an animal reservoir, subclinical human infections may play an important role in maintaining the disease (Manson and Apted, 1982). Person-to-person transmission takes place by means of *Phlebotomus argentipes*, an eminently anthropophilic insect which feeds solely on humans. In India, the number of parasites circulating in human blood was found to be sufficient to infect the vector. Transmission occurs inside houses, which constitute microfoci of infection (Manson and Apted, 1982). In Sudan, the infection has been found in wild rodents of the species *Arvicanthis niloticus* and *Acomys albigena*, domestic rats *Rattus rattus*, and carnivores *Felis philippsi* and *Genetta sangalensis*. It is believed that rodents are the primary hosts for the agent and that carnivores are secondary reservoirs. The vector is *P. orientalis*. Humans develop parasitemia and, under epidemic conditions, can be a source of infection for the vectors.

Numerous investigators believe that visceral leishmaniasis was originally an infection that circulated enzootically among wild animals (canids and perhaps rodents), and that later, domestic dogs were included in its cycle; eventually, the disease became an infection transmitted between humans without the intervention of an animal reservoir, as is the case of kala-azar in India. An argument in favor of this hypothesis is dogs' low degree of adaptation to the parasite and their susceptibility to the clinical disease, which suggests that they are a rather new host in the natural history of the disease. In the Americas, it has been suggested that the fox *Cerdocyon thous*, which becomes infected without becoming ill, could have been the original reservoir. However, more research is needed, especially concerning rate of infection, to confirm that this animal is the original reservoir (Lainson, 1983).

Diagnosis: Confirmation of visceral leishmaniasis is made by identifying the parasite. In the form of visceral leishmaniasis that occurs in the Americas, the parasite can rarely be seen in films of peripheral blood; however, this technique can yield positive results for kala-azar in India. The most sensitive procedure (98% positivity) is splenic aspiration, but this technique entails high risk, especially in patients with anemia and clotting problems. Aspiration of sternal or iliac bone marrow can detect the presence of parasites in 54% to 86% of cases and lymph node aspiration can detect them in 64% of cases (WHO, 1984). In the early stages of the disease, when parasites are scarce, culture in Novy-McNeal-Nicolle or another appropriate medium or intraperitoneal inoculation in hamsters can be used. Often, simultaneous application of both methods yields better results. Polymerase chain reaction has begun to be used more recently. This technique is as sensitive as microscopy of lymph node and bone marrow aspirates in confirmed patients, but it offers the added advantage of confirming the disease in suspected patients who have negative microscopy. Although blood samples on filter paper can be used, the sensitivity of the test increases if lymph node or bone marrow aspirates are used (Osman *et al.*, 1997). In dogs and other canids, the parasites can be observed or isolated by culture or hamster inoculation, using material from cutaneous lesions or the viscera of dead animals.

When the usual methods for detecting the parasite do not produce results or the media needed to perform them are not available, immunologic tests are generally used. The immunofluorescence test is useful, and although cross-reactions with *T. cruzi* are a drawback, these can be avoided by the use of specific antigens. The direct agglutination test to detect visceral leishmaniasis has a sensitivity of over 99% and a specificity of 96% if the appropriate dilution is used (Boelaert *et al.*, 1999). The enzyme-linked immunosorbent assay (ELISA) for IgG antibodies has exhibited 93.4% sensitivity and 93.6% specificity in Sudan (Elassad *et al.*, 1994). In Portugal, the ELISA test showed 100% sensitivity, 90.5% specificity, and 91.4% predictability in man, with an adsorption cut-off value of 0.100; in dogs, it showed 80% sensitivity, 94.3% specificity, and 96.6% predictability, with a cut-off of 0.200. However, the reproducibility of the test was not entirely satisfactory (Mauricio *et al.*, 1995).

Since in active visceral leishmaniasis there is a prevalence of T helper 2 lymphocyte response, which includes the production of IgE, the ELISA test for IgE antibodies can indicate active infection. Atta *et al.* (1998) found these antibodies in 23 patients with visceral leishmaniasis, but did not find them in persons with subclinical *L. chagasi* or *T. cruzi* infections or in healthy individuals. The values fell markedly after treatment. A dot-ELISA test showed 98.5% sensitivity and 96.7% specificity for detecting antigens of *L. donovani* in the circulation, and 98.5% sensitivity and 98.9% specificity for detecting antibodies against *L. infantum*.

Control: Leishmaniasis control measures are directed against the vectors and reservoirs. Application of residual insecticides such as DDT in and around dwellings produced excellent results when use of this insecticide was permitted. The incidence of kala-azar in India decreased markedly in the wake of the antimalaria campaign, and the infection has virtually disappeared from the districts that were sprayed. Spraying should not be limited to dwellings, but should also be done around animal dens, stone walls, refuse dumps, and other places where the vector breeds.

In regions in which the infection is of zoonotic origin, it is considered important to systematically eliminate infected dogs and, to the extent possible, control the fox population. On the Greek island of Crete, destroying infected dogs brought down the incidence of the disease in humans significantly. However, vigorous campaigns in northeastern Brazil have not borne out the effectiveness of controlling dog populations and experimental studies have shown that eliminating dogs does not reduce the incidence of human infection (Dietze *et al.*, 1997). As no other important reservoirs of *L. chagasi* have been found in those areas, the human infection apparently comes from other humans. In regions in which the infection is of human origin, human cases should be detected and treated. Although vaccination against leishmaniasis is considered impractical because the infection inhibits immunity, experimental studies have demonstrated that partial protection was achieved in mice injected with *L. donovani* promastigote antigens incorporated into liposomes (Ali and Afrin, 1997). Mathematical models suggest that the most effective method for controlling visceral leishmaniasis is insecticide application when the vector is accessible. The next most effective control method is reduction of host susceptibility through improved nutrition for children and vaccination of people and dogs. Elimination or treatment of dogs that serve as reservoirs is considerably less effective than either of these methods (Dye, 1996).

Bibliography

Ali, N., F. Afrin. Protection of mice against visceral leishmaniasis by immunization with promastigote antigen incorporated in liposomes. *J Parasitol* 83(1):70–75, 1997.

Altes, J., A. Salas, M. Riera, *et al.* Visceral leishmaniasis: Another HIV-associated opportunistic infection? Report of eight cases and review of the literature. *AIDS* 5(2):201–207, 1991.

Ashford, D.A., J.R. David, M. Freire, *et al.* Studies on control of visceral leishmaniasis: Impact of dog control on canine and human visceral leishmaniasis in Jacobina, Bahia, Brazil. *Am J Trop Med Hyg* 59(1):53–57, 1998.

Atta, A.M., D. Oliveira, J. Correa, M.L. Atta, R.P. Almeida, E.M. Carvalho. Anti-leishmanial IgE antibodies: A marker of active disease in visceral leishmaniasis. *Am J Trop Med Hyg* 59(3):426–430, 1998.

Baneth, G., G. Dank, E. Keren-Kornblatt, *et al.* Emergence of visceral leishmaniasis in central Israel. *Am J Trop Med Hyg* 59(5):722–725, 1998.

Barral, A., D. Pedral-Sampaio, G. Grimaldi Jr., *et al.* Leishmaniasis in Bahia, Brazil: Evidence that *Leishmania amazonensis* produces a wide spectrum of clinical disease. *Am J Trop Med Hyg* 44(5):536–546, 1991.

Barriga, O.O. *Veterinary Parasitology for Practitioners*, 2nd ed. Edina: Burgess International Group; 1997.

Berenguer, J., F. Gómez-Campdera, B. Padilla, *et al.* Visceral leishmaniasis (Kala-Azar) in transplant recipients: Case report and review. *Transplantation* 65(10):1401–1404, 1998.

Bhattacharya, A., T.N. Ghosh. A search for leishmania in vertebrates from kala-azar-affected areas of Bihar, India. *Trans R Soc Trop Med Hyg* 77(6):874–875, 1983.

Boelaert, M., S. El Safi, D. Jacquet, A. de Muynck, P. van der Stuyft, D. Le Ray. Operational validation of the direct agglutination test for diagnosis of visceral leishmaniasis. *Am J Trop Med Hyg* 60(1):129–134, 1999.

Cunha, S., M. Freire, C. Eulalio, *et al.* Visceral leishmaniasis in a new ecological niche near a major metropolitan area of Brazil. *Trans R Soc Trop Med Hyg* 89(2):155–158, 1995.

Deane, L.M., M.P. Deane. Visceral leishmaniasis in Brazil: Geographical distribution and transmission. *Rev Inst Med Trop S Paulo* 4:198–212, 1962.

del Giudice, P., P. Marty, J.P. Lacour, *et al.* Cutaneous leishmaniasis due to *Leishmania infantum*. Case reports and literature review. *Arch Dermatol* 134(2):193–198, 1998.

Dietze, R., G.B. Barros, L. Teixeira, *et al.* Effect of eliminating seropositive canines on the transmission of visceral leishmaniasis in Brazil. *Clin Infect Dis* 25(5):1240–1242, 1997.

Dhiman, R.C., A.B. Sen. Epidemiology of kala-azar in rural Bihar (India) using village as a component unit of study. *Indian J Med Res* 93:155–160, 1991.

Dye, C. The logic of visceral leishmaniasis control. *Am J Trop Med Hyg* 55(2):125–130, 1996.

Elassad, A.M., S.A. Younis, M. Siddig, J. Grayson, E. Petersen, H.W. Ghalib. The significance of blood levels of IgM, IgA, IgG and IgG subclasses in Sudanese visceral leishmaniasis patients. *Clin Exp Immunol* 95(2):294–299, 1994.

Garnham, P.C.C. American leishmaniasis. *Bull World Health Organ* 44:521–527, 1971.

Gradoni, L., E. Pozio, S. Bettini, M. Gramiccia. Leishmaniasis in Tuscany (Italy). III. The prevalence of canine leishmaniasis in two foci of Grosseto Province. *Trans R Soc Trop Med Hyg* 74(3):421–422, 1980.

Gradoni, L., R. Pizzuti, A. Scalone, *et al.* Recrudescence of visceral leishmaniasis unrelated to HIV infection in the Campania region of Italy. *Trans R Soc Trop Med Hyg* 90(3):234–235, 1996.

Guan, L.R. Current status of kala-azar and vector control in China. *Bull World Health Organ* 69(5):595–601, 1991.

Hamidi, A.N., A. Nadim, G.H. Edrissian, G. Tahvildar-Bidruni, E. Javadian. Visceral leishmaniasis of jackals and dogs in northern Iran. *Trans R Soc Trop Med Hyg* 76(6):756–757, 1982.

Harrat, Z., F. Pratlong, S. Belazzoug, *et al. Leishmania infantum* and *L. major* in Algeria. *Trans R Soc Trop Med Hyg* 90(6):625–629, 1996.

Hipólito, O., M.O. Freitas, J.B. Figuereido. *Doenças infeto-contagiosas dos animais domésticos.* 4th ed. São Paulo: Melhoramentos; 1965.

Lacerda, M.M. The Brazilian Leishmaniasis Control Program. *Mem Inst Oswaldo Cruz* 89(3):489–495, 1994.

Lagardere, B., B. Chevallier, R. Cheriet. Le kala azar. *Ann Pediatr (Paris)* 39(3):159–164, 1992.

Lainson, R. Leishmaniasis. *In:* Jacobs, L., P. Arámbulo, section eds. Vol. 1: *CRC Handbook Series in Zoonoses.* Boca Raton: CRC Press; 1982.

Lainson, R. The American leishmaniases: Some observations on their ecology and epidemiology. *Trans R Soc Trop Med Hyg* 77:569–596, 1983.

Lainson, R., J.J. Shaw, Z.C. Lins. Leishmaniasis in Brazil. IV. The fox *Cerdocyon thous* (L) as a reservoir of *Leishmania donovani* in Para State, Brazil. *Trans R Soc Trop Med Hyg* 63(6):741–745, 1969.

López-Vélez, R., J.A. Pérez-Molina, A. Guerrero, *et al.* Clinicoepidemiologic characteristics, prognostic factors, and survival analysis of patients coinfected with human immunodeficiency virus and Leishmania in an area of Madrid, Spain. *Am J Trop Med Hyg* 58(4):436–443, 1998.

Manson, P., F.I.C. Apted. *Manson's Tropical Diseases,* 18th ed. London: Ballière Tindall; 1982.

Marinkele, C.J. La lutte contre les leishmanioses. *Bull World Health Organ* 59:189–203, 1981.

Mauricio, I., L. Campino, P. Abranches. Controle de qualidade da técnica de micro-ELISA aplicada ao diagnóstico da leishmaniose visceral humana e canina. *Acta Med Port* 8(11):607–611, 1995.

Mayrink, W., C. De A. Chiari, P.A. Magalhães, C.A. da Costa. Teste do latex no diagnóstico do calazar americano. *Rev Inst Med Trop S Paulo* 14(4):273–276, 1972.

Minodier, P., R. Piarroux, F. Gambarelli, C. Joblet, H. Dumon. Rapid identification of causative species in patients with Old World leishmaniasis. *J Clin Microbiol* 35(10):2551–2555, 1997.

Osman, O.F., L. Oskam, E.E. Zijlstra, *et al.* Evaluation of PCR for diagnosis of visceral leishmaniasis. *J Clin Microbiol* 35(10):2454–2457, 1997.

Paranhos-Silva, M., L.A. Freitas, W.C. Santos, G. Grimaldi Jr., L.C. Pontes-de-Carvalho, A.J. Oliveira-dos-Santos. A cross-sectional serodiagnostic survey of canine leishmaniasis due to *Leishmania chagasi. Am J Trop Med Hyg* 55(1):39–44, 1996.

Ribeiro-de-Jesus, A., R.P. Almeida, H. Lessa, O. Bacellar, E.M. Carvalho. Cytokine profile and pathology in human leishmaniasis. *Braz J Med Biol Res* 31(1):143–148, 1998.

Seaman, J., A.J. Mercer, E. Sondorp. The epidemic of visceral leishmaniasis in western Upper Nile, southern Sudan: Course and impact from 1984 to 1994. *Int J Epidemiol* 25(4):862–871, 1996.

Senaldi, G., H. Xiao-su, D.C. Hoessli, C. Bordier. Serological diagnosis of visceral leishmaniasis by a dot-enzyme immunoassay for the detection of a *Leishmania donovani*-related circulating antigen. *J Immunol Methods* 193(1):9–15, 1996.

Sherlock, I.A., S.P. de Almeida. Notas sobre leishmaniose canina no Estado de Bahia. *Rev Bras Malariol Doencas Trop* 22(2):231–242, 1970.

Silveira, F.T., R. Lainson, J.J. Shaw, M.M. Povoa. Leishmaniasis in Brazil: XVIII. Further evidence incriminating the fox *Cerdocyon thous* (L) as a reservoir of Amazonian visceral leishmaniasis. *Trans R Soc Trop Med Hyg* 76(6):830–832, 1982.

Wilson, M.E., J.A. Streit. Visceral leishmaniasis. *Gastroenterol Clin North Am* 25(3): 535–551, 1996.

World Health Organization (WHO). *The Leishmaniases. Report of a WHO Expert Committee*. Geneva: WHO; 1984. (Technical Report Series 701).

World Health Organization (WHO). The Leishmaniases and *Leishmania*/HIV Co-infections. May 2000. [web page] Available at http://www.who.int/inf-fs/en/fact116.html. Accessed January 2003.

Zijlstra, E.E., A.M. el-Hassan, A. Ismael. Endemic kala-azar in eastern Sudan: Post-kala-azar dermal leishmaniasis. *Am J Trop Med Hyg* 52(4):299–305, 1995.

Section B

HELMINTHIASES

1. Trematodiases

2. Cestodiases

3. Acanthocephaliases
   and Nematodiases

1. Trematodiases

CERCARIAL DERMATITIS

ICD-10 B65.3

Synonyms: Swimmer's itch or dermatitis, bather's dermatitis, clam digger's itch, schistosome dermatitis.

Etiology: The agents of this disease are cercariae of avian schistosomes (mainly species of the genera *Australobilharzia*, *Bilharziella*, *Gigantobilharzia*, *Microbilharzia*, *Ornithobilharzia*, and *Trichobilharzia*) or of nonhuman mammals (species of the genera *Heterobilharzia*, *Orientobilharzia*, *Schistosoma*, and *Schistosomatium*). All belong to the family Schistosomatidae. Man is an aberrant host for these species and does not sustain the development of the parasite beyond its cutaneous site.

Although there are differences in the details, all schistosomes share basically the same life cycle (see the chapter on Schistosomiasis). The eggs contain a pre-adult stage, the miracidium, when they are eliminated with the definitive host's feces or urine. When the egg reaches the water, the miracidium is released and swims in search of an appropriate intermediate host, which is usually a snail belonging to *Bulineus*, *Lymnaea*, *Nassarius*, *Physa*, *Planorbis*, *Stagnicola*, or another genus. The miracidia penetrate the body of the mollusk and invade the digestive gland (hepatopancreas), where they develop into another pre-adult stage, the sporocyst. Another pre-adult stage forms within the sporocyst, the redia, which, in turn, gives rise to yet another pre-adult stage, the cercaria. After several weeks, the fork-tailed cercariae mature and leave the snail, swimming in search of a definitive host. Their infectivity decreases quickly and they generally die if they fail to find a host within 24 hours. Unlike the cercariae of other trematodes, schistosomes do not form meta-cercariae, but rather invade the definitive host's skin directly, at which time they lose their tails and undergo histological changes in their tegument, becoming juvenile parasites called schistosomula. The schistosomula penetrate the blood or lymph vessels and travel to the lungs, where they remain for several days. They then continue on to the liver, where they reach maturity and mate. From there, they migrate to their final site, where they begin laying eggs.

The definitive hosts of the schistosomes that cause cercarial dermatitis in man are generally geese, ducks, and other waterfowl, or domestic or wild mammals, such as raccoons, otters, and rodents. In man, the cercariae are usually destroyed in the skin before reaching the circulatory system. The species of schistosomes specific to man (*Schistosoma haematobium, S. japonicum, S. mansoni*, and others of limited distribution) also cause a cutaneous syndrome as part of the natural infection, but it is generally less serious. Of a group of 28 Dutch tourists who became infected with human schistosomes in Mali (West Africa), 10 (36%) had symptoms of cercarial dermatitis (Visser *et al.*, 1995).

Geographic Distribution and Occurrence: Cercarial dermatitis occurs worldwide in all climates, and in all places where people, through their recreational or occupational activities, come into contact with contaminated waters in rivers, lakes, floodlands, irrigation canals, and oceans near the coast. Swimmers, clam-diggers, washerwomen, fishermen, and rice-field workers are the groups most likely to be exposed. Although cercarial dermatitis normally occurs as isolated cases, epidemics have been reported—for example, an outbreak among 11 children who contracted the disease while swimming in a park in the US (Anon., 1992) and one involving 58 rice-field workers in Thailand (Kullavanijaya and Wongwaisayawan, 1993).

As a precise diagnosis is difficult, many cases are probably never recognized as cercarial dermatitis. However, the disease appears to be much more common than official statistics indicate: in a survey carried out in the area of Lake Michigan, in the US, 317 human cases of cercarial dermatitis were identified in a single summer (Lindblade, 1998); in another survey conducted among 555 swimmers in Lake Geneva in Switzerland, 153 probable cases were identified (Chamot *et al.*, 1998).

The Disease in Man: Cercarial dermatitis is basically a defense reaction to an aberrant parasite, which the host almost always successfully destroys, but which causes allergic sensitization.

When a person is exposed to cercariae for the first time, the symptomatology is usually mild and may pass unnoticed. Between 10 and 30 minutes after exposure, the affected person feels a transitory itching and macules appear but vanish within 10 to 24 hours. After 5 to 14 days, small papules appear, accompanied by temporary itching where the macules had been. As no immunologic reactions are expected in the first few days of a primary infection and the cercariae are destroyed within approximately 30 minutes in the malpighian layer, the symptoms that occur in the first few days are presumed to be the result of the damage caused by the parasite and the chemical substances it releases. The clinical manifestations that appear towards the end of the first week suggest an allergic reaction to the dead parasite. Baskin *et al.* (1997) observed that cercarial dermatitis patients produced four times more IgE than controls without dermatitis. This finding supports the hypothesis that the cause of the disease is an early hypersensitivity reaction.

The secondary response in individuals sensitized by previous exposures is faster and more intense than the primary reaction. The symptomatology varies somewhat, depending on the parasite species and the affected individual's response capacity. First, red spots develop on the exposed skin, which begins to itch within 30 to 90 minutes after infection. After 6 to 12 hours, the individual develops a macular rash and experiences intense itching (Narain *et al.*, 1994). This rash is replaced 10 to 20 hours later by papules or, in some people, by marked urticaria. The papular eruption normally subsides within about a week, though it may last for up to a month. Complications may occur as the result of secondary bacterial infection caused by scratching.

Experiments with ducks and mice infected with cercariae of the avian cercaria *Trichobilharzia szidati* (Horak *et al., 1998*) have shown that the antigens that cause the cutaneous reaction are present in the invasive cercariae but not in the schistosomula that result from their differentiation.

The Disease in Animals: Occasional cases of cercarial dermatitis in cats and dogs have been reported, mostly in association with the occurrence of the disease in their owners. Its occurrence in domestic animals appears to be much less frequent than in man, but this may be because animals are less able to communicate their symptoms and because the lesions are concealed by their fur. Moreover, it is difficult to distinguish cercarial dermatitis from hookworm dermatitis caused by nematodes of the family Ancylostomatidae.

Source of Infection and Mode of Transmission: The sources of infection for man are the banks of bodies of fresh or salt water where the snails that release the cercariae live. Epidemiologists have identified three situations in which the infection typically occurs. In the first, the infection originates in freshwater bodies frequented by waterfowl (geese, ducks, etc.) or wild mammals (raccoons, otters, etc.). In these cases, the parasites are generally species of the genera *Australobilharzia*, *Gigantobilharzia*, or *Trichobilharzia*, which infect fowl and develop in snails of the genera *Lymnaea*, *Nassarius*, or *Physa*, or the genera *Heterobilharzia* or *Schistosomatium*, which infect mammals and develop in *Lymnaea*, *Physa*, or *Stagnicola* snails. In the second situation, the infection is acquired on the banks of saltwater bodies. In these cases, the parasites generally belong to the genera *Australobilharzia*, *Gigantobilharzia*, *Microbilharzia*, or *Ornithobilharzia*, which infect marine or migratory birds and develop in marine snails such as *Ilyanassa*. In the third case, the infection is acquired in rice fields and floodlands inhabited by parasites of domestic animals and wild rodents, such as *Schistosoma spindale*, a species that affects bovines and wild rats (Inder *et al.*, 1997); *Schistosoma bovis*, a bovine schistosome; *Schistosomatium douthitti*, which affects rodents; and *Heterobilharzia americana*, which affects dogs. Often, the intermediate hosts are snails of the family Planorbidae.

The mode of transmission is direct penetration of the cercariae into the host's skin within 24 hours of its formation.

Diagnosis: Diagnosis is difficult and is based mainly on observation of the patient's clinical symptoms and a history of recent exposure to watercourses in which hosts of nonhuman schistosomes exist. As treatment is purely symptomatic and does not exclude the existence of other allergic conditions, successful treatment does not help to confirm the infection. Although various serum immunologic tests can establish the diagnosis (fluorescence test, cercarial Hullen reaction, circumoval precipitation, etc.) (Pilz *et al.*, 1995), all require specimens of the parasite and give positive results only 10 to 14 days after infection. Indirect immunofluorescence and enzyme-linked immunosorbent assay, employing commercially available human schistosome antigens, have been used to diagnose the infection, but the results are less sensitive (Kolarova *et al.*, 1994).

Control: Apart from the obvious risk posed by the presence of definitive and intermediate hosts of the agents of cercarial dermatitis, a study in the area of Lake Michigan (United States) found that the risk of infection depended on the age of the individual, the time of day when he/she was exposed to contaminated water, the month in which the exposure took place, and the high algae content and shallowness of the water (Lindblade, 1998). Few of these elements are really susceptible to modification. The population of snails in pools, rice fields, or irrigation canals can be controlled with molluscicides (Kolarova *et al.*, 1989), but their use in natural watercourses would probably cause too much ecological damage. In the case of small natural ponds, clearing the vegetation from the banks will create a less favorable environment for snails and removing the mud from the bottom will eliminate them. Use of praziquantel baits has been recommended to eliminate the mature parasites of fowl, but three 200 mg doses daily per duck are needed to produce a permanent reduction in the excretion of eggs. During the pre-patent period, one dose of 22.5 mg per duck daily is sufficient to prevent patency permanently (Muller *et al.*, 1993). In Japan, rice-field workers and other individuals have been protected with copper oleate, which is applied to the skin and allowed to evaporate. Dimethyl phthalate cream can also be used for this purpose. It is recommended that swimmers dry off vigorously as soon as they emerge from the water, since the cercariae are better able to penetrate the skin when it is allowed to air dry slowly.

Bibliography

Anonymous. Cercarial dermatitis outbreak at a state park—Delaware, 1991. *MMWR Morb Mortal Wkly Rep* 41:225–228, 1992.

Baskin, B., K.B. Islam, B. Evengard, L. Emtestam, C.I. Smith. Direct and sequential switching from mu to epsilon in patients with *Schistosoma mansoni* infection and atopic dermatitis. *Eur J Immunol* 27:130–135, 1997.

Chamot, E., L. Toscani, A. Rougemont. Public health importance and risk factors for cercarial dermatitis associated with swimming in Lake Leman at Geneva, Switzerland. *Epidemiol Infect* 120:305–314, 1998.

Horak P., L. Kovar, L. Kolarova, J. Nebesarova. Cercaria-schistosomulum surface transformation of *Trichobilharzia szidati* and its putative immunological impact. *Parasitology* (Pt2): 116:139–147, 1998.

Inder Singh, K., M. Krishnasamy, S. Ambu, R. Rasul, N.L. Chong. Studies on animal schistosomes in Peninsular Malaysia: Record of naturally infected animals and additional hosts of *Schistosoma spindale*. *Southeast Asian J Trop Med Public Health* 28:303–307, 1997.

Kolarova, L., V. Gottwaldova, D. Cechoya, M. Seycoya. The occurrence of cercarial dermatitis in Central Bohemia. *Zentralbl Hyg Umweltmed* 189:1–13, 1989.

Kolarova, L., J. Sykora, B.A. Bah. Serodiagnosis of cercarial dermatitis with antigens of *Trichobilharzia szidati* and *Schistosoma mansoni*. *Cent Eur J Public Health* 2:19–22, 1994.

Kullavanijaya, P., H. Wongwaisayawan. Outbreak of cercarial dermatitis in Thailand. *Int J Dermatol* 32:113–115, 1993.

Lindblade, K.A. The epidemiology of cercarial dermatitis and its association with limnological characteristics of a northern Michigan lake. *J Parasitol* 84:19–23, 1998.

Muller, V., P. Kimmig, W. Frank. [The effect of praziquantel on *Trichobilharzia* (Digenea, Schistosomatidae), a cause of swimmer's dermatitis in humans.] *Appl Parasitol* 34:187–201, 1993.

Narain, K., J. Mahanta, R. Dutta, P. Dutta. Paddy field dermatitis in Assam: A cercarial dermatitis. *J Commun Dis* 26:26–30, 1994.

Pilz, J., S. Eisele, R. Disko. [Cercaria dermatitis (swimmer's itch). Case report of cercaria dermatitis caused by *Trichobilharzia* (Digena, Schistosomatidae).] *Hautarzt* 46:335–338, 1995.

Visser, L.G., A.M. Polderman, P.C. Stuiver. Outbreak of schistosomiasis among travelers returning from Mali, West Africa. *Clin Infect Dis* 20:280–285, 1995.

CLONORCHIASIS

ICD-10 B66.1

Synonyms: Chinese liver fluke disease, oriental liver fluke disease, infection due to *Clonorchis sinensis*.

Etiology: *Clonorchis sinensis* is a small trematode measuring 12–20 mm long and 3–5 mm wide, with a reddish, translucent body. It lives in the bile ducts of humans, pigs, cats, dogs, rats, and several other species of fish-eating mammals. Some authors place it in the genus *Opisthorchis* because adults of the genera *Clonorchis* and *Opisthorchis* are similar in appearance, but there are clear differences in the pre-adult stages. Moreover, the name *Clonorchis* has been used in the medical literature since 1907, so retaining it seems justified. The parasite requires two intermediate hosts to complete its life cycle. The first is any of several operculate aquatic snails, such as species of *Alocinma*, *Bulimus*, *Melanoides*, *Parafossarulus*, and *Semisulcospira*. Among them, *P. manchouricus* seems to be the most important host. The second intermediate host is any of more than 100 species of freshwater fish (often members of the family Cyprinidae), only about a dozen of which are regularly consumed by humans. Three species of freshwater shrimp can also serve as second intermediate hosts.

The infected definitive host eliminates fully embryonated eggs in its feces. If the eggs reach fresh water (rivers, lakes, lagoons, reservoirs, ponds) and find appropriate intermediate hosts, their development continues. The snail ingests the eggs, which hatch in the intestine and release ciliated larvae, or miracidia. The miracidium penetrates the intestinal wall, invades the digestive gland (hepatopancreas), and becomes a sporocyst, which produces other larvae, the rediae. After a redia leaves the sporocyst, it produces still other pre-adult larvae, the cercariae. Multiplication of larvae in the pre-adult stages is called pedogenesis, and is characteristic of trematodes. The cercariae—juvenile stage larvae with a tail—emerge from the snail when they are mature and seek a second intermediate host, which they must find within 24–48 hours or they will die. A cercaria penetrates the skin of a fish, loses its tail, and forms a resistant wall around its body. This cyst, called a metacercaria, lodges under the fish's skin or in the connective tissue or underlying muscles. The metacercariae become infective for the definitive host in approximately one month.

When the definitive host consumes infected raw fish, the metacercariae excyst in the host's duodenum. The juvenile parasite penetrates the ampulla of Vater and moves against the bile flow towards the bile ducts. After three to four weeks, the parasite reaches sexual maturity and begins to lay eggs, and the life cycle begins anew. In rats, it has been shown that 32% of the metacercariae that enter the host reach the liver and that the parasite grows quickly during the first 30 days and then slowly during the following 60 days (Kim, 1995). The entire life cycle is completed in around three months, but the mature parasites can live for up to 40 years.

Geographic Distribution: The endemic area of clonorchiasis is limited to China, Japan, Malaysia, Republic of Korea, Singapore, Taiwan, Vietnam, and possibly Cambodia and the Lao People's Democratic Republic. Human cases have also been found in Hawaii, US, among people who had never traveled elsewhere, but those cases may have been due to consumption of infected fish imported from endemic areas. In several countries of the world, sporadic cases have been diagnosed in immigrants from and in people who had visited the endemic area. For example, a prevalence of 26% was found among 150 Chinese immigrants in New York City, US, and the infection rate was 15.5% among 400 immigrants examined in Montreal, Canada (Sun, 1980).

Occurrence: Human infection appears to be ancient, as eggs of the parasite have been found in human remains 2,600 years old. The prevalence among humans is estimated at between 7 and 30 million cases in the endemic area, with some 20 million people believed to be infected in southeastern China alone. In the Chinese province of Hubei, the infection was found in 5.8% of human inhabitants, 36.4% of cats, 16.7% of pigs, 12.2% and 3.8% of two snail species, and 48.1%, 18.2%, and 17.2% of three fish species (Chen *et al.,* 1997). Although the first human case in the Republic of Korea was not diagnosed until 1915, *C. sinensis* is now the most prevalent human parasite there (Rim, 1990). In 1997, stool sample examinations in that country showed a human infection rate of 11.3%, while intradermal tests detected the infection in 27.6% of those examined. Of 25 fish species tested, 7 were infected, with prevalences ranging from 2.8% to 30%. Nevertheless, this situation represents an improvement over that of several decades ago (Joo *et al.*, 1997). In 1987, for example, a study found that 80.3% of a sample of 76 people were excreting an average of 27,781 eggs per gram of feces (Hong *et al.*, 1994). In Vietnam, the infection was found in 13.7% of humans, 13.3% of snails, and 53.4% to 100% of farm-raised fish, and it was determined that the largest fish were most frequently infected (Kino *et al.*, 1998). In some areas of Japan, 20.6% of dogs and 45.5% of cats examined were infected. In all the endemic areas, the infection has been found to be more prevalent among males than females and among adults than children. These findings are attributed to the fact that the most affected groups are those that eat raw fish most often.

The Disease in Man and Animals: The symptomatology of the disease depends on the number of parasites, the length of time the infection has persisted, and whether continuous reinfections have occurred. In general, when the infection is mild and recent, there are no manifestations of disease. When the infection is more intense and of longer duration, the patient may exhibit loss of appetite, diarrhea, a sensation of intra-abdominal pressure, fever, and eosinophilia. In the heaviest and oldest infections, there may also be enlargement and tenderness of the liver, obstruction of the bile ducts, and even cirrhosis, with edema and ascites. Chen *et al.* (1989) described three stages of the infection in cats: an acute stage of up to 5 weeks' duration, in which specific IgM, IgG, and IgA antibodies are found; a subacute stage that lasts up to 28 weeks, during which only IgG and IgA antibodies are present; and a chronic stage, in which only IgG antibodies are detected. Based on these criteria, the authors found that 3.9% of 74 patients examined were in the subacute stage and 96.1% were in the chronic stage.

Light recent infections cause little harm. The principal types of damage produced by chronic clonorchiasis are hyperplasia of the mucus-secreting epithelium of the bile ducts, localized dilation of the ducts, and lymphocytic and eosinophilic inflammation of the periductal region, which eventually leads to fibrosis. The changes are attributed to irritation and to a 24-kD cysteine proteinase produced by the parasite (Park *et al.,* 1995). A common complication is recurrent pyogenic cholangitis, which results from obstruction of the bile ducts. Mild pancreatitis is also frequent. Clonorchiasis is often cited as a predisposing factor for the formation of gallstones, but Hou *et al.* (1989) found no clinical evidence to substantiate this assertion. However, it was demonstrated that the combination of *C. sinensis* infection and excessive alcohol consumption does predispose one to cholangiocarcinoma (Shin *et al.,* 1996).

Source of Infection and Mode of Transmission: Studies conducted in China, where the distribution of the parasitosis is uneven, have shown that human infection with *C. sinensis* depends primarily on the presence of intermediate hosts, the existence of reservoirs of the infection, and the customary consumption of undercooked fish by the population (Fang, 1994). The primary factor limiting the distribution of the disease is availability of the first intermediate host because only a small number of snail species are susceptible to the parasite. *Parafossarulus manchouricus* is the main host in China, Japan, the Republic of Korea, and Vietnam, but some other species are also susceptible. The second intermediate host is less of a limiting factor, since more than 100 species of freshwater fish and several species of shrimp can harbor the developing parasite. The reservoirs of the parasite are humans, swine, cats, dogs, rats, and several other fish-eating mammals. Persistence of the infection in nature is fostered by the presence of these reservoirs in the same ecological environment as the intermediate hosts—without which they would not have become infected—and the fact that they eliminate several thousand eggs per gram of feces every day. The use of human feces to fertilize carp ponds, a common practice in China, has also helped keep the infection active.

Diagnosis: Specific diagnosis of the infection is made by finding the parasite's eggs in fecal matter or by means of a duodenal probe following administration of a strong solution of magnesium sulfate to produce a reflex contraction of the gallbladder. When the parasite burden is light, it is advisable to use egg concentration methods to examine stool samples. Some authors recommend the zinc sulfate flotation method, but many operculate eggs tend to sediment in saline solutions. The parasite burden can be evaluated by counting the eggs in feces by means of the Stoll dilution method (Rim, 1982). In humans, up to 100 eggs per gram of feces constitutes a light infection; between 100 and 1,000 eggs, a moderate infection; and more than 1,000 eggs a heavy infection (Manson and Apted, 1982). The eggs of *C. sinensis* are considered quite characteristic: they are small (28–35 μm long and 12–19 μm wide), oval, operculate, and embryonated, with a thick, yellowish wall and a pronounced border around the operculum. However, several other trematodes in Southeast Asia that occasionally infect man (e.g., *Heterophyes heterophyes, Metagonimus yokogawai,* and *Opisthorchis viverrini,* the first two of which are intestinal parasites) have eggs that are virtually indistinguishable from those of *C. sinensis* (Ditrich *et al.,* 1992). Examination of the surface structure of the egg by electronic microscopy is a more reliable way to identify the parasite but is difficult to perform in the clinical environment.

Clinical imaging studies, such as cholangiography, sonography, and computerized tomography, may show shapes that suggest infection (Lim, 1990). However, the sensitivity and specificity of these techniques, at least in the case of sonography, appear to be inadequate. Using sonography, Hong *et al.* (1998) found 52% positivity among patients who were excreting eggs and 49% positivity among patients with negative stool samples.

The use of several immunodiagnostic tests has been proposed. The intradermal test shows immediate hypersensitivity and is simple, but it does not indicate if the infection is current. In a sample of 3,180 people examined by means of this technique, 26.2% tested positive, but when stool samples from 598 of the latter group were examined, only 21.6% were found to be excreting eggs (Kim *et al.*, 1990). In one study, immunoenzymatic staining and indirect immunofluorescence using frozen sections of the parasite showed sensitivities of 92% and 88%, respectively, and high specificity: 2% false positives with the first technique and 4% with the second (Liu *et al.*, 1993). Cross-reactions with cases of acute schistosomiasis, chronic schistosomiasis, and paragonimiasis were observed in 14%, 5%, and 0% of cases using immunoenzymatic staining, and in 14%, 10%, and 0% using indirect immunofluorescence. In another study (Lin *et al.*, 1995), use of enzyme-linked immunosorbent assay (ELISA) to detect total Ig, IgG, and IgA showed specificity and sensitivity of 100%, 100%, and 87%–90%, respectively. IgA antibodies were found to have decreased significantly after a month of successful treatment, which indicates that this test can be used to evaluate the results of treatment.

Control: The most effective control measure is probably to refrain from eating undercooked fish in endemic areas. Human clonorchiasis does not exist in northern China, where people do not eat raw fish, although it is prevalent in pigs, cats, dogs, and rats in that region. However, it is very difficult to modify deeply ingrained eating habits that are part of the population's culture. Freezing or salting fish is not a very effective control measure because the metacercariae remain infective for 10 to 18 days at –12°C, for 3 to 7 days at –20°C, and for 5 to 7 days in brine (Fan, 1998). The minimum doses of radiation needed to kill metacercariae are 0.05 kGy when they are isolated outside a host and 0.15 kGy when they are in fish (Duan *et al.*, 1993).

Fish infections can be reduced by allowing human fecal matter to ferment for several weeks before it is used to fertilize fish-culture ponds, as the fermentation process kills *C. sinensis* eggs. Treating the population with praziquantel every six months also significantly reduces the passage of eggs into the environment. Hong *et al.* (1998) showed that this treatment reduced the prevalence of infection from 22.7% to 6.3% in 24 months among inhabitants of a community in which the disease was endemic.

Use of molluscicides is not recommended because these chemicals can kill fish. However, elimination of vegetation from the edges of ponds during the spring and summer will benefit predators that eat snail larvae, which in turn will reduce the population of first intermediate hosts. A possible biological control method involves introducing *Notocotylus attenuatus*, an intestinal trematode of ducks, whose cercariae affect the gonads of snails and render them sterile.

Bibliography

Chen, C.Y., J.W. Shin, S.N. Chen, W.C. Hsieh. A preliminary study of clinical staging in clonorchiasis. *Zhonghua Min Guo Wei Sheng Wu Ji Mian Yi Xue Za Zhi* 22:193–200, 1989.

Chen, S., S. Chen, F. Wu, *et al*. Epidemiological survey on *Clonorchiasis sinensis* in Yangxin County of Hubei Province of PR China. *Southeast Asian J Trop Med Public Health* 28 Suppl:51–53, 1997.

Ditrich, O., M. Giboda, T. Scholz, S.A. Beer. Comparative morphology of eggs of the Haplorchiinae (Trematoda: Heterophyidae) and some other medically important heterophyid and opisthorchiid flukes. *Folia Parasitol* (Praha) 39:123–132, 1992.

Duan, Y.F., C.C. Song, G.C. Shou, *et al*. [Effect of gamma-irradiation on infectivity of *Clonorchis sinensis* metacercariae]. *Zhongguo Ji Sheng Chong Xue Yu Ji Sheng Chong Bing Za Zhi* 11:45–49, 1993.

Fan, P.C. Viability of metacercariae of *Clonorchis sinensis* in frozen or salted freshwater fish. *Int J Parasitol* 28:603–605, 1998.

Fang, Y.Y. Epidemiologic characteristics of *Clonorchiasis sinensis* in Guandong Province, China. *Southeast Asian J Trop Med Public Health* 25:291–295, 1994.

Hong, S.J., Y.H. Lee, M.H. Chung, D.H. Lee, H.C. Woo. Egg positive rates of *Clonorchis sinensis* and intestinal helminths among residents in Kagye-ri, Saengbiryang-myon, Sanchong-gun, Kyongsangnam-do. *Korean J Parasitol* 32(4):271–273, 1994.

Hou, M.F., C.G. Ker, P.C. Sheen, E.R. Chen. The ultrasound survey of gallstone diseases of patients infected with *Clonorchis sinensis* in southern Taiwan. *J Trop Med Hyg* 92:108–111, 1989.

Joo, C.Y., M.S. Chung, S.J. Kim, C.M. Kang. Changing patterns of *Clonorchis sinensis* infections in Kyongbuk, Korea. *Korean J Parasitol* 35:155–164, 1997.

Kim, J. Image analytical observation on the growth and development of *Clonorchis sinensis* in rats. *Korean J Parasitol* 33:281–288, 1995.

Kim, S.S., M.H. Han, S.G. Park, H.S. Lim, S.T. Hong. [A survey on the epidemiological factors of clonorchiasis in the Pohang industrial belt along the Hyungsan river, Kyongsangbuk-do]. *Kisaengchunghak Chapchi* 28:213–219, 1990.

Kino, H., H. Inaba, N. Van De, *et al*. Epidemiology of clonorchiasis in Ninh Binh Province, Vietnam. *Southeast Asian J Trop Med Public Health* 29:250–254, 1998.

Lim, J.H. Radiologic findings of clonorchiasis. *AJR Am J Roentgenol* 155:1001–1008, 1990.

Lin, Y.L., E.R. Chen, C.M. Yen. Antibodies in serum of patients with clonorchiasis before and after treatment. *Southeast Asian J Trop Med Public Health* 26:114–119, 1995.

Liu, X.M., W.F. Hu, Z.H. Wang, D.L. Chen, F.N. Xu. [Comparative studies on the diagnosis of clonorchiasis by IEST and IFAT]. *Zhongguo Ji Sheng Chong Xue Yu Ji Sheng Chong Bing Za Zhi* 11:273–275, 1993.

Manson, P., F.I.C. Apted. *Manson's Tropical Diseases*, 18th ed. London: Baillière Tindall; 1982.

Park, H., M.Y. Ko, M.K. Paik, C.T. Soh, J.H. Seo, K.I. Im. Cytotoxicity of a cysteine proteinase of adult *Clonorchis sinensis*. *Korean J Parasitol* 33:211–218, 1995.

Rim, H.J. Clonorchiasis. *In*: Hillyer, G.V., C.E. Hopla, section eds. Vol. 3, Section C: *CRC Handbook Series in Zoonoses*. Boca Raton, Florida: CRC Press; 1982.

Rim, H.J. Clonorchiasis in Korea. *Kisaengchunghak Chapchi* 28 Suppl:63–78, 1990.

Shin, H.R., C.U. Lee, H.J. Park, *et al*. Hepatitis B and C virus, *Clonorchis sinensis* for the risk of liver cancer: A case-control study in Pusan, Korea. *Int J Epidemiol* 25:933–940, 1996.

Sun, T. Clonorchiasis: A report of four cases and discussion of unusual manifestations. *Am J Trop Med Hyg* 29:1223–1227, 1980.

DICROCELIASIS

ICD-10 B66.2

Synonyms: Dicroceliosis, dicrocoeliasis, lancet fluke infection, infection due to *Dicrocoelium dendriticum*.

Etiology: The agents of this disease are *Dicrocoelium dendriticum* (*D. lanceolatum*) and *D. hospes*, small, translucent, lancet-shaped trematodes, measuring 5–15 mm long by 1.5–2.5 mm wide. They live in the bile ducts of sheep, goats, cattle, and, less frequently, other domestic and wild ruminants. They rarely infect pigs, dogs, rabbits, rodents, or humans.

D. dendriticum requires two intermediate hosts for its development. The first is a land snail (38 species, among them *Cionella lubrica* in North America, *Zebrina detrita* and *Helicella candidula* in Europe, and *Bradybaena similaris* in Malaysia), and the second is an ant (12 species, among them *Formica fusca* in Germany and North America, *F. cinerea* and *F. picea* in the Russian Federation, and *F. gigantis* and *F. rufibarbis* in the Middle East).

The adult parasites deposit small oval eggs (38–45 μm x 22–30 μm), which are brown in color, thick-walled, operculate, and embryonated at the time they are excreted by the host. They are transported by bile and fecal matter to the exterior, where the first intermediate host ingests them. The egg, which is quite resistant to desiccation, releases the miracidium only when it is ingested by a snail. The miracidium forms two generations of sporocysts in the digestive gland of the snail, the second of which produces numerous cercariae, which are expelled from the snail through the respiratory chamber after about three to four months. The cercariae that leave the snail are stuck together in the form of a viscous mass ("slime ball"), measuring 1–2 mm in diameter. Infection with the parasite affects the snail's fertility and longevity (Schuster, 1992). Each slime ball may contain 100 to 400 cercariae, which, after being ingested by the second intermediate host, migrate into the ant's coelom and nervous system and become metacercariae. Each ant may contain between 38 and 76 metacercariae, depending on the species and size of the insect (Schuster, 1991).

The presence of metacercariae in the ant's brain often alters its behavior: instead of returning to the nest as dusk approaches and the temperature drops, an infected ant will climb to the top of a blade of grass. It will then bite down and suffer a spasm of the jaw musculature, making it impossible for the ant to let go. Thus trapped high on the vegetation, the ant is likely to be eaten by a definitive host. When herbivores consume infected ants while grazing, the metacercariae excyst in the duodenum and the juvenile parasites travel against the bile flow to the bile ducts. The parasites mature and begin to lay eggs after 10–12 weeks. The life cycle of *D. hospes*, which has been determined more recently, is similar to that of *D. dendriticum*. The first intermediate host is a pulmonate land snail of the genus *Limicolaria*, and the second is an ant of the genus *Camponotus*, in which the metacercariae develop. The definitive hosts are domestic herbivores (cattle, sheep, goats) and probably also wild ruminants (Frank *et al.*, 1984).

Geographic Distribution and Occurrence: *D. dendriticum* is a widely distributed parasite found in many parts of the world, including North Africa (Egypt), South America (Brazil and Colombia), Asia, Australia, the Caribbean islands, Europe, the Middle East, and parts of the eastern US and Canada. Prevalence rates of 40% have been reported in domestic animals in France, 80% in Poland, 46% in Switzerland, 100% in Yugoslavia, and 75% in goats in the Russian Federation. In Greece, parasite eggs were found in 2 of 232 dogs, but there is some doubt as to whether these were true *D. dendriticum* infections (Haralabidis *et al.*, 1988). *D. hospes* is restricted to the sub-Saharan savannas of Africa. In Côte d'Ivoire and Niger, 50% and 94%, respectively, of cattle and sheep have been found to be infected (Frank *et al.*, 1984).

Human dicroceliasis also occurs worldwide. Since 1988, cases have been reported in Saudi Arabia, the former Czechoslovakia, Spain, Kenya, Nigeria, Somalia, the former Soviet Union, and the US, although it is likely that most cases are not reported. The presence of *Dicrocoelium* spp. eggs in human feces is not unusual, though it does not always indicate true infection: in Nigeria, 2 (0.4%) of 479 human stool samples were found to contain *Dicrocoelium* eggs (Reinthaler *et al.*, 1988), and in a hospital in Saudi Arabia, eggs were found in the stools of 208 patients over a three-year period (el-Shiekh Mohamed and Mummery, 1990). However, many of these cases are due to spurious parasites ingested with the infected liver of domestic animals, and the eggs merely pass through the human digestive tract. Of the 208 cases in Saudi Arabia, at least 7 patients had a true infection, while 34 were spurious cases.

The Disease in Man and Animals: Dicroceliasis generally produces no signs of disease in animals, unless the infection is very heavy or of long standing. When this occurs, there is a general decline in health status, the animals tend to remain prostrate, their temperature decreases, and they exhibit some degree of malnutrition and anemia, though it is not certain that the latter is caused by the parasite infection. Theodoridis *et al.* (1991) found no proof of significant loss of blood or plasma protein in experimentally infected sheep with parasite loads of up to 4,000. Liver enzymes and blood biochemistry are generally within normal ranges. Autopsy, however, reveals hundreds or thousands of parasites in the bile ducts and gallbladder, duct inflammation and proliferation, progressive development of fibrosis in the hepatic parenchyma, and, occasionally, granulomas and abscesses (Camara *et al.*, 1996). The disease is more severe in New World camelids (Wenker *et al.*, 1998). Hamsters infected experimentally showed an increase in bile secretion and an accumulation of oxidizing molecules in the liver, which produced liver damage (Sánchez-Campos *et al.*, 1999).

In most human cases, the main symptoms are dyspepsia and flatulence, although there may occasionally be constipation alternating with diarrhea, vomiting, and abdominal pain. Peripheral eosinophilia is seen in some cases. Laboratory analysis of blood and urine generally reveals no abnormalities. Ectopic localization of parasite eggs in the brain may cause neurological symptoms in rare instances.

Source of Infection and Mode of Transmission: The source of infection for both animals and man is ants infected with metacercariae of the parasite. Animals ingest these insects while grazing. Humans are accidental hosts who are occasionally infected by nibbling on grass containing infected ants or by consuming fruits or vegetables contaminated with these insects. In at least one case, an AIDS patient became infected by consuming a drink contaminated with ants. The infection in snails occurs most frequently in the spring, decreases in the summer, and increases again in the fall. Infected ants are found only when the temperature is below 20°C (Schuster and Neumann, 1988).

Diagnosis: Diagnosis is based on the detection of the eggs of the parasite in feces or bile from the individual suspected to have the infection. Examination of the bile is much more sensitive: of 49 bovines with adult *D. dendriticum* in their livers, eggs were found in the bile of 44 (89.8%) but in the feces of only 13 (26.5%) (Braun *et al.,* 1995). Of the techniques available for demonstrating the presence of eggs, flotation of experimentally contaminated sheep feces, using a solution of mercury iodide mixed with potassium iodide with a specific density of 1.44, yielded an egg recovery rate of 91.2±9.4%, regardless of flotation time. In contrast, solutions of zinc sulfate with specific densities of 1.3 and 1.45, or potassium carbonate with a specific density of 1.45 yielded an egg recovery rate of only 9.0±7.1%, 26.7±24.9%, and 13.0±11.6%, respectively, and more than 3–5 minutes of flotation time were needed to improve the yield. Sedimentation revealed 41.2±1.5% of the infections (Rehbein *et al.,* 1999). To distinguish genuine infections from spurious parasites, it is necessary to ensure that the patient does not eat animal liver for several days and then reexamine the feces for eggs during that period. Although the *Dicrocoelium* spp. eggs are considered distinctive, they cannot be differentiated by means of conventional microscopy from the eggs of *Eurytrema pancreaticum,* a trematode of the pancreas of ruminants and monkeys that develops in land snails and grasshoppers. *E. pancreaticum* has been found in humans in China and Japan on approximately eight occasions.

Immunologic techniques have also been used to diagnose the infection in domestic animals. Counterimmunoelectrophoresis, passive hemagglutination, and agar gel precipitation detected 69.8%, 50.0%, and 23.8% of infections, respectively, in sheep and goats (Jithendran *et al.,* 1996).

Control: Control of dicroceliasis in domestic animals is difficult owing to the variety of intermediate host species (38 snail species and 12 ant species) and to their distribution over wide land areas (in contrast to trematodes with aquatic intermediate hosts, which have a more localized distribution on pasturelands). Although pesticides may be used to control mollusks and ants, their cost and the attendant risk of ecological damage make this an impractical solution. A recommended alternative is to destroy the parasites by treating the definitive hosts, but this, too, is expensive and there are still no drugs available that will totally eliminate the parasite. When possible, cultivation of grasslands can eliminate a very high proportion of the snail population. Similarly, it has been recommended that chickens be introduced in infected areas because they eat snails. The low frequency of human infection probably does not justify mass control measures. It should be sufficient simply to educate the population about the risk of eating, nibbling, or sucking on blades of grass that may be contaminated with ants.

Bibliography

Braun, U., R. Wolfensberger, H. Hertzberg. Diagnosis of liver flukes in cows—a comparison of the findings in the liver, in the feces, and in the bile. *Schweiz Arch Tierheilkd* 137:438–444, 1995.

Camara, L., K. Pfister, A. Aeschlimann. Analyse histopathologique de foie de bovin infesté par *Dicrocoelium dendriticum*. *Vet Res* 27:87–92, 1996.

el-Shiekh Mohamed, A.R., V. Mummery. Human dicrocoeliasis. Report on 208 cases from Saudi Arabia. *Trop Geogr Med* 42:1–7, 1990.

Frank, W., R. Lucius, T. Romig. Studies on the biology, pathology, ecology and epidemiology of *Dicrocoelium hospes* (Looss, 1907) in West Africa (Ivory Coast). *In:* Markl, H., A. Bittner, eds. *Recent German Research on Problems of Parasitology, Animal Health and Animal Breeding in the Tropics and Subtropics. Selected reports on DFG supported research.* Tübingen: Institute for Scientific Co-operation; 1984.

Haralabidis, S.T., M.G. Papazachariadou, A.F. Koutinas, T.S. Rallis. A survey on the prevalence of gastrointestinal parasites of dogs in the area of Thessaloniki, Greece. *J Helminthol* 62:45–49, 1988.

Jithendran, K.P., J. Vaid, L. Krishna. Comparative evaluation of agar gel precipitation, counterimmunoelectrophoresis and passive haemagglutination tests for the diagnosis of *Dicrocoelium dendriticum* infection in sheep and goats. *Vet Parasitol* 61:151–156, 1996.

Malek, E.A. Vol. 2: *Snail-transmitted Parasitic Diseases.* Boca Raton: CRC Press; 1980.

Rehbein, S., S. Kokott, T. Lindner. Evaluation of techniques for the enumeration of *Dicrocoelium* eggs in sheep faeces. *Zentralbl Veterinarmed A* 46:133–139, 1999.

Reinthaler, F.F., F. Mascher, G. Klem, W. Sixl. A survey of gastrointestinal parasites in Ogun State, southwest Nigeria. *Ann Trop Med Parasitol* 82:181–184, 1988.

Sánchez-Campos, S., M.J. Tunón, P. González, J. González-Gallego. Oxidative stress and changes in liver antioxidant enzymes induced by experimental dicroceliosis in hamsters. *Parasitol Res* 85:468–474, 1999.

Schuster, R. Factors influencing the metacercarial intensity in ants and the size of *Dicrocoelium dendriticum* metacercarial cysts. *J Helminthol* 65:275–279, 1991.

Schuster, R. Zur Beeinflussung von *Helicella obvia* durch *Dicrocoelium*-Parthenitae. *Angew Parasitol* 33:61–64, 1992.

Schuster, R., B. Neumann. Zum jahreszeitlichen Auftreten von *Dicrocoelium dendriticum* in Zwischenwirten. *Angew Parasitol* 29:31–36, 1988.

Theodoridis, Y., J.L. Duncan, J.M. MacLean, C.A. Himonas. Pathophysiological studies on *Dicrocoelium dendriticum* infection in sheep. *Vet Parasitol* 39:61–66, 1991.

Wenker, C., J.M. Hatt, H. Hertzberg, *et al.* Dikrozoliose bei Neuweltkameliden. *Tierarztl Prax Ausg G Grosstiere Nutztiere* 26:355–361, 1998.

ECHINOSTOMIASIS

ICD-10 B66.8 Other specified fluke infections

Synonym: Echinostomatidosis.

Etiology: The agents of this trematodiasis are various species of several genera of the family Echinostomatidae. They are trematodes of small but variable size, measuring 5–15 mm long, 1–3 mm wide, and 0.5–0.6 mm thick, which live in the intestine of mammals (generally carnivores, swine, or rats), fowl, and, occasionally, humans. The most remarkable morphologic characteristic of the mature parasite is a collar of spines surrounding the dorsal and lateral sides of the oral sucker. The number, size, and position of the spines are taxonomically significant. The eggs are large (85–125 μm x 55–70 μm), thin-walled, and operculate, and are eliminated before the embryo forms. As the nomenclature of the group is still uncertain, studies are examining their nucleic acids to determine the relationships among some members of the family. The family Echinostomatidae comprises approximately 30 genera. Some 16 species, most of the genus *Echinostoma*, have been recovered from humans (Carney, 1991). The most important causes of zoonosis are the species *E. echinatum* (*E. lindoense*), *E. hortense*, *E. ilocanum*, *E. malayanum*, *E. revolutum*, *E. trivolvis*, and *Hypoderaeum conoideum*. Radomyos *et al.* (1994) examined fecal matter from 681 individuals in northern Thailand and found 8.3% to be infected with *E. malayanum*, 8.1% with *E. ilocanum*, and 0.8% with *E. revolutum*.

The life cycle differs from species to species, but in general two intermediate hosts are required. The cercariae always develop in a freshwater snail (first intermediate host), but they may encyst as metacercariae in another snail, a bivalve mollusk, a tadpole, or a freshwater fish (second intermediate host) (Table 1). The definitive host, including man, becomes infected by consuming raw foods (intermediate hosts) containing metacercariae (see Source of Infection and Mode of Transmission).

Geographic Distribution and Occurrence: Human echinostome infections are confined mainly to the Far East. However, sporadic clinical cases occur in countries such as the US, where more than a million immigrants from that region reside (Liu and Harinasuta, 1996).

E. malayanum is found in India, Indonesia (Sumatra), Malaysia, the Philippines, Thailand, and Singapore, where it infects dogs, cats, pigs, mongooses, rats, and, rarely, humans. *E. ilocanum* is distributed in the Philippines, Indonesia (Java and Sulawesi), parts of southern China, India, and Thailand. In addition to man, it infects murid rodents, dogs, and cats. Prevalences of 1% to 50% have been found among humans in the Philippines, and of 14% among dogs in China. *E. hortense* is found in Japan and the Republic of Korea, where the infection was detected in 3 (0.5%) of 642 human stool samples on one occasion and in 11 (9.5%) of 116 samples on another (Son *et al.*, 1994). Their life cycle has been replicated in the laboratory using *Lymnaea* and *Radix* snails as the first intermediate hosts, tadpoles as the second hosts, and rats as the definitive hosts (Lee *et al.*, 1991). *E. revolutum* is distributed in the Far East and Europe, where it infects ducks, geese, and other fowl. Human infections have been diagnosed in Indonesia (Java and Sulawesi), Thailand, and Taiwan. The prevalence of human infection in Taiwan is estimated at 2.8%–6.5%. *E.*

TABLE 3. Intermediate hosts and geographic distribution of the main zoonotic echinostomes.

| Species | Intermediate hosts | | Distribution |
	First	Second	
Echinostoma echinatum (*E. lindoense*)	*Planorbis* snails	Clams, snails	Brazil, India, Indonesia (Java), Malaysia, Philippines
E. hortense	*Lymnaea, Radix* snails	Tadpoles, fish	Japan, Republic of Korea
E. ilocanum	*Gyraulus, Hippeutis* snails	Snails	China, India, Indonesia (Java and Sulawesi), Philippines, Thailand
E. malayanum	*Indoplanorbis, Lymnaea,* and other snail species	Snails, tadpoles, fish	India, Indonesia (Sumatra), Malaysia, Philippines, Singapore, Thailand
E. revolutum	*Lymnaea* snails	Clams	Indonesia (Java and Sulawesi), Taiwan, Thailand
E. trivolvis	*Heliosoma* snails	Snails, clams, tadpoles, fish	North America
Hypoderaeum conoideum	*Lymnaea, Planorbis* snails	Snails, tadpoles	Thailand

trivolvis, which for many years was confused with *E. revolutum*, is found in North America, where it infects 26 fowl species and 13 mammalian species (Marquardt *et al.*, 2000). *E. echinatum* is a parasite of anseriform fowl in Brazil, India, Indonesia (Java), Malaysia, and the Philippines. It used to also be quite prevalent on the island of Sulawesi (24% to 96%), but no human cases have been detected there in recent decades (see Control). *H. conoideum* is a trematode parasite of fowl that is frequently found in the human population of northern Thailand, where people often eat raw snails.

The Disease in Man and Animals: Most human echinostome infections seem to be of little clinical importance. In the Republic of Korea, for example, although human stool sample examinations have revealed *E. hortense* prevalences of 0.4%, 0.5%, and 9.5% (Lee *et al.*, 1994; Son *et al.*, 1994), only 75 cases had been reported in that country as of 1994 (Huh *et al.*, 1994). The disease's clinical features have not been well studied (Huffman and Fried, 1990). In general, echinostomes are not very pathogenic, and mild and moderate infections often go unnoticed. Heavy infections may cause some degree of diarrhea, flatulence, and colic pain, however. In children, anemia and edema have also been reported and, in at least one case, duodenal ulcers have been observed at the site of parasite attachment (Chai *et al.*, 1994). Studies of

E. hortense in rats have demonstrated that, although the parasites remain mostly in the intestinal lumen, the activity of their suckers destroys the epithelium and causes villus atrophy and crypt hyperplasia (Lee *et al.,* 1990). In fowl, severe enteritis due to *E. revolutum* and *H. conoideum* has been reported.

Source of Infection and Mode of Transmission: The first intermediate host of the echinostomes of zoonotic importance is always a freshwater snail (Table 1). The source of infection for man and other definitive hosts is the second intermediate host, which harbors the metacercariae. In many cases, the metacercariae form in snails; in other cases, they may develop in bivalve mollusks or tadpoles and even freshwater fish. Humans acquire the infection by ingesting an undercooked secondary intermediate host. Among the snails that harbor metacercariae, the genera *Pila* and *Viviparus* are important because they are often eaten raw in the Philippines and on the island of Java. Among the bivalves, clams of the genus *Corbicula* are important for the same reason. A wide variety of freshwater fish have been shown to be suitable hosts for echinostome metacercariae.

From the ecological standpoint, echinostomiasis occurs in regions with an abundance of freshwater bodies, which allow the intermediate hosts to survive. The endemicity of the parasitosis is due to the custom of consuming raw mollusks or fish.

Diagnosis: Diagnosis is based on confirmation of the presence of eggs in fecal matter (see the chapter on Dicroceliasis). The size of the eggs differs, depending on the species of equinostome, and these eggs must be distinguished from the unembryonated eggs of other intestinal or biliary trematodes.

Control: The relatively minor clinical importance of this parasitosis does not justify the establishment of special control programs. In endemic areas, it is recommended that the population be educated about the risks of and warned against eating raw or undercooked mollusks or fish, though changing this long-standing eating habit may be difficult. An interesting example of involuntary ecological control that resulted in the disappearance of the human infection occurred in Lake Lindu, on the island of Sulawesi. The incidence of *E. echinatum* in humans ranged between 24% and 96% in some communities in that region, but introduction of the fish *Tilapia mossambica* into the lake interfered with reproduction of the clam *Corbicula lindoensis*, which was the main source of human infection. As a result, the human infection ceased to occur when this species of clam disappeared. However, the wildlife cycle—between rodents as definitive hosts and freshwater snails as intermediate hosts—persists.

Bibliography

Carney, W.P. Echinostomiasis—a snail-borne intestinal trematode zoonosis. *Southeast Asian J Trop Med Public Health* 22 Suppl:206–211, 1991.

Chai, J.Y., S.T. Hong, S.H. Lee, G.C. Lee, Y.I. Min. A case of echinostomiasis with ulcerative lesions in the duodenum. *Korean J Parasitol* 32:201–204, 1994.

Huffman, J.E., B. Fried. Echinostoma and echinostomiasis. *Adv Parasitol* 29:215–269, 1990.

Huh, S., S.U. Lee, S.C. Huh. A follow-up examination of intestinal parasitic infections of the Army soldiers in Whachon-gun, Korea. *Korean J Parasitol* 32:61–63, 1994.

Lee, S.H., S.W. Hwang, W.M. Sohn, et al. [Experimental life history of Echinostoma hortense]. Kisaengchunghak Chapchi 29:161–172, 1991.

Lee, S.H., T.Y. Noh, W.M. Sohn, et al. [Chronological observation of intestinal lesions of rats experimentally infected with Echinostoma hortense]. Kisaengchunghak Chapchi 28:45–52, 1990.

Lee, S.K., B.M. Shin, N.S. Chung, J.Y. Chai, S.H. Lee. [Second report on intestinal parasites among the patients of Seoul Paik Hospital (1984–1992)]. Korean J Parasitol 32:27–33, 1994.

Liu, L.X., K.T. Harinasuta. Liver and intestinal flukes. Gastroenterol Clin North Am 25:627–636, 1996.

Marquardt, W.C., R.S. Demaree, R.B. Grieve, eds. Parasitology and Vector Biology, 2nd ed. San Diego: Academic Press; 2000.

Radomyos, P., B. Radomyos, A. Tungtrongchitr. Multi-infection with helminths in adults from northeast Thailand as determined by post-treatment fecal examination of adult worms. Trop Med Parasitol 45:133–135, 1994.

Son, W.Y., S. Huh, S.U. Lee, H.C. Woo, S.J. Hong. Intestinal trematode infections in the villagers in Koje-myon, Kochang-gun, Kyongsangnam-do, Korea. Korean J Parasitol 32:149–155, 1994.

FASCIOLIASIS

ICD-10 B66.3

Synonyms: Hepatic distomiasis, fasciolosis, sheep liver fluke disease.

Etiology: The agents of this disease are Fasciola hepatica and Fasciola gigantica, trematodes that live in the bile ducts of wild and domestic ruminants and other herbivores and occasionally infect man.

F. hepatica is a flat fluke, shaped like a laurel leaf, which measures 20 to 40 mm long by 10 to 15 mm wide. It is greenish brown in color. The adult parasite lays about 3,000 eggs a day, which are carried to the host intestine by bile and eliminated in feces before they become embryonated. In order to mature, the eggs need to have suitable conditions of humidity, oxygenation, and temperature. They can survive for about two months in feces that are moist but sufficiently compacted to keep out oxygen, but they will not hatch. The eggs can withstand temperatures from 0°C to 37°C, but they only develop at 10°C to 30°C. In freshwater bodies, the first juvenile stage (miracidium) develops and emerges from the egg in 10 to 12 days at temperatures between 20°C and 26°C, but the process takes 60 days or longer at 10°C. Since the energy reserves of the miracidium are limited, once it has been released it has to invade a snail intermediate host within eight hours in order to stay alive. It is guided to its intermediate host in part by the chemical attraction of the snail's mucus.

The intermediate hosts are amphibious snails of the family Lymnaeidae. In the past, most of the species in question were classified under the genus Lymnaea, but a number of these have been reassigned to other genera, including Fossaria,

Pseudosuccinea, and *Stagnicola* (Barriga, 1997). Since traditional morphological classification is difficult with the family Lymnaeidae, molecular methods are being used to study phylogenetic relationships (Bargues and Mas-Coma, 1997). The most important species are *Fossaria bulimoides, Fossaria modicella, Pseudosuccinea columella, S. caperata,* and *S. montanensi* in North America; *Fossaria viatrix* and *L. diaphana* in a large part of South America; *L. tomentosa* in Australia and New Zealand; *L. truncatula* in Africa, Asia, and Europe; and *L. viridis* in Asia, the state of Hawaii (USA), and Papua New Guinea (Boray, 1982). *Fossaria cubensis and P. columella* are the main intermediate hosts in the Caribbean, Colombia, and Venezuela (Cong *et al.,* 1991).

The miracidia take 30 minutes to penetrate the snail using both enzymatic and mechanical means, following which they become sporocysts. Rediae (sometimes two generations) develop within the sporocysts, and within the rediae, cercariae. It takes between three and seven weeks, depending on the temperature of the water, for the sporocyst to develop inside the snail to the point of producing cercariae. This multiplication of preadult parasite stages inside the snail, known as pedogenesis, is characteristic of the trematodes and may compensate for the comparatively few eggs laid by the adults. It has been estimated that a single *F. hepatica* miracidium can produce 320 cercariae, and an average of 418 cercariae are recovered from one infected snail (Barriga, 1997). The cercariae abandon the snail when it becomes more active, often when more fresh water is available following rainfall. Once they are free, the cercariae swim in the water for about two hours and then attach themselves to aquatic plants, where they secrete a protective envelope, or cyst, around them. Some cercariae may encyst in water, where they usually remain suspended, attached to bubbles. This encysted organism is called a metacercaria. It measures about 0.2 mm in diameter and becomes infective for the definitive host in two days. In order to survive, the metacercaria requires a relative humidity level of under 70% and moderate temperatures. Few of them can withstand the ice of winter, and none can survive a hot, dry summer. All of them live for 6 months at temperatures between 12°C and 14°C, but only 5% live for 10 months. Their maximum survival in nature is probably about one year.

The definitive hosts become infected by ingesting metacercariae along with plants or water. The cystic envelope is digested in the small intestine of the host, and the parasite becomes active, traverses the intestinal wall, moves around in the peritoneal cavity for a couple of days, and, finally, penetrates the hepatic parenchyma. The parasite, which is only 0.3 mm long at this stage, continues to pass through the liver for the next six or seven weeks and then invades the biliary canaliculi, by which time it measures 4 mm to 14 mm. The parasite matures and eggs begin to appear in feces between 56 and 90 days after the initial infection. The infection lasts approximately four to six years in sheep and between one and two years in cattle.

F. gigantica has a life cycle similar to that of *F. hepatica.* However, its intermediate hosts are different aquatic snails belonging to the superspecies *Lymnaea (Radix) auricularia,* and which live in larger bodies of water. These snails hibernate but do not tolerate long summers. In India and Pakistan, the intermediate host is *L. a. rufescens*; in Malaysia, *L. a. rubiginosa*; in Iran, *L. a. geodrosiana*; and in Iraq, *L. lagotis euphratica.* The main intermediate host in Africa is *L. a. natalensis* (Malek, 1980). The development cycle of *F. gigantica* is longer than that of *F. hepatica.* In countries where both trematodes exist, such as Pakistan, their co-occurrence is determined by the presence of appropriate intermediate hosts. *F. hepatica* cannot complete its larval cycle in *L. auricularia*, while *F. gigantica* cannot do so in *L. truncatula*. The definitive hosts of *F. gigantica* are cattle, goats, zebras, sheep, and occasionally man. The prepatent period lasts 9 to 12 weeks. This trematode is distinguished from *F. hepatica* by its larger size (25–75 mm by 12 mm), smaller cephalic cone, less prominent shoulders, more transparent body, and slightly larger eggs (156–197 µm by 90–104 µm for *F. gigantica* and 130–150 µm by 63–90 µm for *F. hepatica*).

Geographic Distribution: *F. hepatica* is found in almost all temperate regions where sheep and other ruminants are raised. Virtually all these areas have sufficient humidity and adequate temperature conditions, at least during part of the year, to sustain a snail population. *F. gigantica*, on the other hand, occurs mainly in tropical areas such as Africa, Asia Minor, Southeast Asia, southern Europe, the state of Hawaii (USA), the former USSR, and possibly southern US.

Occurrence in Man: Human fascioliasis caused by *F. hepatica* has been found mainly in Australia, Bolivia, Cuba, Ecuador, England, Egypt, France, Iran, Peru, and Portugal (García and Bruckner, 1997). The frequency of the parasite in animals does not appear to be closely correlated with its occurrence in man. For example, although the infection is common in cattle in western and southeastern US, only one human case has been reported in that country. The situation is similar in China: although the infection is frequently seen in animals, only 44 human cases were known to have occurred as of 1991 (Chen, 1991). Human fascioliasis can occur sporadically or in outbreaks. The largest epidemics on record were in France, near Lyon in 1956–1957, with some 500 cases, and in the Lot Valley in 1957, with about 200 cases. The common source of infection was watercress contaminated with metacercariae (Malek, 1980). In England, the largest known outbreak affected 40 persons in 1972. In Egypt, one study revealed 40 cases in children in one year (el-Karaksy *et al.*, 1999) and another, a 3% infection rate in children (Curtale *et al.*, 1998). The frequency of human infection in Latin America has been underestimated in the literature. In Cuba, over 100 cases were recorded by 1944 (to which numerous subsequent reports should be added), and in Chile, 82 as of 1959. In 1978, 42 clinical cases were diagnosed in the canton of Turrialba in Costa Rica (Mora *et al.,* 1980). A series of 31 surveys conducted in the Bolivian highland plateau revealed an overall prevalence of 15.4%, with local variations ranging from 0% to 68% (Esteban *et al.*, 1999). In a hyperendemic area of that Bolivian region, the prevalence was found to be 75% in children and 41% in adults—probably the highest figures in the world (Esteban *et al.*, 1997). A study carried out in Cuba revealed an outbreak involving 67 persons, 59 of whom had prepatent infections and were identified initially by coproantigenic investigation. None of the prepatent cases had *Fasciola* antigen in the bloodstream (Espino *et al.*, 1998). A study of 5,861 rural subjects in central Chile showed a prevalence of 0.7% in humans, 13.5% in horses, 6.1% in rabbits, and 20.6% in swine (Apt *et al.*, 1992). There is increasing reliance on immunologic diagnosis to study epidemics and find cases in unsuspected contacts (Bechtel *et al.*, 1992).

Occurrence in Animals: Hepatic fascioliasis is a common disease of cattle, goats, and sheep in many parts of the world. It can also affect swine, rabbits, equines, and other mammals. Morbidity and mortality rates vary from one region to another. In endemic areas, it is not usual to find infection rates of 30%, 50%, or even higher. A study conducted in the central highlands of Peru revealed an infection rate of 18.6% in sheep in the foci of origin and 95.8% in the foci of dissemination. In Puerto Rico, 32% of slaughterhouse cattle were found to be infected. The losses caused by hepatic fascioliasis are difficult to calculate, but in the US, it is estimated that US$ 5.5 million are lost each year because of mortality and morbidity, as well as US$ 2.5 million on account of livers that were confiscated because they failed inspection. According to one estimate, the productive efficiency of cattle with mild infections declines by 8% and in cattle with more serious infections, by more than 20%. In the sheep-raising industry, losses in wool production alone can range from 20% to 39%. Indeed, there are losses from delayed development of the animals; reduced wool, milk, and meat production; lower market prices; and the confiscation of livers. Moreover, when the parasites invade an animal's liver, they pave the way for invasion by *Clostridium novyi*, which can cause infectious necrotic hepatitis.

F. gigantica reaches high levels of prevalence in endemic areas. In China, rates of 50% in cattle, 45% in goats, and 33% in buffalo have been reported. In Iraq, rates of 71% were found in buffalo, 27% in cattle, 19% in goats, and 7% in sheep. In Thailand, the average prevalence of infection was 12% in cattle and buffalo, with local variations from 0% to 85% (Srihakim and Pholpark, 1991).

The Disease in Man: The effect of fascioliasis on human health depends on the parasite burden and the duration of the infection. The migration of young fasciolae across the intestinal wall and through the peritoneal cavity does not cause clinical manifestations, but their final journey across the hepatic parenchyma can lead to traumatic, necrotic, and inflammatory lesions, whose severity depends on the number of parasites. In the bile ducts, the adult *Fasciola* produces pericanalicular inflammation and fibrosis, and adenomatous proliferation in the ductal epithelium. Massive infections can cause biliary stasis due to obstruction of the duct, atrophy of the liver, and periportal cirrhosis. Cholecystitis and cholelithiasis occur with some frequency in chronic cases. The most common manifestations during acute fascioliasis, when the young parasites migrate across the hepatic parenchyma, are abdominal pain, fever, hepatomegaly, eosinophilia, and mild anemia. In a study of 53 patients with eosinophilia of probable parasitic origin, 30 of the cases proved to be due to fascioliasis (el Zawawy *et al.*, 1995). Elsewhere, *F. hepatica* was the parasite most frequently associated with reduced hemoglobinemia in a group of highly parasitized individuals (Curtale *et al.*, 1998). This parasite was also found in 24% of 187 patients with fever of unknown origin (Abdel Wahab *et al.*, 1996).

In the chronic phase, which occurs once the parasite has become localized in the bile ducts, the common signs are biliary colic and cholangitis. The acute-phase eosinophilia usually persists, although sometimes the chronic infection can be asymptomatic (el-Nehwihi *et al.*, 1995). In a study of 47 patients in Chile, the main symptoms were abdominal pain, dyspepsia, weight loss, diarrhea, and fever. Ten of the 47 patients had jaundice. The eosinophil count was normal in 9 and elevated in 38 cases (Faiguenbaum *et al.,* 1962). In Spain, the most common symptoms in 6 fascioliasis patients were eosinophilia (100% over 1,000 cells/mm^3), abdominal pain (100%), fever (83%), weight loss (83%), and generalized myalgia (67%) (de Gorgolas *et al.*, 1992).

As they pass through the peritoneal cavity, the larvae may be diverted to aberrant sites in different parts of the body. Hence it is not unusual for patients to have extrahepatic abnormalities, such as pulmonary infiltrates, pleuropericarditis, meningitis, or lymphadenopathy caused by these parasites (Arjona *et al.*, 1995).

The Disease in Animals: Fascioliasis is a disease of herbivores. Sheep are the most susceptible domestic species, followed by cattle. The disease has both an acute and a chronic form (Soulsby, 1982).

The acute form occurs when the sheep ingests a large number of metacercariae at once, with consequent invasion of a multitude of young parasites in the hepatic parenchyma. The migrating parasites destroy the hepatic tissue, causing hemorrhages, hematomas, necrotic tunnels, and peripheral inflammation. In massive infections, the affected sheep may die suddenly without any clinical manifestations, or they may exhibit weakness, loss of appetite, and pain when palpated in the hepatic region and then die a couple of days later. In less acute cases there may be weight loss and accumulation of fluid in the abdomen (ascites). Other frequent manifestations are eosinophilia, anemia, hypoalbuminemia, and high alanine aminotransferase (ALT) and aspartate transaminase (ASL) levels in serum. In sheep harboring *C. novyi* spores in the liver, the invasion of juvenile fasciolae can lead to infectious necrotic hepatitis with fatal outcome. Cattle rarely suffer from acute fascioliasis.

The chronic form occurs when the host ingests moderate but sustained doses of metacercariae. Instead of sudden, massive invasion and destruction of the liver, the parasites accumulate over time and eventually reach a pathogenic number after they are already localized in the bile ducts. The symptoms are progressive anemia, weakness, loss of appetite, submandibular edema ("bottle jaw"), ascites, diarrhea, and weight loss. The symptomatology depends on the parasite burden. In sheep, 200 to 700 parasites cause chronic disease and in some cases death, while 700 to 1,400 cause subacute disease and certain death. In cattle, the manifestations of fascioliasis are usually constipation, diarrhea in extreme cases, weakness, and emaciation, especially in young animals. Cattle are more resistant than sheep and can tolerate a larger parasite burden without having any significant clinical manifestations: about 1,400 parasites will cause symptoms in 60% of the animals and a few deaths (Barriga, 1997). The animals' condition worsens when pasturage is scarce and improves when it is abundant, but they are never cured, and the parasitosis has a cumulative effect over the years. In swine, fascioliasis is usually asymptomatic and becomes clinically apparent when debilitating factors, such as malnutrition or concurrent illnesses, are present. The parasitosis has also been described in equines and rabbits.

The pathogenesis, pathology, and symptomatology of the infection caused by *F. gigantica* are similar to those of the parasitosis caused by *F. hepatica.* Both acute and chronic forms are seen in sheep, but cattle have only the chronic form.

Source of Infection and Mode of Transmission: The ecology of fascioliasis is linked to the presence of water, which enables the snails that serve as intermediate hosts to survive, and appropriate temperatures, which allow the parasites to complete their life cycle. Physiographic characteristics, soil composition, and climatic factors determine the reproduction rate of *Lymnaea* and hence the epidemiologic dynamics of the disease. Specimens of *Lymnaea*, as well as cases of fascioliasis, can be found in pasturelands in widely diverse settings throughout the world, from sea level flatlands to Andean valleys at elevations of over 3,700 meters. From the ecologic standpoint, the habitat of *Lymnaea* can be divided into two broad types: primary foci, or reservoirs, and areas of dissemination. The primary foci are located in permanently wet environments such as streams, lakes, lagoons, or canals. The snails are found near the banks, where water flows slowly. They begin to lay their eggs in springtime when temperatures rise above 10°C and continue to do so as long as the thermometer remains above this level. At 9°C the eggs hatch in one month; at 17°C to 19°C, in 17 to 22 days; and at 25°C, in 8 to 12 days. Since new snails begin to lay eggs at 3 weeks of age, they can produce up to three generations in a single season as long as they have enough water. It has been calculated that a single specimen of *L. truncatula* can produce up to 100,000 new snails in one season.

Many snails die during dry, hot summers, but a few of them estivate and resume their development when the temperature falls and moist conditions return. Many of them also die during very cold winters, but some go into hibernation and resume their development when temperatures once again rise above 10°C. The snails that manage to survive dry conditions, heat, and cold are the seeds for the next season's crop of snails. Temperature above 10°C is a key factor in the epidemiology of fascioliasis because when it is any colder the *Fasciola* eggs fail to develop, the snails do not reproduce, the stages do not develop inside the snail, and the cercaria do not encyst. Areas of dissemination are characterized by the alternation of flooding and droughts, and they have large concentrations of *Lymnaea*. Snails may reach these areas directly from original foci carried by rising waters, or they may be reactivated after estivation during dry spells. Seasonal foci of this kind turn pastures into enzootic areas in which serious outbreaks occur. *Fasciola* eggs transmitted by infected animals in springtime and early summer develop inside the snails and produce cercariae and metacercariae until the end of summer. The animals that ingest them begin to show signs of the disease at the end of autumn and during winter. The eggs transmitted by these animals infect more snails, but eggs do not develop until sufficiently warm temperatures return in the spring. Hence the metacercariae from this new cycle appear at the end of spring or in early summer. When ingested by animals, these metacercariae produce symptoms in summer and autumn.

The most important definitive host is the sheep. It has been estimated that a sheep with a mild subclinical infection can contaminate a pasture with more than 500,000 eggs a day, and one with a moderate infection can shed 2.5 to 3 million eggs a day. Sheep are followed in importance by cattle, but their production of *Fasciola* eggs declines rapidly. Many other species of domestic and wild herbivores, including lagomorphs, can also serve as definitive hosts. However, studies done in Australia suggest that some of these latter animals are only temporary hosts and cannot maintain the cycle by themselves for any length of time. Such would be the case with rabbits, which do not contaminate pastures to any significant extent.

Man is infected mainly by eating watercress *(Nasturtium officinale)* infested with metacercariae. In France, where watercress is a popular salad ingredient (10,000 tons are consumed each year), human infection is more frequent than in other European countries. Sometimes raw lettuce and other contaminated plants that are eaten raw can also be a source of infection, as can water from irrigation ditches or other receptacles. Alfalfa juice has also been implicated in places where people drink this beverage.

Role of Animals in the Epidemiology of the Disease: Man is an accidental host. The infection cycle in nature is maintained between animals (especially sheep and cattle) and snails of the family Lymnaeidae. Animals, therefore, serve primarily as a reservoir of infection for man. The epidemiological picture of human fascioliasis appears to have changed in recent years. In the last two decades, the number of human cases has increased in places that are geographically unrelated to areas in which the animal disease is endemic. Mas-Coma *et al.* (1999) believe that this infection has ceased to be a secondary zoonosis and propose a new classification for the epidemiology of the human infection.

Diagnosis: The disease is suspected on the basis of clinical manifestations (painful and febrile hepatomegaly coupled with eosinophilia) and is confirmed by the finding of characteristic eggs in feces. During the acute phase, no eggs can be seen because the parasites have not yet matured, and therefore immunologic tests are often used. However, positive reactions may not appear at such an early stage. In this phase, it is important to distinguish fascioliasis from acute hepatitides due to other causes. Epidemiologic antecedents (abundance of cases in the area, custom of eating watercress) and the presence of peripheral eosinophilia assist in identification. In animals, the diagnosis of acute fascioliasis is often made at autopsy based on observation of hepatic lesions and the presence of immature parasites. The most effective method for finding eggs in feces is sedimentation. Sometimes the parasite can be seen using biliary endoscopy. Ultrasound does not show the migrating parasites during the acute phase and reveals only 50% of the patent cases (Fawzy *et al.*, 1992).

Consumption of beef or lamb's liver may cause trematode eggs to appear in feces and consequently give a false positive result in the coprologic examination. A correct diagnosis can be made after excluding liver from the patient's diet for several days. If fecal observation is negative, bile can be examined by duodenal probe. In a series comparing the two approaches, coprologic observation revealed 68% of the cases, whereas the study of the bile aspirate identified 98% of the cases. In Latin America, there have been cases of unnecessary and prolonged hospitalization of hepatic patients, and sometimes even surgical interventions have been performed, because differential diagnosis failed to take fascioliasis into account. A number of immunobiologic tests have been used in an effort to diagnose the infection during the prepatent period, including a skin test, complement fixation, immunofluorescence, immunoelectrophoresis, counterimmunoelectrophoresis, enzyme-linked immunosorbent assay (ELISA), and immunoelectrotransfer. The prepatent period of fascioliasis lasts for so long (more than two months in humans), that it is one of the few parasitic diseases in which immunology is useful for diagnosis. The search for appropriate antigens has improved the specificity and sensitivity of these tests, but there are still cross-reactions, especially with schistosomiasis. ELISA, used on cysteine proteinase regurgitated by the parasite, has yielded sensitivity levels of 89% to 95% and specificity levels of 98% to 100% (Cordova *et al.*, 1999). Early diagnosis of fascioliasis makes it possible to start treatment before liver damage is too far advanced.

Control: Individuals can prevent fascioliasis by not eating raw watercress of wild or unknown origin. Watercress can be cultivated under controlled conditions that prevent access by animals, and therefore fecal contamination, as well as infestation by snails. However, most watercress sold in markets has been gathered by persons who are unaware of the sanitary conditions under which the plant was grown. Rinsing the greens for 10 minutes in running water washes away only 50% of the metacercariae, but citric acid (10 ml/L), commercial vinegar (120 ml/L), liquid soap (12 ml/L), or potassium permanganate (24 mg/L) will detach or kill them all (el-Sayad et al., 1997).

A modern plan for the control of animal fascioliasis, which would ultimately forestall human infection, would include: a) preventing the consumption of metacercariae, b) strategically administering fasciolicides to the definitive hosts, and c) eliminating the intermediate hosts. Preventing the ingestion of *Fasciola* metacercariae involves fencing in contaminated areas, which is difficult, expensive, and not very effective. The strategic administration of fasciolicides, unlike curative treatment, is aimed at interrupting the life cycle of the parasite by treating animals according to a regimen that will prevent the initial infection, the formation of eggs, and, finally, contamination of the environment. There are now highly sophisticated methods for calculating the best time to administer such treatments (Yilma and Malone, 1998). Previously, some of the chemical compounds against *Fasciola* killed only the adult or juvenile specimens, but now broad-spectrum treatments are available. Controlling snails involves ecologic, chemical, and biologic methods. The ecologic approach consists of modifying the environment to interrupt the life cycle of the snails. Drainage of the land, where this is technically and economically feasible, is the one permanent way to control or eliminate the mollusks. It is also beneficial to smooth the banks of watercourses and remove marginal vegetation to prevent the formation of backwater pools where the snails flourish. The chemical approach consists of applying molluscicides. Given the impressive capacity of *Limnaea* spp. for reproduction and recuperation, molluscicides should be applied regularly to keep down the snail population. This approach is very costly and therefore cannot be applied on a large scale on most livestock-raising establishments in the developing countries. However, it can be used on small farms. In temperate climates, molluscicides should be applied for the first time in spring, when the snails are beginning to reproduce. Application can be repeated in mid-summer to kill the snails before the cercariae are released, and again in autumn, to reduce the population going into hibernation. In climates with only two seasons (dry and rainy), molluscicides should be applied at the beginning and end of the rainy season. Many traditional molluscicides are inactivated by organic materials and elevated pH levels. The biologic approach involves enlisting the natural enemies of the snails that serve as intermediate hosts. Although there are many known competitors, predators, and parasites of snails, this subject has not been fully studied. Vaccination against *Fasciola* might be an appropriate control method, but most researchers have found that sheep do not produce significant protective immunity against this parasite.

Bibliography

Abdel Wahab, M.F., T.A. Younis, I.A. Fahmy, I.M. el Gindy. Parasitic infections presenting as prolonged fevers. *J Egypt Soc Parasitol* 26:509–516, 1996.

Apt, W., X. Aguilera, F. Vega, *et al.* Prevalencia de fascioliasis en humanos, caballos, cerdos y conejos silvestres, en tres provincias de Chile. *Bol Oficina Sanit Panam* 115:405–414, 1992.

Arjona, R., J.A. Riancho, J.M. Aguado, R. Salesa, J. González-Macías. Fascioliasis in developed countries: A review of classic and aberrant forms of the disease. *Medicine (Baltimore)* 74:13–23, 1995.

Bargues, M.D., S. Mas-Coma. Phylogenetic analysis of lymnaeid snails based on 18S rDNA sequences. *Mol Biol Evol* 14:569–577, 1997.

Barriga, O.O. *Veterinary Parasitology for Practitioners*, 2nd ed. Edina: Burgess International Group; 1997.

Bechtel, U., H.E. Feucht, E. Held, T. Vogl, H.D. Nothdurft. *Fasciola hepatica*—Infektion einer Familie. Diagnostik und Therapie. *Dtsch Med Wochenschr* 117:978–982, 1992.

Boray, J.C. Fascioliasis. *In*: Hillyer, G.V., C.E. Hopla, section eds. Section C, vol. 3: *CRC Handbook Series in Zoonoses*. Boca Raton: CRC Press; 1982.

Chen, M.G. *Fasciola hepatica* infection in China. *Southeast Asian J Trop Med Public Health* 22 Suppl:356–360, 1991.

Cong, M.Y., G. Perera de Puga, J.R. Ferrer López. Identificación conquiológica de moluscos huéspedes de *Fasciola hepatica* en Cuba. *Rev Cubana Med Trop* 43:202–203, 1991.

Cordova, M., L. Reategui, J.R. Espinoza. Immunodiagnosis of human fascioliasis with *Fasciola hepatica* cysteine proteinases. *Trans R Soc Trop Med Hyg* 93:54–57, 1999.

Curtale, F., M. Nabil, A. el Wakeel, M.Y. Shamy. Anaemia and intestinal parasitic infections among school age children in Behera Governorate, Egypt. Behera Survey Team. *J Trop Pediatr* 44:323–328, 1998.

de Gorgolas, M., R. Torres, C. Verdejo, *et al.* Infestación por *Fasciola hepatica*. Biopatología y nuevos aspectos diagnósticos y terapéuticos. *Enferm Infecc Microbiol Clin* 10:514–519, 1992.

Esteban, J.G., A. Flores, R. Angles, W. Strauss, C. Aguirre, S. Mas-Coma. A population-based coprological study of human fascioliasis in a hyperendemic area of the Bolivian Altiplano. *Trop Med Int Health* 2(7):695–699, 1997.

Esteban, J.G., A. Flores, R. Angles, S. Mas-Coma. High endemicity of human fascioliasis between Lake Titicaca and La Paz valley, Bolivia. *Trans R Soc Trop Med Hyg* 93:151–156, 1999.

Espino, A.M., A. Díaz, A. Pérez, C.M. Finlay. Dynamics of antigenemia and coproantigens during a human *Fasciola hepatica* outbreak. *J Clin Microbiol* 36:2723–2726, 1998.

Faiguenbaum, J., A. Feres, R. Doncaster, *et al.* Fascioliasis (distomatosis) hepática humana. *Bol Chile Parasitol* 17:7–12, 1962.

Fawzy, R.K., A.E. Salem, M.M. Osman. Ultrasonographic findings in the gall bladder in human fascioliasis. *J Egypt Soc Parasitol* 22:827–831, 1992.

García, L.S., D.A. Bruckner. *Diagnostic Medical Parasitology*, 3rd ed. Washington, D.C.: ASM Press; 1997.

el-Karaksy, H., B. Hassanein, S. Ocaza, B. Behairy, I. Gadallah. Human fascioliasis in Egyptian children: Successful treatment with triclabendazole. *J Trop Pediatr* 45:135–138, 1999.

Malek, E.A. Vol. 2: *Snail-transmitted Parasitic Diseases*. Boca Raton: CRC Press; 1980.

Mas-Coma, M.S., J.G. Esteban, M.D. Bargues. Epidemiology of human fascioliasis: A review and proposed new classification. *Bull World Health Organ* 77:340–346, 1999.

Mora, J. A., R. Arroyo, S. Molina, L. Troper, E. Irias. Nuevos aportes sobre el valor de la fasciolina. Estudio en un área endémica de Costa Rica. *Bol Oficina Sanit Panam* 89:409–414, 1980.

el-Newihi, H.M., I.A. Waked, A.A. Mihas. Biliary complications of *Fasciola hepatica*: The role of endoscopic retrograde cholangiography in management. *J Clin Gastroenterol* 21:309–311, 1995.

el-Sayad, M.H., A.F. Alam, M.M. Osman. Prevention of human fascioliasis: A study on the role of acids detergents and potassium permenganate in clearing salads from metacercariae. *J Egypt Soc Parasitol* 27:163–169, 1997.

Soulsby, E.J.L. *Helminths, Arthropods and Protozoa of Domesticated Animals*, 7th ed. Philadelphia: Lea and Febiger; 1982.

Srihakim, S., M. Pholpark. Problem of fascioliasis in animal husbandry in Thailand. *Southeast Asian J Trop Med Public Health* 22 Suppl:352–355, 1991.

Yilma, J.M., J.B. Malone. A geographic information system forecast model for strategic control of fasciolosis in Ethiopia. *Vet Parasitol* 78:103–127, 1998.

el Zawawy, L.A., S.F. el Nassery, M.Z. al Azzouni, *et al.* A study on patients with eosinophilia of suspected parasitic origin. *J Egypt Soc Parasitol* 25:245–255, 1995.

FASCIOLOPSIASIS

ICD-10 B66.5

Etiology: The agent of this infection is *Fasciolopsis buski,* a large, thick, reddish trematode (up to 75 mm long, 20 mm wide, and 3 mm thick) that lives attached to the mucosa of the duodenum and jejunum in humans and swine. The eggs eliminated in the feces must incubate for 16 to 18 days in still water at 30°C to form the first juvenile stage (miracidium) (Soulsby, 1982). Studies in China have found that the eggs need oxygen (they do not tolerate anaerobic conditions) and survive for three to four months at 4°C. The miracidium emerges from the mature egg and penetrates small planorbid snails, mainly of the genera *Gyraulus, Segmentina, Helicorbis, Hippeutis*, and *Polypylis*. In mollusks, the miracidium passes through the sporocyst stage and two generations of rediae. The second generation of rediae gives rise to large numbers of cercariae, which emerge from the snails and encyst as metacercariae on aquatic plants. The studies in China have found that almost 4% of the metacercariae encyst in the water. The definitive hosts, humans or swine, become infected by consuming aquatic plants or water with metacercariae. In the intestine, the metacercaria is released from its envelope, and after about three months, the parasite reaches maturity and reinitiates the cycle by oviposition.

Geographic Distribution and Occurrence: The infection is common in southeast Asia (Waikagul, 1991). The parasitosis occurs in Bangladesh, central and southern China, India, the Indochina peninsula, Indonesia, and Taiwan. Cases have also been reported, many of them among immigrants, in the Philippines, Japan, and several Western countries. Some 10 million people are estimated to have this parasite. Prevalence is very variable but generally low in humans and is thought to be higher in the areas where swine are raised. In some Thai villages, the infection affects up to 70% of the population. In several areas of Chekiang and Kiangsi Provinces, China, the prevalence can be as high as 85%; in contrast, in other areas of the country infection rates ranging from less than 1% to 5% are found. The prevalence of *F. buski* and other geohelminthiases (amebiases) has declined strikingly in this country, but the prevalence of foodborne parasites (trichinosis, cysticercosis, clonorchiasis, paragonimiasis) has increased. In a study of 5,479 randomly chosen persons in China in 1995, 0.8% were infected. Approximately half of all human infections are believed to occur in China (Malek, 1980). The most affected age group is 4- to 13-year-olds. A study conducted in an endemic area of Thailand found that the prevalence of infection in humans was similar to that of the swine population. The swine were also found to harbor fewer parasites, which produced fewer eggs than those lodged in the human intestine (Manning and Ratanarat, 1970). In some areas of China with high rates of human infection, the parasitosis in swine has not been confirmed. This would seem to indicate that, at least in some areas, humans are the parasite's preferred host.

The Disease in Man and Animals: This parasite produces few or no symptoms in most hosts. Perhaps because it is the largest trematode affecting man, traumatic, toxic, and obstructive effects have been attributed to it, with epigastric pain, nausea, diarrhea, undigested food in the feces, and edemas of the face, abdomen, and legs. Yet a clinical study of a group of mostly young persons in Thailand who were eliminating *F. buski* eggs and of a control group found that both groups showed mild gastrointestinal symptoms (Plaut *et al.*, 1969). The severe disease described in the literature seemingly corresponds to cases with a large parasite burden (Liu and Harinasuta, 1996).

Only 3 to 12 parasites are usually found in naturally infected pigs. By and large, the health of the pigs is not affected, and the symptoms of the disease occur only in cases of massive parasitosis.

Source of Infection and Mode of Transmission: The source of infection for humans and swine is aquatic plants and water containing metacercariae. Epidemiological research in China suggests that between 10% and 13% of persons and from 35% to 40% of swine are infected more from drinking water contaminated with metacercariae than from eating plants. Endemic areas offer the ecological conditions necessary for the growth of both the intermediate hosts and the edible aquatic plants. In central Thailand, these conditions occur in flooded fields, where edible aquatic plants are cultivated near dwellings. These fields receive human excreta directly from the houses, which are built on pillars. Human and animal excreta promote the development of mollusks and plants and provide the infective material (the parasite's eggs) for the host. The hosts are the snails *Hippeutis umbilicalis* and *Segmentina trochoideus* in Bangladesh, in addition to *Polypylis hemisphaerula* in China, Thailand, and Taiwan (Gilman *et al.*, 1982). It has also been found that *Helicorbis umbilicalis* is an intermediate host in Laos (Ditrich *et al.*, 1992). The epidemiologically important aquatic plants, whose fruits, pods, roots, bulbs, or stems are eaten by humans, are "water chestnuts" (*Eliocharis* spp., *Trapa* spp.), the lotus *Nymphaea lotus*, and others of the genera *Eichhornia, Ipomoea, Neptunia,* and *Zizania*. Certain parts of these plants are eaten raw, and the teeth and lips are often used to peel the pods and bulbs. In areas where people customarily boil the plants or their "fruits" (water chestnuts) before eating them but give them raw to swine, the infection rate is much higher in these animals than in humans. In general, the prevalence of human infection is higher in areas where the aquatic plants are cultivated and lower in distant towns, since metacercariae attached to the plants are not resistant to desiccation when some time elapses between harvest and marketing. The pig is considered a reservoir of the parasite that could maintain the infection in the human population even if the sanitary elimination of human excreta were achieved. In Muslim countries, such as Bangladesh, swine do not play any role as a reservoir; man is practically the only reservoir and only source of infection for snails (Gilman *et al.*, 1982). The infection can be imported by patients into regions where intermediate hosts exist; one study found that 3 of 93 Thai workers in Israel were infected by *F. buski*.

Diagnosis: The infection is suspected on the basis of symptoms and epidemiological conditions and is confirmed by the discovery of *F. buski* eggs in fecal matter. The eggs are very similar to those of *Fasciola gigantica* and *Fasciola hepatica*; experts say that the eggs of *F. buski* (128–140 μm by 78–85 μm) cannot be distinguished from those of *F. hepatica* (128–150 μm by 60–90 μm) (Zeibig, 1997). The parasite itself can easily be identified when found in vomit or fecal matter. There are no reports on attempts at immunological diagnosis, but the parasite has shown cross-reactions in tests for *Fasciola hepatica*, the larva of *Taenia solium*, and *Trichinella spiralis*.

Control: The simplest way to prevent human parasitosis is to refrain from eating fresh or raw aquatic plants, peeling them with the teeth, or drinking water from contaminated areas, but this recommendation requires changing a habit, which is difficult to achieve. Studies conducted in China have shown that immersing contaminated plants in boiling water for 1 to 2 minutes is sufficient to kill the parasite. Other measures to combat the parasitosis, in addition to health education, are to use molluscicides, to treat the affected population, to treat the human excreta in septic tanks or with quicklime, to prevent the fertilization of fields with human feces, and to prohibit swine raising in endemic areas.

Bibliography

Ditrich O., V. Nasincova, T. Scholz, M. Giboda. Larval stages of medically important flukes (*Trematoda*) from Vientiane province, Laos. Part II. Cercariae. *Ann Parasitol Hum Comp* 67(3):75–81, 1992.

Gilman, R.H., G. Mondal, M. Maksud, *et al.* Endemic focus of *Fasciolopsis buski* infection in Bangladesh. *Am J Trop Med Hyg* 31(4):796–802, 1982.

Liu, L.X., K.T. Harinasuta. Liver and intestinal flukes. *Gastroenterol Clin North Am* 25(3):627–636, 1996.

Malek, E.A. Vol. 2: *Snail-transmitted Parasitic Diseases.* Boca Raton: CRC Press; 1980.

Manning, G.S., C. Ratanarat. *Fasciolopsis buski* (Lankester, 1857) in Thailand. *Am J Trop Med Hyg* 19(4):613–619, 1970.

Plaut, A.G., C. Kampanart-Sanyakorn, G.S. Manning. A clinical study of *Fasciolopsis buski* infection in Thailand. *Trans R Soc Trop Med Hyg* 63(4):470–478, 1969.

Soulsby, E.J.L. *Helminths, Arthropods and Protozoa of Domesticated Animals*, 7th ed. Philadelphia: Lea and Febiger; 1982.

Waikagul, J. Intestinal fluke infections in Southeast Asia. *Southeast Asian J Trop Med Public Health 22* Suppl:158–162, 1991.

Zeibig, E.A. *Clinical Parasitology: A Practical Approach.* Philadelphia: W.B. Saunders; 1997.

GASTRODISCOIDIASIS

ICD-10 B66.8 Other specified fluke infections

Synonym: Amphistomiasis.

Etiology: The agent of this infection is *Gastrodiscoides (Amphistomum) hominis*, a bright-pink, pear-shaped trematode 5–14 mm long by 4–66 mm wide; it lives in the cecum and ascending colon of swine and humans, although it has also been found in monkeys and field rats (Soulsby, 1982). The anterior part of the parasite is conical, but the posterior opens into a disc with a suction cup. The eggs leave the host without embryonating and take 16 to 17 days, at 27°C to 34°C, to form the first juvenile stage (miracidium) and hatch (Neva, 1994). In experiments in India, miracidia were able to produce infection in the planorbid snail *Helicorbis coenosus*, which may be the natural intermediate host. Details of development in the snail are not known, but judging from the cycle of other members of the same family, they are presumed to form oocysts, one or two generations of rediae, and cercariae. Depending on the ambient temperature, the cercariae begin to emerge from the snails 28 to 152 days after infection. Like those of other species of Gastrodiscidae, the cercariae are thought to encyst on aquatic plants and develop into metacercariae. The definitive hosts are infected by ingesting the metacercariae. It has been suggested that *G. hominis* in humans and swine could be different strains or varieties.

Geographic Distribution and Occurrence: This parasitosis occurs primarily in India (states of Assam, Bihar, Orissa, and West Bengal) and in Bangladesh, but has also been recorded in the Philippines, the Indochina peninsula, and in animals in Indonesia (Java), Malaysia, Myanmar, and Thailand. It has been observed in Indian immigrants in Guyana. The geographic distribution may be wider, since the parasite was found in a wild boar in Kazakhstan. Human infection rates vary and can be very high, as in a village in Assam, India, where 41% of the population, mostly children, had the parasite's eggs in their stools. Oddly enough, swine are not abundant in this area.

In a slaughterhouse in India, the parasite was found in 27% of 233 pigs examined. The infection is also found in rodents and several species of nonhuman primates in Asia: rhesus monkeys (*Macaca mulatta*) and cynomologus monkeys (*M. fascicularis, M. irus,* and *M. philippinensis*). The infection rate in 1,201 cynomologus monkeys (*M. fascicularis*) was 21.4%. The infection rate in swine in India is higher in late summer and early autumn, reaching its peak between June and September (Roy and Tandon, 1992).

The Disease in Man and Animals: The infection is clinically apparent probably only when the parasite burden is large. In these cases, there reportedly may be alterations of the mucosa of the colon and cecum, colitis, and mucoid diarrhea (Strickland, 1991).

Source of Infection and Mode of Transmission: The natural definitive host appears to be swine, in which high rates of infection have been found. The parasite has also been found in monkeys and rodents. In general, man is considered to be a secondary definitive host. However, the true relationship between the human and animal trematodes is not yet well known, nor has it been determined experimentally whether the animal parasites are transmitted to man. In some areas in India, the human infection occurs without infection in swine. The reverse situation has also been observed (Malek, 1980). The definitive hosts acquire the infection through the digestive tract, perhaps by ingesting aquatic plants or untreated water containing metacercariae.

Diagnosis: Diagnosis is based on detection of the presence of eggs in feces or, more easily, on identification of the trematode following administration of an antihelminthic to the affected person. The eggs of *Gastrodiscoides* (150–170 μm by 60–70 μm) resemble those of *Fasciolopsis buski*, but are narrower and greenish.

Control: Since the lifecycle of the parasite is not known, it is difficult to recommend control measures. Nonetheless, for individual protection it is suggested that people in endemic areas not consume aquatic plants or untreated water. For prevention through treatment of the animal reservoir, the best time is mid-summer, before the infection reaches its highest prevalence (Roy and Tandon, 1992).

Bibliography

Dutt, S.C., H.D. Srivastara. The life history of *Gastrodiscoides hominis* (Lewis and McConnel, 1876) Leiper, 1913—the amphistome parasite of man and pig. *J Helminthol* 46(1):35–46, 1972.

Faust, E.C., P.C. Beaver, R.C. Jung. *Animal Agents and Vectors of Human Disease*, 4th ed. Philadelphia: Lea & Febiger; 1975.

Malek, E.A. Vol. 2: *Snail-transmitted Parasitic Diseases*. Boca Raton: CRC Press; 1980.

Neva, F.A. *Basic Clinical Parasitology*, 6th ed. Norwalk, Connecticut: Appleton & Lange; 1994.

Roy, B., V. Tandon. Seasonal prevalence of some zoonotic trematode infections in cattle and pigs in the north-east montane zone in India. *Vet Parasitol* 41(1–2):69–76, 1992.

Soulsby, E.J.L. *Helminths, Arthropods and Protozoa of Domesticated Animals*, 7th ed. Philadelphia: Lea & Febiger; 1982.

Strickland, G.T., ed. *Hunter's Tropical Medicine*, 7th ed. Philadelphia: Saunders; 1991.

HETEROPHYIASIS

ICD-10 B66.8 Other specified fluke infections

Synonyms: Heterophydiasis, heterophyes infection (small intestine).

Etiology: The agents of this infection are trematodes of the family Heterophyidae, which infect the intestine of man and other vertebrates. As of 1980, Malek (1980) had recognized 10 species in the world that were infective for man, the most common being *Heterophyes heterophyes*, *Heterophyes nocens*, *Metagonimus yokogawai*, and *Stellantchasmus falcatus*. The others on this list were *Cryptocotyle (Tocotrema) lingua*, *Haplorchis calderoni*, *Haplorchis taichui*, *Haplorchis vanissima*, *Haplorchis* *yokogawai*, and *Stamnosoma armatum*. In 1991, Chai and Lee (1991) added six more species that had infected man in the Republic of Korea: *Centrocestus armatus*, *Heterophyes dispar*, *Heterophyopsis continua*, *M. takahashii*, *Pygidiopsis summa*, and *Stictodora fuscatum*. Later *Metagonimus miyatai*, which for a while had been considered a type of *M. yokogawai*, was described in patients in the Republic of Korea and Japan (Saito *et al.*, 1997). Genetic studies have differentiated the two species (Yu *et al.*, 1997). The most important species from the medical standpoint are *H. heterophyes* and *M. yokogawai*. For example, in a study carried out in Korea, 5 patients under treatment produced a total of 3,007 specimens of *M. yokogawai*, 120 of *H. nocens,* and 46 of *S. falcatus* (Chai *et al.*, 1998).

All the heterophyids have a similar biological cycle: the first intermediate host is an appropriate aquatic snail (*Cerithidea, Cleopatra, Melania, Pironella, Semisulcospira, Tympanotomus*), which ingests the mature eggs, and in which the cercariae are produced. In addition, there is a second intermediate host in which the metacercariae are produced—usually one of a large variety of fish that live in fresh or brackish water. The second intermediate hosts of *C. armatus, M. takahashii,* and *M. yokogawai* are freshwater fish; those of *H. continua, H. nocens, P. summa, S. falcatus,* and *S. fuscatum* are found in brackish water (Chai and Lee, 1991); and those of *H. heterophyes*, in estuaries and fresh or brackish water. Because of their public health importance, *H. heterophyes* and *M. yokogawai* are covered here in detail.

H. heterophyes is a very small pyriform trematode measuring 1–1.7 mm long by 0.3–0.4 mm wide that lives in the small intestine of humans, cats, dogs, foxes, and other fish-eating mammals or birds. When observed in host feces, the eggs contain a completely developed miracidium, which must be ingested by an appropriate aquatic snail (first intermediate host) in order to continue its development cycle. Once inside the snail (in Egypt, *Pirenella* spp.; in Japan, *Cerithidea cingulata* and *Semisulcospira libertina*), the miracidia give rise to sporocysts, which in turn give rise to one or two generations of rediae, and the last in turn to cercariae. The cercariae invade the second intermediate host, which may be one of about a dozen species of fish from fresh or brackish water that customarily spawn in brackish or salt water. The cercariae form cysts under the scales or in the musculature of these fish and transform into metacercariae. In Egypt, metacercariae are found primarily in mullet (*Mugil*), *Tilapia*, and a few other species, and in Japan, in several species of goby belonging to the genus *Acanthogobius*. When man or another definitive host eats raw fish containing metacercariae, the parasites are released from the cystic envelope and develop inside the intestine until they turn into adult trematodes, which start to lay eggs in about nine days.

M. yokogawai measures 1–2.5 mm long by 0.4–0.8 mm wide and lives in the small intestine of humans, dogs, cats, swine, pelicans, and possibly other piscivorous birds. The development cycle is similar to that of *H. heterophyes*. The first intermediate hosts are snails of the genera *Semisulcospira, Hua,* or *Thiara*; the second intermediate hosts are fish belonging to the salmon and trout families.

Geographic Distribution and Occurrence: *H. heterophyes*, and probably *H. dispar*, are found in Southeast Asia, the Near and Middle East, Turkey, the Balkans, and Spain. The largest endemic focus is in the Nile Delta, where conditions are especially favorable for propagation of this parasitosis: enormous numbers of *Pirenella* snails live at the bottom of the delta's brackish lagoons, mullet is abundant, the population traditionally eats raw fish, and facilities for sanitary waste disposal are inadequate. Most of the mullet contain metacercariae, with counts as high as 6,000 metacercariae per fish, and almost all the dogs and cats are infected. In one locality, it was estimated that 65% of the schoolchildren had parasites. In addition to the endemic and hyperendemic areas already mentioned, a very low prevalence of *H. heterophyes* has been recorded in western Africa.

A high prevalence of *H. nocens* was reported in Yamaguchi Prefecture in Japan. However, subsequent surveys in other prefectures showed prevalence rates of less than 1% (Malek, 1980). In 1994, Chai *et al.* (1994) found a large focus of *H. nocens* in the Republic of Korea: 43% of 98 persons were infected.

M. yokogawai is found primarily in the Far East and the northern provinces of Siberia. It is seen less often in central Europe and has also been reported in Spain. In a hospital in Seoul, Korea, a total of 52,552 fecal samples were examined between 1984 and 1992, and the only heterophyid observed was *M. yokogawai*, which was present in 1.2% of the samples (Lee *et al.*, 1994). Also, a 1991 study in Korea found *Metagonimus* spp. in 12% of the males and 6% of the females examined, with more intense infections in males. The prevalence was higher in persons over 30 years old, but there was no correlation between age and intensity. Eight species of freshwater fish were found to be infected with metacercariae. In 1993, 465 persons and 68 fish were studied along the Hantan River in Korea and it was determined that 3.4% of the people and 21% of the fish were infected with *M. miyatai* (Park *et al.*, 1993). Ahn (1993) found *Metagonimus* infection in 7.8% of 1,067 individuals examined in Korea, with rates ranging between 3.8% and 12.8% in 5 different riverbank areas. In fish, the infection rate was 81% in the 318 specimens studied.

The range of *S. falcatus* includes Australia, Hawaii (USA), Indonesia, Japan, the Philippines, Thailand, and the Middle East.

The Disease in Man and Animals: Mild infections are usually asymptomatic. A large parasite burden can cause irritation of the intestinal mucosa with excessive secretion of mucus, superficial necrosis of the epithelium, chronic diarrhea, colic, and nausea. Aberrant eggs of the parasite sometimes enter the bloodstream and produce granulomatous foci in various tissues and organs, including the myocardium and brain. In the Philippines, it is believed that 15% of the cases of fatal myocarditis may be caused by the eggs of these parasites (García and Bruckner, 1997). Nevertheless, most human cases are benign. In *M. yokogawai* infections, parasites have been found both free-living in the lumen and encrusted in the intervillous spaces. Other observations have included massive infiltrations of lymphocytes, plasmocytes, and eosinophils in the stroma, erosion of neighboring enterocytes, depletion of globet cells, and occasionally, edema of the villi (Chi *et al.*, 1988).

The picture is similar in animals. The infection is clinically apparent only when the number of parasites is large. In 1962, a metacercarial organism similar to *S. falcatus*, provisionally labeled "agent SF," was isolated in Japan from dogs in which it was causing mild disease. It is now known that the RNA sequences of this agent are 99.1% homologous with *Ehrlichia risticii*, the organism that causes Potomac horse fever, and 98.7% homologous with *E. sennetsu*, which infects humans in western Japan (Wen *et al.*, 1996). Its transmission would be similar to that of the canine rickettsia *Neorickettsia helminthoeca* via the trematode *Nanophyetus salmincola* (Soulsby, 1982).

Source of Infection and Mode of Transmission: The source of infection for man, other mammals, and birds is fish (from fresh, brackish, or salt water) infected with the parasite metacercariae. The custom of eating raw or undercooked fish is the main cause of the human infection. The critical host, because of its specificity, is the snail. The parasite is less selective regarding the second intermediate host, which can be one of a number of fish species found in fresh, brackish, or salt water, and even certain shrimp. Contamination of the water with human or animal excreta ensures completion of the parasite's development cycle. The primary definitive hosts vary depending on the parasite species: for some it is piscivorous birds; for others, dogs, cats, or man. Other definitive hosts include numerous species of birds and wild animals that feed on fish.

Diagnosis: Diagnosis is based on the microscopic observation of parasite eggs in fecal matter. The eggs of *H. heterophyes* and *M. yokogawai* (Zeibig, 1997), as well as those of *Clonorchis* and *Opisthorchis*, are all virtually indistinguishable. The surface structure of the eggs is a more reliable criterion than traditional morphology, but it is more difficult to visualize (Ditrich *et al.*, 1992). The species can be identified by examining the adult trematodes following anthelminthic treatment. There is no information on the diagnosis of heterophyiasis using immunologic tests, but experimental infection has demonstrated cross-reactions: 10% with antigens of schistosome eggs, and 35% with raw extract of *Fasciola* (Hassan *et al.*, 1989).

Control: The human infection can be prevented through education aimed at promoting the thorough cooking of fish and the proper disposal of excreta. Metacercariae survive up to seven days in fish preserved in brine and for several days if they are marinated in vinegar. Dogs and cats should not be fed raw fish or scraps containing raw fish because they can become infected, contaminate the environment, and thus maintain an ongoing infection cycle.

Bibliography

Ahn, Y.K. [Intestinal flukes of genus *Metagonimus* and their second intermediate hosts in Kangwon-do]. *Korean J Parasitol* 31:331–340, 1993.

Chai, J.Y., S.H. Lee. Intestinal trematodes infecting humans in Korea. *Southeast Asian J Trop Med Public Health* 22 Suppl:163–170, 1991.

Chai, J.Y., H.K. Nam, J. Kook, S.H. Lee. The first discovery of an endemic focus of *Heterophyes nocens* (Heterophyidae) infection in Korea. *Korean J Parasitol* 32:157–161, 1994.

Chai, J.Y., T.E. Song, E.T. Han, *et al.* Two endemic foci of heterophyids and other intestinal fluke infections in southern and western coastal areas in Korea. *Korean J Parasitol* 36:155–161, 1998.

Chi, J.G., C.W. Kim, J.R. Kim, S.T. Hong, S.H. Lee. Intestinal pathology in human metagonimiasis with ultrastructural observations of parasites. *J Korean Med Sci* 3:171–177, 1988.

Ditrich, O., M. Giboda, T. Scholz, S.A. Beer. Comparative morphology of eggs of the Haplorchiinae (Trematoda: Heterophyidae) and some other medically important heterophyid and opisthorchiid flukes. *Folia Parasitol (Praha)* 39:123–132, 1992.

García, L.S., D.A. Bruckner. *Diagnostic Medical Parasitology,* 3rd ed. Washington, D.C.: ASM Press; 1997.

Hassan, M.M., A.M. Farghaly, R.L. el-Gamal, A.M. el-Ridi. Cross-reactions in immunodiagnosis of patients infected with *Schistosoma, Fasciola* and *Heterophyes* using ELISA. *J Egypt Soc Parasitol* 19(2 Suppl):845–851, 1989.

Hong, S.J., C.K. Chung, D.H. Lee, H.C. Woo. One human case of natural infection by *Heterophyopsis continua* and three other species of intestinal trematodes. *Korean J Parasitol* 34:87–89, 1996.

Lee, S.K., B.M. Shin, N.S. Chung, J.Y. Chai, S.H. Lee. [Second report on intestinal parasites among the patients of Seoul Paik Hospital, 1984–1992]. *Korean J Parasitol* 32:27–33, 1994.

Malek, E.A. Vol. 2: *Snail-transmitted Parasitic Diseases.* Boca Raton: CRC Press; 1980.

Park, M.S., S.W. Kim, Y.S. Yang, *et al.* Intestinal parasite infections in the inhabitants along the Hantan River, Chorwon-Gun. *Korean J Parasitol* 31:375–378, 1993.

Saito, S., J.Y. Chai, K.H. Kim, S.H. Lee, H.J. Rim. *Metagonimus miyatai* sp. nov. (Digenea: Heterophyidae), a new intestinal trematode transmitted by freshwater fish in Japan and Korea. *Korean J Parasitol* 35:223–232, 1997.

Soulsby, E.J.L. *Helminths, Arthropods and Protozoa of Domesticated Animals,* 7th ed. Philadelphia: Lea & Febiger; 1982.

Yu, J.R., J.S. Chung, J.Y Chai. Different RAPD patterns between *Metagonimus yokogawai* and *Metagonimus Miyata* type. *Korean J Parasitol* 35:295–298, 1977.

Wen, B., Y. Rikihisa, S. Yamamoto, N. Kawabata, P.A. Fuerst. Characterization of the SF agent, an *Ehrlichia* sp. isolated from the fluke *Stellantchasmus falcatus,* by 16S rRNA base sequence, serological, and morphological analyses. *Int J Syst Bacteriol* 46:149–154, 1996.

Zeibig, E.A. *Clinical Parasitology: A Practical Approach.* Philadelphia: Saunders; 1997.

NANOPHYETIASIS

ICD-10 B66.8 Other specified fluke infections

Synonyms: Elokomin fluke fever, salmon poisoning (in animals).

Etiology: The agent of this disease is *Nanophyetus* (*Troglotrema*) *salmincola,* a small digenetic intestinal trematode of several carnivores that also infects man. On the basis of several biological differences and their geographic distribution, two sub-species are recognized: *N. salmincola salmincola* in the northwestern US and *N. salmincola schikhobalowi* in Siberia, Russian Federation.

The adult trematode lives in the small intestine of coyotes, cats, lynxes, raccoons, nutrias, dogs, minks, foxes, and other carnivores. It can also infect fish-eating birds and humans. Thirty-two species can be natural or experimental hosts of the trematode. The parasites are tiny (0.8–2.5 mm by 0.3–0.5 mm) and require two intermediate hosts to develop. The first is a snail of the family Pleuroceridae. In the US, it has been identified as *Goniobasis plicifera, Juga* sp., *Oxytrema plicifer* var. *silicula,* and *O. silicula,* but its classification still appears uncertain. In Siberia, it has been identified as *Semisulcospira cancellata, S. laevigata,* and *Juga* sp. (Besprozvannykh, 1994). The second host is a specimen of the salmon family (*Onchorhynchus, Salmo, Salvelinus,* etc.) and, less frequently, of other families (Cottidae, Cyprinidae, lampreys, and even the Pacific giant salamander) (Soulsby, 1982). The eggs eliminated in the feces of the definitive hosts are not embryonated and must remain in the water for 87 to 200 days for the miracidium to form completely. It then leaves the egg, penetrates a snail, and multiplies through two generations of rediae to form the cercariae that leave the snail. These swim around and penetrate the skin of an appropriate fish and ultimately encyst in the kidneys, muscles, fins, and secondarily, any other organ. The metacercariae measure between 0.11 mm and 0.25 mm in diameter, become infective to the definitive host in 10 or 11 days, and can survive up to five years in live fish. When a definitive host ingests raw fish with metacercariae, they de-encyst, reach maturity in the intestine, and begin oviposition in five to eight days.

Geographic Distribution and Occurrence: *N. s. salmincola* is distributed along the Pacific coast of the US, mainly in Oregon. Until 1989, about a dozen human cases had been reported in that country (Fritsche *et al.*, 1989). *N. s. schikhobalowi* is distributed in the northern part of Sakhalin Island and along the mountain tributaries of the Amur River in eastern Siberia. The rate of human infection in some of the villages along these tributaries can reach 98%. The distribution of nanophyetiasis is determined by the presence of the species of the first intermediate host, the snail. In the US, the snail is *Oxytrema silicula*, and in Siberia, *Semisulcospira cancellata* and *S. laevigata*.

The Disease in Man: The infection causes clinical manifestations only when there are abundant parasites (Fang *et al.*, 1991). Half of the patients studied by Fritsche *et al.* (1989) showed only eosinophilia, but the other half complained of gastrointestinal symptoms. The most frequent symptoms were chronic diarrhea, nausea, abdominal pain, and high peripheral eosinophilia (Harrell and Deardorff, 1990).

Mild infections by *N. s. schikhobalowi* are asymptomatic. Patients with a parasite burden of 500 or more flukes experience diarrhea (43%), gastric pain (32%), constipation (16%), and nocturnal salivation (16%).

The Disease in Animals: In canines the de-encysted parasite attaches to the mucosa of the small intestine. In the US, different parasites can produce superficial enteritis that could even cause bleeding, but they commonly cause few or no symptoms. The principal significance of the parasite in the US, however, is that in all of its states it can harbor the agent of "salmon poisoning" or Elokomin fluke fever.

The name "salmon poisoning" is unfortunate because the disease is actually a rickettsiosis caused by *Neorickettsia helminthoeca*, not a poisoning. This rickettsia affects only canines. The organism is released when the parasite de-encysts and attaches to the canine intestine, but the eggs of the trematode emerge infected and maintain the infection until the metacercariae form and while they remain in the fish. In dogs, the disease manifests itself 5 to 7 days after infection with high fever, complete anorexia, vomiting, bloody diarrhea, thrombocytopenia, general lymphadenopathy, severe weight loss, and mortality of up to 90% in 7 to 10 days if not treated in time.

Elokomin fluke fever affects canines, ferrets, raccoons, and bears, and can occur in conjunction with "salmon poisoning." It is caused by the *Neorickettsia elokominica* rickettsia, which is antigenically distinct from *N. helminthoeca*, although it is transmitted the same way. Although weight loss is also severe, adenopathy is more prevalent than diarrhea, and the mortality among untreated cases is only 10%.

In Siberia, according to observations by Russian researchers, the infection in cats, dogs, brown rats, and badgers by *N. s. schikhobalowi* can cause a severe, fatal disease. On the other hand, it is not known whether the parasites in Siberia transmit any other microorganism.

Fish infected with the trematode can also become sick. Different species of salmonids experimentally exposed to *N. salmincola* showed different degrees of susceptibility. In general, species from the enzootic area were more resistant than those from other areas. Death among fish subjected to massive infections occurred mainly in the first 24 hours, in other words, during the penetration and migration of the cercariae. Although gradual infection probably does not cause as much pathology, most researchers agree that the parasites have pathological effects on fish, especially if vital organs such as the heart and gills are invaded by a large number of migrating cercariae. Infected fish also show stunted development and an impairment in swimming ability (Millemann and Knapp, 1970).

Source of Infection and Mode of Transmission: Both humans and animals contract *N. salmincola* infection by ingesting raw or undercooked fish, especially salmonids, infected with metacercariae of the parasite. Yet there is at least one case of infection from the handling of infected fish, without evidence that there was ingestion (Harrell and Deardorff, 1990).

The source of "salmon poisoning" and Elokomin fluke fever infection is fish infected by the trematode, which in turn is infected by the respective rickettsiae. As indicated, these infections occur only in the US. In areas in both the Russian Federation and the US where the trematode exists, a high rate of infection by metacercariae is found in fish, especially in salmonids.

Diagnosis: Diagnosis is confirmed by observation of the parasite eggs in human or animal feces. The eggs measure 87–97 µm by 35–55 µm, and have a small, indistinct operculum and a small lobe in the opposite end. Rickettsial infections are confirmed by a microscopic examination of biopsies of affected lymphatic ganglia, where intracellular bodies with the typical structure of rickettsiae are seen.

Control: The main prevention measure is to educate the population not to consume undercooked fish or give it to their dogs. Salting or pickling fish does not appear to be very effective because the metacercariae are very resistant: they can survive up to 165 days in fish kept at 3°C.

Bibliography

Besprozvannykh, V.V. [The epizootiological problems of trematodiases in the Maritime Territory]. *Med Parazitol (Mosk)* 3:28–31, 1994.

Fang, G., V. Araujo, R.L Guerrant. Enteric infections associated with exposure to animals or animal products. *Infect Dis Clin North Am* 5:681–701, 1991.

Fritsche, T.R., R.L. Eastburn, L.H. Wiggins, C.A. Terhune, Jr. Praziquantel for treatment of human *Nanophyetus salmincola* (*Troglotrema salmincola*) infection. *J Infect Dis* 160(5):896–899, 1989.

Harrell, L.W., T.L. Deardorff. Human nanophyetiasis: Transmission by handling naturally infected coho salmon (*Oncorhynchus kisutch*). *J Infect Dis* 161(1):146–148, 1990.

Malek, E.A. Vol. 2: *Snail-transmitted Parasitic Diseases*. Boca Raton: CRC Press; 1980.

Millemann, R.E., S.E. Knapp. Biology of *Nanophyetus salmincola* and "salmon poisoning" disease. *Adv Parasitol* 8:1–41, 1970.

Soulsby, E.J.L. *Helminths, Arthropods and Protozoa of Domesticated Animals*, 7th ed. Philadelphia: Lea & Febiger; 1982.

OPISTHORCHIASIS

ICD-10 B66.0

Etiology: The agents of this disease are *Opisthorchis viverrini, O. felineus*, and *Amphimerus pseudofelineus (Opisthorchis guayaquilensis)*, trematodes that lodge in the bile ducts of humans, cats, dogs, and other animals that eat raw fish. It is often difficult to differentiate between the genera *Opisthorchis* and *Clonorchis* and between the species *O. viverrini* and *O. felineus* because the adult specimens are indistinguishable. However, there are clear differences in the excretory system during the preadult stages. The development cycle of *Opisthorchis* is similar to that of *Clonorchis* (see Clonorchiasis), requiring two intermediate hosts: aquatic snails are the first, and various species of freshwater fish are the second.

O. viverrini measures 7–12 mm by 1.5–2.5 mm and is reddish in color when it is fresh. The eggs, each of which contains a fully formed miracidium when it leaves the adult parasite, must be ingested by an appropriate first intermediate host, in which they form rediae and cercariae within four to six weeks (Adam *et al.*, 1995). The first intermediate host may be any of four species of snails: *Bithynia siamensis goniomphalus, B. s. siamensis, B. (Digoniostoma) funniculata*, or *B. laevis*. The cercariae, which average about 280 per snail, swim until they find a second intermediate host and penetrate its skin. They then become encysted, mainly in subcutaneous tissues and often at the base of the fins, in the form of metacercariae. By the end of six weeks, they are infective for the definitive host. The role of the second intermediate host is assumed by any of several cyprinid fish (carp), such as *Cyclocheilicthys, Hampala*, and *Puntius*. The definitive hosts of this species are man, the civet *Felis viverrina*, dogs, domestic and wild cats, and other animals that eat fish or fish scraps. When these hosts ingest a fish containing metacercariae, the parasites excyst inside the duodenum and new juvenile parasites migrate via the choledochus to the smaller bile ducts, where they mature and begin to lay eggs within four weeks. They can live for up to 20 years.

O. felineus cannot be distinguished from *O. viverrini* in the adult stage. Its life cycle is similar to that species, but it uses the snails *Bithynia (Bulimus) leachi, B. infata*, or possibly *B. tentaculata* as its first intermediate host. Freshwater fish of the genera *Barbus, Blicca, Leuciscus*, or *Tinca* serve as the second intermediate host. The definitive hosts are humans, swine, cats, dogs, and foxes.

A. pseudofelineus measures 4 mm in length by 2 mm in width. The definitive hosts are the coyote *(Canis latrans)*, dogs, and cats.

Geographical Distribution and Occurrence: *O. viverrini* is found in Laos, northeastern Thailand, and Viet Nam, where it affects some 8 million individuals

(Khamboonruang *et al.*, 1997). In northeastern Thailand, an estimated 3.5 million people were infected with *O. viverrini* in 1965; 5.4 million in 1981 (Bunnag and Harinasuta, 1984); and 6–7 million in 1991 (Loaharanu and Sornmani, 1991). In some hyperendemic regions, the infection rates have reached as high as 72%–87% of the population. In 1981, the prevalence of human opisthorchiasis in northeastern Thailand was 35%; however, a decade after the establishment in 1988 of a national control program involving diagnosis, treatment, and education, the rate had fallen to 18.5%, with fluctuations ranging from 5% to 56% in different localities (Jongsuksuntigul and Imsomboon, 1997). In Laos, a study conducted in the early 1990s showed that 90% of the males in the villages surveyed were infected with the adult parasite, as were 36% of the domestic or stray cats tested, while 0.5% of the snails *B. s. goniomphalus* had cercariae and 7 species of carp had metacercariae. Only 0.6% of the human infections were serious, while 66% were mild (Giboda *et al.*, 1991). In a subsequent study, it was found that 37.5% of 128 children in the villages of southeastern Laos were infected (Kobayashi *et al.*, 1996).

   O. felineus is found near lakes and in river basins of the former USSR, such as those of central Siberia, Kazakhstan, the lower Dnieper, and the Kama River. There are smaller foci in eastern, southern, and central Europe, the Democratic People's Republic of Korea, and possibly India, Japan, and the Philippines. It is estimated that more than 1 million people are infected with this trematode. In some hyperendemic areas, such as Siberia, the infection rate is very high not only in the nomadic population but also among people living in some urban areas. A study carried out in the city of Tobolsk (Siberia) a few years after World War II estimated that 83% of the human population was infected, as were 100% of the cats and 90% of the dogs tested. In Kazakhstan, 100% of the specimens of some species of fish were found to have metacercariae. The snails that serve as the first intermediate host are very abundant in certain endemic regions, and their infection rate is high. A study carried out in the Ural region between 1986 and 1991 revealed infections in 10% to 30% of the human population tested, 0.2% of the snails of the genus *Codiella*, and 12% to 73% of the carp (Tsybina, 1994).

   A. pseudofelineus was first found in humans and described as *Opisthorchis guayaquilensis* in Pedro P. Gómez Parish, Manabí Province, Ecuador. Eggs of the parasite were found in 7.3% of fecal samples from 245 persons in the area (with the rate ranging from 4% in the town center to 32% in peripheral outlying locations). In the same parish, 3 of 100 dogs examined had parasites, whereas none of 80 swine tested had the parasite. The trematode has been found in several animal species in Brazil (Santa Catarina), Ecuador, Panama, and the US (Artigas and Pérez, 1962), but since 1988, there have been no further reports of this species.

The Disease in Man and Animals: The infection causes hepatomegaly, and in most cases, pericholangitis. These changes are restricted to the medium-sized and large bile ducts, which are the sites occupied by the parasite. The small interlobular ducts do not exhibit changes. The most common damage is dilation of the ducts, with hyperplasia, desquamation, proliferation, and adenomatous transformation of the epithelial cells, and infiltration of the wall with connective tissue. Dilation of the gallbladder, chronic cholecystitis, and carcinomas occur only in adults (Riganti *et al.*, 1989). The symptomatology of the disease is similar to that of the hepatic distomiasis caused by *Clonorchis sinensis* and depends on both the parasite burden and the duration of the infection. In general, when only a few parasites are present, the infection is asymptomatic, even though there may be appreciable damage to the bile capillaries. With a parasitosis of medium intensity there is fever, diarrhea, flatulence, moderate jaundice, asthenia, cephalalgia, hepatomegaly, and passive congestion of the spleen. In chronic cases with a large parasite burden, there may be mechanical obstruction and biliary stasis, as well as secondary infections with cholangitis, cholangiohepatitis, and formation of micro- and macroabscesses. When the parasitosis is massive, there may also be invasion of the pancreas, producing catarrhal inflammation of the pancreatic ducts. Infections caused by *O. felineus* often produce erythematous papular eruptions. It is thought that *Opisthorchis* may play a role in the development of hepatic carcinomas, especially cholangiocarcinomas. Although a close correlation has been observed between the infection and this type of cancer in the parasite's endemic areas, there are also areas with high prevalence of the cancer in which the parasite is not present (Sinawat *et al.*, 1991; Holzinger *et al.*, 1999). In a study conducted in an endemic area, the levels of antibody to the parasite were lower in individuals who had parasite eggs in their feces than in those who were not shedding eggs. This finding was interpreted as evidence that the infection produces protective immunity (Akai *et al.*, 1994). However, the prevalence rate, number of eggs in feces, and number of parasites in the liver become stabilized in adults (Sithithaworn *et al.*, 1991) rather than decline with age, as might be expected if there were protective immunity.

Source of Infection and Mode of Transmission: Man and other definitive hosts become infected by eating raw or undercooked fish containing metacercariae. Human opisthorchiasis occurs only where appropriate intermediate hosts, especially snails, are found, and where people customarily eat raw, lightly salted, or sun-dried fish. However, infected travelers can carry the parasite to other areas. High rates of infection have been found among Thai workers in other Asian countries. In the US, a 1987 study revealed a 0.6% prevalence of *Opisthorchis* and *Clonorchis* infections in 216,275 fecal examinations (Kappus *et al.*, 1991). In highly endemic areas, it is thought that man is primarily responsible for maintaining the cycle, since people contaminate rivers and lakes with fecal matter containing the eggs of the parasite. The main species of fish that transmit *O. felineus* to man, and those that also have the highest prevalence of metacercariae, are *Idus melanotus, Tinca tinca,* and *T. vulgaris.* In Thailand, the fish most often found to be infected with *O. viverrini* metacercariae are *Cyclocheilicthys siaja, Hampala dispar,* and *Puntius orphoides,* with infection rates ranging from 51% (in the first species) to 74% (in the second).

Animals can maintain a natural cycle independent of man. In one area in the former USSR, 85% of the cats examined were found to be infected, but no cases were detected in the human population, since the people there do not eat raw fish. Fecal matter deposited by animals on riverbanks is washed into watercourses by rain.

Diagnosis: Laboratory diagnosis is based on demonstrating the presence of parasite eggs in feces either by sedimentation techniques or by duodenal probe. *Opisthorchis* eggs are rather heavy (specific gravity: 1.2814) and do not float readily in a saturated solution of sodium nitrate, which has a higher specific gravity (1.4) (Harnnoi *et al.*, 1998). Of the immunologic tests, enzyme-linked immunosorbent assay (ELISA) is used most often. Assays to detect circulating antibodies for *O. viverrini* have shown moderately high sensitivity (91% to 92%), but specificity of only 70% to 80%. Cross-reactions have been seen in patients with a wide range of other infections: *Ascaris lumbricoides, Blastocystis hominis, Paragonimus heterotremus, Plasmodium* spp., *Schistosoma* spp., *Strongyloides stercoralis, Taenia* spp., *Trichinella spiralis,* and *Trichuris trichiura,* as well as ancylostomes and yeasts (Sakolvaree *et al.,* 1997). The use of monoclonal antibodies in an ELISA test to detect an *O. viverrini* metabolic antigen in stool samples yielded slightly greater sensitivity than the observation of eggs in feces and proved to be capable of detecting infections on the basis of a single specimen (Sirisinha *et al.,* 1995).

Control: Opisthorchiasis is an infection that needs to be controlled. It is estimated that in Thailand, one-third of the population (6–7 million individuals) are infected, of whom 60% are 15- to 60-year-olds in the workforce. The income lost by this population is estimated at US$ 65 million a year, and the direct cost in terms of medical care has been calculated at US$ 19.4 million (Loaharanu and Sornmani, 1991).

Control of opisthorchiasis entails three interrelated strategies: diagnosis and treatment of patients with symptomatic infections to reduce contamination of the environment; health education of the population at risk to discourage the consumption of raw fish and unsanitary disposal of feces; and the improvement of facilities for the adequate disposal of excreta (Jongsuksuntigul and Imsomboon, 1998). These strategies have been applied in endemic areas in the northern and northeastern parts of Thailand. Although prevalence of the infections was reduced in the northeast from 35% in 1981 to 18.5% in 1991, with variations ranging from 5% to 56% (Jongsuksuntigul and Imsomboon, 1997), it increased considerably in the north. The weakest link appears to be education: the regular consumption of raw fish declined from 14% to 7% of the population between 1990 and 1994, but 42% continued to eat it occasionally. Another weak link is the continued lack of sanitary excreta disposal systems, since opisthorchiasis predominates in low-income rural areas where it is difficult to implement this strategy.

For individual protection, the cooking of fish is effective. Temperatures of –10°C and lower kill the metacercariae within 5 days, and saline solutions of 5%, 10%, or 15% destroy them in 10 to 3 days, depending on the strength. Russian investigators have reported that incubation of carp in 6% acetic acid (household vinegar) for four hours prior to salting considerably increases the capacity of salt to kill the metacercariae of *O. felineus.* It has also been proposed to irradiate fish with a radioactive dose of 0.1 kGy, which has been shown to be effective in destroying the cercariae without affecting the organoleptic properties of the food (Loaharanu and Sornmani, 1991). On the other hand, since humans are often reinfected soon after treatment, Hinz *et al.* (1994) propose that therapy be administered during the month of March, when the risk of infection is minimal.

Bibliography

Adam, R., H. Arnold, E. Hinz, V. Storch. Morphology and ultrastructure of the redia and pre-emergent cercaria of *Opisthorchis viverrini* (Trematoda: Digenea) in the intermediate host *Bithynia siamensis goniomphalus* (Prosobranchia: Bithyniidae). *Appl Parasitol* 36:136–154, 1995.

Akai, P.S., S. Pungpak, V. Kitikoon, D. Bunnag, A.D. Befus. Possible protective immunity in human opisthorchiasis. *Parasite Immunol* 16:279–288, 1994.

Artigas, P. de T., M.D. Pérez. Considerações sôbre *Opisthorchis pricei,* Foster, 1939, *O. guayaquilensis,* Rodrigues, Gómez e Montalván, 1949, e *O. pseudofelineus,* Ward, 1901. Descrição de *Amphimerus pseudofelineus minutus* n. sub. sp. *Mem Inst Butantan* 30:157–166, 1962.

Bunnag, D., T. Harinasuta. Opisthorchiasis, clonorchiasis and paragonimiasis. *In:* Warren, K.S., A.A.F. Mahmoud, eds. *Tropical and Geographical Medicine.* New York: McGraw-Hill; 1984.

Giboda, M., O. Ditrich, T. Scholz, T. Viengsay, S. Bouaphanh. Current status of food-borne parasitic zoonoses in Laos. *Southeast Asian J Trop Med Public Health* 22 Suppl:56–61, 1991.

Harnnoi, T., A. Wijit, N. Morakote, V. Pipitgool, W. Maleewong. Specific gravity of *Opisthorchis viverrini* eggs. *J Helminthol* 72:359–361, 1998.

Hinz, E., S. Saowakontha, V. Pipitgool. Opisthorchiasis control in northeast Thailand: Proposal for a new approach. *Appl Parasitol* 35:118–124, 1994.

Holzinger, F., K. Z'graggen, M.W. Buchler. Mechanisms of biliary carcinogenesis: A pathogenetic multi-stage cascade towards cholangiocarcinoma. *Ann Oncol* 10 Suppl 4:122–126, 1999.

Jongsuksuntigul, P., T. Imsomboon. The impact of a decade long opisthorchiasis control program in northeastern Thailand. *Southeast Asian J Trop Med Public Health* 28:551–557, 1997.

Jongsuksuntigul, P., T. Imsomboon. Epidemiology of opisthorchiasis and national control program in Thailand. *Southeast Asian J Trop Med Public Health* 29:327–332, 1998.

Kappus, K.K., D.D. Juranek, J.M. Roberts. Results of testing for intestinal parasites by state diagnostic laboratories, United States, 1987. *MMWR CDC Surveill Summ* 40:25–45, 1991.

Khamboonruang, C., R. Keawvichit, K. Wongworapat, *et al.* Application of hazard analysis critical control point (HACCP) as a possible control measure for *Opisthorchis viverrini* infection in cultured carp (*Puntius gonionotus*). *Southeast Asian J Trop Med Public Health* 28 Suppl 1:65–72, 1997.

Kobayashi, J., B. Vannachone, A. Xeutvongsa, *et al.* Prevalence of intestinal parasitic infection among children in two villages in Lao PDR. *Southeast Asian J Trop Med Public Health* 27:562–565, 1996.

Loaharanu, P., S. Sornmani. Preliminary estimates of economic impact of liver fluke infection in Thailand and the feasibility of irradiation as a control measure. *Southeast Asian J Trop Med Public Health* 22 Suppl:384–390, 1991.

Riganti, M., S. Pungpak, B. Punpoowong, D. Bunnag, T. Harinasuta. Human pathology of *Opisthorchis viverrini* infection: A comparison of adults and children. *Southeast Asian J Trop Med Public Health* 20:95–100, 1989.

Sakolvaree, Y., L. Ibáñez, W. Chaicumpa. Parasites elicited cross-reacting antibodies to *Opisthorchis viverrini. Asian Pac J Allergy Immunol* 15:115–122, 1997.

Sinawat, P., V. Hemsrichart. A histopathologic study of 61 cases of peripheral intrahepatic cholangiocarcinoma. *J Med Assoc Thai* 74:448–453, 1991.

Sirisinha, S., R. Chawengkirttikul, M.R. Haswell-Elkins, *et al.* Evaluation of a monoclonal antibody-based enzyme linked immunosorbent assay for the diagnosis of *Opisthorchis viverrini* infection in an endemic area. *Am J Trop Med Hyg* 52:521–524, 1995.

Sithithaworn, P., S. Tesana, V. Pipitgool, *et al.* Quantitative post-mortem study of *Opisthorchis viverrini* in man in north-east Thailand. *Trans R Soc Trop Med Hyg* 85:765–768, 1991.

Tsybina, T.N. [The ecological-epidemiological characteristics of opisthorchiasis in Sverdlovsk Province]. *Med Parazitol (Mosk)* 3:45–50, 1994.

PARAGONIMIASIS

ICD-10 B66.4

Synonyms: Pulmonary distomiasis, endemic hemoptysis, lung fluke disease, infection due to *Paragonimus* species.

Etiology: This disease is caused by trematodes of the genus *Paragonimus*. In a highly detailed review, Blair *et al.* (1999) refer to 50 species in this genus, although not all of them are valid. The following nine species of *Paragonimus* have been reported in humans:

1. *P. africanus*, in Cameroon, Côte d'Ivoire, Equatorial Guinea, and Nigeria, since 1976; it also parasitizes monkeys and, experimentally, dogs and rodents.

2. *P. heterotremus*, in China, Lao People's Democratic Republic, and Thailand, since 1970; it also parasitizes cats, rodents, and, experimentally, dogs and rabbits.

3. *P. kellicotti*, in the US, since 1986; it also parasitizes canids, felids, other carnivores, swine, goats, and, experimentally, rodents.

4. *P. mexicanus* (synonyms: *P. peruvianus, P. ecuadoriensis*), in Colombia, Costa Rica, Ecuador, El Salvador, Guatemala, Honduras, Mexico, Nicaragua, Panama, Peru, and Venezuela, since 1983; it also parasitizes marsupials, monkeys, wild carnivores, and, experimentally, dogs and cats.

5. *P. miyazakii*, in Japan, since 1992; it also parasitizes wild carnivores, swine, and, experimentally, dogs, cats, and rodents.

6. *P. ohirai*, in Japan, since 1988; it also parasitizes wild carnivores, swine, and, experimentally, dogs, cats, rodents, and rabbits.

7. *P. skrjabini*, in China, since 1975; it also parasitizes monkeys, wild carnivores, and, experimentally, dogs, cats, and rodents.

8. *P. uterobilateralis*, in Cameroon, Côte d'Ivoire, Gabon, Guinea, Liberia, and Nigeria, since 1973; it also parasitizes monkeys, dogs, wild carnivores, and, experimentally, dogs, cats, and rodents.

9. *P. westermani* (partial synonym: *P. philippinensis*), in China, Gabon, India, Indonesia, Japan, Lao People's Democratic Republic, Nepal, Papua New Guinea, the Philippines, Republic of Korea, Russian Federation, Samoa, Taiwan, and Viet Nam, since the nineteenth century; it also parasitizes macaques, wild and domestic carnivores, swine, rodents, galliform and anseriform birds, and, experimentally, rabbits.

Most of these species were described in the 1960s, and their association with man has been recognized since the 1970s and 1980s, and, in one case, the 1990s. The notable exception is *P. westermani*, which was recognized as a human parasite in 1880. The fact that *P. westermani* was discovered so early reflects its greater abundance and also explains why most of the information on human paragonimiasis refers to this species. Because of its wide distribution, high prevalence, and notable pathogenicity, *P. westermani* is considered the *Paragonimus* species of greatest importance for human health. It is followed by *P. heterotremus*, and, in third place with somewhat lower frequency, by *P. mexicanus* (García and Bruckner, 1997). However, there are still species that remain to be assessed in terms of their importance. For example, a recent study in western Africa found four species of *Paragonimus* in humans: *P. africanus, P. uterobilateralis*, a specimen similar to *P. westermani*, and a previously unrecognized species of the genus *Euparagonimus*

(Cabaret *et al.*, 1999). Moreover, diploid and triploid forms of *P. westermani* have been observed in Asia, and it has yet not been determined whether they constitute different species (Blair *et al.*, 1999). Finally, DNA sequence analysis has revealed that there are two groups within the species *P. westermani*, a northeastern one found in China, Japan, Republic of Korea, and Taiwan, and a southern one found in Malaysia, the Philippines, and Thailand (Blair *et al.*, 1997).

Paragonimus trematodes are reddish brown, oval parasites measuring about 4–8 mm wide, 7–16 mm long, and 2–5 mm thick, which lodge in the lungs of the definitive hosts. Their development cycle requires two intermediate hosts: the first is a snail, and the second, an appropriate freshwater crab or crayfish. Man and other mammals, particularly carnivores, are the definitive hosts, and they harbor the parasite in their lungs. The parasite lays 1,000–2,000 eggs a day, which are shed via expectoration, or in feces if bronchial secretions are swallowed. If the eggs reach water, they continue to develop and form a ciliated larva, or miracidium, which hatches in about three weeks and swims around in search of a snail in which to carry on its cycle. Only certain species of snails allow the cycle to continue: for *P. westermani*, they are species of the genera *Semisulcospira*, *Brotia*, and *Melanopides* in Southeast Asia and *Juga* in the Russian Federation; for *P. heterotremus*, the genera *Oncomelania* and *Neotricula* in Thailand and the genus *Tricula* in China; and for *P. mexicanus*, the genera *Oncomelania* and *Aroapyrgus* in Costa Rica, Ecuador, Mexico, and Peru.

Since the miracidium usually invades the snail by active means, it needs to find an intermediate host within a day or two before its energy is exhausted. Once it penetrates an appropriate snail, the miracidium is transformed into a sac called a sporocyst, within which juvenile trematodes, referred to as rediae, are generated. The rediae give rise to a second generation of rediae inside the first, and from the latter, new juvenile forms, called cercariae, emerge. This multiplication of juvenile stages within the snail, referred to as pedogenesis, greatly increases the number of parasites produced by each egg, and hence its biotic potential. A large number of parasites can be lethal for the snail. The cercariae abandon the snail after 9 to 13 weeks, depending on the temperature and humidity, and seek a crustacean in which to encyst. For *P. westermani,* it can be a species from the genera *Cambaroides*, *Candidiopotamon*, *Ceylonthelphusa*, *Eriocheir*, *Geothelphusa*, *Huananpotamon*, *Isolapotamon*, *Macrobrachium*, *Malayapotamon*, *Oziothelphusa*, *Parapotamon*, *Parathelphusa*, *Potamiscus*, *Potamon*, *Procambarus*, *Siamthelphusa*, *Sinopotamon*, *Sundathelphusa*, or *Varuna*; for *P. heterotremus,* the genera *Esanthelphusa*, *Larnaudia*, *Malayapotamon*, *Potamiscus*, *Potamon*, *Siamthelphusa*, or *Sinopotamon*; for *P. mexicanus*, the genera *Hypolobocera*, *Odontothelphusa*, *Pseudothelphusa*, *Ptychophallus*, or *Zilchiopsis*. In rare cases, metacercariae of *P. skrjabini*, which is infective for dogs and cats, have been found in the frog *Rana boulengeri* in China. The cercariae can actively penetrate the crustacean, and the crustacean can also become infected from eating infected snails. Once lodged in the muscles or gills of the crustacean, the parasite surrounds itself with a resistant envelope and turns into a metacercaria. It remains there for several weeks until it becomes infective for the definitive host.

The definitive host becomes infected upon eating freshwater crabs or crayfish that contain metacercariae. Once in the intestine, the metacercariae are released from their envelope and penetrate the intestinal wall, remain in the peritoneal cavity for several days, and then migrate through the diaphragm into the pleural cavity. There they form pairs and invade the lungs, where they encyst in the conjunctival tissue of the airways and begin to lay eggs 8 to 10 weeks after the initial infection. Although *Paragonimus* trematodes are morphologically hermaphroditic, functionally they are unisexual and, with the exception of the triploid forms of *P. westermani*, they do not self-fertilize. Juveniles that do not find a mate usually continue to move around in the pleural cavity or the lungs and cause further damage, while the adults in the pulmonary cysts are usually found in pairs. When metacercariae are ingested by an inappropriate host—for example, a wild boar, rabbit, or rodent—the parasites remain inside without developing further and utilize the animal as a transfer, or paratenic, host. The wild boar (*Sus scrofa leucomystax*) appears to serve as a paratenic host for *P. westermani* and *P. miyazakii*. On the island of Kyushu in Japan, the human infection has been attributed to the ingestion of raw wild boar meat containing juvenile forms of the parasite (WHO, 1979).

Geographic Distribution and Occurrence: *Paragonimus* is found throughout the world. Human infections occur in Africa, the Americas, and Asia. The geographic distribution of species that affect humans is indicated above in the section on etiology. The most important endemic areas are East and Southeast Asia, China, Japan, Lao People's Democratic Republic, the Philippines, Republic of Korea, Thailand, Taiwan, and the maritime provinces of the former USSR, and there are also isolated foci in India and Viet Nam. The main etiologic agent in all these areas is *P. westermani,* but in some countries, other species occur either concurrently or separately. Toscano *et al.* (1995) have calculated that 20 million people in the world are infected, several million of them in Asia. In the Republic of Korea, the infected population was estimated at 1 to 1.5 million. A study conducted in several provinces of Thailand revealed an infection rate of 6.5% in 503 persons examined. In Taiwan, the average infection rate in schoolchildren was 1.6% (Malek, 1980). A sizable endemic area was identified in Vietnam, in which 44 of 155 patients (28%) with chronic pulmonary disease were found to be infected with *Paragonimus* (Queuche *et al.*, 1997). The prevalence in Japan, which rose during World War II and immediately thereafter, has declined sharply (Nawa, 1991). In a survey conducted in an endemic region of Cameroon, examination of sputum or feces revealed *P. africanus* eggs in 5.6% of 900 persons examined, with the highest rates in the population under 20 years of age (Kum and Nchinda, 1982). In eastern Nigeria, cases of *P. uterobilateralis* infection tend to occur sporadically, but the number of paragonimiasis cases increased considerably during and after the civil war of 1967–1970, and 100 cases were diagnosed in one university hospital (Nwokolo, 1972). Sputum specimens from 69 patients revealed that 66 had eggs of *P. uterobilateralis* and 3 had eggs of *P. africanus* (Voelker and Nwokolo, 1973). Isolated cases have been observed in Liberia and Guinea.

The main species that infects man in Latin America is *P. mexicanus*. Human cases of the disease have been seen in Colombia, Costa Rica, Ecuador, El Salvador, Honduras, Mexico, and Peru (in Cajamarca and along the coast north of Lima). In Ecuador, between 1921 and 1969, a total of 511 cases were reported, and between 1972 and 1976, there were 316 cases in four provinces of that country, most of them in the province of Manabí (Arzube and Voelker, 1978). In a study carried out in northwestern Ecuador, 43% of the crayfish examined were found to be infected, and 62% of the streams proved to be harboring infected crustaceans (Vieira, 1992). About 20 cases have been diagnosed in Cajamarca, Peru, and some have been also reported in Mexico.

The parasite's range of distribution in lower mammals is much broader than the corresponding human infection, since the spread of human infection depends on the eating habits of the population.

The Disease in Man: *Paragonimus* trematodes reside mainly in the lungs. A long time elapses between the ingestion of metacercariae and the appearance of symptoms, though the duration of this period is variable. The parasites can cause damage as they migrate toward the lungs and seek a mate in the pleural cavity, while they are encysted in the lungs, and sometimes when they become lodged in ectopic sites. Indeed, experimental studies in dogs have shown that migration toward the lungs can produce considerable damage. During this phase, there can be abdominal pain, fever, and diarrhea. Pleural pathology, often with effusion, is common in *P. westermani* infections. The prominent symptoms of pulmonary paragonimiasis are chronic productive cough, thoracic pain, blood-tinged viscous sputum, and sometimes fever (Im *et al.*, 1993; Kagawa, 1997). Intense physical exercise can induce hemoptysis, which is the most notable sign. Eosinophilia is common. Small numbers of parasites in the lungs do not significantly affect the health of the patient and do not interfere with routine activity. The triploid forms of *P. westermani* are larger, produce bigger cysts, and cause more damage. About two-thirds of the shadows revealed by radiography are located in the middle and lower portions of the lungs; they are rarely seen in the apex. The most frequent and serious ectopic localization of *P. westermani* is the brain, but the parasite may also be found in the spinal cord, thoracic muscles, subcutaneous tissue, and abdominal cavity and organs. According to reports of cases in the Americas, the brain has also been parasitized by species other than *P. westermani*. In the Republic of Korea, which is a hyperendemic area, an estimated 5,000 cases of cerebral paragonimiasis occur each year. The symptomatology is similar to that of cerebral cysticercosis, with cephalalgia, convulsions, jacksonian epilepsy, hemiplegia, paresis, and visual disorders. Abdominal paragonimiasis produces a dull pain in that region, which may be accompanied by mucosanguineous diarrhea when the intestinal mucosa is ulcerated. In other localizations, the symptomatology varies depending on the organ affected.

The subcutaneous nodular form, characterized by intense eosinophilia, is predominant in infections caused by *P. skrjabini* in China and *P. heterotremus* in Thailand. This form is clinically similar to cutaneous larva migrans. In addition to migratory subcutaneous nodules, the most common manifestations of *P. skrjabini* infection in China are pleural, ocular, cerebral, pericardial, and hepatic lesions, while pulmonary symptoms are relatively infrequent. Cases of ectopic paragonimiasis in the brain, liver, and perivesical and cutaneous fat have been observed in Latin America. Twelve cases of cutaneous paragonimiasis occurred in the same family in Ecuador; in addition, there was a single isolated case in that country and another in Honduras (Brenes *et al.*, 1983).

The Disease in Animals: Animals parasitized by *P. westermani* frequently have cysts in the lungs, which pass to the respiratory tract and the pleural cavity. The symptoms are similar to those of human pulmonary paragonimiasis, with coughing and bloody sputum.

In the laboratory, trematodes appear in the lungs of dogs 23 to 35 days after experimental infection. The parasitosis begins as pneumonitis and catarrhal bronchitis, which are followed by interstitial pneumonia and the formation of cysts.

Source of Infection and Mode of Transmission: The source of *Paragonimus* infection for man and other definitive hosts is freshwater crabs and crayfish containing parasite metacercariae. Transmission results from the ingestion of raw or undercooked crustaceans, raw crabs marinated in wine ("drunken crabs"), or crustacean juices. Paragonimiasis is a public health problem in countries where it is customary to eat raw crustaceans or use them for supposedly therapeutic purposes. However, the disease is a problem in Japan as well, even though crustaceans are well cooked before they are eaten; in this case, the main source of infection is hands and cooking utensils contaminated during the preparation of crustaceans.

It is possible that man may also become infected by eating meat from animals that are paratenic hosts carrying immature parasites, as evidenced by cases on the island of Kyushu, Japan, that occurred following the consumption of raw wild boar meat. The hypothesis that there are paratenic hosts is reinforced by the fact that paragonims have been observed in carnivores such as tigers and leopards that do not eat crustaceans (Malek, 1980). Wars and internal conflicts that force people to relocate and cause shortages of normal protein food sources can also contribute to sharp increases in the prevalence of the infection, as was seen in Nigeria during its civil war and in Japan during World War II (see Geographic Distribution and Occurrence).

Transmission is always cyclic—the infection cannot be transmitted directly from one definitive host to another. The parasite must complete its natural cycle, and in order for this to happen the two intermediate hosts must be present—appropriate species of both snails and crustaceans.

The reservoir of *Paragonimus* spp. comprises man, domestic animals, and many species of wild animals (see Etiology). In endemic areas of eastern Asia, the human infection rate is high enough that man can maintain the infection cycle alone through ongoing contamination of freshwater bodies with human feces. In such areas, the role of animal definitive hosts may be of secondary importance. In certain areas of Japan, mass administration of bithionol to the human population led to a considerable reduction in the infection rate in crustaceans (WHO, 1979). This experience bears out the importance of human infection in maintaining the endemic. In other parts of Asia, wild animals have been parasitized by *P. westermani* in areas where there were no known human cases, which suggests that there may be a wild cycle independent of the domestic one. On the other hand, in several parts of Africa, Latin America, and Asia, wild animals are more important than man or domestic animals in maintaining the infection cycle. For example, the main natural reservoir of *P. uterobilateralis* is the African civet (*Viverra civetta*): parasite eggs were found in 26 of 28 fecal specimens examined (Sachs and Voelker, 1982).

Diagnosis: In endemic areas, paragonimiasis may be suspected if the typical symptoms are present and the consumption of raw or undercooked crustaceans is a local custom. Radiographic examination is useful, but the findings may be negative even in symptomatic patients. Moreover, interpretation of the results can be difficult in nonendemic areas because the images may be mistaken for those of tuberculosis. Computerized tomography may give a more reliable view of the lesions (Im *et al.*, 1993; Kagawa, 1997). Specific diagnosis of pulmonary paragonimiasis is based on the identification of eggs in sputum, fecal matter, pleural effusions, or biopsies. The eggs are reddish brown, operculate, and enlarged at the end opposite the operculum. Published sources report the following egg sizes: *P. westermani*, 85 μm by 47 μm, with abopercular enlargement; *P. heterotremus,* 86 μm by 48 μm, with no enlargement; *P. mexicanus,* 79 μm by 48 μm, with an undulated shell; *P. africanus,* 92 μm by 48 μm, with an undulated shell; *P. miyazakii,* 75 μm by 43 μm, with no enlargement; *P. skrjabini,* 80 μm by 48 μm, with no enlargement; and *P. uterobilateralis,* 68 μm by 41 μm, with abopercular enlargement. It is important to differentiate the eggs of *Paragonimus* from those of other trematodes, as well as cestodes of the order Pseudophyllidea, such as *Diphyllobothrium.* The cerebral forms can be mistaken for tumors or cysticercosis, and the cutaneous forms, for other migratory larvae—hence the interest in developing indirect tests. An intradermal test that was only weakly sensitive and of questionable specificity was widely used in the past for epidemiologic purposes. In a province of China, a 1961 study found that 24% of the persons examined had positive skin tests, and almost half of those cases were confirmed. In 1991, following a control campaign, 9% of the cases were positive and only 0.4% of them were confirmed. Currently, the most common test is the enzyme-linked immunosorbent assay (ELISA) using 32 and 35 kDa specific antigens. This assay can distinguish infections caused by different species of *Paragonimus* (Kong *et al.,* 1998). In addition, the polymerase chain reaction is being used to diagnose paragonimiasis (Maleewong, 1997).

Control: In endemic areas, control efforts should be directed at interrupting the infection cycle by the following means: a) education of people to prevent the consumption of raw or undercooked crabs or crayfish; b) mass treatment of the population to reduce the reservoir of infection; c) elimination of stray dogs and cats for the same purpose; d) sanitary disposal of sputum and fecal matter to prevent the contamination of rivers; and e) controlling snails with molluscicides in areas where this approach is feasible. For a control program to be effective, it should encompass the entire watershed area and adjacent regions.

In Latin America, where the transmission cycle appears to occur predominantly in wildlife and where human cases are sporadic, the only practical measure is to educate and warn the population about the danger of eating raw or undercooked crustaceans. A study in China investigated the possibility of destroying metacercariae in crustaceans by irradiation with cobalt-60. No parasites could be recovered from mice infected with metacercariae irradiated at 2.5 kGy, but the fact that the mice developed antibodies indicates that the parasites had managed to colonize their tissues. Some of the metacercariae irradiated at 2 kGy excysted and survived in the mice for up to 30 days. Metacercariae irradiated at 0.1 kGy did not reach the adult stage in cats (Song *et al.,* 1992).

Bibliography

Arzube, M.E., J. Voelker. Uber das Vorkommen menschlicher Paragonimiasis in Ecuador (1972–1976). *Tropenmed Parasitol* 29:275–277, 1978.

Blair, D., T. Agatsuma, T. Watanobe, M. Okamoto, A. Ito. Geographical genetic structure within the human lung fluke, *Paragonimus westermani,* detected from DNA sequences. *Parasitology* 115 (Pt4):411–417, 1997.

Blair, D., Z.B. Xu, T. Agatsuma. Paragonimiasis and the genus *Paragonimus. Adv Parasitol* 42:113–222, 1999.

Brenes, R.R., M.D. Little, O. Raudales, G. Muñoz, C. Ponce. Cutaneous paragonimiasis in man in Honduras. *Am J Trop Med Hyg* 32:376–378, 1983.

Cabaret, J., C. Bayssade-Dufour, G. Tami, J.L. Albaret. Identification of African Paragonimidae by multivariate analysis of the eggs. *Acta Trop* 72:79–89, 1999.

García, L.S., D.A. Bruckner. *Diagnostic Medical Parasitology*, 3rd ed. Washington, D.C.: ASM Press; 1997.

Im, J.G., Y. Kong, Y.M. Shin, *et al.* Pulmonary paragonimiasis: Clinical and experimental studies. *Radiographics* 13:575–586, 1993.

Kagawa, F.T. Pulmonary paragonimiasis. *Semin Respir Infect* 12:49–58, 1997.

Kong, Y., A. Ito, H.J. Yang, *et al.* Immunoglobulin G (IgG) subclass and IgE responses in human paragonimiases caused by three different species. *Clin Diag Lab Immunol* 5:474–478, 1998.

Kum, P.N., T.C. Nchinda. Pulmonary paragonimiasis in Cameroon. *Trans R Soc Trop Med Hyg* 76:768–772, 1982.

Maleewong, W. Recent advances in diagnosis of paragonimiasis. *Southeast Asian J Trop Med Public Health* 28 Supp 1:134–138, 1997.

Malek, E.A. Vol. 2: *Snail-transmitted Parasitic Diseases*. Boca Raton: CRC Press; 1980.

Miyazaki, I. Paragonimiasis. *In*: Hillyer, G.V., C.E. Hopla, section eds. Section C, Vol. 3: *CRC Handbook Series in Zoonoses*. Boca Raton: CRC Press; 1982.

Nawa, Y. Recent trends of paragonimiasis westermani in Miyazaki Prefecture, Japan. *Southeast Asian J Trop Med Public Health* 22 Suppl:342–344, 1991.

Nwokolo, C. Endemic paragonimiasis in Eastern Nigeria. Clinical features and epidemiology of the recent outbreak following the Nigerian civil war. *Trop Geogr Med* 24:138–147, 1972.

Queuche, F., Cao Van Vien, Le Dang Ha. Un foyer de paragonimose au Viet Nam. *Sante* 7:155–159, 1997.

Sachs, R., J. Voelker. Human paragonimiasis caused by *Paragonimus uterobilateralis* in Liberia and Guinea, West Africa. *Tropenmed Parasitol* 33:15–16, 1982.

Song, C.C., Y.F. Duan, G.C. Shou, H. Zhu. Effect of cobalt-60 irradiation on the infectivity of *Paragonimus westermani* metacercariae. *J Parasitol* 78:869–871, 1992.

Toscano, C., S.H. Yu, P. Nunn, *et al.* Paragonimiasis and tuberculosis, diagnostic confusion: A review of the literature. *Trop Dis Bull* 92:R1–R26, 1995.

Vieira, J.C., H.D. Blankespoor, P.J. Cooper, *et al.* Paragonimiasis in Ecuador: Prevalence and geographical distribution of parasitisation of second intermediate hosts with *Paragonimus mexicanus* in Esmeraldas province. *Trop Med Parasitol* 43:249–252, 1992.

Voelker, J., C. Nwokolo. Human paragonimiasis in Eastern Nigeria by *Paragonimus uterobilateralis*. *Z Tropenmed Parasitol* 24:323–328, 1973.

World Health Organization (WHO). *Parasitic Zoonoses. Report of a WHO Expert Committee, with the Participation of FAO*. Geneva: WHO; 1979. (Technical Report Series 637).

SCHISTOSOMIASIS

ICD-10 B65

Synonyms: Bilharziasis, Katayama syndrome (acute schistosomiasis).

Etiology: The primary agents of human schistosomiasis are the small blood trematodes *Schistosoma mansoni*, *S. japonicum*, and *S. haematobium*, which measure 0.5–2.5 cm in length and live in pairs inside blood vessels. In certain restricted geographic areas, the species *S. intercalatum, S. mekongi,* and *S. malayensis* also affect humans. There have also been reports of human infections caused by the bovine parasite *S. mattheei,* although most of these may be caused by the hybridization of *S. mattheei* and *S. haematobium* (Kruger and Evans, 1990). *S. mansoni* and *S. haematobium* are considered strictly human species, although *S. mansoni* has occasionally been observed in rodents, monkeys, and insectivores, and *S. haematobium* has been seen in monkeys. *S. japonicum* can infect seven other mammalian orders, including domestic herbivores and carnivores, swine, and rats; *S. mekongi* can infect dogs; *S. malayensis* affects wild rats (Greer *et al.,* 1989); *S. intercalatum* is a primary parasite of ruminants; and the bovine *S. mattheei* also infects other ruminants and rodents. DNA comparisons have demonstrated that *S. mekongi* is closely related to *S. japonicum* and *S. malayensis,* and observations in nature have shown that *S. intercalatum* and *S. mattheei* can hybridize with *S. haematobium* and produce fertile offspring (Jusot *et al.,* 1997; Tchuem Tchuente *et al.,* 1997). This phenomenon raises doubts regarding the specificity of these species (WHO, 1980). There are 19 recognized species of *Schistosoma,* but their phylogenetic relationships are complex (Rollinson *et al.,* 1997).

Unlike the other digenic trematodes, which are hermaphrodites, the schistosomes have both male and female forms. The males are shorter and broader than the females, and they have a gynecophoral canal running along the ventral surface in which the female, which is long and thin, is permanently accommodated. Adults live in the venous system of their definitive hosts, where they mate and lay 100 to 3,500 eggs a day, depending on the species. Although all the species have a similar life cycle, there are variations in their required intermediate hosts and in the final localization of the adults in the circulatory system. *S. mansoni* is found primarily in the mesenteric veins that drain the large intestine, especially in the sigmoid branches; *S. japonicum* is found mainly in the mesenteric venules of the small intestine; *S. haematobium,* in the plexuses of the vena cava system that drains the bladder, pelvis, and uterus; and *S. intercalatum* and *S. mekongi,* the portal and mesenteric veins. In man, *S. mattheei* granulomas are found in the large intestine and the liver, but the eggs may be found in both feces and urine.

The eggs are transported by the venous circulation until they form a thrombus, at which point they secrete enzymes that enable them to traverse the wall of the organ and take up residence in the lumen. From the lumen they are eliminated in feces, urine, or other secretions or excretions of the affected organ. The eggs are deposited with a zygote inside, and before leaving the host they develop a larva (miracidium). When they reach water, most of the eggs hatch within eight hours, stimulated by light and water temperatures of 5°C to 36°C (Ye *et al.,* 1997). The released miracidia swim in search of a suitable intermediate host, but they lose their infectivity if they fail to find one within about 10 hours. The snail intermediate hosts belong to the following genera: *Biomphalaria* and *Tropicorbis* in the case of *S. mansoni; Oncomelania* for *S. japonicum; Bulinus, Physopsis,* and *Planorbarius* for *S. haematobium* (Marquardt *et al.,* 2000), *S. mattheei,* and *S. intercalatum; Tricula* and *Lithoglyphopsys* for *S. mekongi;* and *Robertsiella* for *S. malayensis.* The miracidium penetrates the snail and turns into a mother sporocyst, which forms daughter sporocysts inside it, and the latter, in turn, produce fork-tailed cercariae. The time lapse between penetration of the miracidium and emergence of cercariae can be as short as 20 days, but it is usually 4 to 7 weeks. The number of cercariae produced depends on the parasite and snail species in question, as well as the size of the snail: *Biomphalaria glabrata* can generate between 30,000 and 180,000 cercariae of *S. mansoni*; *Bulinus globosus*, 12,000 to 24,000 cercariae of *S. haematobium*; and *Oncomelania*, 450 to 9,000 cercariae of *S. japonicum* (Marquardt *et al.*, 2000).

Unlike the cercariae of other digenic trematodes, the schistosome cercariae do not form a metacercaria but instead invade the skin of the definitive host directly, often penetrating via the hair follicles or sebaceous glands by enzymatic and mechanical means. This process has to be completed within 36 hours or the cercaria loses its infectivity. Penetration takes only a matter of minutes; the cercaria drops its tail in the course of penetration, and within a few hours, it transforms into a juvenile schistosome (schistosomulum), which differs from the cercaria in morphology, antigenicity, and physiology. The schistosomula travel through the bloodstream to the lungs, where they stop briefly, and then move through the circulatory and porta systems to the liver, where they reach sexual maturity and mate. About three weeks after the initial infection, the parasites travel against the blood flow to the mesenteric, vesical, or pelvic venules, depending on the species. Oviposition begins at 5 to 7 weeks (*S. japonicum*), 7 to 8 weeks (*S. mansoni*), or 10 to 12 weeks (*S. haematobium*). The parasites live for several years, and there have been reports of infections lasting up to 30 years.

Geographic Distribution and Occurrence: Schistosomiasis is endemic in 74 developing countries, and more than 80% of the infected persons live in sub-Saharan Africa (WHO, 2003a). Direct mortality is relatively low, but the infection poses a public health problem because of the chronic pathology and disability that it produces. Despite control efforts in a number of countries, approximately 200 million people are still infected, of whom 120 million are symptomatic and 20 million have severe disease (WHO, 2003b).

S. mansoni has the widest geographic distribution; it is found in 52 countries of Africa (western and central parts of the continent, Egypt, and almost all the countries south of the Sahara except for a strip on the west running from Cameroon to South Africa), the Eastern Mediterranean, the Caribbean, and parts of South America. The range of *S. mansoni* is coextensive with that of *S. haematobium* in large areas. In Senegal, for example, there are places in which the prevalence of *S. mansoni* infection is nearly 100% and that of *S. haematobium* is 28% (De Clercq *et al.*, 1999). There are also isolated foci in Egypt, Saudi Arabia, and Yemen. *S. haematobium* infection is found on some islands of the Lesser Antilles, the eastern coast of Brazil (north of São Paulo), and the coast of Venezuela, and in the Dominican Republic and Puerto Rico. It is believed that schistosomiasis was introduced to the Americas by slaves from Africa. *S. haematobium,* the agent of vesical schistosomiasis, is endemic in 53 countries of Africa as well as the Middle East, Madagascar, the southwestern Arabian peninsula, and along the Tigris and Euphrates rivers. In Tanzania, it is the most abundant helminth in children (Booth *et al.*, 1998). *S. japonicum* infection is found in eight countries of Southeast Asia and the Western Pacific (Cambodia, China, Indonesia, the Philippines, and several small foci in Japan, Laos, Malaysia, and Thailand). *S. intercalatum* infection occurs in Cameroon, the Democratic Republic of Congo, Gabon, and other parts of central and western Africa, and prevalence in different areas ranges from 2.5% to 21.2%. The parasite causes bleeding intestinal lesions (Jusot *et al.*, 1997; Tchuem Tchuente *et al.*, 1997). Since its intermediate hosts (*Bulinus globosus, B. forskalii*) are found throughout

Africa, this species has been tending to spread. *S. mekongi* occurs in northern Cambodia, Laos, and Thailand, especially along the Mekong River, where in one area the prevalence was 40% in a group of 2,391 schoolchildren and 49.3% in 1,396 persons in the general population. Young persons 10 to 14 years of age were most affected, and the pathology was often severe (Stich *et al.*, 1999). *S. malayensis* occurs in the Malay Peninsula (Greer *et al.*, 1989). Human infection caused by *S. mattheei* has been reported in South Africa. Eggs of this parasite are often found in human feces and urine, with infection rates as high as 40% (WHO, 1979).

In China, infection caused by *S. japonicum* is found in the Yangtze River valley and to its south over an area inhabited by 100 million people, most of whom work in the rice fields. Before the current control program was undertaken, it was estimated that more than 10 million people were infected. In Japan, the human infection is largely under control and only a few hundred carriers remain. In the Philippines, an estimated 600,000 people are infected.

In the Americas, Brazil alone has an estimated 8 to 12 million infected individuals. In that country, tests carried out during preparations for its schistosomiasis control program revealed a positivity rate of 22.8% in 739,995 fecal samples from schoolchildren in 6 endemic states (Machado, 1982). In some localities in northeastern Minas Gerais, Brazil, 100% of the population was found to be infected. In the Caribbean area, the rates per 100,000 population in 1972 were 4.8 in the Dominican Republic, 39.2 in Guadeloupe, 1.3 in Puerto Rico, and 375.7 in Saint Lucia. In the US, an average of 170 imported cases were reported annually between 1969 and 1972, most of them from the Caribbean islands. Mahmoud (1977) estimated that, even though the parasitosis is not transmitted in the US for lack of intermediate hosts, some 400,000 infected persons were living there. The infection has spread in some areas because of new irrigation projects and the migration of infected populations. In Brazil, schistosomiasis has spread to the states of Goiás, Maranhão, Pará, Paraná, Santa Catarina, São Paulo (where there are several isolated foci), and from the northeast to southern Minas Gerais (Katz and Carvalho, 1983). In Paraguay, there have been no reports of infection, but more than 100 *S. mansoni*-infected Brazilian immigrants have been found, and the snail *Biomphalaria tenagophila*, which could serve as an intermediate host, is present there.

Despite the fact that several countries have managed to reduce the occurrence of schistosomiasis through vigorous control programs, its prevalence has changed little in recent decades because of the expansion of irrigation and the human migrations mentioned earlier. Reports published in 1999, based on research in selected communities from different countries, gave the following prevalence ranges for *S. mansoni*: 34%–58% in Egypt, 1% in Puerto Rico (down from 21% in 1993), 53%–76% in Senegal, 88% in Tanzania, 2% in Togo, 30%–84% in Uganda, and 1.4% in Venezuela (down from 14% in 1943). In addition, there were an estimated 2 million infected persons in Madagascar. For *S. haematobium*, the ranges were as follows: 7%–11% in Egypt, 97% in Kenya, 46% in Niger, 17% in Nigeria, 53%–64% in Senegal, and 25% in Togo. In addition, there are an estimated half million infected persons in Madagascar. In 1998, two surveys carried out in different municipalities of São Paulo State in Brazil showed 0.4% and 43% positive serology for *S. mansoni*, but only 4.3% and 8.5% of the individuals were shedding eggs.

With regard to the infection in animals, in Brazil *S. mansoni* infection has been found in many rodents, other wild species, and cattle; in eastern Africa, in baboons, rodents, and dogs; and in Egypt, in gerbils (genus *Gerbillus*) and Nile rats. The infection rates are often quite high. In some areas of eastern Africa infection rates of more than 50% have been seen in baboons (WHO, 1979). Natural infection with *S. japonicum,* in turn, has been found in many animal species, and in some areas the rates are high (see Source of Infection and Mode of Transmission). *S. haematobium* has been known to infect nonhuman primates, rodents, and swine on rare occasions, and the prevalence has been low (WHO, 1979).

The Disease in Man: Approximately 90% of schistosome infections in humans are asymptomatic. However, some patients suffer acute respiratory abnormalities with radiographic signs and unspecific symptoms similar to those of influenza. There can be more significant morbidity, and even mortality, from fibrotic reactions to parasite eggs laid in host tissue, leading especially to portal hypertension in the case of *S. mansoni* or *S. japonicum,* and urinary tract obstruction in the case of *S. haematobium* (El-Garem, 1998). However, the disease's clinical presentation has changed over the last 10 to 15 years thanks to specific chemotherapy for schistosomiasis and to environmental changes in many countries, and its earlier hepatosplenic and other manifestations (ascites, gastric hemorrhage, splenomegaly, cor pulmonale, glomerulopathy) are now less severe (Andrade, 1998). Between 6% and 27% of infected women suffer from genital lesions, but the nature and treatment of these lesions is not yet understood (Feldmeier, 1998). In less than 5% of those infected with *S. mansoni*, the obstruction of pulmonary circulation causes pulmonary hypertension and cor pulmonale (Morris and Knauer, 1997). Occasionally, the eggs reach the central nervous system and produce a granulomatous reaction. When there are only a few eggs and they are widely scattered, no signs are observed, but large granulomas can cause increased intracranial pressure and focalized signs, often in the lumbosacral spinal cord (Ferrari, 1999; Pittella, 1997).

The seriousness of the disease is dictated by the parasite burden and the length of time the patient has been infected; both factors affect the number of eggs that settle in host tissues, which is the main determinant of chronic pathology. School-age children and occupational groups that spend time frequently and for long periods in water, such as fishermen and rice growers, have more intense infections because of the accumulation of parasites from repeated infections. However, there is a limit to this accumulation because the schistosomes generate concomitant immunity; in other words, the adult forms of the parasite partially protect against new infections by schistosomula.

The symptomatology of schistosomiasis may be divided into four phases, according to the evolution of the parasitosis. The first phase corresponds to the penetration of cercariae. It is commonly manifested by a cutaneous allergy to the parasite's products, which occurs with greater frequency and intensity in reinfections. At first there are petechiae with edema and pruritus; these are followed by urticaria, which can become vesicular and last from 36 hours to 10 days. Unlike birds, humans do not always have cutaneous manifestations. The second phase occurs when the schistosomula invade the pulmonary capillaries. In most cases there are no clinical manifestations, although massive infections can produce pneumonitis with coughing and asthma-like crises, along with eosinophilic infiltration. The third phase develops when the parasite matures inside the liver and oviposition begins to take place in the corresponding venules. This phase does not usually produce damage to the tissues or clinical manifestations, but in the case of massive infections there may be fever, diarrhea, abdominal pain, urticaria, and prostration. It is believed that these symptoms represent an acute immune response to antigens released by the eggs, with the formation of abundant cytokines. The fourth, or chronic or granulomatous phase, reflects the tissue response to the deposition of eggs. The antigens of the eggs that are retained in the tissues generate a cell-mediated immune response that forms granulomas around the eggs. When the granulomas become abundant in a tissue, they converge and can invade an important part of the organ. Prior stimulation of the patient by antigens of the adult parasite and the intervention of tumor necrosis factor alpha seem to play an important role in the formation of granulomas (Leptak and McKerrow, 1997).

In *S. mansoni* infection, the main lesions are found in the intestinal wall. Over time, they spread to the liver and produce interlobular fibrosis and portal hypertension, ascites, and splenomegaly. In advanced stages, there may be pulmonary lesions and respiratory symptoms. In the chronic phase, the following clinical forms can be distinguished: intestinal, hepatointestinal, hepatosplenic, and pulmonary. In a study of *S. mansoni* morbidity in three rural villages on an island off Tanzania, prevalence was 86% and the average parasite burden was 176 eggs per gram of feces, while 80% of those infected had abdominal pain, 43% had melena, and 35% had diarrhea. The disease was more serious in children and adolescents. Ultrasound revealed hepatomegaly in 35% of the infected individuals and splenomegaly in 80%, both of which were associated with a high parasite burden and were less notable in those who had already been treated with praziquantel. Mild periportal fibrosis was common, and signs of portal hypertension were observed in 2% of the subjects. Serum procollagen-IV-peptide levels were elevated in patients with severe periportal fibrosis, suggesting that this might be a marker of hepatic schistosomiasis (Kardorff *et al.*, 1997). The most indicative signs of acute *S. mansoni* infection are fever, diarrhea, abdominal pain, weight loss, and eosinophilia. The signs of chronic disease are usually persistent diarrhea and abdominal pain with hepatomegaly or splenomegaly.

The symptoms of disease caused by *S. japonicum* are similar to those caused by *S. mansoni*, but they are usually more severe, the period of incubation is shorter, and the early lesions are typically located in the small intestine rather than the colon. Intestinal and hepatic fibrosis develop much more rapidly because *S. japonicum* lays more eggs.

In infections caused by *S. haematobium,* the lesions and symptoms correspond primarily to the urogenital tract, and, to a lesser degree, the intestine. Papillomatous folds, pseudoabscesses, and miliary pseudotubercles develop in the wall of the bladder, and sometimes there is total fibrosis of the organ. Obstruction of the urethra and the ureters is common. The main symptoms are painful and frequent urination, terminal hematuria, suprapubic pain, and recurrent urinary infections. The hepatopathies are less serious than those seen in *S. mansoni* infections. The eggs may also travel to the intestine, especially the venules that drain the rectum, and they may be eliminated in the feces. Evidence suggests that vesical schistosomiasis may be a predisposing condition for malignant tumors because of the continuous irritation produced by the eggs. In a survey of more than 1,000 persons infected with *S. haematobium* in two hyperendemic localities in Mali, half the subjects did not have clinical manifestations and only 30% had pathologic lesions. Both infection and morbidity rates were higher in children aged 7 to 14 years old. Use of the dipstick test to measure microhematuria proved to be more sensitive in detecting the disease than the infection. Treatment with praziquantel resolved more than 80% of the urinary tract lesions within a year (Traore, 1998).

In human infections caused by *S. mattheei* or *S. intercalatum*, the lesions and symptoms are usually mild. As a rule, *S. mattheei* is found in persons simultaneously infected by *S. mansoni* or *S. haematobium*. Infection caused by *S. intercalatum* occurs primarily in young people and tends to gradually disappear in older age groups as the population acquires resistance to the parasite. About 90% of patients infected by *S. intercalatum* complain of intestinal disorders, and some 70% have bloody feces. Hepatomegaly occurs in approximately 50% of the cases, but portal hypertension is not seen. Other species of nonhuman schistosomes, such as *S. bovis* and *S. rodhaini*, produce an abortive infection in man because the parasite does not reach maturity.

There is also an acute form of schistosomiasis, often referred to as Katayama fever, which develops four to six weeks after a massive primary infection with *S. japonicum*, and sometimes, *S. mansoni*. The clinical manifestations are similar in some respects to those of serum disease: fever, eosinophilia, lymphadenopathy, hepatosplenomegaly, and sometimes dysentery. Because of the clinical manifestations and the fact that the disease occurs at the beginning of oviposition, it is believed that this syndrome is caused by the formation of antigen-antibody complexes in the bloodstream.

The Disease in Animals: Schistosomiasis can be quite common in animals. Prevalence rates in cattle have been found to be as high as 62% (Bangladesh), 90% (Sudan), and 92% (Zimbabwe). The species that are most pathogenic for domestic ruminants are *S. bovis* and *S. japonicum*. *S. mattheei* and *S. spindale* are less pathogenic, and sometimes the former is eliminated spontaneously over time. As in man, schistosomiasis in cattle has an acute phase, caused when recently matured parasites release large quantities of eggs in the intestinal mucosa, and a chronic phase, during which the damage is caused by the reaction to antigens produced by eggs trapped inside tissues. The former, referred to as the intestinal syndrome, occurs seven to nine weeks after a massive initial infection and causes severe hemorrhagic lesions in the intestinal mucosa, with infiltration of eosinophils, lymphocytes, macrophages, and plasmocytes, along with profuse diarrhea or dysentery, dehydration, anorexia, anemia, hypoalbuminemia, weight loss, and retarded development. The duration of the disease varies depending on the parasite burden, and recovery is spontaneous. The chronic phase, or hepatic syndrome, is a cell-mediated immune response to antigens from the trapped eggs. As in man, the reaction leads to the formation of inflammatory foci, granulomas, fibroses, and ultimately, the obstruction of portal irrigation. The chronic disease occurs in animals that have been repeatedly exposed to infections with large numbers of cercariae, and the principal manifestations are emaciation, anemia, eosinophilia, and hypoalbuminemia (Soulsby, 1982). Unlike man, animals do not appear to be susceptible to splenomegaly or esophageal varices, but the presence of dead parasites can cause them to develop enlarged follicles or lymph nodes, as well as venous thromboses, with infarct of the organ. In addition to the liver, the schistosome eggs can settle in the intestinal wall, lungs, kidneys, bladder, and other organs, where they cause damage and symptoms in proportion to the parasite burden. Cattle have also been reported to have obstructive phlebitis caused by the presence of adult parasites in the veins.

Source of Infection and Mode of Transmission: Schistosomiasis is one of the main human parasitoses and is very important to public health because of its debilitating effect on people throughout large areas of the world. Geographic distribution of the infection appears to be undergoing a change. While some areas are making progress through vigorous control campaigns, the infection is spreading to others in the wake of new irrigation projects or carried by individuals. Moreover, the geographic range of the intermediate hosts is greater than that of the human infection. The Aswan Dam in Egypt provides an example of how environmental change can impact on the disease. Although construction of the dam has resulted in important economic benefits for the country, it has also brought about profound ecological changes in the region and created favorable conditions for the survival of the mollusks that act as intermediate hosts of *S. mansoni*, but not for those of *S. haematobium*. Before construction of the dam, *S. mansoni* schistosomiasis was common in the Nile Delta but infrequent in the region from Cairo to Khartoum, Sudan. The dam reduced the flow rate of the Lower Nile and held back the alluvial sediment, thereby favoring penetration of the mollusks by the miracidia and also facilitating human contact with the cercariae that emerge from them. At the same time, there was an increase in human activities, such as fishing and washing clothes and utensils, along the Nile River. All these factors contributed to an increase in the prevalence of *S. mansoni* infection in Upper Egypt. The ecology of Lower Egypt (the Nile Delta) also underwent changes favorable to the vectors of this parasitosis. The absence of alluvial sediment promoted the growth and spread of aquatic plants as well as the microflora on which the mollusks feed, with a consequent increase in their population and greater possibility of transmission of the parasite to the human host (Malek, 1975). The situation in Egypt, which has been repeated in several other countries of Africa, the Americas, and Asia, shows that knowledge of ecological conditions is essential to understanding the variability of the human infection. The growing rate at which dams are being constructed in the developing countries, sometimes without prior ecologic and epidemiologic studies to serve as a basis for implementing disease prevention measures, is helping to bring about the spread and intensification of schistosomiasis.

The primary intermediate hosts of *S. mansoni (Biomphalaria)* and *S. haematobium (Bulinus)* are aquatic snails that flourish in irrigation canals, lagoons, river backwaters, and small shaded natural pools of water under 2 meters deep with a flow rate of less than 15 m per minute. *Bulinus*, unlike *Biomphalaria*, can survive in mud after the water has dried up. The intermediate host of *S. japonicum (Oncomelania)*, on the other hand, is an amphibious snail that can live for several months in a relatively dry environment, maintaining the larval stages of the parasite. These mollusks become infected when their water becomes contaminated with fecal matter from definitive hosts, especially humans, or urine in the case of *S. haematobium*.

Man acquires the infection by the cutaneous route by entering water that contains mollusks infected with the parasite. For this reason, schistosomiasis is essentially a rural infection. Studies in endemic areas have shown that the prevalence of infection in the snails concerned is generally lower than 5% and that the density of free-living cercariae is extremely low because they are dispersed over a large volume of water. Moreover, the latter are infective for only a few hours. These low rates suggest that the intense infections needed to cause disease require relatively prolonged exposure to contaminated water. Thus, it follows that the population likely to have the highest prevalence rates and parasite burdens (and consequently more severe disease) is children and young adults aged 5 to 25 years, who spend the most time in water. In some regions, schistosomiasis is also an occupational disease of farm laborers who work in irrigated fields (rice, sugarcane) and fisherman who work in fish culture ponds and rivers. Another highly exposed group is the village women who wash clothing and utensils along the banks of lakes and streams. The infection can also be contracted while bathing, swimming, or playing in the water.

Man is the main definitive host of *S. mansoni*. Patent *S. mansoni* infections have also been seen in rodents, monkeys, and insectivores. Studies in the Americas have shown that rodents alone cannot maintain prolonged environmental contamination, but perhaps baboons (*Papio* spp.) in Africa can do so. Nevertheless, for epidemiologic purposes, *S. mansoni* is regarded as an exclusively human species. *S. haematobium* is also an exclusively human parasite; observations of infection in monkeys have been scarce and epidemiologically insignificant. However, *S. japonicum* is an entirely different matter: at least 31 mammalian species belonging to seven orders, including virtually all domestic animals, are capable of having patent infections caused by this parasite. These species play an important epidemiologic role because they contaminate the water, enabling man to become infected. In Taiwan, there is a strain of *S. japonicum* that is widespread in rodents and domestic animals, but it causes only an abortive infection in man because the parasite does not reach maturity. In addition, *S. mekongi* can infect dogs, and *S. malayensis* is a parasite of wild rats (Greer *et al.*, 1989), but the precise influence of the animal reservoir on human infection is unknown in both instances. *S. intercalatum* and *S. mattheei* are animal parasites that secondarily infect man (the former is a parasite, *inter alia*, of sheep, goats, and rats, and the latter, of cattle, sheep, goats, equines, and rodents). They are usually found in mixed infections along with *S. mansoni* or *S. haematobium*, so that the true importance of these species for human health is unclear. DNA comparisons have shown that *S. mekongi* is closely related to *S. japonicum* and *S. malayensis*, and observations in nature have shown that *S. intercalatum* and *S. mattheei* can hybridize with *S. haematobium* and produce fertile offspring (Jusot *et al.*, 1997; Tchuem Tchuente *et al.*, 1997).

It has been observed that persons infected with abortive animal schistosomes or those that have little pathogenicity for man develop a degree of cross-resistance that protects them against subsequent human schistosome infections. It is even thought that resistance produced by abortive infections of the zoonotic strain *S. japonicum* in Taiwan has spared the island from being invaded by the human strain. In light of this heterologous or cross-immunity, some researchers have proposed vaccinating humans with the antigens or parasites of animal species (zooprophylaxis).

The influence of factors involving the parasite, host, and environment on the persistence of schistosomiasis has been studied using *S. mansoni* in rats (Morand *et al.*, 1999).

Diagnosis: Schistosomiasis is suspected when the characteristic symptoms occur in an epidemiologic environment that facilitates its transmission. Specific diagnosis is based on demonstrating the presence of *S. mansoni* or *S. japonicum* eggs in feces and those of *S. haematobium* in either feces or urine. The eggs of all the human schistosome species are long and nonoperculate. Those of *S. mansoni* are brownish-yellow, measure 110–180 µ long by 40–70 µ wide, and have a characteristic lateral spine. Those of *S. haematobium* are about the same size and have a very pronounced terminal spine, while those of *S. japonicum* are smaller and have a rudimentary sub-terminal spine. *S. intercalatum* eggs are difficult to differentiate from those of *S. haematobium* (Almeda *et al.*, 1996). The eggs may begin to appear five weeks after the initial infection. The ease with which their presence is confirmed depends on the intensity and duration of the infection; mild and long-standing infections produce few eggs. Whenever schistosomiasis is suspected, samples should be examined over a period of several days, since the passage of eggs is not continuous. Direct, unen-riched examination of the samples is not a very sensitive method. The Kato-Katz thick smear technique offers a good balance between simplicity and sensitivity, and it is commonly used in the field (Borel *et al.*, 1999).

Among the feces concentration techniques, formalin-ether sedimentation is con-sidered one of the most efficient. In chronic cases with scant passage of eggs, the rectal mucosa can be biopsied for high-pressure microscopy. Also, the eclosion test, in which the feces are diluted in unchlorinated water and incubated for about four hours in a centrifuge tube lined with dark paper, can be used. At the end of this time, the upper part of the tube is illuminated in order to concentrate the miracidia, which can be observed with a magnifying glass. In addition to the mere presence of eggs, it is important to determine whether or not the miracidia are alive (which can be seen from the movement of the miracidium or its cilia) because the immune response that leads to fibrosis is triggered by antigens produced by the miracidium. In cases of prepatent, mild, or long-standing infection, the presence of eggs is difficult to demonstrate, and diagnosis therefore usually relies on finding specific antigens or antibodies (Tsang and Wilkins, 1997). However, searching for parasite antigens is not a very efficient approach when the live parasite burden is low. The circumoval precipitation, cercarien-Hullen reaction, miracidial immobilization, and cercarial fluorescent antibody tests are reasonably sensitive and specific, but they are rarely used because they require live parasites. The enzyme-linked immunosorbent assay (ELISA) and immunotransference (Western blot) tests are now preferred. A recom-binant protein of *S. mansoni* (Sm22.3) has been produced that recognizes antibod-ies to *S. mansoni* or *S. haematobium* with 80% sensitivity and 95% specificity, but it still cross-reacts with serum from malaria infections (Hancock *et al.*, 1997). IgM and IgG antibodies from all acute patients recognized the *S. mansoni* SM31/32 anti-gen, but only 10% of the IgM antibodies from chronic patients reacted. Hence, the reaction of this antigen to IgM antibodies may be a marker of acute disease (Valli *et al.*, 1999).

A questionnaire administered to students and teachers from schools in urinary schistosomiasis endemic areas revealed a surprisingly large number of *S. haemato-bium* infections (Partnership for Child Development, 1999). In many cases, cen-trifugation and examination of the urine sediment is sufficient to find eggs, although filtration in microporous membranes is more sensitive. Examination of the urine sediment for eosinophils reveals more than 80% of all infections. The use of strips dipped in urine to detect blood or proteins also reveals a high number of infections, even though the test is nonspecific. Also, there are now strips impregnated with spe-cific antibodies that reveal the presence of *S. haematobium* antigens when dipped in a urine specimen (Bosompem *et al.*, 1997). Although this method is less sensitive than the ELISA test, it is easy to use in mass studies. Searching for antibodies or antigens in serum was substantially more sensitive than looking for eggs in urine (Al-Sherbiny *et al.*, 1999).

Control: The measures available for controlling schistosomiasis are: 1) diagnosis and treatment of patients; 2) selective or mass chemotherapy; 3) health education; 4) control of the intermediate hosts; 5) adequate water supply and sanitary excreta disposal systems; and 6) modification of the environment.

Chemotherapy of infected individuals is not only curative but also preventive in that it halts the production of eggs that contaminate the environment. Clinical trials with praziquantel to treat *S. mansoni* infection in Brazil, *S. haematobium* in Zambia, and *S. japonicum* in the Philippines and Japan have given excellent results in terms of both parasitologic cure and the reduction of eggs being eliminated (WHO, 1980). In a three-year study carried out in Madagascar, 289 individuals from a village in which *S. mansoni* was hyperendemic were treated systematically with praziquantel and prevalence declined from 66%, with an average of 202 eggs per gram of feces, to 19% and 27 eggs per gram (Boisier *et al.*, 1998). In most cases, it is not recommended to treat the entire community; a more effective approach is to perform parasitologic examinations and treat only the infected individuals. When the intensity of infection declines in a given population, it may be necessary to resort to serologic diagnosis, which is more sensitive. In communities that have a high prevalence of infection but limited economic resources, treatment can be restricted to the groups with the highest parasite burdens, such as children between 7 and 14 years old. In the case of schistosomiasis caused by *S. japonicum*, however, Olds *et al.* (1996) recommend mass treatment or treatment aimed at large, high-risk groups because there are many animal reservoirs, parasitologic diagnosis is not very sensitive, the disease is more serious, and there is no apparent correlation between severity of the disease and parasite burden.

Health education consists essentially in teaching people to avoid contact with contaminated water and not to contaminate water with their own excreta. However, many of the populations most affected by schistosomiasis are communities with low levels of schooling and such limited resources that they often have no alternative but to use contaminated water or to contaminate the environment with their excreta. The intermediate hosts have been controlled in a number of areas by draining or filling in swampland, removing vegetation from water bodies, and improving irrigation systems. In Japan, excellent results were achieved by lining irrigation canals with concrete. The use of molluscicides, though expensive, is a rapid and effective means of reducing transmission if it is combined with other prevention measures, especially chemotherapy. The cost-benefit ratio is more favorable where the volume of water to be treated is small, and for rivers or lakes where transmission is focal (limited to a relatively small habitat). Selection of the molluscicide to be used should take into account the nature of the snail's habitat, the cost of the chemical compound, and any harmful effects it might have on fish and other forms of aquatic life. The introduction of snails that compete with the intermediate hosts of the schistosome has been successful in some areas. In Puerto Rico, for example, introduction of the snail *Marisa cornuarietis,* coupled with chemical control, has eliminated *B. glabrata* almost entirely from the nearby island of Vieques. However, *M. cornuarietis* is not effective in ecosystems with dense vegetation or in swamps or rivers (WHO, 1980). In Saint Lucia, *B. glabrata* was apparently eliminated from swampy areas and streams between 6 and 22 months after the introduction of *Tiara granifera*, a snail from Southeast Asia. Unfortunately, this snail can serve as the intermediate host of *Paragonimus westermani* (Prentice, 1983). Environmental sanitation (especially the provision of potable water and sanitary waste elimination systems) in rural areas is costly and therefore difficult to implement in the short term and on the needed scale. Moreover, changing the environment entails an improved standard of living for the population, more education, and healthier surroundings—objectives that are difficult to achieve.

The measures described above are useful when they are incorporated realistically within the framework of a control program. In Venezuela, the Schistosomiasis Control Program was launched in 1945 and prevalence of the infection has fallen from 14% in 1943 to 1.4% in 1996. Up until 1982, active cases were diagnosed by fecal examination, which was then followed by treatment, but starting that year, serologic surveys were added because many infections were too mild to be diagnosed by parasitology. Nevertheless, the true prevalence is believed to be underestimated. Given that 80% of infected individuals pass fewer than 100 eggs per gram of feces, it is possible that these people maintain foci of infection, thereby undermining control efforts. Biological control using snails that compete with the intermediate hosts has not been totally successful, since B. glabrata has managed to reinfect some areas and increase the prevalence of infection in others. Indeed, infected snails have been found over an expanse of approximately 15,000 km^2 in which the infection was believed to have been eradicated several years ago. As a result, the entire schistosomiasis control strategy in Venezuela has been revised (Alarcón de Noya et al., 1999). In Brazil, chemotherapy has been a very important tool for reducing morbidity, incidence, and prevalence in endemic areas, but the provision of potable water, sanitary disposal of excreta, and health education still remain the essential requirements for definitive and permanent control (Katz, 1998).

Although chemotherapy has been very successful in controlling schistosomiasis, reinfection makes it necessary for people to take the treatment often, sometimes annually. Hence the search for a vaccine. Despite reasonable success in domestic and laboratory animals, vaccines for human use are still far from being effective, both because man does not respond to vaccination the same way that animals do and because the methods used with animals (such as infection with irradiated cercariae) are not directly applicable to man. Indeed, vaccination was not considered a viable alternative for the control of schistosomiasis until recently, when the identification of certain protective antigens and the possibility of producing them as recombinant molecules raised hopes for success in this endeavor (Bergquist, 1998).

Bibliography

Alarcón de Noya, B., C. Balzán, C. Arteaga, I. Cesari, O. Noya. The last fifteen years of schistosomiasis in Venezuela: Features and evolution. Mem Inst Oswaldo Cruz 94:139–146, 1999.

Almeda, J., C. Ascaso, G.A. Marcal, et al. Morphometric variability of Schistosoma intercalatum eggs: A diagnostic dilemma. J Helminthol 70:97–102, 1996.

Al-Sherbiny, M.M., A.M. Osman, K. Hancock, A.M. Deelder, V.C. Tsang. Application of immunodiagnostic assays: Detection of antibodies and circulating antigens in human schistosomiasis and correlation with clinical findings. Am J Trop Med Hyg 60:960–966, 1999.

Andrade, Z.A. The situation of hepatosplenic schistosomiasis in Brazil today. Mem Inst Oswaldo Cruz 93 Suppl 1:313–316, 1998.

Bergquist, N.R. Schistosomiasis vaccine development: Progress and prospects. Mem Inst Oswaldo Cruz 93 Suppl 1:95–101, 1998.

Boisier, P., C.E. Ramarokoto, V.E. Ravaoalimalala, *et al.* Reversibility of *Schistosoma mansoni*-associated morbidity after yearly mass praziquantel therapy: Ultrasonographic assessment. *Trans R Soc Trop Med Hyg* 92:451–453, 1998.

Booth, M., C. Mayombana, P. Kilima. The population biology and epidemiology of schistosome and geohelminth infections among school children in Tanzania. *Trans R Soc Trop Med Hyg* 92:491–495, 1998.

Borel, E., J.F. Etard, A. Addo, M. Diakite. Comparison of a digestion-sedimentation technique with the Kato-Katz technique in the detection and quantification of *S. mansoni* eggs in light to moderate infections. *Parasite* 6:175–178, 1999.

Bosompem K.M., I. Ayi, W.K. Anyan, *et al.* A monoclonal antibody-based dipstick assay for diagnosis of urinary schistosomiasis. *Trans R Soc Trop Med Hyg* 91:554–556, 1997.

De Clercq, D., J. Vercruysse, M. Picquet, *et al.* The epidemiology of a recent focus of mixed *Schistosoma haematobium* and *Schistosoma mansoni* infections around the 'Lac de Guiers' in the Senegal River Basin, Senegal. *Trop Med Int Health* 4:544–550, 1999.

El-Garem, A.A. Schistosomiasis. *Digestion* 59:589–605, 1998.

Ferrari, T.C. Spinal cord schistosomiasis. A report of 2 cases and review emphasizing clinical aspects. *Medicine (Baltimore)* 78:176–190, 1999.

Feldmeier, H., R.C. Daccal, M.J. Martins, V. Soares, R. Martins. Genital manifestations of schistosomiasis *mansoni* in women: Important but neglected. *Mem Inst Oswaldo Cruz* 93 Suppl 1:127–133, 1998.

Greer, G.J., D.T. Dennis, P.F. Lai, H. Anuar. Malaysian schistosomiasis: Description of a population at risk. *J Trop Med Hyg* 2:203–208, 1989.

Hancock, K., Y.B. Mohamed, X. Haichou, *et al.* A recombinant protein from *Schistosoma mansoni* useful for the detection of *S. mansoni* and *Schistosoma haematobium* antibodies. *J Parasitol* 83:612–618, 1997.

Jusot, J.F., P.P. Simarro, A. De Muynck. La bilharziose à *Schistosoma intercalatum*: considerations cliniques et epidemiologiques. *Med Trop (Mars)* 57:280–288, 1997.

Kardorff, R., R.M. Gabone, C. Mugashe, *et al. Schistosoma mansoni*-related morbidity on Ukerewe Island, Tanzania: Clinical, ultrasonographical and biochemical parameters. *Trop Med Int Health* 2:230–239, 1997.

Katz, N. Schistosomiasis control in Brazil. *Mem Inst Oswaldo Cruz* 93 Suppl 1:33–35, 1998.

Katz, N., O.S. Carvalho. Introdução recente de esquistossomose *mansoni* no Sul do Estado de Minas Gerais, Brasil. *Mem Inst Oswaldo Cruz* 78:281–284, 1983.

Kruger, F.J., A.C. Evans. Do all human urinary infections with *Schistosoma mattheei* represent hybridization between *S. haematobium* and *S. mattheei*? *J Helminthol* 64:330–332, 1990.

Leptak, C.L., J.H. McKerrow. Schistosome egg granulomas and hepatic expression of TNF-alpha are dependent on immune priming during parasite maturation. *J Immunol* 158:301–307, 1997.

Machado, P.H. The Brazilian program for schistosomiasis control, 1975–1979. *Am J Trop Med Hyg* 31:76–86, 1982.

Mahmoud, A.A. Schistosomiasis. *New Engl J Med* 297(24):1329–1331, 1977.

Mahmoud, A.A. Schistosomiasis. *In:* Warren, K.S., A.A. Mahmoud, eds. *Tropical and Geographical Medicine.* New York: McGraw-Hill; 1984.

Malek, E.A. Effect of the Aswan high dam on prevalence of schistosomiasis in Egypt. *Trop Geogr Med* 27:359–364, 1975.

Marquardt, W.C., R.S. Demaree, Jr., R.B. Grieve, eds. *Parasitology and Vector Biology,* 2nd ed. San Diego: Academic Press; 2000.

Morand, S., J.P. Pointier, A. Theron. Population biology of *Schistosoma mansoni* in the black rat: Host regulation and basic transmission rate. *Int J Parasitol* 29:673–684, 1999.

Morris, W., C.M. Knauer. Cardiopulmonary manifestations of schistosomiasis. *Semin Respir Infect* 12:159–170, 1997.

Ndamba, J., O. Makura, P.R. Gwatirisa, N. Makaza, K.C. Kaondera. A cost effective two step rapid diagnosis of urinary schistosomiasis in Zimbabwe. *Cent Afr J Med* 44:167–171, 1998.

Olds, G.R., R. Olveda, G. Wu, *et al.* Immunity and morbidity in schistosomiasis *japonicum* infection. *Am J Trop Med Hyg* 55(Suppl 5):121–126, 1996.

Partnership for Child Development. Self-diagnosis as a possible basis for treating urinary schistosomiasis: A study of schoolchildren in a rural area of the United Republic of Tanzania. *Bull World Health Organ* 77:477–483, 1999.

Pittella, J.E. Neuroschistosomiasis. *Brain Patol* 7:649–662, 1997.

Prentice, M.A. Displacement of *Biomphalaria glabrata* by the snail *Thiara granifera* in field habitats in St. Lucia, West Indies. *Ann Trop Med Parasitol* 77:51–59, 1983.

Rollinson, D., A. Kaukas, D.A. Johnston, A.J. Simpson, M. Tanaka. Some molecular insights into schistosome evolution. *Int J Parasitol* 27:11–28, 1997.

Soulsby, E.J.L. *Helminths, Arthropods and Protozoa of Domesticated Animals*, 7th ed. Philadelphia: Lea and Febiger; 1982.

Stich, A.H., S. Biays, P. Odermatt, *et al.* Foci of *Schistosomiasis mekongi*, Northern Cambodia: II. Distribution of infection and morbidity. *Trop Med Int Health* 674–685, 1999.

Tchuem Tchuente, L.A., V.R. Southgate, J. Vercruysse, *et al.* Epidemiological and genetic observations on human schistosomiasis in Kinshasa, Zaire. *Trans R Soc Trop Med Hyg* 91:263–269, 1997.

Traore, M., H.A. Traore, R. Kardorff, *et al.* The public health significance of urinary schistosomiasis as a cause of morbidity in two districts in Mali. *Am J Trop Med Hyg* 59:407–413, 1998.

Tsang, V.C., P.P. Wilkins. Immunodiagnosis of schistosomiasis. *Immunol Invest* 26:175–188, 1997.

Valli, L.C., H.Y. Kanamura, R.M. Da Silva, R. Ribeiro Rodríguez, R. Dietze. Schistosomiasis *mansoni*: Immunoblot analysis to diagnose and differentiate recent and chronic infection. *Am J Trop Med Hyg* 61:302–307, 1999.

Williams, S.A., D.A. Johnston. Helminth genome analysis: The current status of the filarial and schistosome genome projects. *Parasitology* 118 Suppl:S19–38, 1999.

World Health Organization (WHO). *Parasitic Zoonoses. Report of a WHO Expert Committee, with the Participation of FAO.* Geneva: WHO; 1979. (Technical Report Series 637).

World Health Organization (WHO). *Epidemiology and Control of Schistosomiasis. Report of a WHO Expert Committee.* Geneva: WHO; 1980. (Technical Report Series 643).

World Health Organization (WHO). *Schistosomiasis. Disease information* [Web page]. Available at www.who.int/tdr/diseases/schisto/diseaseinfo.htm. Accessed 14 February 2003.

World Health Organization (WHO). *Schistosomiasis.* [Web page]. Available at www.who.int/ctd/schisto/index.html. Accessed 14 February 2003.

Ye, X.P., Y.L. Fu, Z.X. Wu, R.M. Anderson, A. Agnew. The effects of temperature, light and water upon the hatching of the ova of *Schistosoma japonicum*. *Southeast Asian J Trop Med Public Health* 8:575–580, 1997.

2. Cestodiases

BERTIELLIASIS

ICD-10 B71.9 Cestode infection, unspecified

Etiology: *Bertiella studeri* (*B. satyri*) and *B. mucronata* are anoplocephalid cestodes whose natural definitive hosts are nonhuman primates. Differentiation of the two species is based on the size of the glandular portion of the vagina, the eggs and their pyriform apparatus, and the number of testes. Some specialists think that these differences are not sufficient to separate *B. studeri* from *B. mucronata,* and accept only the former species name. Others accept geographic and host segregation as additional valid criteria (Denegri *et al.*, 1998). Adult cestodes are 10 to 30 cm long and 1 cm wide. The gravid proglottids (segments) are much wider than they are long, detach in groups of about 20, and are eliminated in the feces of the primates. The intermediate hosts are oribatid mites of the genera *Dometorina, Achipteria, Galumna, Scheloribates,* and *Scutovertex.* These mites are about 0.5 mm long, live in the soil and humus, and, since they feed on organic matter, can become infected by ingesting cestode eggs found in soil contaminated by the fecal matter of infected monkeys. The embryo travels to the mites' body cavity and forms a larva known as cysticercoid. When a monkey ingests an infected mite with its food, digestion of the mite releases the cysticercoids, which mature into adult cestodes in the host's intestine.

Geographic Distribution and Occurrence: This parasitosis is rare in man. Up to 1999, 56 cases in humans had been reported: 45 cases of infection by *B. studeri,* 7 by *B. mucronata,* and 4 by *Bertiella* sp. (Ando *et al.*, 1996; Denegri and Perez-Serrano, 1997). The cases caused by *B. studeri* occurred in east Africa, Gabon, India, Indonesia, the island of Mauritius, the Philippines, the Russian Federation, Saint Kitts in the Lesser Antilles, Singapore, Spain, Thailand, the US (state of Minnesota), and Yemen. At least two of the three cases caused by *B. studeri* in the New World seem to be associated with Old World monkeys: the monkeys on Saint Kitts are of African origin, and the case in Spain was apparently acquired in Kenya. Three cases caused by *B. mucronata* were reported in Argentina, two in Brazil, one in Cuba, and one in Paraguay. The cases caused by *Bertiella* sp. occurred in the Democratic Republic of the Congo, Great Britain, India, and Saudi Arabia. The natural hosts of *B. studeri* belong to the genera *Simya, Anthropithecus, Hylobates,*

Cercopithecus, Troglodytes, Macaca, Pan, and *Papio*; the natural hosts of *B. mucronata* belong to the genera *Allouata, Callicebus, Cebus,* and *Callithrix.* Infection in monkeys is common. Prevalences of 3.6% to 14.0% have been reported in rhesus monkeys, 1.4% to 5.3% in cynomolgus monkeys, 7.1% in Japanese macaques, and 7.7% in baboons (Flynn, 1973).

The Disease in Man and Animals: The infection causes neither symptoms nor lesions in monkeys (Owen, 1992). It is generally also asymptomatic in man, but some cases with abdominal pain, intermittent diarrhea, anorexia, constipation, and weight loss have been reported. These symptoms seem to be more common in children. In rare cases, severe abdominal pain and intermittent vomiting have been described.

Source of Infection and Mode of Transmission: Nonhuman primates, which constitute the natural reservoir of the cestode, acquire the parasitosis by ingesting infected oribatid mites with their food. Man can become infected by accidental ingestion of food contaminated with soil containing infected mites. This occurs when people are in close contact with monkeys kept at home or in zoos, or when there are large numbers of monkeys in the peridomestic environment.

Diagnosis: Preliminary diagnosis is based on observation of the proglottids eliminated in the feces and is subsequently confirmed by microscopic examination of the eggs obtained from the proglottids. The eggs are slightly oval and thin-shelled, and the embryo is encased in a capsule or pyriform apparatus with two blunt horns. The eggs of *B. studeri* are 49–60 by 40–46 μm and the eggs of *B. mucronata* are 40–46 by 36–40 μm.

Control: Since human infection is accidental and infrequent, its prevention is difficult. Ingestion of food contaminated with soil from environments where monkeys are numerous should be avoided.

Bibliography

Ando, K., T. Ito, K. Miura, H. Matsuoka, Y. Chinzei. Infection of an adult in Mie Prefecture, Japan by *Bertiella studeri. Southeast Asian J Trop Med Public Health* 27:200–201, 1996.

Denegri, G.M., J. Perez-Serrano. Bertiellosis in man: A review of cases. *Rev Inst Med Trop Sao Paulo* 39:123–127, 1997.

Denegri, G.M., W. Bernadina, J. Perez-Serrano, F. Rodriguez-Caabeiro. Anoplocephalid cestodes of veterinary and medical significance: A review. *Folia Parasitol (Praha)* 45:1–8, 1998.

Flynn, R.J. *Parasites of Laboratory Animals.* Ames: Iowa State University Press; 1973.

Owen, D.G. *Parasites of Laboratory Animals.* London: Royal Society of Medicine Services; 1992.

Turner, J.A. Other cestode infections. *In:* Hubbert, W.T., W.F. McCulloch, P.R. Schnurrenberger, eds. *Diseases Transmitted from Animals to Man,* 6th ed. Springfield: Thomas; 1975.

COENUROSIS

ICD-10 B71.9 Cestode infection, unspecified

Synonyms: Coenuriasis, vertigo, gid, sturdy.

Etiology: *Coenurus cerebralis, C. serialis,* and *C. brauni* are larval stages of the cestodes *Taenia multiceps, T. serialis,* and *T. brauni,* respectively. While those names do not correspond to the species of the parasite, and therefore should not be written in italics or in Latin with the first letter capitalized, the custom goes back to the time when the relationship between the larval and adult stages of cestodes was not known. Those species used to be assigned to the genus *Multiceps,* whose identifying characteristic is that the larval stage is a coenurus. Since this property is not evident when the adult cestodes are examined, and since they are morphologically indistinguishable from cestodes of the genus *Taenia,* they are currently assigned to the genus *Taenia.* However, certain authors still reserve the subgenus *Multiceps* for those larval stages (Barriga, 1997). Parasitologists disagree about how to differentiate these species: some attribute the morphological differences observed, especially in the larvae, to factors inherent in the host. For example, Lachberg *et al.* (1990) developed a *C. serialis* that seemed to be a racemose cysticercus in an immunodeficient mouse; Bohrmann (1990) found muscular coenuri in a gazelle, despite the belief that coenuri in ruminants are forms of *T. multiceps* and are almost always found in the central nervous system. Currently, new molecular biology techniques are being used to study cestodes, and these questions will probably be resolved in the near future (Gasser and Chilton, 1995).

The definitive hosts are domestic dogs or wild canids such as coyotes, foxes, and jackals, which harbor the tapeworms in their small intestines. The intermediate hosts of *T. multiceps* are domestic herbivores, mainly sheep. The larval stage, *C. cerebralis,* is found in the central nervous system of these animals, in particular the brain and spinal cord. It is believed that goats can develop this coenurus in the subcutaneous or intermuscular tissue or in other organs. In the past, this parasite was identified in goats as *T. gaigeri,* but the taxonomy of cestodes that form coenuri is too complicated to allow for the acceptance of new species without strong arguments. The intermediate hosts of *T. serialis* are lagomorphs and rodents, especially the domestic rabbit and the hare. The *C. serialis* larva develops in the subcutaneous and intermuscular connective tissue. However, at least one case of fatal infection caused by the *T. serialis* larva in the brain of a cat has been described (Huss *et al.,* 1994). The intermediate hosts of *T. brauni* are wild rodents. The *C. brauni* coenuri also develop in the subcutaneous connective tissue.

The life cycle starts with the expulsion of gravid proglottids or eggs with the feces of the definitive host. Intermediate hosts are infected by ingesting the eggs deposited in grass or in water. The oncospheres (embryos) penetrate the wall of the small intestine and, through the blood vessels, are distributed to different tissues and organs. *C. cerebralis* reaches maturity only in the central nervous system; the coenuri of the other two species develop in connective tissue. The only morphological difference between *C. cerebralis* and *C. serialis* is that the former has 500 to 700 scolices distributed in non-linear groups and the latter has 400 to 500 scolices distributed in radial lines (Barriga, 1997). The coenurus reaches full development in the brain in six to eight months and can grow to a size of 5 cm or more; it forms a cyst that contains a considerable amount of liquid and has a germinal membrane with several hundred scolices. The cycle is completed when a dog or wild canid ingests tissue or an organ containing coenuri. Each coenurus can give rise to numerous tapeworms, which develop in the small intestine of the canids. There is no reliable morphological criterion for distinguishing the species in the adult stage.

Geographic Distribution and Occurrence: *T. multiceps* and its larval stage, *C. cerebralis,* are cosmopolitan in cattle-raising areas but occur primarily in temperate climates. While up until 1950 just five cases of infection with the larva were recognized in man, by 1990, some 55 human cases of cerebral coenurosis had been recorded in the world, most in Africa or South America. There were also a few cases in the US and in the sheep raising areas of western Europe (Pau *et al.*, 1990). Up until 1998, six cases were recorded in the US (Ing *et al.*, 1998). A study carried out in Ethiopia found that 37 of 37 sheep (100%) that were apparently sick with coenurosis and 5 of 183 sheep (2.7%) that were apparently healthy had *T. multiceps* larvae with diameters ranging from 0.8 cm to 6.5 cm. In 96% of the cases, the larvae were in the brain, and in the rest of the cases they were in the cerebellum. Prediction of the localization of the coenurus based on the direction of the parasite's circular movements or gid or the deviation of the head were accurate in just 62% of the cases. A retrospective study showed that the local prevalence of coenurosis in sheep was 2.3% to 4.5% and that the prevalence of taeniasis in autopsied stray dogs was 47%. Seventy-two percent of infections in sheep occurred when the animals were between the ages of 6 and 24 months (Achenef *et al.*, 1999). In Iran, 738 of 7,992 sheep (9.8%) studied were infected with *T. multiceps* larvae (Oryan *et al.*, 1994). In Great Britain, *T. multiceps* was found in 4 (0.5%) and *T. serialis* was found in 5 (0.6%) of 875 foxhounds, *T. multiceps* was found in 15 (1.7%) and *T. serialis* was found in 3 (0.3%) of 882 farm dogs, and *T. serialis* was found in 1 of 197 foxes (0.5%) (Jones and Walter, 1992). In Germany, *T. multiceps* was found in 3.3% of 397 foxes (Ballek *et al.*, 1992), and in Peru, it was found in 20% of 20 foxes (Moro *et al.*, 1998).

T. serialis and its larval stage, *C. serialis,* are also cosmopolitan. Human infection is rare; about 10 cases have been recognized, mostly in Africa (Faust *et al.*, 1974). In man, the coenuri may invade the connective tissue and central nervous system. The frequency of coenurosis in leporids is not known.

T. brauni and its larval stage, *C. brauni,* occur in tropical Africa (central and eastern) and also in South Africa. In central Africa, where this is the only species found, about 25 human cases of coenurosis in connective tissue have been described, as well as one case with ocular localization. The frequency of coenurosis in wild rodents is not known.

The Disease in Man: Most human infections are located in the brain, less frequently, they are subcutaneous, and, in rare cases, they are ocular or peritoneal. The cerebral form is the most serious (Ing *et al.*, 1998). Several years may pass between infection and the appearance of symptoms, and the symptomatology varies with the neuroanatomic localization of the coenurus: cerebral coenurosis is manifested by signs of intracranial hypertension, and the disease is very difficult to distinguish clinically from neurocysticercosis or cerebral hydatidosis. Symptoms that may be observed consist of headache, vomiting, paraplegia, hemiplegia, aphasia, and epileptiform seizures. Papilloedema is a sign of increased intracranial pressure. The coenurus can also develop in the vitreous humor and may affect the retina and choroid. The degree of damage to vision depends on the size of the coenurus and the extent of the choroidoretinal lesion. The prognosis for coenurosis of the nervous tissue is always serious and the only treatment is surgery, although recently, the testing of treatment with praziquantel or albendazole has begun.

Coenurosis of the connective tissue caused by *C. brauni,* which is seen primarily in tropical Africa, is the most benign form. The subcutaneous cysts resemble lipomas or sebaceous cysts.

Interestingly, researchers have discovered that coenuri produce certain components that interfere with the host's immunity and may be responsible for the host's relative tolerance of the larva (Rakha *et al.*, 1997).

The Disease in Animals: Cerebral coenurosis occurs primarily in sheep, although it may also occur in goats, cattle, and horses. Two phases can be distinguished in the symptomatology of cerebral coenurosis in sheep. The first phase is associated with the invasion and migration of the parasite. Massive numbers of larva can migrate simultaneously and cause meningoencephalitis and the death of the animal. This acute form is not frequent and occurs mainly in lambs. The second phase corresponds to the establishment of the coenurus in the cerebral tissue. In general, symptoms are not observed until the parasite reaches a certain size and begins to exert pressure on the nervous tissue. Symptoms vary with the location of the parasite and may include circular movements or gid, incoordination, paralysis, convulsions, excitability, and prostration. Mortality is high. Softening of the cranial wall was observed in 42% of 62 sheep with coenurosis. This change occurs most often in young animals and when the coenuri are situated on the surface of the brain.

Source of Infection and Mode of Transmission: The transmission cycle of infection by *T. multiceps* takes place between dogs and domestic herbivores. Man is an accidental host and does not play any role in the epidemiology of the disease. The main factor in maintaining the parasitosis in nature is access by dogs to the brains of dead or slaughtered domestic herbivores that were infected with coenuri. The life cycle of the other two species of *Taenia* that form coenuri depends on predation by dogs on leporids and rodents.

Taenia eggs expelled in the feces of infected dogs or other canids are the source of infection for man and for the other intermediate hosts. In general, the eggs are eliminated by the definitive host in the proglottids. Since these dry out rapidly and are destroyed outside the host, the eggs are released and dispersed by the wind, rain, irrigation, and waterways.

Diagnosis: Diagnosis in the definitive hosts can be made only by recovery and examination of the parasite; even so, identification of the species is doubtful. Neither the proglottids nor the eggs are distinguishable from those of other species of *Taenia*. Diagnosis in the intermediate hosts can be made only by recovery and examination of the parasite. The morphological differences between *C. cerebralis* and *C. serialis* are explained above. The presumptive diagnosis in man is generally made by establishing the existence of a lesion that occupies space; however, since coenurosis is much less common than hydatidosis, coenurosis is rarely considered before the parasite is recovered (Pierre *et al.*, 1998). Because of the relative infrequency of human coenurosis, there has been no incentive to develop immunological diagnostic techniques. However, the tests that are currently available indicate that cross-reactions with other cestodes are common (Dyson and Linklater, 1979).

Control: For man, individual prophylaxis consists of avoiding the ingestion of raw food or water that may be contaminated with dog feces. General preventive measures for cestodiases consist of preventing infection in the definitive host so that it cannot contaminate the environment, preventing infection in the intermediate host so that it cannot infect the definitive host, or changing the environment so that both actors are not found in nature. Some details on the application of these measures for the control of coenurosis can be found in the chapter on Hydatidosis, which has a similar epidemiology.

Bibliography

Achenef, M., T. Markos, G. Feseha, A. Hibret, S. Tembely. *Coenurus cerebralis* infection in Ethiopian highland sheep: Incidence and observations on pathogenesis and clinical signs. *Trop Anim Health Prod* 31:15–24, 1999.

Ballek, D., M. Takla, S. Ising-Volmer, M. Stoye. [The helminth fauna of red foxes (*Vulpes vulpes Linnaeus* 1758) in north Hesse and east Westphalia. 1. Cestodes]. *Dtsch Tierarztl Wochenschr* 99:362–365, 1992.

Barriga, O.O. *Veterinary Parasitology for Practitioners*, 2nd ed. Edina: Burgess International Group; 1997.

Bohrmann, R. *Coenurus* in the muscles of a gemsbok (*Oryx gazella*). *Vet Parasitol* 36:353–356, 1990.

Dyson, D.A., K.A. Linklater. Problems in the diagnosis of acute coenurosis in sheep. *Vet Rec* 104:528–529, 1979.

Faust, E.C., P.F. Russell, R.C. Jung. *Craig and Faust's Clinical Parasitology*, 8th ed. Philadelphia: Lea & Febiger; 1970.

Gasser, R.B., N.B. Chilton. Characterisation of taeniid cestode species by PCR-RFLP of ITS2 ribosomal DNA. *Acta Trop* 59:31–40, 1995.

Huss, B.T., M.A. Miller, R.M. Corwin, E.P. Hoberg, D.P. O'Brien. Fatal cerebral coenurosis in a cat. *J Am Vet Med Assoc* 205:69–71, 1994.

Ing, M.B., P.M. Schantz, J.A. Turner. Human coenurosis in North America: Case reports and review. *Clinic Infect Dis* 27:519–523, 1998.

Jones, A., T.M. Walters. A survey of taeniid cestodes in farm dogs in mid-Wales. *Ann Trop Med Parasitol* 86:137–142, 1992.

Lachberg, S., R.C. Thompson, A.J. Lymbery. A contribution to the etiology of racemose cysticercosis. *J Parasitol* 76:592–594, 1990.

Moro, P.L., J. Ballarta, R.H. Gilman, G. Leguia, M. Rojas, G. Montes. Intestinal parasites of the grey fox (*Pseudalopex culpaeus*) in the central Peruvian Andes. *J Helminthol* 72:87–89, 1998.

Oryan, A., N. Moghaddar, S.N. Gaur. Metacestodes of sheep with special reference to their epidemiological status, pathogenesis and economic implications in Fars Province, Iran. *Vet Parasitol* 51:231–240, 1994.

Pau, A., C. Perria, S. Turtas, *et al.* Long-term follow-up of the surgical treatment of intracranial coenurosis. *Br J Neurosurg* 4:39–43, 1990.

Pierre, C., M. Civatte, A. Chevalier, J.P. Terrier, P. Gros, E. Carloz. Le diagnostic des helminthes en anatomie pathologique. *Med Trop (Mars)* 58:85–97, 1998.

Rakha, N.K., J.B. Dixon, S.D. Carter. Immunological activities of a lymphocyte mitogen isolated from coenurus fluid of *Taenia multiceps* (Cestoda). *Parasite* 4:9–16, 1997.

CYSTICERCOSIS

ICD-10 B69

Etiology: The agent of this disease is the larval form or cysticercus of *Taenia solium* and *T. crassiceps*. Observation of the *T. solium* larva in man was reported as far back as the sixteenth century; the *T. crassiceps* larva was reported just five times. The *T. saginata* larva does not seem to occur in man (see below). Before the relationship between taeniae and their cysticerci was understood, the larval stages were described with their own scientific names, as if they were separate species. Thus, the *T. solium* larva was called *Cysticercus cellulosae*, the *T. crassiceps* larva was *C. longicollis*, and the *T. saginata* larva was *C. bovis*. This unfortunate situation still exists today.

The definitive host of the *T. solium* and *T. saginata* cysticerci is man; the definitive hosts of *T. crassiceps* are the fox and other wild canids. The natural intermediate hosts of the *T. solium* cysticercus are the domestic pig and the wild boar. These cysticerci are also occasionally found in dogs, cats, sheep, deer, camels, monkeys, and humans. The intermediate hosts of the *T. crassiceps* cysticerci are wild rodents, but the cysticercus has also been found in man and in one dog. The natural hosts of the adult larvae of *T. saginata* are domesticated cattle and, rarely, wild artiodactyls. In the past, cases of human infection by cysticerci with unarmed rostella—identified as *T. saginata (C. bovis)*—have been described. Currently, this is not considered a valid criterion for identifying the species because the hooks can detach due to the host's reaction. Current expert opinion holds that there is no reliable proof of human parasitism caused by the larval stages of *T. saginata*. Accordingly, cases of human cysticercosis caused by *C. bovis* have not been mentioned in the literature during the last decade. Individual cases of human infection with the cysticercus of *T. ovis* have been reported in the spinal cord of man in the former Soviet Union and with the cysticercus of *T. taeniaeformis* in the liver of a boy in Argentina; a case of infection with the cysticercus of *T. hydatigena* in the liver has also been reported.

The adult stage of *T. solium* lives in the small intestine of man and regularly eliminates gravid proglottids, which are generally expelled to the external environment with the feces; there they dry out and release the eggs. The eggs remain near the droppings or are disseminated by the wind, rain, or other climatic phenomena, contaminating water or food which may be consumed by pigs or man (for further details, see the chapter on Taeniasis). The eggs are infective from the time they leave the intestine. When a pig or a person ingests them, the hexacanth embryo is activated inside the egg then released from it; it then penetrates the intestinal mucosa, and is spread via the bloodstream. Once lodged in its preferred tissue, the embryo is transformed into a cysticercus which looks like an ovoid vesicle approximately 5 mm by 8–10 mm and contains the scolex of the invaginated adult taenia. The scolex of the cysticercus, like that of the adult taenia, has four suckers and two different-sized rows of hooks. This larva becomes infective for a new definitive host in 60 to 70 days. In pigs, the cysticerci preferentially locate in striated or cardiac muscle; in man, the majority of cysticerci found are located in the nervous system or subcutaneous tissue, although they have also been found in the eye socket, musculature, heart, liver, lungs, abdominal cavity, and almost any other area. The diversity of human localizations may be due more to the ease of detecting the cysticercus in the infected individual than to an actual tropism. Rarely, a multilobular larva that resembles a bunch of grapes has been found, but with vesicles that have no scolices, at the base of the infected person's brain; it has been designated *Cysticercus racemosus*. The histology of the parasite indicates that it is a taenia larva, and most authors believe it is a degenerative state of *C. cellulosae*, perhaps due to the localization. However, others have posited that it may be a form of coenurus (see the chapter on Coenurosis).

T. crassiceps is a taenia found in wild animals. Its cysticerci are found in foxes and can affect other wild canids, such as coyotes. The adult stage of *T. crassiceps* has been identified in hamsters and mice treated with corticoids. The cysticerci are found in the subcutaneous tissue or the peritoneal or pleural cavities of wild rodents and, very rarely, in man. One case of the adult larva of *T. crassiceps* has been described in a dog.

T. crassiceps seems to be so closely related to *T. solium* that the antigens of the former are used for serologic diagnosis of and vaccination against the latter.

Geographic Distribution: Distribution of the *T. solium* cysticercus is worldwide and coincides with the distribution of infection with the adult taenia (see the chapter on Taeniasis). Human cysticercosis caused by *T. crassiceps* larvae has been reported only in Austria, Canada, France, and Germany, but infection with the adult parasite—and, therefore, the opportunity for human infection with the larva—occurs where foxes are present.

Occurrence in Man: Human cysticercosis occurs worldwide, but is especially important in the rural areas of developing countries, including those of Latin America. Obviously, its prevalence is parallel to that of the adult *T. solium* parasite (see the chapter on Taeniasis). In some areas, the prevalence is very high; for example, cysticercus antibodies were found in 14.9% of 222 blood donors in Mozambique (Vilhena *et al.*, 1999), 17% and 10% of the populations of two communities in Guatemala (García-Noval *et al.*, 1996), 22% of 41 rural residents and 16% of 363 urban residents in Honduras (Sánchez *et al.*, 1998), 9% of 9,254 individuals in Ecuador (Escalante *et al.*, 1995), 3.2% of 2,180 people in five Brazilian counties (Lonardoni *et al.*, 1996), and 9%, 4.5%, and 2% of 438 inhabitants of three Bolivian settlements (Jafri *et al.*, 1998). A recent study conducted in Cuzco, Peru, showed a prevalence of 13% in 365 people and 43% in 89 pigs with the inmuno-electrotransfer test (Western blot) (García *et al.*, 1999). Another study carried out in Honduras in 1991 showed 30% positive serology for porcine cysticercosis and 2% of human feces positive for taenia. Four years later, the prevalence of porcine cysticercosis was 35% and that of taeniasis was 1.5% (Sánchez *et al.*, 1997). A study carried out in Brazil found that the clinical prevalence of human cysticercosis ranged from 0.1% to 9% and that the serologic prevalence fluctuated between 0.7% and 5.2% (Agapejev, 1996).

Neurocysticercosis, the most serious form of the disease, has been observed in 17 Latin American countries. A 0.43% rate of neurocysticercosis was found in the course of 123,826 autopsies in nine countries that account for two-thirds of the population of Latin America. It has been estimated that out of every 100,000 inhabitants, 100 suffer from neurocysticercosis and as many as 30 from ocular or periocular cysticercosis. The highest morbidity rates are found in Brazil, Chile, El Salvador, Guatemala, Mexico, and Peru (WHO, 1979). The prevalence of neurocysticercosis seems to be especially high in Central America and Mexico. It was estimated that cysticercosis was the cause of 1% of all deaths in the general hospitals of Mexico City and 25% of the intracranial tumors. Autopsies carried out from 1946 to 1979 on 21,597 individuals who died in general hospitals in Mexico found cerebral cysticercosis in 2.9%, leading to the conclusion that about 3% of the general population was affected by this parasitosis (Mateos, 1982). In the Triângulo Mineiro, Minas Gerais, Brazil, a rate of 2.4% of cysticercosis was found in 2,306 autopsies; of these, 66% were cases of neurocysticercosis, 26.8% had cardiac localization, 25% had musculoskeletal localization, and 7.1% had cutaneous localization (Gobbi et al., 1980).

In India, cerebral cysticercosis is second in importance, after tuberculosis, as a cause of expansive diseases of the skull, and is one of the principal causes of epilepsy. Neurocysticercosis is also common in Indonesia. On the other hand, human cysticercosis has disappeared in western and central Europe; it is also disappearing in eastern and southern Europe.

Just four cases of human cysticercosis caused by *T. crassiceps* larvae have been reported since 1992: one in the anterior chamber of the eye of an apparently healthy girl in Austria (Arocker-Mettinger et al., 1992), another in the subcutaneous tissue of an AIDS patient in Germany (Klinker et al., 1992), and twice in France (Chermette et al., 1995; François et al., 1998), both in AIDS patients. Apparently an intraocular case was reported earlier in Canada.

Occurrence in Animals: Information on swine cysticercosis comes from veterinary inspection records at slaughterhouses and packing plants. However, it must be borne in mind that usual inspection methods, which consist of cutting the meat at sites where the parasite preferentially locates, reveal only a portion of infected animals. It is also important to point out that swine raised on small family farms, where they have a greater opportunity to ingest human feces, are generally slaughtered by their owners without veterinary inspection or are sold without restrictions in local markets.

For obvious reasons, in all areas where human taeniasis exists, animal cysticercosis is also found, with variations in prevalence from region to region. In the Americas, only some countries and islands in the Caribbean have not recorded this parasitosis. In Brazil, which accounts for more than 65% of the total swine population in Latin America, 0.83% of 12 million pigs slaughtered in 10 states during 1970–1972 were found to be infected with *C. cellulosae*. Similar rates have been observed in Mexico and several South American countries, such as Chile (0.7%) and Colombia. In a survey conducted in Mexico, 17 of 75 (23%) swine examined were found to be positive for cysticercosis by palpation of the tongue and 26 (35%) by serology (Rodríguez-Canul et al., 1999). In Cuzco, Peru, a prevalence of 43% was found in 89 pigs by immunoelectrotransfer (García et al., 1999). Another survey conducted in Honduras showed 30% positive serology for porcine cysticercosis (Sánchez et al., 1997).

In South Africa, the only African country with more than a million swine, the infection rate in slaughterhouses was under 1.5%. In the Democratic Republic of the Congo, the rate ranges from 0.1% to 8.1%, depending on the region. In Asia, information on the prevalence of animal infection is scarce. Porcine cysticercosis is disappearing in Europe. In the former Soviet Union, the rate of cysticerci in swine was

0.14% in 1962 and only 0.004% in 1970. Similar figures have been reported from Hungary and other countries of eastern Europe. At present, very few endemic foci are found on that continent, as a consequence of modernized swine-raising practices. Economic losses due to the confiscation of bovine and swine carcasses infected by cysticercosis can be significant. In 1963, swine cysticercosis was the reason for 68% of all confiscations in six slaughterhouses in Central America, causing an estimated loss of one-half million dollars. During 1980, 264,000 swine carcasses were confiscated in Mexico, and total losses due to swine cysticercosis were estimated at more than US$ 43 million. Losses due to bovine cysticercosis in Latin America are possibly even greater than those due to swine cysticercosis. The economic impact consists of not only the losses caused by the animal parasitosis, but also the cost of treating human neurocysticercosis, which involves significant expenses for surgery, hospitalization, and work days lost. The cost of medical care in Mexico for a patient with neurocysticercosis has been estimated at more than US$ 2,000.

No information is available on the prevalence of the *T. crassiceps* cysticercus in rodents. In the past decade, the adult parasite was found in 18% to 29% of several thousand red foxes examined in France, Germany, and Spain; cysticercus was also found in Greece, and reported in less than 10% of arctic foxes examined in the state of Alaska, US.

The Disease in Man: Cysticercosis is a disease which varies in severity according to the localization of the parasite. Man can harbor from one to several hundred cysticerci in various tissues and organs. The localization that most often prompts a medical consultation is the central nervous system (neurocysticercosis), followed by the eye and its surrounding tissues (ocular and periocular cysticercosis). Localization in muscles and subcutaneous connective tissue is generally not clinically apparent unless large numbers of cysticerci are involved, causing muscular pain, cramps, and fatigue.

The symptomatology of neurocysticercosis varies with the number of cysticerci, their stage of development (young, mature, intact, degenerate), morphology (vesicular or racemose), location in the central nervous system, and the reaction of the patient. The cysticerci locate most frequently in the meninges, cerebral cortex, and ventricles, and less frequently in the parenchyma. The symptoms generally appear several years after the infection, when the death of the larva causes inflammatory reactions. The symptoms are often not well defined and may resemble those of a cerebral tumor, basal meningitis, encephalitis, intracranial hypertension, and hysteria. In a study of 119 cases, Sousa *et al.* (1998) found that 64% of the patients consulted a doctor because of epileptiform attacks and 22% because of headaches; two patients had an altered mental state. Computerized tomography showed that 44% of the patients had more than five cysticerci and that the parietal lobe was the site most often affected. However, there was no relationship between the severity of the symptoms and the radiographic findings. Of 54 patients under the age of 17 studied in Ecuador (del Brutto, 1999), 89% had convulsions and just 3 had increased intracranial pressure. Computerized tomography revealed parenchymatous cysticerci in 52 patients, 19 (36%) with a single cysticercus. In 122 children in Mexico, the main symptoms were convulsions, intracranial hypertension, and learning difficulties (Ruíz-García *et al.*, 1997). A study in Brazil found that the most common clinical characteristics were epileptic syndrome (22.92%), intracranial hypertension (19% to 89%), and psychiatric symptoms (9% to 23%); 6% of the clinical patients and 48.5% of the autopsies represented asymptomatic cases (Agapejev, 1996). The presence of cysticerci in the central nervous system does not always give rise to clinical symptoms. Rodríguez-Canul et al. (1999) identified five asymptomatic cases serologically. Chimelli et al. (1998) reviewed 2,522 autopsies in Brazil and found 38 (1.5%) cases of cysticercosis. Of these, 22 (58%) had not been previously diagnosed, and 21 (55%) had been asymptomatic. Data from several Latin American countries show that in 46.8% of the cases in which cysticerci were found in the central nervous system during autopsy, the individual had had no clinical manifestations of the parasitosis during his life.

Ocular and periocular cysticercosis is less frequent, accounting for some 20% of cases. The cysticerci locate primarily in the vitreous humor, subretinal tissue, and the anterior chamber of the eye. The parasitosis may cause uveitis, iritis, and retinitis, as well as palpebral conjunctivitis, and may affect the motor muscles of the eye.

Until recently, no effective chemotherapy was available for cysticercosis. Surgery was the only treatment, and it presented serious risks in the case of neurocysticercosis and was often only palliative. It has been estimated that more than 30% of such patients die during the operation or in the postoperative period. The advent of new drugs, especially praziquantel, in recent years, has resulted in up to a 68% rate of cure or clinical improvement with medical treatment (Robles et al., 1997).

The clinical manifestations of cysticercosis are determined by a strong inflammatory reaction that seems to occur only during and after the death of the parasite. While the cysticercus generates significant immune responses, the inflammation around viable cysticerci is quite moderate. It is now known that the live cysticercus produces taeniaestatin and paramyosin, which inhibit complement activation, and sulfated polysaccharides, which activate complement at sites distant from the parasite and may inhibit the proliferation of lymphocytes and macrophages (White et al., 1997). These actions probably limit the inflammatory reaction while the parasite is alive.

Cases of human cysticercosis caused by T. crassiceps are so scarce that there is no general picture of their symptomatology. The François et al. case (1998) was a subcutaneous and intermuscular tumor of the arm, fluctuating and painful, in an AIDS patient. The lesion contained cysticerci that resemble small vesicles surrounded by a granulomatous reaction with fibrocollagenous tissue contained in a caseous material. The Klinker et al. case (1992) involved a paravertebral pseudohematoma in an AIDS patient that spread to most of the back in the following weeks and caused a deficiency of clotting factor V and local bleeding that required transfusions. The lesion ruptured spontaneously, releasing blood and spherules 2 to 3 mm in diameter, which were identified as cysticerci of the parasite. Treatment with a combination of mebendazole and praziquantel reduced the lesion and coagulation returned to normal, but the patient suffered a relapse four months later. In this case, there appears to have been asexual multiplication of the cysticerci, as was described in rodents, which are natural intermediate hosts.

The Disease in Animals: Cysticercosis in swine does not usually manifest itself clinically. In isolated cases, infected swine may experience hypersensitivity of the snout, paralysis of the tongue, and epileptiform convulsions, but the useful life of swine is usually too short for neurologic manifestations to appear. Dogs that ingest human feces and become infected with the eggs of *T. solium* sometimes show symptoms of cerebral cysticercosis which may be confused with those of rabies. Experimental infection of cattle with a high dose of *T. saginata* eggs can produce fever, weakness, sialorrhea, anorexia, and muscular stiffness. Death may occur as a result of degenerative myocarditis.

Source of Infection and Mode of Transmission: Man acquires cysticercosis through *Cysticercus cellulosae* infestation by consuming water or food (e.g., vegetables or fruits) contaminated with *T. solium* eggs that were released into the environment by gravid proglottids eliminated by an infected person. Such contamination also allows for the infection of swine by coprophagy. A person's hands may be contaminated by contact with contaminated soil or water or from eggs from his own feces, and thus transmitted to others. *T. solium* eggs only survive for a few weeks or months outside the host, but, since the taeniae can live for many years in the human intestine and eliminate several hundred thousand eggs every day, environmental contamination can continue for a long time. The risk is particularly high in the rural areas of developing countries, where the lack of adequate excreta disposal systems promotes outdoor defecation and consequent contamination of peridomestic areas. Moreover, taeniae eggs can be spread by rain, wind, and, possibly, by coprophagous insects, and transported over long distances by watercourses and, possibly, also in the intestines of gulls and other birds. Such dispersion facilitates the contamination of produce from the family garden, either through contamination of the area around the house or through irrigation with water that was contaminated farther upstream. In addition, the lack of potable water supply hinders the effective washing of hands and foods. This situation often generates a cycle of autoinfection in the family: it has been shown that the most important risk factor for cysticercosis is the presence of a family member who is infected with taenia. A study of soldiers and their relatives in Mexico, for example, showed that 12.2% of the soldiers had cysticercosis and 0.5% had taeniasis, and that 12% of the soldiers' relatives with cysticercosis had eliminated proglottids in the past. Just 3.7% of the relatives in an uninfected control group had eliminated proglottids in the past (García-García *et al.*, 1999).

It is also common for poor peasants to raise some swine under very primitive conditions and sell them locally or slaughter them for big celebrations. Those animals have many opportunities to become infected through human feces and, since they are consumed without veterinary inspection, they are often the source of taeniasis infection in the community. *T. solium* cysticerci can survive for several years in the swine and for more than a month in the carcass.

Food handlers can be of vital importance in transmission: thus, in a Peruvian village, it was found that 3% of the general population was infected with taeniasis and 24% was infected with cysticercosis, while 8.6% of the vendors of a locally-prepared pork dish had taeniasis and 23.3% had cysticercosis (García *et al.*, 1998). A survey in Honduras found a 16% to 22% prevalence of human cysticercosis, and it was determined that the most important risk factors were hog-raising in the area around the house, lack of potable water, lack of sanitary excreta disposal, existence of a dirt floor in the house, general lack of education, and ignorance of the parasite's biology (Sánchez *et al.*, 1998). In a study in Mexico, the main human risk factors for acquiring cysticercosis were the consumption of cysticercosis-infected swine and proximity to a taeniasis-infected person. A study on Reunion Island in the Indian Ocean showed that household swine raising—a common practice there—can maintain significant levels of human cysticercosis even if levels of taeniasis are low: 14 of 993 (1.4%) individuals examined serologically for cysticercosis were positive, even though just 0.02% had taeniasis and no swine with cysticercosis were found in the island's slaughterhouses (Chamouillet et al., 1997). In addition to these risk factors, a study in China determined that the risk factors for human cysticercosis also included: poor personal hygiene, lack of knowledge about the infection in swine, poor swine breeding practices, and a history of taeniasis.

For swine, the greatest risk of acquiring cysticercosis comes from livestock-raising practices that allow the animals to roam freely and expose them to human feces. Animals confined in corrals had a much lower risk of acquiring the infection than free-roaming swine (Rodríguez-Canul et al., 1999).

Likewise, it has been suggested that the gravid proglottids of the taenia could be carried by reversed peristalsis to the stomach, where the eggs could be activated, and from there, once again be carried to the intestine, where the oncosphere would be liberated and give rise to cysticercosis. Despite the fact that most authors rejected that possibility, the recent finding of the oral expulsion of a T. saginata in a patient (Gupta et al., 1997) necessitates review of this opinion.

Diagnosis: Apart from subcutaneous and intraocular cysticercosis and some cysticercoses of the central nervous system, most cysticercus infections are clinically inapparent. Diagnosis of subcutaneous cysticercosis can be made by biopsy of the nodules or by radiography. Ocular cysticerci may be discovered by ophthalmoscopy. Neurological imaging, and especially computerized tomography, are very useful in the diagnosis of neurocysticercosis because this procedure allows lesions of various densities to be distinguished and absorption coefficients of different tissues to be quantified (Carpio et al., 1998). In a study carried out in Ecuador, that procedure discovered 8 cases in 46 subjects examined (17%) in a rural population and 35 cases in 147 subjects examined (24%) in an urban population. In contrast, inmunoelectrotransfer discovered 6 of 42 cases (14%) in the rural population and 28 of 124 cases (23%) in the urban population (Cruz et al., 1999). Since the course of treatment of cysticercosis depends on the interpretation of the clinical manifestations, the findings on imaging, and the immunological results, del Brutto et al. (1996) developed protocols for diagnosing individual cases as possible, probable, or definite.

The cerebrospinal fluid of those affected by neurocysticercosis shows an increase in the level of proteins, especially the gammaglobulin fraction, and a marked cellular reaction with a high percentage of plasmocytes and eosinophils. Eosinophilia is also generally present.

Serologic tests can be valuable when used in conjunction with other diagnostic procedures. Although some laboratories still recommend the hemagglutination reaction test, the enzyme-linked immunosorbent assay (ELISA) and the immunoelectrotransfer test are more sensitive, particularly with selected antigens. In a study of sera that were positive with ELISA, just 85.4% were positive with hemagglutination (Ferreira et al., 1997). Immunoelectrotransfer with 8 kDa and 26 kDa antigens is considered sensitive and specific (Rodríguez-Canul et al., 1999). Using the ELISA with recombinant antigens, 96.3% sensitivity and 91.5% specificity have been obtained (Hubert et al., 1999). However, serology is not the preferred method of clinical diagnosis because it indicates contact with the parasite but not necessarily an active infection. In fact, most seropositive individuals are asymptomatic. *T. solium* and *T. crassiceps* share antigens, to the point that the use of *T. crassiceps* antigens to diagnose or vaccinate against *T. solium* is under study.

Diagnosis of swine cysticercosis can be made antemortem by palpation of the tongue, where the cysticerci are felt in cases of intense infection. More often, it is made by study of the cysticerci during postmortem examination in slaughterhouses and packing plants. This method, which only examines certain muscles where the cysticercus commonly locates, is a compromise between cost and efficiency, and many cases of mild infection are not detected. While there is not much incentive for developing serologic methods of diagnosing the swine infection, Rodríguez-Canul *et al.* (1999) used immunoelectrotransfer of 8 kDa and 26 kDa antigens with the swine infection and achieved 93% sensitivity and 100% specificity.

Control: Health education for at-risk populations is the foundation of cysticercosis prevention. A study in China (see Source of Infection and Mode of Transmission) established that control of human cysticercosis required a combination of health education and treatment of taeniases (Cao *et al.*, 1997). A study in Mexico evaluated the effects of health education about the disease by measuring the change in knowledge and habits and in the prevalence of swine cysticercosis before and after an education program that promoted knowledge about transmission of the parasite and the appropriate hygiene practices for preventing transmission. After program execution, there were significant changes in knowledge of the parasite's biology, but behavioral changes were short-lived and less impressive. The incidence of human taeniasis decreased from 5.2% to 1.2% (Sarti *et al.*, 1997).

In addition to individual protective measures for humans, control measures for cysticercosis consist of interrupting the chain of transmission of the parasite at any of the following intervention points: the production of eggs by an infected person, the dissemination of eggs to the environment, the ingestion of eggs by the intermediate host, the development of the cysticercus in the intermediate host, and the dissemination of the cysticerci to the definitive host (Barriga, 1997). For more details on control, see the chapter on Taeniasis.

Recently, successful attempts have been made to provide mass treatment to a human population with human taeniasis: in an area of Guatemala where *T. solium* is endemic, the prevalence of human taeniasis decreased from 3.5% to 1%, and that of swine cysticercosis decreased from 55% to 7% after 10 months of treatment (Allan *et al.*, 1997). García *et al.* (1999) found that cases of human and swine cysticercosis tend to be associated in geographic groups and that their serologies were positively correlated. Swine serology, therefore, is a suitable indicator of environmental contamination by *T. solium* and should be used to estimate the risk of human infection.

Bibliography

Agapejev, S. Epidemiology of neurocysticercosis in Brazil. *Rev Inst Med Trop Sao Paulo* 38:207–216, 1996.

Allan, J.C., M. Velásquez-Tohom, C. Fletes, *et al.* Mass chemotherapy for intestinal *Taenia solium* infection: Effect on prevalence in humans and pigs. *Trans R Soc Trop Med Hyg* 91:595–598, 1997.

Arocker-Mettinger, E., V. Huber-Spitzy, H. Auer, G. Grabner, M. Stur. *Taenia crassiceps* in der Vorderkammer des menschlichen Auges. Ein Fallbericht. *Klin Monatsbl Augenheilkd* 201:34–37, 1992.

Barriga, O.O. *Veterinary Parasitology for Practitioners*, 2nd ed. Edina: Burgess International Group; 1997.

Cao, W., C.P. van der Ploeg, J. Xu, C. Gao, L. Ge, J.D. Habbema. Risk factors for human cysticercosis morbidity: A population-based case-control study. *Epidemiol Infect* 119:231–235, 1997.

Carpio, A., A. Escobar, W.A. Hauser. Cysticercosis and epilepsy: A critical review. *Epilepsia* 39:1025–1040, 1998.

Chamouillet, H., B. Bouteille, H. Isautier, A. Begue, M. Lecadieu. Seroprévalence de la cysticercose, taeniasis et ladrerie porcine, à La Réunion en 1992. *Med Trop (Mars)* 57:41–46, 1997.

Chermette, R., J. Bussieras, J. Marionneau, *et al.* Cysticercose envahissante à *Taenia crassiceps* chez un patient atteint de sida. *Bull Acad Natl Med* 179:777–780, 1995.

Chimelli, L., A.F. Lovalho, O.M. Takayanagui. Neurocysticercie. Contribuição da necropsia na consolidação da notificação compulsória em Ribeirão Preto-SP. *Arq Neuropsiquiatr* 56:577–584, 1998.

Cruz, M.E., P.M. Preux, C. Debrock, *et al.* Épidémiologie de la cysticercose cérébrale dans une communauté des Andes en Equateur. *Bull Soc Pathol Exot* 92:38–41, 1999.

Cruz, M.E., P.M. Schantz, I. Cruz, *et al.* Epilepsy and neurocysticercosis in an Andean community. *Internat J Epidemiol* 28:799–803, 1999.

del Brutto, O.H. Neurocysticercosis en niños: análisis clínico, radiológico y de factores pronósticos en 54 pacientes. *Rev Neurol* 25:1681–1684, 1997.

del Brutto, O.H., N.H. Wadia, M. Dumas, M. Cruz, V.C. Tsang, P.M. Schantz. Proposal of diagnostic criteria for human cysticercosis and neurocysticercosis. *J Neurol Sci* 142:6, 1996.

Eom, K.S., H.J. Rim. Morphologic descriptions of *Taenia asiatica* sp. n. *Korean J Parasitol* 31:1–6, 1993.

Escalante, L., E.C. Rowland, M.R. Powell. Prevalence of anti-*Taenia solium* antibodies in sera from outpatients in an Andean region of Ecuador. *Mem Inst Oswaldo Cruz* 90:715–719, 1995.

Ferreira, A.P., A.J. Vaz, P.M. Nakamura, A.T. Sasaki, A.W. Ferreira, J.A. Livramento. Hemagglutination test for the diagnosis of human neurocysticercosis: Development of a stable reagent using homologous and heterologous antigens. *Rev Inst Med Trop Sao Paulo* 39:29–33, 1997.

Flisser, A., J.P. Williams, C. Laclette, *et al.*, eds. *Cysticercosis: Present state of knowledge and perspectives. Proceedings of an International Workshop on Cysticercosis held in San Miguel de Allende, Guanajuato, Mexico, on November 16–18, 1981.* New York: Academic Press; 1982.

François, A., L. Favennec, C. Cambon-Michot, *et al. Taenia crassiceps* invasive cysticercosis: A new human pathogen in acquired immunodeficiency syndrome? *Am J Surg Pathol* 22:488–492, 1998.

García, H.H., R. Araoz, R.H. Gilman, *et al.* Increased prevalence of cysticercosis and taeniasis among professional fried pork vendors and the general population of a village in the Peruvian highlands. Cysticercosis Working Group in Peru. *Am J Trop Med Hyg* 59:902–905, 1998.

García, H.H., R. Gilman, A.E. González, R. Pacheco, M. Verastegui, V.C. Tsang. Human and porcine *Taenia solium* infection in a village in the highlands of Cusco, Peru. The Cysticercosis Working Group in Peru. *Acta Trop* 3:31–36, 1999.

García-García, M.L., M. Torres, D. Correa, *et al.* Prevalence and risk of cysticercosis and taeniasis in an urban population of soldiers and their relatives. *Am J Trop Med Hyg* 61:386–389, 1999.

García-Noval, J., J.C. Allan, C. Fletes, *et al.* Epidemiology of *Taenia solium* taeniasis and cysticercosis in two rural Guatemalan communities. *Am J Trop Med Hyg* 55:282–289, 1996.

Gobbi, H., S.J. Adad, R.R. Neves, *et al.* Ocorrência de cisticercose *(Cysticercus cellulosae)* em Uberaba, M.G. *Rev Pat Trop (Goiana, Brazil)* 9:51–59, 1980.

Gupta, R.L., V. Agrawal, S. Kumar, Monika. Oral expulsion of *Taenia saginata. Indian J Gastroenterol* 16:70–71, 1997.

Hubert, K., A. Andriantsimahavandy, A. Michault, M. Frosch, F.A. Muhlschlegel. Serological diagnosis of human cysticercosis by use of recombinant antigens from *Taenia solium* cysticerci. *Clin Diagn Lab Immunol* 6:479–482, 1999.

Jafri, H.S., F. Torrico, J.C. Noh, *et al.* Application of the enzyme-linked immunoelectro-transfer blot to filter paper blood spots to estimate seroprevalence of cysticercosis in Bolivia. *Am J Trop Med Hyg* 58:313–315, 1998.

Klinker, H., K. Tintelnot, R. Joeres, *et al. Taenia-crassiceps*-Infektion bei AIDS. *Dtsch Med Wochenschr* 117:133–138, 1992.

Lonardoni, M.V., D.A. Bertolini, T.G. Silveira, *et al.* Frequência de anticorpos anti-*Cysticercus cellulosae* em indivíduos de cinco munícipios da região Norte do Estado do Paraná-Brazil. *Rev Saude Publica* 30:273–279, 1996.

Mateos Gómez, J. H. La cysticercosis cerebral en Mexico. II. Frecuencia. *Gac Med Mex* 118:2–4, 1982.

Robles, C., N. Vargas-Tentori, A.M. Sedano. Quimioterapia de la cysticercosis. Resultados de 10 años o más después del seguimiento. *Gac Med Mex* 133:127–139, 1997.

Rodríguez-Canul, R., A. Fraser, J.C. Allan, J.L. Domínguez-Alpizar, F. Argaez-Rodríguez, P.S. Craig. Epidemiological study of *Taenia solium* taeniasis/cysticercosis in a rural village in Yucatan state, Mexico. *Ann Trop Med Parasitol* 93:57–67, 1999.

Ruíz-García, M., A. González-Astiazaran, F. Rueda-Franco. Neurocysticercosis in children. Clinical experience in 122 patients. *Childs Nerv Syst* 13:608–612, 1997.

Sánchez, A.L., O. Gómez, P. Allebeck, H. Cosenza, L. Ljungstrom. Epidemiological study of *Taenia solium* infections in a rural village in Honduras. *Ann Trop Med Parasitol* 91:163–171, 1997.

Sánchez, A.L., M.T. Medina, I. Ljungstrom. Prevalence of taeniasis and cysticercosis in a population of urban residence in Honduras. *Acta Trop* 69:141–149, 1998.

Sarti, E., A. Flisser, P.M. Schantz, *et al.* Development and evaluation of a health education intervention against *Taenia solium* in a rural community in Mexico. *Am J Trop Med Hyg* 56:127–132, 1997.

Sousa, A.Q., H.L. Sa, T.R. Queiroz, W.G. Horta, R.D. Pearson. Neurocysticercosis in Ceará State, northeastern Brazil: A review of 119 cases. *Am J Trop Med Hyg* 58:759–762, 1998.

Vilhena, M., M. Santos, J. Torgal. Seroprevalence of human cysticercosis in Maputo, Mozambique. *Am J Trop Med Hyg* 61:59–62, 1999.

White, A.C., Jr., P. Robinson, R. Kuhn. *Taenia solium* cysticercosis: Host-parasite interactions and the immune response. *Chem Immunol* 66:209–230, 1997.

World Health Organization (WHO). *Parasitic Zoonoses. Report of a WHO Expert Committee, with the Participation of FAO.* Geneva: WHO; 1979. (Technical Report Series 637.)

DIPHYLLOBOTHRIASIS

ICD-10 B70.0

Synonyms: Bothriocephaliasis, bothriocephalosis, dibothriocephaliasis, broad tapeworm infection, fish tapeworm infection.

Etiology: The agent of this disease is a cestode of various species of the genus *Diphyllobothrium* (synonyms *Bothriocephalus, Dibothriocephalus*). Nomenclature within the genus is still imprecise because the limits of intraspecific morphologic variation and the factors associated with that variation are not known. The type species, and most important one, is *D. latum*. Some of the species currently considered valid are: a dwarf form of *Diphyllobothrium*, described as *D. parvum* in 1908 and subsequently confirmed as *D. latum*, *D. parvum* type in two human cases in the Republic of Korea; *D. nihonkaiense*, one of the most common parasites from fish in Japan (Ohnishi and Murata, 1993); *D. klebanovskii*, a highly prevalent species (0.07%) in the northeastern part of the former Soviet Union (Muratov *et al.*, 1992); and *D. yonagoense*, which has been reported in human cases in the Republic of Korea. The following species have been described in human cases found in arctic and subarctic communities: *D. dendriticum*, which is found farther north than *D. latum*; *D. ursi* in northern Canada and in Alaska, US; *D. dalliae* in Alaska and Siberia; and *D. klebanovskii* in Siberia (Curtis and Bylund, 1991). *D. pacificum* has been described in Chile and Peru, and *D. dendriticum* has been described in Argentina and Chile.

In this section, *D. latum* is used to describe the life cycle of the cestode. The parasite requires two intermediate hosts: the first of these is a copepod (small, planktonic crustacean); the second, a freshwater fish from one of several species. The adult or strobilar form of the parasite lives in the small intestine of man, dogs, cats, bears, and other wild animals; it has a scolex without hooks or suckers with two sucking grooves or bothria, measures 3 to 12 m long and 10 to 20 mm at its widest part, and may have 3,000 to 4,000 proglottids. The gravid proglottids expel eggs from the intestine through a uterine pore, along with chains of proglottids that are empty or contain just a few eggs, which detach and are eliminated with the feces. A single parasite can shed up to a million eggs per day. The eggs eliminated in the host's feces contain an immature embryo which, after incubating in fresh water for 10 to 15 days at 15–25 °C, forms a ciliated embryo called a coracidium. The coracidium, some 50–100 μm in diameter, emerges from the egg and remains in the water until it is ingested by the first intermediate host, a copepod crustacean. Ingestion must occur within 24 hours of eclosion because the coracidium loses its infectiveness rapidly; however, the embryo of the species that use marine fish as intermediate hosts can tolerate the semi-brackish water of estuaries or briny sea water. This embryo lodges in the coelomic cavity of the crustacean and, in 10 to 20 days, turns into a procercoid, a solid, elongated larva 6 to 10 mm long with a circular caudal appendage. When the crustacean and larva are ingested by the second intermediate host, any one of a variety of fish, the procercoid migrates to the muscles and other organs of the fish and becomes a plerocercoid or sparganum in about a month. If the first fish is eaten by a larger fish, the transport or paratenic host, the plerocercoid simply migrates from one fish to the other. A large fish can harbor up to 1,000 plerocercoids. When the infected fish is eaten by a definitive host, the plerocercoid lodges in the small intestine and starts to grow until it matures, and it begins to release eggs after 25 to 30 days. Human infections have been known to last up to 30 years (Marquardt *et al.*, 2000).

The first intermediate host is an almost-microscopic copepod crustacean of the genera *Diaptomus* (the Americas), *Eudiaptomus* (Asia and Europe), *Acanthodiaptomus* (Alpine region, the Carpathians, Scandinavia, Tibet, and Turkestan), *Arctodiaptomus* (Ural Mountains region), *Eurytemora* (North America), *Boeckella* (Australia), or *Cyclops* (Africa, Asia, and Europe) (von Bonsdorff, 1977). The most important fish that act as second intermediate hosts in the transmission of *D. latum* to man are the pike (*Esox* spp.); the perches (*Perca* spp. and *Stizostedion* spp.); the burbot (*Lota* spp.); and the acerina (*Acerina cernua*). In Chile the agents of *D. latum* transmission are the salmonids introduced from Europe: rainbow trout (*Salmo gairdneri*) and brown trout (*Salmo trutta*), as well as certain autochthonous fish species. Salmon of the genus *Oncorhynchus* are a source of infection in the US, Eurasia, and Japan. The larvae of *D. dendriticum* are found mainly in salmonid fish and have never been found in pike or perch. In contrast, *D. latum* is rarely found in salmonids. *D. ursi* and *D. klebanovskii* predominate in Pacific salmon. *D. klebanovskii* is found in the eastern part of the former Soviet Union, the Sea of Japan, and the Bering Sea. The usual definitive hosts are carnivores and the intermediate hosts are fish of the genera *Oncorhynchus* and *Salvelinus* (Muratov, 1990). *D. dalliae* has an affinity for local fish, such as the Alaska blackfish (Curtis and Bylund, 1991). In southern Argentina, Revenga (1993) found that 9% of brook trout are hosts to *D. latum* and 27% are hosts to *D. dendriticum*; rainbow trout are also hosts to both species, but perch are host only to *D. latum* (19%), and the mackerel were not infected with any species.

D. latum seems to be a primary human parasite, because it is in humans where the parasite reaches its greatest size and the infections are the most protracted; this appears to be an ancient illness, since eggs thought to be from *D. latum* have been found in Paleolithic mummies. But it also infects other fish-eating mammals, such as dogs, cats, swine, bears, and wild carnivores. The other diphyllobothrids seem to be predominantly zoophilic, because infections in man generally persist a few months and the cestode is expelled by itself. While the most important definitive hosts for *D. dendriticum* are gulls, this role can also be played by other birds and mammals, such as dogs, cats, rats, or man. *D. pacificum* is found on the Pacific coast of the Americas. Its natural definitive hosts are pinnipeds such as the sea lion *Otaria byronia* (*O. flavescens*) on the Peruvian coast. The intermediate hosts, as yet unidentified, would be planktonic copepods and marine fish. The species has also been found in other pinnipeds of the family Otariidae along the northern Pacific coast and in fur seals (*Arctocephalus australis*) on San Juan Fernández Island, Chile. Plerocercoid larvae of *Diphyllobothrium* spp. have been found off the coast of Peru in the following species of marine fish: croakers (*Sciaena deliciosa*), cocos (*Paralonchurus peruanus*), *Trachinotus paitensis*, and others (Tantaleán, 1975). The intermediate hosts definitive for *D. ursi* in Alaska, US, and British Columbia, Canada, are the bears *Ursus arctos* and *U. americanus* and, occasionally, man. The second intermediate host is the salmon *Oncorhynchus*. Other human cases in Alaska and northeastern Siberia are attributed to *D. dalliae,* a diphyllobothrid of dogs, foxes, and gulls, whose plerocercoids are found in the blackfish *Dallia pectoralis*.

Geographic Distribution and Occurrence: *D. latum* is a cosmopolitan species found in the temperate zones, between the subarctic and subtropical, particularly in lacustrine regions. The most appropriate biotopes are lakes, river banks, and reservoirs, where the cestode finds the intermediate hosts it needs to continue its life cycle; but for humans to become infected they must eat raw or undercooked fish. The areas of greatest prevalence of this parasitosis are eastern and northeastern Finland, northern Norway, and northern Sweden. The prevalence of infection has decreased notably in almost all Eurasian countries. In Finland, where the prevalence was about 20% in the 1940s, a rate of 1.8% was found in the period 1969–1972. Notwithstanding, it was estimated that in 1973 more than 9 million persons were infected worldwide (5 million in Europe, 4 million in Asia, and 0.1 million in the Americas) (von Bonsdorff, 1977; WHO, 1979). Another endemic area is Karelia, Estonia, and St. Petersburg, Russian Federation, where lakes are abundant; important foci are also found in Siberia. In Hawaii, US, where the parasite does not exist, a case of human infection was found in a boy who had never been off the Islands and who apparently contracted it from imported fish (Hutchinson *et al.*, 1997). In the Republic of Korea, 37 cases of diphyllobothriasis were reported in 1997, in addition to 21 cases in which the eggs were found in feces (Chung *et al.*, 1997). Examination of the feces of 52,552 patients between 1984 and 1992 in a hospital in Seoul, Republic of Korea, revealed that 0.004% were infected with *D. latum* (Lee *et al.*, 1994). In Australia, the cestode has been found only in European immigrants and, apparently, the parasite does not occur naturally in that country.

D. latum appears to have been introduced into North and South America by European immigrants. In North America, the highest prevalence of diphyllobothriasis is found among Eskimos, with rates between 30% and 80% in some localities. The infection is probably caused by several species of *Diphyllobothrium*. Plerocercoids have been found in several species of fish in the Great Lakes in North America, but the infection does not seem to exist in the area. The infection in humans has been described in several areas of the US and in Montreal and Toronto, Canada. The first confirmed case in Cuba was described in 1990 (Bouza Suárez *et al.*, 1990). In Peru, the human infection is caused by *D. pacificum*; it was found in 136 of 314 patients with cestodiasis examined between 1962 and 1976. Semenas and Úbeda (1997) reported on 13 cases diagnosed in Patagonia, Argentina between 1986 and 1995. In northern Chile, 13 cases of infection by *D. pacificum* were diagnosed; in addition, plerocercoids of *D. dendriticum* were found in fish, and the adult parasite in gulls in the lake region of the south (Torres, 1982). In the Valdivia River Basin in southern Chile, Torres *et al.* (1989) found a prevalence of 1.2% in 1,295 individuals. All the parasites recovered after treatment were identified as *D. latum*. A study of 1,450 fish revealed plerocercoids of *D. latum* or *D. dendriticum* in two species of imported fish (*Salmo gairdneri* and *Salmo trutta*) and in a few autochthonous species. A retrospective study of 10,758 patients (over a 10-year period) also found, in the Valdivia River area, 11 cases of diphyllobothriasis (Kurte *et al.*, 1990).

With respect to animals, in Alaska, US, cestodes of the genus *Diphyllobothrium* spp. were found in 57 of 97 autopsied dogs. Torres *et al.* (1989) found *D. latum* in 5.3% to 9.8% of dogs, but none in cats or swine. They subsequently examined the feces of 159 people, 17 dogs, 19 swine, and 4 cats, and found just one infected cat. Abo-Shehada and Ziyadeh (1991) found *D. latum* in 1.5% of 756 dogs in Jordan. In

1992, Muratov reported the presence of *D. klebanovskii* in 47% of brown bears, 1 of 2 black bears, 1.7% of wolves, 1.6% of dogs, 0.3% of otters, and 2.8% of swine in the northeastern Russian Federation; he believes that the natural definitive hosts are brown and black bears.

The Disease in Man: While humans generally host just a single specimen, multiple parasitism is not uncommon. *D. latum* attaches itself to the mucosa of the ileum and less frequently to that of the jejunum. In most cases, the parasitosis is asymptomatic. When symptoms occur, they generally consist of diarrhea, epigastric pain, nausea, and vomiting (Curtis and Bylund, 1991). Some patients who harbor a large number of parasites may suffer mechanical obstruction of the intestine. The most serious complication of diphyllobothriasis is megaloblastic anemia; in the Baltic countries it occurs in less than 2% of persons with *D. latum* parasites, mainly in individuals with parasites localized in the jejunum. The symptomatology is similar to that of pernicious anemia. It stems from the parasites blocking and competing for the absorption of vitamin B_{12}. The parasite interferes with that vitamin's combination with the intrinsic factor (a normal component of the gastric juice), thus resulting in vitamin B_{12} deficiency. Patients frequently manifest slight jaundice, fever, glossitis, edema, hemorrhage, debility, and paresthesia in the legs. The illness occurs mainly in persons 20 to 40 years of age. Megaloblastic anemia seems to be rare among individuals with diphyllobothriasis in Latin America. For example, Frisancho *et al.* (1994) failed to find the parasite in 45 patients with megaloblastic anemia of unknown etiology studied in Peru. There are no reports of cases of anemia due to diphyllobothriasis other than those caused by *D. latum*.

The Disease in Animals: Infection by *Diphyllobothrium* is not clinically apparent in dogs and cats. Several epizootics in trout have been described in Great Britain and Ireland; they were caused by infection with a large number of diphyllobothrid plerocercoids that may not have been *D. latum*. In general, infection with a small number of larvae causes no major damage, but invasion by a large number of larvae may cause death.

Source of Infection and Mode of Transmission: The cycle of infection is maintained in nature by the contamination of rivers, lakes, and reservoirs with the feces of humans and other fish-eating mammals. Contamination of water with feces containing *D. latum* eggs allows the initial infection of copepods and subsequent infection of fish. Humans become infected by eating fish or its roe or liver raw, lightly salted, or smoked without sufficient heat. An example of the relationship between eating habits and prevalence of the parasite is provided in Finland. While human diphyllobothriasis is common in eastern Finland, where consuming raw fish is an ancestral habit, in western Finland this practice is not followed and infection is infrequent in spite of the existence of similar ecologic conditions (von Bonsdorff, 1977). *Ceviche*, a popular dish made of fish with lemon juice, salt, and hot peppers, which is consumed in several Latin American countries, can be a source of infection for man. The multiple cases of *D. pacificum* infection in Peru are attributed to *ceviche* prepared with marine fish. The Japanese dish sushi, which is also made with raw fish, gave rise to four cases of diphyllobothriasis in California (CDC, 1981). Human infection is not limited to the endemic areas, but can be extended by transport and consumption of refrigerated infected fish. One case of human infection was found in Hawaii, US, where the autochthonous parasite does not exist. The infection was apparently contracted through imported fish (Hutchinson *et al.*, 1997).

Humans are the principal definitive host for *D. latum,* but in their absence other fish-eating mammals can maintain the cycle by a similar transmission mechanism.

There are indications that anadromous fish (which migrate annually from the ocean to fresh water) could serve as a common source of infection by plerocercoids of various species of *Diphyllobothrium* for both land and marine mammals. In this way, freshwater fish that feed on anadromous fish could acquire larvae of marine origin, and land mammals could become infected by eating these fish raw.

Diagnosis: Specific diagnosis is carried out by identifying the eggs of the cestode (55–75 by 40–55 µm, operculate, unembryonated, and with a small lobe on the abopercular end) in the fecal matter. It is not possible to distinguish the species by examining the eggs, but attempts can be made to differentiate them by studying the proglottids passed spontaneously or after treatment. While formalin-ether sedimentation gives the best results in connection with the concentration of eggs in fecal matter, the number of eggs the parasite produces is so high that it is rarely necessary to concentrate them.

Control: Prevention of the infection in humans is based on the following: a) educating the population to abstain from eating raw or undercooked fish and contaminating the lakes with their feces; b) treating cestode carriers to prevent contamination of the environment; c) in endemic areas, cooking fish to 56 °C for 5 minutes or freezing it to –10 °C for 48 hours or to –18 °C for 24 hours to kill the plerocercoids; and d) taking steps to control fecal contamination of lakes and rivers, which is often difficult because of economic conditions in the affected areas. Treatment of domestic dogs in the area of lakes or rivers where fishing occurs may be useful, as may refraining from feeding dogs or cats scraps of raw fish. Most tests show, however, that humans are the principal reservoir of *D. latum* for other humans.

Bibliography

Abo-Shehada, M.N., Y. Ziyadeh. Prevalence of endoparasites in dog faecal deposits in Jordan. *J Helminthol* 65:313–314, 1991.

Bouza Suárez, M., G. Hormilla Manso, B. Dumenigo Ripoll, R. Quintana Olmos, R. Cordovi Prado. Primer caso de certeza de *Diphyllobothrium latum* en Cuba. *Rev Cubana Med Trop* 42:9–12, 1990.

Chung, P.R., W.M. Sohn, Y. Jung, S.H. Pai, M.S. Nam. [Five human cases of *Diphyllobothrium latum* infection through eating raw flesh of redlip mullet, *Liza haematocheila*]. *Korean J Parasitol* 35:283–289, 1997.

Curtis, M.A., G. Bylund. Diphyllobothriasis: Fish tapeworm disease in the circumpolar north. *Arctic Med Res* 50:18–24, 1991.

Frisancho, O., V. Ulloa, W. Ruíz, *et al.* Anemia megaloblástica asociada a diarrea crónica. Estudio prospectivo y multicéntrico en Lima. *Rev Gastroenterol Peru* 14:189–195, 1994.

Hutchinson, J.W., J.W. Bass, D.M. Demers, G.B. Myers. Diphyllobothriasis after eating raw salmon. *Hawaii Med J* 56:176–177, 1997.

Kurte, C., M. Silva, E. Gajardo, P. Torres. Nuevos casos de difilobotriasis humana en Panguipulli, Chile. *Bol Chil Parasitol* 45:59–61, 1990.

Lee, S.K., B.M. Shin, N.S. Chung, J.Y. Chai, S.H. Lee. [Second report on intestinal parasites among the patients of Seoul Paik Hospital (1984–1992)]. *Korean J Parasitol* 32:27–33, 1994.

Marquardt, W.C., R.S. Demaree, R.B. Grieve. *Parasitology and Vector Biology*, 2nd ed. San Diego: Academic Press; 2000.

Muratov, I.V. [Diphyllobothriasis in the Far East of the USSR]. *Med Parazitol (Mosk)* (6):54–58, 1990.

Muratov, I.V., P.S. Posokhov, N.A. Romanenko, A.S. Zimin, G.F. Glazyrina. [The epidemiological characteristics of diphyllobothriasis caused by *Diphyllobothrium klebanovskii* in the Amur River basin]. *Med Parazitol (Mosk)* 3:46–47, 1992.

Ohnishi, K., M. Murata. Single dose treatment with praziquantel for human *Diphyllobothrium nihonkaiense* infections. *Trans R Soc Trop Med Hyg* 87:482–483, 1993.

Revenga, J.E. *Diphyllobothrium dendriticum* and *Diphyllobothrium latum* in fishes from southern Argentina: Association, abundance, distribution, pathological effects, and risk of human infection. *J Parasitol* 79:379–383, 1993.

Semenas, L., C. Úbeda. Difilobotriasis humana en la Patagonia, Argentina. *Rev Saude Publica* 31:302–307, 1997.

Tantaleán, N. Hallazgo de larvas plerocercoides de *Diphyllobothriidae luhe*, 1910 (Cestoda) en peces del mar peruano. *Bol Chile Parasit* 30:18–20, 1975.

Torres, P. Estado actual de la investigación sobre cestodos del género *Diphyllobothrium cobbold* en Chile. *Rev Med Chil* 110:463–470, 1982.

Torres, P., R. Franjola, J. Pérez, *et al.* Epidemiología de la difilobotriasis en la cuenca del Río Valdivia, Chile. *Rev Saude Publica* 23:45–57, 1989.

United States of America, Department of Health and Human Services, Centers for Disease Control and Prevention (CDC). *Diphyllobothriasis* associated with salmon—United States. *MMWR Morb Mortal Wkly Rep* 30:331–337, 1981.

von Bonsdorff, B. *Diphyllobothriasis in Man.* London, New York: Academic Press; 1977.

World Health Organization. *Parasitic Zoonoses. Report of a WHO Expert Committee, with the Participation of FAO.* Geneva: WHO; 1979. (Technical Report Series 637).

DIPYLIDIASIS

ICD-10 B71.1

Synonyms: Dipylidiosis, dog cestode infection, dog tapeworm infection.

Etiology: *Dipylidium caninum* is a cestode 10 to 70 cm long and 3 mm at its widest part, with 60 to 175 proglottids; its definitive hosts are the dog, cat, and some wild felids and canids. The intermediate hosts are mainly dog fleas (*Ctenocephalides canis*) and cat fleas (*C. felis*). The human flea (*Pulex irritans*) and the dog louse (*Trichodectes canis*) can occasionally serve as intermediate hosts. The gravid proglottids detach singly or in groups from the strobila or chain of segments or proglottids that make up the body of the cestode; they are mobile and pass to the exterior on their own or with the feces. The proglottids disintegrate in the environment, releasing the eggs, which must be ingested by the flea larvae to continue their development to adulthood. The eggs hatch in the intestine of the flea larva, and the embryos (oncospheres) penetrate the celomic cavity; there they turn into cysticercoids. During this development of the parasite, the flea larva continues its own development until it becomes an adult insect. Hinaidy (1991) conducted a study in Austria of 9,134 fleas from 198 cats and 182 dogs, and found that 98.5% of the cat fleas and 77.5% of the dog fleas were *C. felis*, and that 2.3% of the cat fleas and 1.6% of the dog fleas contained, on average, not more than two or three cysticercoids per flea. When a dog or cat ingests an infected flea, the cysticercoid is released in the small intestine through digestion, establishes itself in the mucosa, and becomes an adult parasite in about 20 days. The longest survival time recorded for the parasite in cats is three years.

Geographic Distribution: The parasite exists wherever there are dogs and fleas.

Occurrence in Man: There are fewer than 150 cases of human infection reported in the literature; most are in young children, especially in the US and Europe. In Latin America, the infection has been observed in Chile (17 cases), Argentina, Uruguay, Brazil, Venezuela, Guatemala, Mexico, and Puerto Rico. The infection is so rare in humans that, when single cases occur, they are reported in almost all countries (Wijesundera and Ranaweera, 1989; Raitiere, 1992; Reid *et al.*, 1992; Neafie and Marty, 1993; Brandstetter and Auer, 1994).

The Disease in Animals: *D. caninum* is the most common dog cestode in urban areas due to the almost universal presence of the intermediate host, the flea. The prevalence of infection with *D. caninum* in dogs is high, but varies worldwide. Prevalences of 45% were reported in 156 dogs autopsied in Nairobi (Wachira *et al.*, 1993); 19.8% in 756 samples of dog droppings in Jordan (Abo-Shehada and Ziyadeh, 1991); 13.2% in 303 rural dogs in Uruguay (Cabrera *et al.*, 1996); 9.2% in 315 rural dogs in Great Britain (Jones and Walters, 1992); and 1.1% in 3,329 dogs in Germany (Epe *et al.*, 1993); also, it was found sporadically in 371 stray dogs in Switzerland (Deplazes *et al.*, 1995). Several surveys of foxes conducted in Europe found a prevalence of 0.2% to 3.8%. The infection in cats is as prevalent as or more prevalent than in dogs, but is also variable. Prevalences of 23.8% were found in samples of the droppings of 52 cats in Nigeria (Umeche and Ima, 1988); 23% in 1,502 cats autopsied in South Africa (Baker *et al.*, 1989); 20.7% in 58 cats autopsied in Spain (Calvete *et al.*, 1998); and 1.4% in fecal samples of 1,147 cats in Germany (Epe *et al.*, 1993).

The Disease in Man: Because of its epidemiological characteristics, human dipylidiasis affects mainly infants and young children. The symptomatology consists of digestive disorders, such as diarrhea and colic, irritability, erratic appetite, and insomnia; the infection is often asymptomatic. In a series of patients studied in Chile (Belmar, 1963), abdominal distension was almost always seen. Elimination of motile proglottids is the sign usually noticed by the patients' parents, and is sometimes the only manifestation of the infection. In about 25% of the cases, more than one parasite has been found.

The Disease in Animals: Dipylidiasis, like other cestodiases of dogs and cats, rarely has clinical manifestations. During an epidemiological survey, Barriga (1997) collected 1.1 kg of *D. caninum* upon purging an asymptomatic 13 kg dog with arecoline. Anal irritation or itching has often been attributed to the movement of gravid proglottids in the anal area, because some infected animals rub themselves on the ground as if trying to scratch themselves; however, the presence of inflamed anal sacs, which also causes similar symptoms, has not been confirmed.

Source of Infection and Mode of Transmission: Dogs and cats generally defend themselves against fleas by biting them and, frequently, by ingesting them. This behavior ensures continuation of the parasite's life cycle. Man is also infected by ingesting fleas infected with cysticercoids of *D. caninum*. Almost all cases of human infection are in very young children who live in homes with infected dogs or cats. The child accidentally eats the flea when kissing or biting the pet, or when the flea drops into his food or attaches itself to a wet pacifier.

Diagnosis: In humans and animals, diagnosis is based on microscopic observation of the gravid proglottids. These cestodes have, as a unique characteristic, two genital pores, one on each side of the proglottid. No other human cestode has this characteristic. *D. caninum* is whitish and resembles a melon seed (when expanded) or a grain of boiled rice (when contracted); it is highly motile and can often be seen crawling on the coat of infected animals or on the skin, diapers, or feces of an infected baby. Each proglottid contains a large number of eggs typical of cestodes, but arranged in groups of 5 to 20 in sacs known as oviferous capsules. For observing proglottids or eggs, better results are achieved by examining material collected from the perianal region than by examining the fecal matter.

Control: Prophylactic measures consist of eliminating fleas from the home and cestodes from pets. While recommended, watching small children to keep them from ingesting fleas is difficult.

Bibliography

Abo-Shehada, M.N., Y. Ziyadeh. Prevalence of endoparasites in dog faecal deposits in Jordan. *J Helminthol* 65:313–314, 1991.

Baker, M.K., L. Lange, A. Verster, S. van der Plaat. A survey of helminths in domestic cats in the Pretoria area of Transvaal, Republic of South Africa. Part 1: The prevalence and comparison of burdens of helminths in adult and juvenile cats. *J S Afr Vet Assoc* 60:139–142, 1989.

Barriga, O.O. *Veterinary Parasitology for Practitioners*, 2nd ed. Edina: Burgess International Group; 1997.

Belmar, R. *Dipylidium caninum* en niños. Comunicación de 13 casos y tratamiento con un derivado de salicilamida. *Bol Chile Parasitol* 18:63–67, 1963.

Brandstetter, W., H. Auer. *Dipylidium caninum*, ein seltener Parasit des Menschen. [*Dipylidium caninum*, a rare parasite in man]. *Wien Klin Wochenschr* 106:115–116, 1994.

Cabrera, P.A., S. Parietti, G. Haran, *et al.* Rates of reinfection with *Echinococcus granulosus, Taenia hydatigena, taenia ovis* and other cestodes in a rural dog population in Uruguay. *Int J Parasitol* 26:79–83, 1996.

Calvete, C., J. Lucientes, J.A. Castillo, *et al.* Gastrointestinal helminth parasites in stray cats from the mid-Ebro Valley, Spain. *Vet Parasitol* 75:235–240, 1998.

Deplazes, P., F. Guscetti, E. Wunderlin, H. Bucklar, J. Skaggs, K. Wolff. Endoparasitenbefall bei Findel- und Verzicht-Hunden in der Sudschweiz. [Endoparasite infection in stray and abandoned dogs in southern Switzerland]. *Schweiz Arch Tierheilkd* 137:172–179, 1995.

Epe, C., S. Ising-Volmer, M. Stoye. Ergebnisse parasitologischer Kotuntersuchungen von Equiden, Hunden, Katzen und Igeln der Jahre 1984–1991. [Parasitological fecal studies of equids, dogs, cats and hedgehogs during the years 1984–1991]. *Dtsch Tierarztl Wochenschr* 100:426–428, 1993.

Jones, A., T.M. Walters. A survey of taeniid cestodes in farm dogs in mid-Wales. *Ann Trop Med Parasitol* 86:137–142, 1992.

Hinaidy, H.K. Beitrag zur Biologie des Dipylidium caninum. 2. Mitteilung. [The biology of Dipylidium caninum. Part 2]. *Zentralbl Veterinarmed [B]* 38:329–336, 1991.

Marx, M.B. Parasites, pets, and people. *Prim Care* 18:153–165, 1991.

Neafie, R.C., A.M. Marty. Unusual infections in humans. *Clin Microbiol Rev* 6:34–56, 1993.

Raitiere, C.R. Dog tapeworm (*Dipylidium caninum*) infestation in a 6-month-old infant. *J Fam Pract* 34:101–102, 1992.

Reid, C.J., F.M. Perry, N. Evans. *Dipylidium caninum* in an infant. *Europ J Pediatr* 151:502–503, 1992.

Tanowitz, H.B., L.M. Weiss, M. Wittner. Diagnosis and treatment of intestinal helminths. Common intestinal cestodes. *Gastroenterologist* 1:265–273, 1993.

Umeche, N., A.E. Ima. Intestinal helminthic infections of cats in Calabar, Nigeria. *Folia Parasitol (Praha)* 35:165–168, 1988.

Wachira, T.M., M. Sattran, E. Zeyhle, M.K. Njenga. Intestinal helminths of public health importance in dogs in Nairobi. *East Afr Med J* 70:617–619, 1993.

Wijesundera, M.D., R.L. Ranaweera. Case reports of *Dipylidium caninum*; a pet associated infection. *Ceylon Med J* 34:27–30, 1989.

HYDATIDOSIS

ICD-10 B67 Echinococcosis

Synonyms: Echinococciasis, hydatid disease, hydatid cyst.

Etiology: The agent of this disease is the hydatid or larval stage of the cestodes *Echinococcus granulosus*, *Echinococcus multilocularis*, *Echinococcus oligarthrus*, and *Echinococcus vogeli*. While other species and subspecies of *Echinococcus* have occasionally appeared in the literature, their taxonomic status is doubtful or uncertain. The definitive hosts of *E. granulosus* are domestic dogs and some wild canids. The adult cestode lives attached deep inside the mucosal crypts of the definitive host's small intestine and is 3 to 6 mm long; it has 22 large hooks and 18 small hooks on the scolex and usually has just 3 proglottids, of which only the last is gravid. The gravid proglottid, containing several hundred eggs, detaches from the strobila, is expelled with the feces, and disintegrates in the environment. Each egg contains an embryo (oncosphere) with six hooks (hexacanth), which must be ingested by an intermediate host to continue its development. Intermediate hosts are sheep, bovines, swine, goats, equines, camelids (Asian and American), cervids, and man. The oncosphere is released in the small intestine of the intermediate host, passes through the intestinal wall, and is carried by the bloodstream to various organs, where it undifferentiates and then differentiates again to develop the larval stage, called the hydatid. After three weeks the hydatid measures 250 µm in diameter and has a central cavity. Around the fifth month, it measures approximately 1 cm and it is apparent that its wall consists of two layers: an external, cuticular or laminar layer, formed by numerous thin nacreous lamina that resemble the cross-section of an onion, and another, internal layer, germinative or proligerous, which is a delicate cellular syncytium. The larval form of *E. granulosus* typically consists of a single cavity (is unilocular). The interior of the hydatid is filled with liquid. During the same period, brood capsules bud off from the germinative layer, and invaginated protoscolices, which constitute the infective agent of the parasite, develop within them. These capsules either adhere to the wall by means of a peduncle or float freely in the hydatid fluid. The capsules and the protoscolices that float freely in the hydatid fluid are known as "hydatid sand." Some hydatids do not form capsules, and sometimes the capsules do not form protoscolices: these are sterile larvae. In contrast, daughter hydatids with a two-layer wall like that of the mother sometimes form inside the hydatid. As the larva develops and the tissues of the host are compressed, the host responds with a fibrotic reaction, surrounding the larva with dense connective tissue, the adventitial layer. The hydatid surrounded by this connective tissue is the hydatid cyst. The most common localizations of these cysts are the liver (in about two-thirds of the cases) and the lungs (in about a fourth of the cases); on rare occasions they may become situated in some other organ, such as the kidneys, spleen, bones, and brain. The cycle is completed when a dog or other canid ingests the viscera of an intermediate host in which there are fertile hydatid cysts. The scolex attaches to the wall of the dog's small intestine and develops into an adult cestode that begins to produce infective eggs 47 to 61 days after infection. A single cyst can give rise to thousands of adult cestodes because of the large number of scolices. The species *E. granulosus* is polytypic, and morphological, biochemical, and biological variants have been found in different parts of the world. For example, in Great Britain, two strains occur: an equine strain whose development cycle involves horses and dogs, and an ovine strain that circulates between sheep and dogs. In addition to the differences in morphology and development in the different intermediate hosts, the two strains also differ in biochemical and physiological characteristics. Even though dogs are definitive hosts for both, it seems that the equine strain is not transmitted to sheep and vice versa. Doubts also exist about the equine strain's infectivity for man. In Latin America, except around Santa María, Rio Grande do Sul, Brazil, horses are rarely affected by the larval form of *E. granulosus*, in spite of their close contact with dogs. In the boreal region of the northern hemisphere, the strain of *E. granulosus* that circulates between wolves and the large deer *Rangifer* and *Alces* is transmitted with difficulty to domestic ungulates (Schantz, 1982). In Australia, three strains are distinguished; one circulates between the dingo and macropodid marsupials (wallabies, kangaroos), and the other two (one continental and the other from Tasmania) circulate between dogs and sheep but differ in some biochemical, morphological, and biological properties (Thompson and Kumaratilake, 1982). Studies in the former Soviet Union have shown that the strain circulating between dogs and sheep is not infective for swine, and the strain circulating between dogs and swine is not transmitted to sheep. Recent molecular biology studies have confirmed the presence of four genotypes in Argentina: the ovine, circulating between sheep and humans; the ovine from Tasmania, circulating in sheep and humans; the porcine in swine; and the camelid in humans (Rozenzvit *et al.*, 1999). Similar work is being carried out on the other species (Rinder *et al.*, 1997).

    The adult form of *E. multilocularis*, sometimes identified as *Echinococcus alveolaris* or *Echinococcus sibiricensis*, measuring 1.2 to 3.7 mm, is somewhat smaller than that of *E. granulosus*. It has 27 large hooks and 23 small hooks on the scolex. The species are distinguished by subtle characteristics of the mature proglottid and by the number and shape of the hooks on the scolex. The natural definitive hosts are foxes, chiefly the arctic fox (*Alopex lagopus*) and the red fox (*Vulpes vulpes*). The intermediate hosts are wild rodents, primarily species of the genera *Microtus*, *Clethrionomys*, and *Lemmus*. Domestic dogs and cats may also serve as definitive hosts when they enter the cycle by feeding on infected wild rodents. The rodents develop the hydatid in the liver after ingesting eggs deposited with the fecal matter of definitive hosts; in about 60 days, the hydatid contains infective protoscolices. Unlike the larva of *E. granulosus*, this hydatid has a weak cuticular layer that enables it to constantly form small exogenous brood capsules that invade and destroy the surrounding tissue. The vesicles are filled with a gelatinous liquid and generally lack protoscolices in humans. Due to its spongelike morphology, the cyst of *E. multilocularis* is commonly called a "multilocular" or "alveolar" cyst. The absence of protoscolices seems to indicate that man is not a satisfactory host because, when a cyst is transplanted from man to a suitable rodent, the cyst begins to produce them. When a fox, dog, or cat ingests an infected rodent, the protoscolices give rise to the development of adult cestodes, which begin producing infective eggs that are eliminated in the fecal matter in about 33 days.

The adult form of *E. oligarthrus* is about 2 to 3 mm long and consists of a scolex with 33 large hooks and 26 small hooks, an immature proglottid, a mature proglottid, and a terminal gravid proglottid. The definitive hosts are wild felids such as pumas, jaguars, jaguarundis, and lynxes. The intermediate hosts are wild rodents such as the agouti *Dasyprocta* and possibly other rodents as well. The hydatid of *E. oligarthrus* also forms daughter larvae, which are external, larger, and filled with liquid, with abundant protoscolices in man, and not invasive like those of *E. multilocularis*. This noninvasive cyst, which has multiple external compartments and abundant protoscolices, is generally called "polycystic."

The adult form of *E. vogeli* is 3.9 to 5.6 mm long, has 42 large hooks and 33 small hooks, and has been found in a wild canid (*Speothos venaticus*), which ranges from Panama to northern Argentina. The intermediate host is the local rodent *Cuniculus paca*, known as paca. The hydatid of *E. vogeli* is also polycystic and is differentiated from the hydatid of *E. oligarthrus* by the number and shape of the hooks on the protoscolices.

Geographic Distribution: *E. granulosus* is the most widespread of the species, with areas of high endemicity in southern South America (Argentina, southern Brazil, Chile, Peru, and Uruguay); the Mediterranean coast, especially Bulgaria, Cyprus, southern France, Greece, Italy, Portugal, Romania, Spain, and Yugoslavia; the southern part of the former Soviet Union; the Middle East; southwestern Asia (Iran, Iraq, and Turkey); northern Africa (Algeria, Morocco, and Tunisia); Australia; New Zealand; Kenya; and Uganda. In some of these countries, the incidence has recently diminished notably because of control programs.

The distribution of *E. multilocularis* is limited to the northern hemisphere. The parasitosis occurs in central and eastern Europe, the former Soviet Union, Turkey, Iraq, northern India, central China, some islands of Japan, several provinces of Canada, Alaska, and several north central states of the US. The most important endemic areas are the northern tundras of Europe and Asia and their American extension, as well as central Siberia, the central Asian republics of the former Soviet Union, and central China. In Europe, infection with *E. multilocularis* occurs in Austria, Belgium, France, Germany, Liechtenstein, Luxembourg, Poland, and Switzerland (Eckert, 1996). Infections caused by *E. granulosus* and *E. multilocularis* may occur together in the same areas, as happens, for example, in some parts of the former Soviet Union, Alaska (US), and Canada.

   E. oligarthrus and *E. vogeli* are present only in South and Central America. Although the areas of infection coincide, since the definitive host of *E. vogeli* exists only from Panama to northern Argentina, cases of polycystic hydatidosis outside this area are probably imported or due to *E. oligarthrus*. Moreover, this species was identified recently in northeastern Mexico (Salinas-López *et al.*, 1996), and this is the first available report on it in North America.

   Occurrence in Man: The prevalence of classic unilocular hydatidosis caused by *E. granulosus* varies considerably between geographic areas. The highest infection rates are recorded in countries with livestock industries, especially sheep raising, in rural areas, and among people of limited economic and cultural means. Information on the prevalence of human hydatidosis is often based on doctors' reports. But studies from Chile (Serra Canales *et al.*, 1999) have shown that doctors' reports could represent just a quarter of the cases found by studying hospital admission or surgery records. Consequently, the published figures should be used advisedly. Moreover, it is necessary to distinguish between the infection, which may be asymptomatic, and the disease, which, by definition, is symptomatic. The most reliable sources of information on the incidence of the disease are the hospital records of surgical operations. In Latin America, the highest concentration of cases occurs in the Southern Cone of South America (Argentina, southern Brazil, the mountains of Peru, and Uruguay) (Arámbulo, 1997). In the 1960s, the annual incidence of surgical cases per 100,000 inhabitants was 1.0 in Peru, 2.0 in Argentina, 7.8 to 7.9 in Chile, and approximately 20 in Uruguay. However, these data paint an unrealistic picture, because prevalence refers to the total population of the country and not the rural population, which is the population at real risk for the infection. The prevalence of infection caused by *E. granulosus* in an endemic area of the Peruvian Andes was 9.1% in 407 individuals examined by imaging and immunoelectrotransfer (Western blot), 87% in 117 slaughterhouse sheep, and 32% in 104 dogs. The prevalence of human cases was five times higher than that reported in 1980, when a control program was suspended (Moro *et al.*, 1997). In the IX Region of Chile, in the vicinity of the 38th south parallel, between 18 and 48 per 100,000 inhabitants have the human infection, and the prevalence in local slaughterhouses is about 40% for sheep and cattle and 15% for swine. The cost of treatment alone comes to US$ 300,000 a year (Gutierrez *et al.*, 1992). According to official sources, the incidence of hydatidosis in Chile has declined in recent years, but a critical study of hospital cases found that the actual incidence in the period 1985–1994 fluctuated between 6.5 and 11.4 per 100,000 inhabitants. In other words, it was four times higher than the official figures reported (Serra Canales *et al.*, 1999). The authors believe the apparent decrease is the result of problems in the reporting system. In southern Argentina, a 1994 survey found 16 cases (26.7 per 100,000), with a human serological prevalence of 1.3% and a parasitological prevalence of 2.3% in dogs (Larrieu *et al.*, 1996). In southern Uruguay, 156 cases (1.6%) of cystic hydatidosis were recently diagnosed in 9,515 individuals examined by ultrasound and serology (Carmona et al., 1998). The prevalence of infection in the general population can be determined by various diagnostic methods. In Chile, a series of 115,819 autopsies performed between 1947 and 1970 uncovered 359 cases of human hydatidosis (310 per 100,000), and 108 (204 per 100,000) in 53,014 autopsies of individuals who died violent deaths. These figures on the prevalence of the infection are 25 to 40 times higher than the estimated prevalence of the disease for the same period. In the other Latin American countries, hydatidosis is not a health problem; some countries have sporadic cases and others have not reported the disease in humans. There are endemic pockets in the US among inhabitants of Basque origin who breed sheep in the northern California area, among Eskimos in Alaska, and among the indigenous peoples of Arizona and New Mexico. However, a significant percentage of the cases in California may be imported; Donovan et al. (1995) found that 25 of 28 patients (89%) in Los Angeles had been born abroad and 19 were immigrants from the Near East or central Asia. The Mediterranean coast of Europe constitutes one of the areas of highest prevalence, comparable only to the Southern Cone of South America. In Asia, the highest prevalences of infection are found in the southwest (Iraq and Turkey), in the southern republics of the former Soviet Union, and in China and Japan. In six provinces of China, 26,065 surgical cases of cystic hydatidosis were reported between 1951 and 1990, the majority after 1980. An extensive survey in agricultural areas found rates of infection of 0.5% to 4.5% in humans by imaging, 3.3% to 90% in sheep, and 7% to 71% in dogs (Chai, 1995). A serologic study in northwestern Mongolia found a 5.2% rate of infection in 334 seminomadic shepherds (Watson-Jones et al., 1997). In Africa, the areas with the highest rates of infection are in Kenya and in the northwestern part of the continent. A recent survey carried out in Libya with ultrasound techniques found 339 abdominal infections in 20,220 individuals (1.7%); 233 (69%) of them were also positive with the enzyme-linked immunosorbent assay (ELISA) (Shambesh et al., 1999). Oceania is another area of high prevalence; the morbidity rate in humans in Australia is estimated at 1.2 per 100,000 inhabitants and 2.3 per 100,000 inhabitants in New Zealand before control programs were set up.

Occurrence of the human infection caused by E. multilocularis was thought to be sporadic, with low endemicity. From 1970 to 1980, 91 cases were diagnosed in France, equaling a prevalence rate comparable to the prevalences in Germany and Switzerland. The only region with a high prevalence (1% of the population) was Rebun Island, Japan, where effective control measures were established. However, since 1990 there has been a significant increase in the prevalence of human infection caused by this parasite in the northern part of Eurasia (Romig et al., 1999). In Europe, the prevalence of E. multilocularis in foxes is 1% to 50%. The infection in dogs and cats is rare (<1%), and the prevalence in humans is 0.02 to 1.4 cases per 100,000 persons in most cases. Although it is not a very common infection, it is considered very important because mortality is higher than 90% without treatment, and treatment is very expensive (Eckert, 1996). In 1990, a study of 606 individuals drawn from the general population of the province of Gansu, China, found 8.8% with positive serology for the parasite. A study using ultrasonography and serology conducted the following year confirmed the infection in 65 of 1,312 people (5%). Examination of domestic dogs found E. multilocularis in 10% (Graig et al., 1992). Subsequently, 584 cases were diagnosed in seven provinces of China; it is estimated that the prevalence ranges from 2.8% to 19.2%, and morbidity ranges from 2.4% to 5% (Jiang, 1998).

Up to 1998, 86 cases of human polycystic hydatidosis had been diagnosed in Latin America, in the region between Nicaragua and Argentina; 32 were attributed to *E. vogeli*, 3 to *E. oligarthrus* (2 orbital cases in Suriname and Venezuela, and 1 cardiac in Brazil), and 51 whose causal agent could not be determined because the hooks of the protoscolices were not found (Basset *et al.*, 1998). The cases of human polycystic hydatidosis reported in Argentina, Chile, Costa Rica, Nicaragua, and Uruguay are probably caused by *E. oligarthrus* or are imported cases of *E. vogeli,* because the definitive host of the latter species does not exist in those countries (D'Alessandro, 1997).

Occurrence in Animals: In all areas where the prevalence of human infection by *E. granulosus* is high, a high rate of parasitism in animals, both the intermediate and definitive hosts, is to be expected. Some specific examples were mentioned in the previous section. In dogs in endemic areas, infection rates greater than 30% are commonly found. In sheep, the most important intermediate host in many parts of the world, rates of infection are also high. The rate of hydatid cysts found in slaughterhouses in hyperendemic areas of Latin America varies from 20% to 95% of sacrificed animals. The highest rates are found in rural slaughterhouses, where older animals are slaughtered. High prevalence rates are also found in cattle, swine, and goats. In Argentina and Uruguay, hydatid cysts have not been found in horses; in Chile, the prevalence is low (0.29%), while in an area of Rio Grande do Sul, Brazil, it is about 20%. According to some parasitologists, the strain that parasitizes horses is a special biotype of *E. granulosus* that has adapted itself to this animal species (see Etiology). In other parts of the world, such as the Middle East, in addition to high rates in sheep, a high prevalence is found in camels, which are intermediate hosts, and in dogs, jackals, and wolves, which are definitive hosts. Buffaloes are important intermediate hosts in some countries.

The prevalence of the infection caused by *E. multilocularis* in the natural definitive host, the fox, can reach high percentages in some localities; in dogs in Alaska, US, it is almost 6%. In rodents, the intermediate hosts of *E. multilocularis*, the infection rate is relatively low and varies from 2% to 10%.

Little is known of the prevalence of *E. oligarthrus* infection in wild felids (the definitive hosts) and rodents (the intermediate hosts). Infection by *E. vogeli* was found in 96 of 425 pacas (*Cuniculus paca*), the main intermediate host, caught in Colombia (Rausch *et al.*, 1981).

The Disease in Man: The hexacanth embryo of *E. granulosus* generally travels in the bloodstream until it colonizes a part of the liver or lung, and remains there for years, growing slowly and silently, without causing major tissular reactions or clinical signs. The symptoms generally appear when the larva grows large enough to compress or erode the neighboring tissues or ducts and interfere with their function. Absorption of parasitic antigens by the host often sensitizes the individual and may cause hypersensitivity phenomena. Because the *E. granulosus* cyst generally has a single compartment, as opposed to those of the other species, human infection by this parasite is usually called "cystic" or "unilocular" hydatidosis. Many cysts are asymptomatic throughout the infected individual's life and are discovered only at autopsy, during surgery, or in radiographs, all related to other causes. A review of almost 190,000 autopsies performed in Chile from 1947 to 1984 found that 363 of 568 cases of cerebral hydatidosis (64%) and 79 of 116 cases of cerebral cysticerco- sis (68%) had been discovered during these autopsies. From this it is clear that the symptomatology of unilocular or cystic hydatidosis depends on the location of the cyst and its size. The most common location is the liver (65% to 70% of cases), fol- lowed by the lungs (about 25% of cases). There are indications that the localization of the hydatids may depend on the strain of *E. granulosus*. Thus, in the case of wild *E. granulosus* of the boreal region, which circulates between wild cervids and wolves, the lung localization predominates in humans, and the disease is generally more benign than that caused by the *E. granulosus* strain of the domestic cycle. In a small percentage of patients, the cysts localize in other organs or tissue. In loca- tions where growth of the cyst is not restricted by anatomical structures, it can reach a very large size and contain several liters of fluid. For example, rupture of the cyst by external trauma in hypersensitive patients can result in anaphylactic shock and pulmonary edema caused by rapid absorption of the antigen through the peritoneal or pleural serosa. Another serious consequence of cyst rupture is hydatid seeding within the abdominal or pleural cavity, and the formation of many new cysts in the serosa. Rupture of a cyst can also cause arterial embolisms in the lungs and some- times in other organs. Early diagnosis in man is important for prevention of com- plications and rupture of the cyst, with its consequent seeding in multiple locations. For inoperable cases, treatment with mebendazole for several years is used, result- ing in reduction of the cysts in several cases.

In hepatic hydatidosis, most cysts (approximately 75%) are located in the right lobe; they may be situated either deep in the parenchyma or superficially, below Glisson's capsule. The intraparenchymatous cysts cause atrophy of the surrounding tissue and, through pressure on the veins and biliary passages, provoke congestion and biliary sta- sis, which may be complicated by a secondary infection. A subcapsular cyst may grow upward (anterosuperior cyst) and adhere to the diaphragm, and the cyst may even cross the diaphragm and open into the thoracic cavity, or it may grow toward the peritoneal cavity, where it can adhere to and empty into the hollow abdominal viscera. In a study of 677 patients who had surgery for hepatic hydatid cysts, Hernando *et al.* (1996) found that the most common clinical manifestations were dyspepsic symptoms (60%), hepatomegaly or a palpable mass in the right hypochondrium (58%), and pain (46%). Most cysts were solitary (66%) and in the right lobe (65%). The most common com- plication of surgery was a biliary fistula; the average period of hospitalization was 25 days and the mortality rate was 1.6%. The average age of the patients was about 39 and the prevalence was the same in both sexes.

The second most common location is the lungs. The cyst is generally located in the lower lobe, and more frequently in the right lung than in the left. In the lung, as in the liver, a cyst's presence may be asymptomatic, or it may be manifested by symptoms such as pain in the affected side of the chest (especially if the cyst is peripheral), dry cough, hemoptysis, vomiting if the cyst ruptures, and sometimes deformation of the thorax. Expectoration of the cyst (hydatid vomica) occurs with some frequency in pulmonary hydatidosis and may be followed by recovery. Hueto Pérez de Heredia *et al.* (1999) studied the clinical and epidemiological characteris- tics of 40 patients with thoracic hydatidosis, 32 of whom had pulmonary cysts.

Bone hydatidosis causes destruction of the trabeculae, necrosis, and spontaneous fracture. This localization is estimated to occur in 1% of the cases. Hydatidosis of vital organs, such as the central nervous system, heart, and kidneys, has a grave prognosis. The latency period of cerebral hydatidosis is relatively short, about eight months in the general population and four months in children. In Spain (Jiménez-Mejías *et al.*, 1991), most patients (74%) had a solitary cyst, 74% in the right lobe, and in half the cases the cyst was intraparenchymatous.

The disease caused by *E. multilocularis*, or alveolar hydatidosis, is progressive and malignant. In the vast majority of cases, the multilocular cyst is located in the liver and rarely in other organs. In general, the cyst starts as a small vesicle, which, by exogenous and endogenous proliferation of the germinative membrane, forms multiple vesicles in all directions, producing its multilocular appearance. After a time, the center necroses and the cyst becomes a spongy mass consisting of small irregular cavities filled with a gelatinous substance. Metastasis can occur, giving rise to secondary cysts in different organs. The symptomatology is similar to that of a slowly developing mucinoid carcinoma of the liver. Alveolar hydatidosis is afebrile if there is no secondary infection, but causes hepatomegaly and often splenomegaly. In more advanced stages, ascites and jaundice appear as a consequence of intrahepatic portal hypertension. The course of the disease is always slow, and signs and symptoms appear after many years. The average age in a group of 33 cases in Alaskan (US) Eskimos was 53 years, and the investigators (Wilson and Rausch, 1980) estimate that 30 years had passed from the time of infection to the appearance of symptoms. The most common objective signs were hepatomegaly and a palpable abdominal mass derived from the liver. By the time symptoms were apparent, the majority of the patients could not be operated on. The disease is usually fatal without an organ transplant.

In a study of 72 human cases of *E. vogeli* or *E. oligarthrus* polycystic hydatidosis, D'Alessandro (1997) found that in 80% of the cases the lesions were limited to the liver or other organs. The most frequent signs were palpable, hard, round masses in the liver, hepatomegaly, bulging abdomen, pain, significant weight loss, and fever. All the cases were fatal, and in 25% there were signs of portal hypertension; 10% of the cases were asymptomatic. In a study of seven human cases of polycystic hydatidosis caused by *E. vogeli*, Meneghelli *et al.* (1992) found that the most common signs were abdominal pain, hepatomegaly, jaundice, weight loss, anemia, fever, hemoptysis, palpable abdominal masses, and portal hypertension. In four cases, hepatic calcifications were observed. The most frequent localizations were the liver (six cases), the lungs (two), the mesentery (two), the spleen (one), and the pancreas (one).

To appreciate the importance of hydatidosis in public health, it should be remembered that the principal treatment is surgery, and hospitalization is lengthy; about 60% of those operated on cannot return to work until about four months after leaving the hospital, and approximately 40% are incapacitated for six or more months.

The Disease in Animals: Clinical symptoms are not seen in dogs parasitized by the adult form of *E. granulosus*. Barriga and Al-Khalidi (1986) obtained more than 5,000 parasites from the intestine of an asymptomatic 8.5-kg dog. Infection with a large number of parasites probably causes enteritis. In the domestic intermediate hosts of *E. granulosus*, no definite clinical symptomatology has been found, even in cases of multiple cysts in the liver and lungs. In contrast, some studies indicate that parasitized sheep become fatter, which would make them more attractive to predators and hinder their escape.

The confiscation of viscera with hydatid cysts, especially livers, accounts for significant economic losses. This procedure results in the loss of an estimated 1,500,000 pounds of viscera annually in New Zealand. In Uruguay, approximately 60% of all beef livers are confiscated because of hydatidosis and fascioliasis. It has been estimated that the viscera of 2 million cattle and 3.5 million sheep are confiscated every year in the Southern Cone, causing losses estimated at US$ 6.3 million in Argentina and US$ 2.5 million in Chile. The costs of medical and surgical care of human patients must be added to the losses suffered by the livestock economy. Hospitalization is usually lengthy (about seven weeks). The cost of hospitalization for a surgical case of hydatidosis, without complications, is from US$ 1,500 to $2,000 in Argentina and Chile.

Foxes infected by *E. multilocularis* do not manifest clinical symptoms, even when harboring an enormous number of parasites in their intestines. On the other hand, infection by the larval form in arvicoline rodents is often fatal when the cystic burden is large (Schantz, 1982).

Source of Infection and Mode of Transmission: The dog-sheep-dog cycle is the most important cycle for maintenance of the parasitism in the endemic areas of the southern part of South America and many other areas of the world. Sheep are the most important intermediate hosts of unilocular hydatidosis caused by *E. granulosus* for several reasons: the infection rate is generally high among these animals, 90% or more of their cysts are fertile, they live in close association with dogs, and, since they are often sacrificed for household consumption on ranches, the viscera are customarily fed to dogs. Also the Southern Cone of South America is a region with a high concentration of sheep: approximately 50% of the total sheep population lives on 10% of the total land area of the continent. Finally, the number of dogs on sheep ranches is high.

Sheep and other intermediate hosts contract hydatidosis by grazing on pastures contaminated with dog feces containing eggs of the cestode. Those eggs are deposited directly on the grazing land or are carried by rain or wind. The dogs in turn are infected by eating viscera that contain fertile cysts (with viable protoscolices). Man is an intermediate host and plays no role in the transmission of the parasite, unless he is eaten by a carnivore. Nevertheless, his sanitary habits make him the main agent responsible for perpetuating the infection by feeding dogs viscera that contain hydatid cysts. The adult cestode of *E. granulosus* can live in a dog's intestine for about a year, but it remains fertile for just 6 to 10 months. Therefore, theoretically the infection would die out if man ceased reinfecting dogs by feeding them raw viscera. Domestic animals that serve as secondary hosts could still become infected for a time, since the eggs of *Echinococcus* are resistant to environmental factors, but the infection cycle would be halted if dogs were prevented access to the infected viscera.

A gravid proglottid of *E. granulosus* contains a very small number of eggs (from 200 to 800) compared with those of other tapeworms, which contain many thousands. It is estimated that only one segment of *E. granulosus* is eliminated every two weeks (Lawson and Gemmell, 1983). This low biotic potential of *E. granulosus* is compensated for by the high rate and intensity of infection in the definitive host and by the asexual multiplication of the larva in the intermediate host. The survival time and dispersion of the eggs are of great epidemiological interest. The eggs have little resistance to desiccation and extreme temperatures. In the laboratory, the eggs of *E. granulosus* can survive in water or damp sand for three weeks at 30°C, 225 days at 6°C, and 32 days at 10–21°C (Lawson and Gemmell, 1983). After 10 days, radial dispersion up to 80 m from the place the feces were deposited has been confirmed for eggs of other taeniids; they may be able to disperse even greater distances with the aid of mechanical vectors such as carrion birds and arthropods. The physical composition of the soil, its porosity, and the kind of vegetation cover also help determine the length of time that the eggs survive.

As we have said, man is an accidental host, and his direct contact with dogs is important. The gravid proglottids are found primarily on the surface of fecal matter, and they can accumulate in the perianal region, where they disintegrate and release the eggs. The dog carries the eggs on its tongue and snout to different parts of its body, and a person's hands can become contaminated by touching the animal. Close contact with dogs and deficient personal hygiene practices, such as failure to wash the hands before eating, are important factors in the transmission of the infection from dogs to humans. Another important source of human infection can be vegetables and water contaminated with infected dog feces. Coprophagic flies may also serve as mechanical vectors of the eggs.

Although hydatidosis is usually an infection of the rural population, infected dogs and human cases of the disease occur in urban areas. The difference in infection rates between religious and ethnic groups is merely a reflection of their relationship with dogs. In Lebanon, for example, a higher prevalence of hydatidosis has been observed among Christians than among Moslems because the Koran asserts that dogs are "dirty" animals. Long-standing cultural and religious habits account for the high and unusual incidence of hydatidosis among the members of the Turkana tribe of northwestern Kenya. This pastoral tribe, which includes about 150,000 persons, has attracted the attention of researchers. A large number of dogs live with the members of this tribe, and the dogs have a high rate of infection. The Turkana use dog feces as a lubricant and as medicine, and they either do not bury dead persons or cover them only with a thin layer of earth, making it possible for the dogs to eat the cadavers (Macpherson, 1983). More than 1,500 Turkana with hydatidosis were operated on between 1965 and 1980; annual incidence, based on hospitalized cases of the disease, varies from 220 per 100,000 inhabitants in the northern part of the district to 18 per 100,000 in the southern part (French and Nelson, 1982). In contrast to findings in 111 patients with pulmonary hydatidosis in Uruguay (Yarzábal and Capron, 1971), whose cysts did not contain protoscolices, 60% of 154 cysts in Turkana patients were fertile.

In the Holarctic region of North America—Alaska (US) and Canada—unilocular hydatidosis exists in a wild cycle that develops between the wolf (*Canis lupus*) and several cervid species. Another wild cycle independent of the domestic cycle has been described in Australia between dingoes and marsupials such as wallabies and kangaroos. The strobilar form of *E. granulosus* has been found in Argentina in three species of foxes of the genus *Dusicyon*, and the larval form has been found in the European hare. In contrast to what is occurring in the northern region of the Americas, wildlife infection in Argentina appears to derive from the domestic cycle.

Alveolar hydatidosis (*E. multilocularis*) has many natural foci in the northern hemisphere; the parasite circulates between foxes of the genera *Alopex* and *Vulpes*, the definitive hosts, and arvicoline and microtine rodents, the intermediate hosts.

Man can come into accidental contact with the eggs of the cestode when handling dead foxes or drinking water from streams contaminated with the feces of infected foxes. Domestic dogs and cats can carry the infection into the home when they hunt wild rodents. A community in which arvicoline rodents and dogs abound can become a hyperendemic focus, as has happened in some Eskimo villages of the North American boreal tundra. Coprophagous flies can act as mechanical transfer hosts of the eggs. A study carried out in Auvergne, France, found the infection in 2.4% of 943 captured *Arvicola terrestris scherman* rodents. In the area where they were captured, the prevalence varied from 0% to 4.6%, which suggests that the distribution is focal. Only 2 of the 23 animals (8.7%) had fertile larvae. In the same region, 8.5% of 70 foxes (*Vulpes vulpes*) harbored the strobilar form, and five human cases occurred in 10 years (Pétavy and Deblock, 1983).

The cycles of *E. vogeli* and *E. oligarthrus* are exclusively wild. Man probably becomes infected accidentally by eggs of *E. vogeli* through the feces of dogs that are fed the viscera of the paca or with eggs of *E. oligarthrus* from the feces of cats that eat infested rodents.

Diagnosis: A diagnosis of human hydatidosis is suspected based on the clinical symptoms and epidemiological circumstances. Imaging methods such as radiography, computerized tomography, ultrasonography, and scintigraphy are used. While they do not confirm the diagnosis, they are very helpful to the specialist. Ultrasonography is the first choice because it is economical, noninvasive, simple, and accurate and reveals developing cysts that generally cannot be found with X-rays (Suwan, 1995). Numerous immunobiologic tests have been used in the diagnosis of human hydatidosis by *E. granulosus*, among them Casoni's intradermal test, complement fixation, indirect hemagglutination, latex agglutination, inmunoelectrophoresis, electrosyneresis, and double diffusion to detect antibodies against the arc 5 antigen. Practically all have been displaced by ELISA and the immunoelectrotransfer or Western blot test. Casoni's intradermal test is not very sensitive and is nonspecific for the diagnosis. While it was once used for epidemiological surveys, the collection of drops of blood on filter paper now makes it possible to use serologic techniques that are much more sensitive and specific on a large scale. The complement fixation, indirect hemagglutination, and latex agglutination tests have no operational advantage over ELISA and are much less specific or sensitive. The techniques based on observation of arc 5 were abandoned when it was found that the respective antigen was specific not for *Echinococcus* but for many cestodes. Navarrete *et al.* (1995) found that ELISA diagnosed 96.6% of hydatidosis patients but cross-reacted with taeniasis and ascariasis; indirect hemagglutination diagnosed 86% of patients but also gave cross-reactions, and the double diffusion test for arc 5 diagnosed 79% of patients but did not give false positives. Only ELISA gave false positives. Moreover, the test with selected antigens is not only highly sensitive and specific but can also distinguish among infections caused by different species of *Echinococcus*. ELISA for *E. multilocularis*, for example, showed a sensitivity of 93% and a specificity of 97%, in contrast to another ELISA for *E. granulosus* that showed a sensitivity of 89% and a specificity of 99% (Helbig *et al.*, 1993). But there seem to be wide variations in the sensitivity and specificity of the test among different laboratories. For example, Navarrete *et al.* (1995) found, in Valdivia, Chile, that 28 of 29 patients (96.5%) with hydatidosis confirmed by surgery showed positive reactions to ELISA, and taeniasis and ascariasis patients showed false positives; but Arienti *et al.* (1996) reported that ELISA was positive in just 62 of 176 surgery patients (35.2%) in Córdoba, Argentina, and they found no false positives. The differences do not seem to be due to a variation in the methods or composition of the antigenic extracts used (Coltorti and Cammarieri, 1993). More recent reports compared ELISA with antigen electrotransfer and attributed an 82% specificity to ELISA and a 94% to 97% specificity to the transfer test (Poretti *et al.*, 1999). More recently, the polymerase chain reaction has also been used to detect nucleic acids from the parasite in patients' bloodstreams (Kern *et al.*, 1995).

Results of all the tests vary according to the location of the cyst and its physiological state. The immunodiagnostic tests seem to be less sensitive for detecting pulmonary than hepatic hydatidosis. Several investigators are looking for antigens characteristic of fertile or live cysts, since these cysts are the only ones that can cause secondary hydatidosis. Knowledge of whether a cyst is sterile or dead enables the doctor to be more conservative in treatment.

Even though there is no reason why the immunological methods for diagnosing cysts cannot be adapted to domestic animals, there apparently has been no incentive to do so. The traditional method of diagnosing hydatidosis in these species is postmortem examination in slaughterhouses or packing plants.

Intestinal echinococcosis in the definitive hosts is traditionally diagnosed by administering a strong purgative, generally arecoline hydrobromide, and searching for the parasite in the feces. The maximum effectiveness of this technique is about 65% if both the feces and the vomit are examined. Besides being slow and tedious, this method is dangerous because the eggs of *Echinococcus* are infective when they are eliminated. There is evidence that intradermic reactions may be positive in infected dogs (Barriga and Al-Khalidi, 1986), but the discovery, using ELISA, of circulating antibodies has a sensitivity of just 61% (Gasser *et al.*, 1994). In recent years, investigators have attempted to find antigens to the parasite in droppings (coproantigens) by using ELISA with monoclonal antibodies and through polymerase chain reactions. The specificity and sensitivity of the former test were 95% to 99% and 80% to 93%, respectively. The specificity and sensitivity of the latter were 100% and 94%, respectively (Deplazes and Eckert, 1996).

Control: At present, conventional control measures consist of: 1) educating the rural population about hydatidosis and its control; 2) centralizing the slaughtering of animals for food in units with veterinary control; 3) ensuring sanitary conditions for slaughtering done on ranches and preventing dogs' access to raw viscera; 4) reducing the number of dogs on the ranches and treating them for *Echinococcus* on a regular basis. A fifth measure has recently been added: looking for human hydatidosis during primary health care visits. This has made it possible to diagnose many unsuspected cases and interest the population in the control campaign. Recently, joint and coordinated implementation of these health measures, both medical and veterinary, has resulted in noteworthy improvement in the results of the control campaigns.

One of the first examples of organized control was the campaign on Cyprus, which was carried out only in the area controlled by the Government of Cyprus; certain areas of the island remained uncontrolled. The activity was initiated in 1971 with a vigorous attack phase directed essentially at dogs: in two years, two-thirds of the estimated 45,000 dogs were sacrificed, and the rest were treated 3 or 4 times a year. The parasite disappeared, and the campaign was suspended in 1985. Studies carried out in the period 1993–1996 showed that the parasite had returned in 20% of the communities checked. A consolidation campaign was then initiated, this time emphasizing both control of the intermediate hosts and treatment of dogs. The campaign carried out in Tasmania, Australia, reduced the rate of infection in dogs from 12.6% in 1965–1966 to 0.09% in 1981–1982, and the rate in sheep from 52.2% in 1966–1967 to 0.7% in 1981–1982. New cases of human hydatidosis fell from 19 in 1966 to 4 in 1982; in practice, the disease was no longer found in young people (Australia, 1973). In 1991, however, hydatid cysts were found in cattle in the northern part of the state, where the parasitism was thought to have been eradicated. In Iceland, health education and a highly motivated population were the main factors in the success of the campaign to eradicate the infection. The main objective of the program was to develop an understanding of the problem and a sense of responsibility in the people. The campaign that resulted in the eradication of E. granulosus in New Zealand has been described by Gemmell (1990). Campaigns for control on islands, such as Cyprus, Iceland, New Zealand, and Tasmania, in Australia, have shown that the area under control must remain totally closed to the introduction of new definitive or intermediate hosts; otherwise, the initial phase of attacking the problem must be followed by a permanent, indefinite consolidation phase (Economides et al., 1998). Observations in Bulgaria also indicate that, even if complete eradication is achieved, control activities should continue to ensure that the infection does not recur. The annual incidence of human hydatidosis in Bulgaria in 1950–1962 was 6.5 per 1,000 inhabitants; that provided the impetus for a control campaign from 1971 to 1982, which decreased the figure to 2 per 100,000. Administrative and economic problems between 1983 and 1995 necessitated suspension of the control measures, and the incidence returned to the previous levels (Todorov and Boeva, 1999). In Peru, suspension of the control programs in a hyperendemic area was associated with a five-fold increase in the incidence of the human infection (Moro et al., 1997).

In Latin America and other developing areas where socioeconomic and cultural conditions differ from those in Iceland, New Zealand, and Tasmania (Australia), the relative effect of each known control procedure must be evaluated to adapt them to the environment, or new procedures must be found. Regional programs for the control of hydatidosis are being carried out in four Latin American countries (Argentina, Chile, Peru, and Uruguay). Programs have been organized in several Argentine provinces. For example, in the control program being carried out in Río Negro, in the southern part of the country, the canine population is subject to diagnostic treatment or deparasitization, the infection in sheep is being detected and controlled in the slaughterhouses, classes are being taught in the schools, community health education is being promoted through the media, and human cases are being sought out, reported, and treated. Between 1979 and 1992, canine echinococcosis was reduced from 41.5% to 4.2%, ovine hydatidosis from 61% to 13%, and the human infection in children age 10 and younger from 64 per 100,000 to 4.5 per 100,000 (Larrieu et al., 1994). China officially initiated a national program for the control of hydatic disease between 1992 and 1995, based on education, improvement of sanitation in slaughtering livestock, and deparasitization of dogs (Chai, 1995).

While the control of hydatidosis does not include the benefit of a system of immunization of the hosts, a vaccine against development of the larva in intermediate hosts is in the final stages of evaluation (Lightowlers *et al.*, 1996). This vaccine is highly effective, but marketing problems have created a roadblock to its widespread use.

With regard to individual human protection, the following are recommended: avoiding close contact with dogs that may carry the eggs of the parasite on their tongues or coats and avoiding ingestion of raw vegetables and water that may have been contaminated with the feces of infected dogs. This is particularly important in the household gardens of sheep ranches where local dogs roam and sometimes defecate.

Bibliography

Arámbulo, P., III. Public health importance of cystic echinococcosis in Latin America. *Acta Trop* 67:113–124, 1997.

Arienti, H.M., S.I. Guignard, D.E. Rinaldi, O.C. Elbarcha. Comparación de dos métodos serológicos para el diagnóstico de hidatidosis. *Bol Of Sanit Panam* 121:221–227, 1996.

Australia, Department of Health Services, Department of Agriculture. *Tasmanian Hydatid Disease Newsletter.* Nov. 1973.

Barriga, O.O., N.W. Al-Kalidi. Humoral immunity in the prepatent primary infection of dogs with *Echinococcus granulosus*. *Vet Immunol Immunopathol* 11:375–389, 1986.

Basset, D., C. Girou, I.P. Nozais, *et al.* Neotropical echinococcosis in Suriname: *Echinococcus oligarthrus* in the orbit and *Echinococcus vogeli* in the abdomen. *Am J Trop Med Hyg* 59:787–790, 1998.

Carmona, C., R. Perdomo, A. Carbo, *et al.* Risk factors associated with human cystic echinococcosis in Florida, Uruguay: Results of a mass screening study using ultrasound and serology. *Am J Trop Med Hyg* 58:599–605, 1998.

Chai, J.J. Epidemiological studies on cystic echinococcosis in China—a review. *Biomed Environ Sci* 8:122–136, 1995.

Coltorti, E., G. Cammarieri. Inmunodiagnóstico de hidatidosis: evaluación de antígenos de líquido hidatidíco y de líquido vesicular de cisticerco de *Taenia crassiceps*. *Rev Inst Med Trop Sao Paulo* 35:155–162, 1993.

Craig, P.S., L. Deshan, C.N. Macpherson, *et al.* A large focus of alveolar echinococcosis in central China. *Lancet* 340:826–831, 1992.

D'Alessandro, A. Polycystic echinococcosis in tropical America: *Echinococcus vogeli* and *E. oligarthrus*. *Acta Trop* 67:43–65, 1997.

Deplazes, P., J. Eckert. Diagnosis of the *Echinococcus multilocularis* infection in final hosts. *Appl Parasitol* 37:245–252, 1996.

Donovan, S.M., N. Mickiewicz, R.D. Meyer, C.B. Panosian. Imported echinococcosis in southern California. *Am J Trop Med Hyg* 53:668–671, 1995.

Eckert, J. [The "dangerous fox tapeworm" (*Echinococcus multilocularis*) and alveolar echinococcosis of humans in central Europe]. *Berl Munch Tierarztl Wochenschr* 109:202–210, 1996.

Economides, P., G. Christofi, M.A. Gemmell. Control of *Echinococcus granulosus* in Cyprus and comparison with other island models. *Vet Parasitol* 79:151–163, 1998.

French, C.M., G.S. Nelson. Hydatid disease in the Turkane District of Kenya. II. A study in medical geography. *Ann Trop Med Parasitol* 76:439–457, 1982.

Gasser, R.B., L. Parada, A. Acuña, *et al.* Immunological assessment of exposure to *Echinococcus granulosus* in a rural dog population in Uruguay. *Acta Trop* 58:179–185, 1994.

Gemmell, M.A. Australasian contributions to an understanding of the epidemiology and control of hydatid disease caused by *Echinococcus granulosus*—past, present and future. *Int J Parasitol* 20:431–456, 1990.

Gutierrez, R., J. Inostroza, C. Oberg, *et al.* Hidatidosis en la IX Region de Chile. Un problema y desafío regional. *Rev Med Chile* 120:311–316, 1992.

Helbig, M., P. Frosch, P. Kern, M. Frosh. Serological differentiation between cystic and alveolar echinococcosis by use of recombinant larval antigens. *J Clin Microbiol* 31:3211–3215, 1993.

Hernando, E., J.L. García Calleja, E. Córdoba, L. Lahuerta, F. del Río, V. Ferreira. Hidatidosis hepática. Revisión de una serie de 677 pacientes intervenidos quirúrgicamente. *Gastroenterol Hepatol* 19:140–145, 1996.

Hueto Pérez de Heredia, J., M. Pérez de las Casas, J. Domínguez del Valle, *et al.* Hidatidosis torácica. Nuestra experiencia en los últimos quince años. *Rev Clin Española* 199:13–17, 1999.

Jiang, C. Alveolar echinococcosis in China. *Chin Med J (Engl)* 111:470–475, 1998.

Jiménez-Mejías, M.E., E. Castillo-Ojeda, J.A. Cuello Contreras, *et al.* Hidatidosis cerebral. Análisis de una serie de 23 casos. *Med Clin Barc* 97:125–132, 1991.

Kern, P., P. Frosch, M. Helbig, *et al.* Diagnosis of *Echinococcus multilocularis* infection by reverse-transcription polymerase chain reaction. *Gastroenterology* 109:596–600, 1995.

Larrieu, E., M.T. Costa, G. Cantoni, *et al.* Control de la hidatidosis en la provincia de Río Negro, Argentina: evaluación de actividades de atención veterinaria (1). *Rev Sanid Hig Publica* 68:197–202, 1994.

Larrieu, E., R. Lamberti, J. Casaza, *et al.* Hidatidosis/equinococosis en el área de General Acha, Provincia de la Pampa, Argentina. *Bol Chil Parasitol* 51:95–97, 1996.

Lawson, J.R., M.A. Gemmell. Hydatidosis and cysticercosis: the dynamics of transmission. *Adv Parasitol* 22:261–308, 1983.

Lightowlers, M.W., S.B. Lawrence, C.G. Gauci, *et al.* Vaccination against hydatidosis using a defined recombinant antigen. *Parasite Immunol* 18:457–462, 1996.

Macpherson, C.N. An active intermediate host role for man in the life cycle of *Echinococcus granulosus* in Turkane, Kenya. *Am J Trop Med Hyg* 32:397–404, 1983.

Meneghelli, U.G., A.L. Martinelli, M.A. Llorach Velludo, A.D. Bellucci, J.E. Magro, M.L. Barbo. Polycystic hydatid disease (*Echinococcus vogeli*). Clinical, laboratory and morphological findings in nine Brazilian patients. *J Hepatol* 14:203–210, 1992.

Moro, P.L., J. McDonald, R.H. Gilman, *et al.* Epidemiology of *Echinococcus granulosus* infection in the central Peruvian Andes. *Bull World Health Organ* 75:553–561, 1997.

Navarrete, N., M.I. Jersic, R. Denis. Comparación de tres técnicas en el diagnóstico serológico de la hidatidosis humana. *Bol Chil Parasitol* 50:97–100, 1995.

Pétavy, A.F., S. Deblock. [The Auvergnan focus of alveolar echinococcosis. Research on the intermediate host, description of the lesions]. *Ann Parasitol Hum Comp* 58:439–453, 1983.

Poretti, D., E. Felleisen, F. Grimm, *et al.* Differential immunodiagnosis between cystic hydatid disease and other cross-reactive pathologies. *Am J Trop Med Hyg* 60:193–198, 1999.

Rausch, R.L., A. D'Alessandro, V.R. Rausch. Characteristics of the larval *Echinococcus vogeli* Rausch and Bernstein, 1972 in the natural intermediate host, the paca, *Cuniculus paca* L. (Rodentia: Dasyproctidae). *Am J Trop Med Hyg* 30:1043–1052, 1981.

Rinder, H., R.L. Rausch, K. Takahashi, H. Kopp, A. Thomschke, T. Loscher. Limited range of genetic variation in *Echinococcus multilocularis*. *J Parasitol* 83:1045–1050, 1997.

Romig, T., B. Bilger, U. Mackenstedt. [Current spread and epidemiology of *Echinococcus multilocularis*]. *Dtsch Tierarztl Wochenschr* 106:352–357, 1999.

Rozenzvit, M.C., L.H. Zhang, L. Kamenetzky, S.G. Canova, E.A. Guarnera, D.P. McManus. Genetic variation and epidemiology of *Echinococcus granulosus* in Argentina. *Parasitology* 118 (Pt 5):523–530, 1999.

Salinas-López, N., F. Jiménez-Guzman, A. Cruz-Reyes. Presence of *Echinococcus oligarthrus* (Diesing, 1863) Luhe, 1910 in *Lynx rufus texensis* Allen, 1895 from San Fernando, Tamaulipas state, in north-east Mexico. *Int J Parasitol* 26:793–796, 1996.

Sánchez, G.A., C. De Bernard, O.E. Sousa. Hidatidosis poliquística hepática. Informe clínico e histopatológico del segundo caso de equinococosis autóctono en la Republica de Panama. *Rev Med Panama* 17:3–11, 1992.

Schantz, P.M. Echinococcosis. *In*: Jacobs, L., P. Arámbulo III, section eds. Section C, vol. 1: *CRC Handbook Series in Zoonoses*. Boca Raton: CRC Press; 1982.

Serra Canales, I., V. García L., A. Pizarro G., A. Luzoro V., G. Cavada C., J. López C. Un método universal para corregir la subnotificación en enfermedades transmisibles. Incidencia real de la hidatidosis humana en Chile: 1985–1994. *Rev Med Chile* 127:485–492, 1999.

Shambesh, M.A., P.S. Craig, C.N. Macpherson, M.T. Rogan, A.M. Gusbi, E.F. Echtuish. An extensive ultrasound and serologic study to investigate the prevalence of human cystic echinococcosis in northern Libya. *Am Trop Med Hyg* 60:462–468, 1999.

Suwan, Z. Sonographic findings in hydatid disease of the liver: Comparison with other imaging methods. *Ann Trop Med Parasitol* 89:261–269, 1995.

Thompson, R.C., L.M. Kumaratilake. Intraspecific variation in *Echinococcus granulosus*: the Australian situation and perspectives for the future. *Trans R Soc Trop Med Hyg* 76:13–16, 1982.

Todorov, T., V. Boeva. Human echinococcosis in Bulgaria: A comparative epidemiological analysis. *Bull World Health Organ* 77:110–118, 1999.

Watson-Jones, D.L., P.S. Craig, D. Badamochir, M.T. Rogan, H. Wen, B. Hind. A pilot, serological survey for cystic echinococcosis in north-western Mongolia. *Ann Trop Med Parasitol* 91:173–177, 1997.

Wilson, J.F., R.L. Rausch. Alveolar hydatid disease. A review of clinical features of 33 indigenous cases *of Echinococcus multilocularis*. Infection in Alaskan Eskimos. *Am J Trop Med Hyg* 29:1340–1355, 1980.

Yarzábal, L.A., A. Capron. Aportes de la inmunoelectroforesis al diagnóstico inmunológico de la hidatidosis. *Torax* 20:168–174, 1971.

HYMENOLEPIASIS

ICD-10 B71.0

Etiology: The agents of this disease are the cestodes *Hymenolepis nana* and *Hymenolepis diminuta*. Divergent opinions exist among parasitologists with respect to the nomenclature of *H. nana*, which infects man as well as rodents, particularly mice. Some consider *H. nana* in mice a subspecies and assign it the name *H. nana* var. *fraterna*, and *H. nana* var. *nana* in humans; others maintain that both parasites are biological strains of a single species, physiologically adapted to particular hosts but capable of causing cross-infections. Experimental and epidemiological observations support a noteworthy host specificity in both the human and murine parasite. Although children have been infected experimentally with the parasite of rodent origin and rodents have been infected with the parasite of human origin, human infection always occurs more easily with the human cestode. From the epidemiological standpoint, most human infections with *H. nana* come from other people. In fact, there does not seem to be strong evidence of transmission of the infection from rodents to man in nature. Moreover, there is no correlation between the rates of human and rodent infection in the same region. Over the last decade, the names *H. nana* var. *fraterna* and *H. fraterna* have hardly appeared in the literature.

The cycle of *H. nana* is direct in most human infections, not requiring the intervention of an intermediate host. In these cases, man acts as both definitive and intermediate host. The adult parasite is small, very narrow, 2.5 to 4 cm long by 1 mm wide, and translucent, so it is difficult to see. The scolex has hooks (is "armed"), and the body is composed of some 200 proglottids wider than they are long. The terminal gravid proglottids contain 80 to 180 eggs each. These proglottids disintegrate in the intestine of the host, and the eggs, now infective, are carried with the feces to the external environment. When another human host ingests the embryonated eggs, the oncosphere (hexacanth embryo) is released in the upper part of the small intestine, penetrates the villi, and, in about four days, changes into a cysticercoid larva. The larva has an invaginated scolex like the cysticercus, but it is microscopic and solid, not vesicular like the cysticercus. The cysticercoid ruptures the villus, travels to the lumen of the intestine, and attaches itself to the upper ileum, where it reaches the adult phase about 30 days after infection. It then begins to release eggs, reinitiating the cycle. The size of the adult parasites is partly determined by the number of parasites coexisting in the intestine: the more parasites, the smaller is each individual. This is attributed to competition for essential nutrients and is known as the crowding effect. While the adult larva of *H. nana* lives just a few weeks, the infection can continue because the cestode is replaced with new infections or by autoinfection. Endogenous autoinfection is believed to be a common mode of re-infection for man: some of the cestode's eggs hatch inside the intestine, producing cysticercoids which give rise to new adults; the entire cycle occurs without the larva leaving the host. But the actual occurrence of autoinfection in man requires study because it does not occur in rodents (see below). When the eggs eliminated with the feces of a definitive host are eaten by the larvae of fleas or cereal or flour beetles, the cysticercoid develops in the intestine of those arthropods. These intermediate hosts continue their development with the cestode larva, which is infective for the person or rodent that eats it. *H. nana* in rodents grows especially well in mice, with more difficulty in rats, and has the same life cycle described above.

H. diminuta is a cestode of rodents, in particular rats, and, rarely, man. The adult is found in the small intestine of rats and, more rarely, mice. It has a hookless scolex (is unarmed) and approximately 1,000 proglottids, wider than they are long, and measures 20 to 60 mm long and 4 mm wide in the distal portion. The embryonated eggs are eliminated with rodent fecal matter and must be ingested by an intermediate host for the oncosphere to develop further. The principal intermediate hosts are larvae of fleas (*Nosopsyllus* and *Xenopsyllus*) and of cereal beetles (*Tribolium* and *Tenebrio*), but different coprophilic arthropods, as well as several species of coleopterans, lepidopterans, myriapods, and cockroaches can support the larva's development. The egg hatches in the intestine of these arthropods, and the oncosphere penetrates the coelomic cavity, where it changes into a cysticercoid larva. When the infected arthropod is ingested by a rodent, the cysticercoid disinvaginates its scolex, attaches to the mucosa of the small intestine, and develops into an adult cestode in about three weeks.

Geographic Distribution and Occurrence: The two species of *Hymenolepis* that infect man have worldwide distributions. The hymenolepiasis caused by *H. nana* is the most prevalent human cestodiasis in the world. In Chile, 49.6% of 2,426 intestinal cestodiases confirmed between 1961 and 1971 were caused by *H. nana*. However, its prevalence is highly variable. A random sample of reports obtained from all over the world in the last decade yielded the following findings: 24% of the infections in 315 rural children and 18% in 351 urban children examined in Zimbabwe (Mason and Patterson, 1994), 21% in 110 preschool children in Peru (Rodríguez and Calderón, 1991), 16% in 1,800 children in Egypt (Khalil *et al.*, 1991), 8.8% in 147 children in daycare centers in Botucatu, São Paulo, Brazil (Guimarães *et al.*, 1995), 8.7% in 381 apparently healthy people in Bolivia (Cancrini *et al.*, 1988), 8% in 266 rural children in Honduras (Kaminsky, 1991), 2% in 100 children in orphanages in Egypt (Makhlouf *et al.*, 1994), 2% in 146 children in a hospital in Canada (Kabani *et al.*, 1995), 0.4% in 280 samples from the general population in Nigeria (Agi, 1995), 0.4% in 219 school children in Chile (Navarrete and Torres, 1994), 0.4% in 216,275 fecal samples sent for parasitological examination in the US (Kappus *et al.*, 1991), 0.03% in 52,552 patients in a hospital in Seoul, Republic of Korea (Lee *et al.*, 1994), and 0.008% in more than 3 million fecal samples taken in Cuba between 1981 and 1995 (Suárez Hernández *et al.*, 1998).

In general, the prevalence is higher in urban than in rural environments, and in children's institutions, such as orphanages, daycare centers, boarding schools, and other schools where children are crowded together and at risk for acquiring the infection from their companions. The prevalence in rodents can also be high in certain places: in Santiago, Chile, it was found that 7.8% of 128 samples examined were infected, and in Bombay, India, that 14.5% were infected. But the correlation between the rates of murine and human infection has not been proven.

H. diminuta is a common cestode in rats, less common in mice, and infrequent in man. In the Republic of Korea, the parasite was found in 14 of 43 captured *Rattus norvegicus* (33%). Most texts indicate that about 200 cases of hymenolepiasis caused by *H. diminuta* in man have been reported worldwide. Between 1989 and 1999, six human cases were reported in the literature, one each in India, Italy, Jamaica, Spain, the US, and Yugoslavia. During that same period, one case was found in Chile in more than 70,000 fecal examinations, but prevalences of 0.3% were reported in 1,050 examinations in São Tomé and Príncipe in western Africa, and 4% in 900 examinations in Minas Gerais, Brazil.

The Disease in Man and Animals: Hymenolepiasis occurs mainly in children. The parasitosis is asymptomatic in some cases, but in others it produces clinical signs. Of 200 infected children in Egypt, 84% had symptoms; in 62% of these cases, the patient's body weight was below the third percentile (Khalil *et al.*, 1991). A study of 325 infected children in Mexico found that the most important and consistent symptoms in the children infected only by *H. nana* were abdominal pain, decreased appetite, and irritability, but weight loss, meteorism, and flatulence were also present. The symptoms varied very little with the parasite load. In cases of concomitant parasitism with *Giardia intestinalis*, one of the most common symptoms is diarrhea (Romero-Cabello *et al.*, 1991). In 250 infected children in Cuba, the major symptoms were abdominal pain, diarrhea, and anorexia (Suárez Hernández *et al.*, 1998). Anxiety, restless sleep, and anal or nasal pruritus are frequently attributed to *H. nana* infections; eosinophilia greater than 5% has been observed in about 30% of the cases. The prepatent period lasts from 2 to 4 weeks.

In human infections, *H. diminuta* appears to be less pathogenic than *H. nana*. The parasitosis does not seem to markedly affect the health of rodents. A large number of parasites may cause catarrhal enteritis.

Source of Infection and Mode of Transmission: The most important risk factors found in infected children were contamination of the environment with human feces, lack of drinking water (Kaminsky, 1991), poor environmental hygiene, and the presence of another infected person in the home (Mason and Patterson, 1994). The reservoir of *H. nana* for human infection is man himself, and transmission between humans occurs by the fecal-oral route. The infection is more common in children because of their deficient hygiene habits, particularly in overcrowded conditions, as in orphanages, boarding schools, and other schools. Autoinfection is believed to be common in man, although studies with rodents do not support this opinion (see Control). The role played by rodents in the epidemiology of the human parasitosis is not well known, but it is thought that, under natural conditions, they play a very limited role. While it has been shown experimentally that animal strains can infect man and vice versa, there is no correlation between the prevalence of human and murine infections in the same area; also, the higher risks of human infection point to infection acquired from another person (see above). Nevertheless, rodents may play a role in fecal contamination of food. Accidental ingestion of arthropods infected with cysticercoids (for example, cereal and flour beetles such as *Tenebrio* and *Tribolium*) is a possible, but probably very rare, mechanism of infection.

H. nana is transmitted among rodents by the fecal-oral route, as it is in man. Coprophagia contributes significantly to the spread of the parasitosis. Ingestion of infected arthropods is probably a more important mechanism among rodents than among human beings.

The natural reservoirs of *H. diminuta* are rodents, mainly rats. Man is infected only accidentally by ingesting insects infected with the cysticercoid, particularly insects that contaminate precooked cereals. Since the parasite's eggs are infective only for arthropods, interhuman transmission of the cestode does not occur. This explains the rarity of human infection. The parasitosis can become established in laboratory rodent colonies, which may create great difficulties in experimentation.

Diagnosis: Infection is suspected on the basis of the symptomatology and the epidemiological circumstances. Specific diagnosis is made by detecting the characteristic eggs in the feces. A single fecal examination is not conclusive and, in the event of a negative result, the examination should be repeated up to three times, with samples taken on alternate days. The eggs of *H. nana* are clear, thin-shelled, oval or round, and 38 μm to 45 μm in diameter; the embryo has small projections, with filaments, on each end. The eggs of *H. diminuta* are 60 μm to 79 μm in diameter and have no filaments. The space between the shell and the embryo is empty and resembles the white of a fried egg; the embryo resembles the yolk.

Inasmuch as fecal examination is simple and unequivocally demonstrates the presence of the parasite, there has been no interest in developing immunological diagnostic tests. However, immunological diagnoses would be possible because the study of antigens of *H. nana* and other cestodes has shown that the parasite has antigens in common with the other helminths as well as exclusive antigens (Montenegro *et al.*, 1994). In fact, Castillo *et al.* (1991) showed that the enzyme-linked immunosorbent assay (ELISA) for *H. nana* antibodies in the serum has a sensitivity of 79% and a specificity of 83%. But cross-reactions were quite common: the most frequent occurred with the sera of cysticercosis (28%) or hydatidosis (35%) patients, and the antibodies disappeared 90 days after successful treatment of the infection. ELISAs to detect *Taenia* spp. antigens in the feces (coproantigens) did not show cross-reactivity with the feces of rodents infected with certain species of murine *Hymenolepis*, including *H. diminuta*, but reacted at low dilutions with the feces of patients with *H. nana* (Allan *et al.*, 1990).

Control: Since hymenolepiasis caused by *H. nana* is basically an infection due to contamination of the environment with human feces, prevention of the infection consists of avoiding contamination of the environment and, secondarily, avoiding contact of individuals with eggs from the contaminated environment. Kosoff *et al.* (1989) showed, in Costa Rica, that the infection was significantly more prevalent in poor communities without access to sewer systems than in communities with easy access to them. Mason and Patterson (1994) studied the epidemiological characteristics of groups of patients in urban and rural areas of Zimbabwe and found that, while all indicators suggested that the infection was intrafamiliar in urban patients, the same phenomenon was not present in rural patients.

One dose of praziquantel probably cures 75% to 80% of infections. This level of efficacy, along with the fact that the parasite's eggs survive for just a short time (less than two weeks) in the external environment, indicates that treatment of infected persons would have a strong effect on preventing new infections. However, the periodic treatment of school children with effective anthelminthics has decreased the prevalence of other parasites, but has not definitively reduced the rates of infection with *H. nana* or *G. intestinalis* in the respective groups. Most *H. nana* infections are probably produced through the anus-hand-hand-mouth cycle, as occurs with *Enterobius vermicularis*, so the infective eggs remain in the external environment for a short time. Under these circumstances, consistent hand washing before eating can be of great importance. While there is no information on the role of mechanical vectors in the dissemination of *H. nana* eggs, protection of food from flies, cockroaches, and other arthropods is a good general hygiene practice. Protection of food and water for human consumption to prevent access by rodents is probably more important in the case of *H. diminuta* than in the case of *H. nana*.

Although attempts to vaccinate people at risk for *H. nana* have not been published, this seems to be a possibility, since studies in murines have shown that infection with eggs produces strong, rapid immunity against homologous infections and less rapid immunity against cysticercoid infection. That immunity prevents autoinfection in immunocompetent rodents (Ito, 1997) and raises questions about the occurrence of autoinfection in man.

Bibliography

Agi, P.I. Pattern of infection of intestinal parasites in Sagbama community of the Niger Delta, Nigeria. *W Afr J Med* 14:39–42, 1995.

Allan, J.C., G. Ávila, J. García Noval, A. Flisser, P.S. Craig. Immunodiagnosis of taeniasis by coproantigen detection. *Parasitology* 101 Pt 3:473–477, 1990.

Cancrini, G., A. Bartoloni, L. Núñez, F. Paradisi. Intestinal parasites in the Camiri, Gutierrez and Boyuibe areas, Santa Cruz Department, Bolivia. *Parasitologia* 30:263–269, 1988.

Castillo, R.M., P. Grados, C. Carcamo, et al. Effect of treatment on serum antibody to *Hymenolepis nana* detected by enzyme-linked immunosorbent assay. *J Clin Microbiol* 29:413–414, 1991.

Ferreti, O., F. Gabriele, C. Palmas. Development of human and mouse strain of *Hymenolepis nana* in mice. *Int J Parasitol* 11:425–430, 1981.

Guimarães, S., M.I. Sogayar. Occurrence of *Giardia lamblia* in children of municipal daycare centers from Botucatu, São Paulo State, Brazil. *Rev Inst Med Trop Sao Paulo* 37:501–506, 1995.

Ito, A. Basic and applied immunology in cestode infections: from *Hymenolepis* to *Taenia* and *Echinococcus*. *Int J Parasitol* 27:1203–1211, 1997.

Kabani, A., G. Cadrain, C. Trevenen, T. Jadavji, D.L. Church. Practice guidelines for ordering stool ova and parasite testing in a pediatric population. The Alberta Children's Hospital. *Am J Clin Pathol* 104:272–278, 1995.

Kaminsky, R.G. Parasitism and diarrhoea in children from two rural communities and marginal barrio in Honduras. *Trans R Soc Trop Med Hyg* 85:70–73, 1991.

Kappus, K.K., D.D. Juranek, J.M. Roberts. Results of testing for intestinal parasites by state diagnostic laboratories, United States, 1987. *Morb Mortal Wkly Rep CDC Surveill Summ* 40:25–45, 1991.

Khalil, H.M., S. el Shimi, M.A. Sarwat, A.F. Fawzy, A.O. el Sorougy. Recent study of *Hymenolepis nana* infection in Egyptian children. *J Egyp Soc Parasitol* 21:293–300, 1991.

Kosoff, P., F. Hernandez, V. Pardo, M. Visconti, M. Zimmerman. Urban helminthiasis in two socioeconomically distinct Costa Rican communities. *Rev Biol Trop* 37:181–186, 1989.

Lee, S.K., B.M. Shin, N.S. Chung, J.Y. Chai, S.H. Lee. [Second report on intestinal parasites among the patients of Seoul Paik Hospital, 1984–1992]. *Korean J Parasitol* 32:27–33, 1994.

Makhlouf, S.A., M.A. Sarwat, D.M. Mahmoud, A.A. Mohamad. Parasitic infection among children living in two orphanages in Cairo. *J Egyp Soc Parasitol* 24:137–145, 1994.

Mason, P.R., B.A. Patterson. Epidemiology of *Hymenolepis nana* infections in primary school children in urban and rural communities in Zimbabwe. *J Parasitol* 80:245–250, 1994.

Montenegro, T., R.H. Gilman, R. Castillo, et al. The diagnostic importance of species specific and cross-reactive components of *Taenia solium, Echinococcus granulosus,* and *Hymenolepis nana*. *Rev Inst Med Trop Sao Paulo* 36:327–334, 1994.

Navarrete, N., P. Torres. Prevalencia de infección por protozoos y helmintos intestinales en escolares de un sector costero de la provincia de Valdivia, Chile. *Bol Chil Parasitol* 49:79–80, 1994.

Rodríguez, J., J. Calderón. Parasitosis intestinal en pre-escolares de Tarapoto. *Rev Gastroenterol Peru* 11:153–160, 1991.

Romero-Cabello, R., L. Godínez-Hana, M. Gutiérrez-Quiroz. Aspectos clínicos de la himenolepiasis en pediatría. *Bol Med Hosp Infant Mex* 48:101–105, 1991.

Suárez Hernández, M., E. Bonet Couce, M. Díaz González, I. Ocampo Ruiz, I. Vidal García. Estudio epidemiológico de la infección por *Hymenolepis nana* en la provincia de Ciego de Ávila, Cuba. *Bol Chil Parasitol* 53:31–34, 1998.

INERMICAPSIFERIASIS

ICD-10 B71.9 Cestode infection, unspecified

Etiology: The agent of this infection is *Inermicapsifer madagascariensis* (synonyms: *Inermicapsifer cubensis* and *Inermicapsifer arvicanthidis*). The cestode is 27 cm to 42 cm long and its maximum width is 2.3 mm; it has 350 proglottids. *Inermicapsifer* is distinguished from *Raillietina* (see the chapter on Raillietiniasis) by its hookless (unarmed) scolex and sucker. The gravid segments, in which egg capsules take the place of a uterus, are longer than they are wide (in contrast to the nongravid segments, which are wider than they are long). Each gravid segment encloses 150 to 175 capsules 49 μm to 53 μm in diameter, each containing six or more eggs. Its life cycle is unknown, but by analogy to related parasites of the genus *Raillietina,* it is believed that an arthropod acts as intermediate host. Kourí *et al.* (1963) discuss this rare parasite in detail.

Geographic Distribution and Occurrence: *I. madagascariensis* is a parasite of rodents (*Arvicanthis*) in eastern Africa, where it very occasionally affects man. Outside Africa, it may be exclusively a human parasite. Human cases have been recorded in the Democratic Republic of the Congo, Kenya, Madagascar, Mauritius, Philippines, Puerto Rico, Thailand, and Venezuela. The highest number of cases (more than 100 up until 1949) has been recorded in Cuba, mainly in children 1 to 2 years old. Since 1989, two more cases have been reported in a Havana hospital (González Núñez *et al.*, 1996).

The Disease and Diagnosis: The parasitosis is generally unaccompanied by clinical symptoms. Specific diagnosis is based on microscopic examination of the proglottids. To differentiate *Inermicapsifer* from *Raillietina,* the scolex of the cestode, which may be expelled spontaneously or following treatment, must be examined.

Source of Infection and Mode of Transmission: The intermediate host is not known, but, by extension of what occurs in related genera, is probably an arthropod. The larval stage would develop in an arthropod that ingests cestode eggs deposited with the fecal matter of the definitive host (rodent or man). The cycle would be completed when the definitive host ingests an intermediate host infected with the larva. In Africa, the transmission cycle would be rodent-arthropod-rodent, and, rarely, rodent-arthropod-man. Outside the African continent, transmission would occur from human to arthropod to human.

Control: Since the life cycle of the parasite and consequently the mode of transmission are unknown, the only preventive measures that can be recommended consist of rodent control and personal and environmental hygiene.

Bibliography

Belding, D.L. *Textbook of Clinical Parasitology*, 3rd ed. New York: Appleton-Century-Crofts; 1965.

Faust, E.C., P.F. Russell, R.C. Jung. *Craig and Faust's Clinical Parasitology*, 8th ed. Philadelphia: Lea & Febiger; 1970.

González Núñez, I., M. Díaz Jidy, F. Núñez Fernández. Infección por *Inermicapsifer madagascariensis* (Davaine, 1870); Baer, 1956. Presentación de 2 casos. *Rev Cubana Med Trop* 48:224–226, 1996.

Kourí, P., J.G. Basnuevo, F. Sotolongo. *Manual de parasitología*. Tomo I: *Helmintología humana*. Havana; 1963.

MESOCESTOIDIASIS

ICD-10 B71.9 Cestode infection, unspecified

Etiology: The agents of mesocestoidiasis are the cestodes *Mesocestoides lineatus* and *Mesocestoides variabilis*. Their life cycle is not well known. The adult parasites measure 40 cm or longer and not more than 2 mm wide, with proglottids shaped like melon seeds, similar to those of *Dipylidium caninum*, but with each one having a single set of reproductive organs. The nomenclature of the genus is uncertain because there is a great deal of variation and the morphological characteristics are not well established. The definitive hosts are foxes, dogs, cats, and different species of wild carnivores. The first intermediate host may be a coprophagous arthropod that ingests the eggs of the gravid proglottids eliminated by the definitive host. Oribatid arthropods have been experimentally infected and have developed cysticercoids. The second intermediate hosts harbor a larval form known as tetrathyridium in the peritoneal or pleural cavities, liver, or lungs. The tetrathyridium is similar to a plerocercoid, thin with variable length, but the scolex has four acetabula or invaginated suckers on the thicker end, instead of the plerocercoid's two bothria (grooved suckers). Moreover, the tetrathyridium can multiply asexually in the host by dividing lengthwise. The intermediate hosts are mainly rodents, but also dogs, cats, birds, amphibians, and reptiles. Some mammals, such as cats and dogs, can harbor both the adult cestode and the tetrathyridium. When a definitive host ingests the meat of an animal infected with the larval form, the larval form develops into an adult cestode in the host's intestine in two to four weeks.

Geographic Distribution and Occurrence: *M. variabilis* occurs in Central and North America; *M. lineatus* is found in Africa, Asia, and Europe. Mesocestoidiasis is rare in man: about 20 cases have been described, including 7 in Japan, 2 in the US, 2 in Rwanda and Burundi, 1 in Greenland, and 1 in the Republic of Korea. Just two human cases have been reported since 1989: one in the Republic of Korea (Eom *et al.*, 1992) and the other in the US (Schultz *et al.*, 1992). The limited space devoted to it by textbooks on veterinary medicine notwithstanding, infection caused by adult *Mesocestoides* in carnivores, especially red foxes, seems to be common. In Malawi, *Mesocestoides* spp. was found in 34% of 120 native dogs at autopsy (Fitzsimmons, 1967). Between 1997 and 1999, *Mesocestoides* sp. was found in the intestines of 73% of 342 red foxes in Greece, 54% of 1,300 in Germany, 24% of 68 in the Netherlands, and 23% of 201 in Spain. In eight localities in Alaska, US, infection rates of 0% to

58% were found in 254 arctic foxes; in Spain, 37% of 8 lynxes were found to be infected at autopsy, as were 14% of 58 autopsied stray cats. In endemic areas, peritoneal infection caused by tetrathyridia is common in domestic animals (Crosbie *et al.*, 1998) as well as snakes and frogs. Massive infection can cause illness.

The Disease and Diagnosis: In man, the main symptoms are digestive disturbances, abdominal pain, diarrhea, and a massive discharge of small proglottids, a constant reminder to the patient that he has a foreign living being inside him (Eom *et al.*, 1992). The adult parasite does not produce symptoms in dogs and cats. Diagnosis is based on microscopic examination of the gravid proglottids. These segments are barrel-shaped, like those of *Dipylidium caninum*, but with a single set of reproductive organs, and they contain eggs with a double membrane grouped in a central, thick-walled parauterine organ. A large number of larval forms in the serous cavities can cause peritonitis and edema in cats and dogs. The clinical symptoms of the peritoneal infections in 11 dogs were recently published (Crosbie *et al.*, 1998). The animals had distended abdomens and dysuria; while lesions were not found with radiography, ultrasonography did show abnormal structures; microscopic examination of the abdominal fluid showed structures compatible with the tetrathyridium, and polymerase chain reaction confirmed the diagnosis.

Source of Infection and Mode of Transmission: Dogs, cats, and wild carnivores contract the parasitosis by eating birds, amphibians, reptiles, and small mammals infected with the tetrathyridium. Man is occasionally infected by the same mechanism when he eats the meat of insufficiently cooked intermediate hosts. In Japan, several cases were caused by eating the raw livers of snakes, to which popular belief attributes curative powers. The human case that occurred in Africa was probably due to ingestion of raw partridge meat. In the same locality, tetrathyridium infection was found in chickens, guinea fowl, and partridge; the case that occurred in the Republic of Korea was probably due to the ingestion of chicken viscera.

Control: Human infection is so infrequent that large-scale control measures are not a consideration. Individual control of human infection in endemic areas consists of not eating the raw or insufficiently cooked meat of wild animals. Tetrathyridium infections should be eradicated as quickly as possible to prevent multiplication in the tissues.

Bibliography

Crosbie, P.R., W.M. Boyce, E.G. Platzer, S.A. Nadler, C. Kerner. Diagnostic procedures and treatment of eleven dogs with peritoneal infections caused by *Mesocestoides* spp. *J Am Vet Med Assoc* 213:1578–1583, 1998.

Eom, K.S., S.H. Kim, H.J. Rim. Second case of human infection with *Mesocestoides lineatus* in Korea. *Kisaengchunghak Chapchi* 30:147–150, 1992.

Fitzsimmons, W.P. A survey of the parasites of native dogs in Southern Malawi with remarks on their medical and veterinary importance. *J Helminthol* 41:15–18, 1967.

Schultz, L.V., R.R. Roberto, G.W. Rutherford III, B. Hummert, I. Lubell. *Mesocestoides* (Cestoda) infection in a California child. *Pediatr Infect Dis J* 11:332–334, 1992.

RAILLIETINIASIS

ICD-10 B71.9 Cestode infection, unspecified

Etiology: *Raillietina celebensis* and *Raillietina demerariensis* are the main species described as agents of the disease in man. The other species of the genus *Raillietina* found in man, such as *R. asiatica*, *R. formosana*, *R. garrisoni*, *R. madagascariensis*, and *R. siriraji*, are thought to be identical to one of these two. The natural definitive hosts of *R. celebensis* are rodents, especially rats. It measures up to 40 cm in length by 2.5 mm wide, at a maximum, and has more than 500 proglottids. The suckers are not spinose, which is uncommon in this genus. The gravid proglottids contain 300 to 400 egg capsules with up to 4 eggs each. *R. demerariensis* has been found in both rodents and howling monkeys. The original specimen described in the first human case (1895, in Guyana) measured 23 cm and had 320 proglottids. The specimens mentioned most often in the literature are those recovered in 1925 in Ecuador: they measured up to 12 m and had up to 5,000 proglottids. The gravid proglottids are shaped like grains of rice; they contain 75 to 250 egg capsules with 7 to 9, and sometimes up to 12, eggs each. The length of this parasite is unusual for the genus *Raillietina*. The biological cycle of the species that affect man is not known, but the intermediate host is assumed to be an arthropod, probably an ant or beetle, as it is for other species of the genus. About 225 species of *Raillietina* parasitize birds and mammals. The intermediate hosts of the species for which the life cycle is known are beetles, flies, and ants. When these insects ingest the *Raillietina* eggs, they develop into cysticercoids in their tissues and generate new adult worms when a suitable definitive host eats the insect.

Geographic Distribution and Occurrence: *R. celebensis* has been recovered from children in southeastern Africa, Australia, Iran, Japan, Mauritius, the Philippines, Taiwan, Thailand, and the Turkestan region of Asia. Some 20 human cases have been reported in the Philippines, and 11 in Thailand. The infection is common in rodents: 54% of *Rattus norvegicus* and 9% of *Rattus rattus* in Taiwan were found to be infected, as were 5% of *R. rattus* and 7% of *Bandicota bengalensis* in Bombay, India. The situation does not seem to have changed in recent years; 37% of rats in Thailand were infected in 1997.

R. demerariensis is a neotropical species that has been found in human infections in Cuba, Ecuador, Guyana, and Honduras. *Raillietina quitensis*, *Raillietina equatoriensis*, *Raillietina leoni*, and *Raillietina luisaleoni* are considered to be synonymous with this species. The largest endemic focus is found in the parish of Tumbaco, near Quito, Ecuador, where the infection rate in school-age children varied from 4% to 12.5% during the period 1933 to 1961. The parasitosis was diagnosed in 0.14% of 8,148 children in the Children's Homes in Quito and in 0.08% of the patients in another hospital in the same city. Outside of Ecuador, human infection is very rare.

The Disease in Man: The infection occurs primarily in children. In Ecuador, the symptomatology attributed to this parasitosis consists of digestive upsets (nausea, vomiting, diarrhea, colic), nervous disorders (headaches, personality changes, convulsions), circulatory problems (tachycardia, arrhythmia, lipothymia), and general disorders (weight loss and retarded growth). Observations in the Philippines indicated that the human infection is usually asymptomatic and the parasite is expelled spontaneously by the infected individual.

Source of Infection and Mode of Transmission: Rodents are the reservoirs of the infection. By analogy with infections caused by *Raillietina* in other animal species, it is thought that man becomes infected by accidentally ingesting food contaminated with an arthropod infected with cysticercoids.

Diagnosis: Proglottids can be observed in the fecal matter; they resemble grains of rice and are frequently mistaken for such. The gravid proglottids of *R. celebensis* have 300 to 400 egg capsules, each containing 1 to 4 oval eggs measuring 99 µm by 46 µm in diameter. The gravid proglottids of *R. demerariensis* have 75 to 250 egg capsules, each with 7 to 12 subspherical eggs measuring 25 µm to 40 µm in diameter. Free capsules can be found in the feces as a result of disintegration of the proglottid. The proglottids of *Raillietina* are similar to those of *Inermicapsifer*. The two genera are easily differentiated on the basis of the scolex: the scolex of *Raillietina* has hooks, while the scolex of *Inermicapsifer* is unarmed.

Control: The human infection is so infrequent that large-scale control actions are not warranted. However, it has been shown that burning and annual treatment of fields where the cotton rat (*Sigmodon hispidus*) lives can significantly reduce the prevalence and intensity of infection with *Raillietina* sp. in rodents. Individual control measures should include hygienic handling of food, in particular, to prevent its contamination by infected insects.

Bibliography

Belding, D.L. *Textbook of Parasitology*, 3rd ed. New York: Appleton-Century-Crofts; 1965.

Boggs, J.F., S.T. McMurry, D.M. Leslie, Jr., D.M. Engle, R.L. Lochmiller. Influence of habitat modification on the community of gastrointestinal helminths of cotton rats. *J Wildl Dis* 27:584–593, 1991.

Faust, E.C., P.R. Russell. *Craig and Faust's Clinical Parasitology*, 7th ed. Philadelphia: Lea & Febiger; 1964.

Jueco, N.L. *Raillietina* infection. *In*: Jacobs, L., P. Arámbulo III, eds. Section C, Vol. 1: *CRC Handbook Series in Zoonoses*. Boca Raton: CRC Press; 1982.

León, L.A. Un foco endémico de raillietiniasis observado a través de treinta años. *Rev Medicina (México)* 44:342–348, 1964.

Namue, C., C. Wongsawad. A survey of helminth infection in rats (*Rattus* spp.) from Chiang Mai Moat. *Southeast Asian J Trop Med Public Health* 28 Suppl(1):179–183, 1997.

Niphadkar, S.M., S.R. Rao. On the occurrence of *Raillietina* (R) *celebensis* (Jericki, 1902) in rats of Bombay with special reference to its zoonotic importance. *Ind Vet J* 46:816–818, 1969.

SPARGANOSIS

ICD-10 B70.1

Synonyms: Larval diphyllobothriasis, spirometrosis, plerocercoid infection.

Etiology: The agent of this zoonosis is the second larval stage (plerocercoid or sparganum) of the pseudophyllidean cestode of the genus *Spirometra* (*Diphyllobothrium, Lueheela*). Several species of medical interest have been described: *Spirometra mansoni, Spirometra mansonoides, Spirometra erinaceieuropaei,* and *Spirometra proliferum.* But, because taxonomic recognition of plerocercoids in man is extraordinarily difficult (Rego and Schaffer, 1992), there is uncertainty as to whether these names actually correspond to different species. There has been a tendency recently to identify the parasites occurring in the Far East as *S. mansoni,* those of the Americas as *S. mansonoides,* and those of Australia as *S. erinaceieuropaei.* Studies of nucleic acids have made it possible to differentiate *S. erinacei* from *S. mansonoides* (Lee *et al.,* 1997). *S. proliferum* is a rare form of branched plerocercoid whose definitive host is unknown; it produces lateral buds and multiplies in the host's tissues. Serologically, it seems to be related to *S. erinacei* (Nakamura *et al.,* 1990). Noya *et al.* (1992) have studied its structure.

The definitive hosts of sparganum are domestic and wild canids and felids. The development cycle requires two intermediate hosts: the first is a copepod (planktonic crustacean) of the genus *Cyclops,* which ingests coracidia (free, ciliated embryos) that develop from *Spirometra* eggs when they reach the water with the feces of the definitive host. In the tissues of the copepod, the coracidium turns into the first larva, or procercoid. When a second intermediate host ingests an infected crustacean, the procercoid develops into a second larval form, the plerocercoid or sparganum. According to some researchers, the natural second intermediate hosts would be amphibians, although they may also be other vertebrates, including reptiles, birds, small mammals (rodents and insectivores), swine, nonhuman primates, and man. Fish are not satisfactory hosts for plerocercoids. Numerous species of vertebrates become infected with plerocercoids by feeding on amphibians, but they may also develop plerocercoids after ingesting water with copepods infected by procercoids. Several animal species that are not generally definitive hosts function as paratenic or transport hosts, since the larvae they acquire by feeding on animals infected with plerocercoids encyst again, after passing through the intestinal wall and migrating to other tissues, waiting for a definitive host. This transfer process is undoubtedly important in the life cycle, but the fact that many species that act as secondary hosts can be infected directly by ingestion of copepods containing procercoids is probably no less important. When the sparganum reaches the intestine of the definitive host, it attaches to the mucosa; in 10 to 30 days, it matures into an adult cestode and begins to produce eggs.

The adult parasite reaches about 25 cm in length in the intestine of the definitive hosts: cats, dogs, and wild carnivores. The sparganum varies from 4 to 10 cm long in tissues of the secondary intermediate hosts and the paratenic hosts, including man.

Geographic Distribution and Occurrence: Worldwide. Human cases have been described in Argentina, Australia, Belize, Brazil, China, Colombia, Ecuador,

Guyana, India, Japan, Malaysia, Mexico, Paraguay, Puerto Rico, the Republic of Korea, Sri Lanka, Taiwan, the US, Venezuela, and Viet Nam. But human infection is rare: probably fewer than 500 cases have been reported, mostly in Southeast Asia, China, and the Republic of Korea. Up to 1996, 62 cases had been reported in the US (Griffin et al., 1996). Approximately 30 cases have been diagnosed in Africa.

Infections caused by the adult cestode and by plerocercoid larvae are frequent in some areas. Some time ago, surveys in Japan indicated that 95% of the cats and 20% of the dogs were infected with Spirometra in some areas; a recent study of 916 dogs over eight years showed that just 0.7% were infected. In Australia, it was found that 15% of the cats were infected. In Maracay, Venezuela, about 3% of the cats were found to be infected, and in other Latin American countries, the adult parasite has been recognized in domestic animals and several wild species, such as foxes, felids, and marsupials.

Sparganosis (infection by the plerocercoid) can be found in a great variety of animal species. In some localities of Florida (US), infection with plerocercoids was found in 50% to 90% of the water snakes. On the outskirts of Brisbane, Australia, 25% of the frogs (Hyla coeruela) were found to be infected. In that country, during the period 1971–1972, 100% of the wild pigs captured and fattened for human consumption in a slaughterhouse in New South Wales were confiscated because they contained spargana. Moreover, the infection has been found in crocodile meat for human consumption. A high prevalence of sparganosis has also been found in Yugoslavia. Spargana were found in 49% of 37 Leptodactylus ocellatus frogs and in five of six Philodryas patagoniense snakes in Uruguay. In Asian countries where parasitological studies were conducted, high rates of infection were found in frogs and snakes.

The Disease in Man: The incubation period, determined in a study of 10 patients who ate raw frog meat, lasts from 20 days to 14 months (Bi et al., 1983). The localizations of the sparganum in man include the brain, spinal cord, subcutaneous tissue, breast, scrotum, urinary bladder, abdominal cavity, eye, and intestinal wall. The most common localization seems to be the subcutaneous connective tissue and superficial muscles, where the initial lesion is nodular, develops slowly, and can be found on any part of the body. The main symptom is pruritus and, sometimes, urticaria. The lesion is painful when there is inflammation. The patient may feel discomfort when the larva migrates from one location to another. In a recent clinical study of 22 cases of sparganosis in the province of Hunan, China, half the patients suffered from migratory subcutaneous nodules, which disappeared and reappeared as the sparganum migrated (Bi et al., 1983). The subcutaneous lesion resembles a lipoma, fibroma, or sebaceous cyst (Tsou and Huang, 1993). Ocular sparganosis occurs mainly in Thailand, Viet Nam, and parts of China. Its main symptoms consist of a painful edema of the eyelids, with lacrimation and pruritus. A nodule measuring 1 to 3 cm forms after three to five months, usually on the upper eyelid.

Migration of the sparganum to internal organs can give rise to the visceral form of the disease. The preferred localizations are the intestinal wall, perirenal fat, and the mesentery; vital organs are rarely affected. When the plerocercoid invades the lymphatic system, it produces a clinical picture similar to that of elephantiasis. Eosinophils are abundant in the areas near the parasite; examination of blood samples reveals mild leukocytosis and increased eosinophilia.

An infrequent but serious form is proliferative sparganosis caused by *S. proliferum*. The sparganum of *S. proliferum* is pleomorphic, with irregular branches and proliferative buds that detach from the larva and migrate to different tissues in the host, where they repeat the process and invade other organs. The life cycle of *S. proliferum* is not known. Nine confirmed and three suspected cases of this clinical form have been described: seven in Japan (Nakamura *et al.*, 1990), one in the US, and one in Venezuela; in the three suspected cases the larvae were too undifferentiated for positive identification.

The cerebral form is reported with some degree of frequency in the Republic of Korea. It is especially prevalent in inhabitants of rural areas who have eaten frogs or snakes, it is chronic, and the most common symptoms are convulsions, hemiparesis, and headache (Chang *et al.*, 1992; Kim *et al.*, 1996).

The Disease in Animals: The adult cestode, which lodges in the intestine of the definitive host, generally does not affect the health of the animal. In cats, however, it may produce weight loss, irritability, and emaciation, together with an abnormal or exaggerated appetite. Infection by the larvae or spargana can be clinically apparent when their number is large and especially when they invade vital organs. In the intermediate host, the disease is almost always asymptomatic if the number of parasites is relatively small. It has often been noted that rats infected with spargana become extremely fat. This is because the plerocercoid produces a growth factor that, while not equivalent to the mammalian growth hormone, combines with that hormone's receptors and imitates its effect (Phares, 1996).

Source of Infection and Mode of Transmission: Sparganosis is maintained in nature primarily by contamination of natural or artificial bodies of water (lagoons, marshes, lakes, and so forth) with feces from felids and canids infected with *Spirometra* spp. Contamination of water with eggs of *Spirometra* spp. leads to the infection of copepods and of the second intermediate hosts that ingest these crustaceans. An important means of infection is transfer of the second larva (sparganum, plerocercoid) from one secondary host to another, which increases the number of animal species and individuals infected. The infection is acquired through the ingestion of infected meat; various mammal and bird species become infected by feeding on parasitized frogs or snakes. The high rate of infection in wild pigs in Australia may be due to this mechanism, although it may also stem from ingesting copepods in the drinking water from lagoons. In any case, contamination of the water is assured by wild canids that share the habitat.

The infection rate in man is low compared to the rate in other animals. Man acquires sparganosis mainly by ingesting larvae contained in the raw or undercooked meat of animals infected with spargana, such as amphibians, reptiles, birds, and wild mammals. Another mode of infection, also by larval transfer, is by contact. In Thailand and Viet Nam, frogs are popularly believed to have an antiphlogistic effect, and they are applied as poultices. This custom is responsible for ocular sparganosis. It is also probable that man can acquire sparganosis via drinking water, by ingesting copepods infected with procercoids (first larvae).

Man is an accidental host and does not play a role in the life cycle of the parasite. However, under certain ecologic conditions, such as those in some regions of central Africa, it is suspected that man may act as an intermediate host in the epidemiological chain. In those regions, hyenas are the definitive hosts of *Spirometra* and man is apparently the only host infected with spargana. In these circumstances, the infection cycle is maintained as a result of a tribal custom of letting hyenas devour human corpses.

Diagnosis: Diagnosis is confirmed through the symptoms of the infection and the epidemiological history of the patient. Although magnetic resonance imaging is better than computerized tomography for the clinical study of sparganosis, neither of these techniques is diagnostic (Chang and Han, 1998). Nishiyama *et al.* (1994) showed that enzyme-linked immunosorbent assay (ELISA) serologic studies have high sensitivity and specificity for sparganosis *mansoni* in humans; however, specific diagnosis can be made only by removing the lesion and confirming the presence of the plerocercoid. Sparganum looks like a bright white ribbon with the undulating movement typical of a pseudosegmented cestode and with an invagination at the oral end. Attempts have been made to identify the species of *Spirometra* by infecting dogs and cats via the digestive route, but most of those attempts have not produced adult parasites. Diagnosis in definitive hosts infected with adult cestodes can be made by coprologic examination or autopsy.

Control: Human sparganosis can be prevented by: 1) avoiding ingestion of water contaminated with copepods that may be infected, unless it is first boiled or filtered; 2) making sure that meat that may contain spargana is sufficiently cooked; and 3) avoiding compresses, poultices, or dressings prepared with the meat of frogs, snakes, or other poikilotherms that may be infected.

Bibliography

Bi, W.T., *et al.* [A report of 22 cases of *Sparganosis mansoni* in Hunan Province]. *Chin J Pediatr* 21:355, 1983.

Chang, K.H., M.H. Han. MRI of CNS parasitic diseases. *J Magn Reson Imaging* 8:297–307, 1998.

Chang, K.H., J.G. Chi, S.Y. Cho, M.H. Han, D.H. Han, M.C. Han. Cerebral sparganosis: Analysis of 34 cases with emphasis on CT features. *Neuroradiology* 34:1–8, 1992.

Griffin, M.P., K.J. Tompkins, M.T. Ryan. Cutaneous sparganosis. *Am J Dermatopathol* 18:70–72, 1996.

Kim, D.G., S.H. Paek, K.H. Chang, *et al.* Cerebral sparganosis: Clinical manifestations, treatment, and outcome. *J Neurosurg* 85:1066–1071, 1996.

Lee, S.U., S. Huh, C.K. Phares. Genetic comparison between *Spirometra erinacei* and *S. mansonoides* using PCR-RFLP analysis. *Korean J Parasitol* 35:277–282, 1997.

Mueller, J.F., O.M. Froes, T. Fernández. On the occurrence of *Spirometra mansonoides* in South America. *J Parasitol* 61:774–775, 1975.

Nakamura, T., M. Hara, M. Matsuoka, M. Kawabata, M. Tsuji. Human proliferative sparganosis. A new Japanese case. *Am J Clin Pathol* 94:224–228, 1990.

Nishiyama, T., T. Ide, S. R. Himes, Jr., S. Ishizaka, T. Araki. Immunodiagnosis of human sparganosis *mansoni* by micro-chemiluminescence enzyme-linked immunosorbent assay. *Trans R Soc Trop Med Hyg* 88:663–665, 1994.

Noya, O., B. Alarcón de Noya, H. Arrechedera, J. Torres, C. Arguello. *Sparganum proliferum*: An overview of its structure and ultrastructure. *Int J Parasitol* 22:631–640, 1992.

Phares, K. An unusual host-parasite relationship: The growth hormone-like factor from plerocercoids of spirometrid tapeworms. *Int J Parasitol* 26:575–588, 1996.

Rego, A.A., G.V. Schaffer. Esparganose em alguns vertebrados do Brasil. Dificuldades na identificação das espécies de *Luheella* (*Spirometra*). *Mem Inst Oswaldo Cruz* 87(Suppl 1):213–216, 1992.

Tsou, M.H., T.W. Huang. Pathology of subcutaneous sparganosis: Report of two cases. *J Formos Med Assoc* 92:649–653, 1993.

TAENIASIS

ICD-10 B68.0 *Taenia solium* taeniasis;
B68.1 *Taenia saginata* taeniasis

Etiology: The cestodes *Taenia solium, T. saginata,* and *T. asiatica. T. solium* and *T. saginata* have been known as human parasites for more than 300 years (Shulman, 1982). *T. asiatica*, a species closely resembling *T. saginata*, was described as a new species in 1993 (Eom and Rim, 1993), although most authors consider *T. asiatica* to be a subspecies of *T. saginata* rather than a new species, and call it *T. saginata asiatica*. This section will use the specific name only to differentiate it from *T. saginata saginata*.

The definitive host of these taeniae is man, in whose small intestine the adult stage lodges. The natural intermediate hosts of *T. solium* are the domestic pig and the wild boar, although dogs, cats, sheep, deer, camels, monkeys, and individuals infected with the larva or cysticercus have occasionally been found (human cysticercus infection is presented in the chapter on Cysticercosis). The natural intermediate hosts of *T. saginata* are bovines of the family Bovidae and some members of the family Cervidae. The natural intermediate hosts of *T. asiatica* are domestic and wild swine (Fan *et al.*, 1990a; Fan *et al.*, 1990b).

T. solium, or swine taenia, measures 2 to 4 m in length and is made up of 800 to 1,000 proglottids or segments. The gravid proglottids detach from the strobila in groups of 5 or 6, are somewhat motile, are expelled with the feces, and contain from 30,000 to 50,000 eggs. Pigs, because of their coprophagic habits, may ingest a large number of eggs, both those contained in the proglottids and those existing free in fecal matter. The embryos (oncospheres) are released from the egg in the pig's intestine, penetrate the intestinal wall, and within 24 to 72 hours, spread via the circulatory system to different tissues and organs of the body. Complete development of the larva or cysticercus (which was called *Cysticercus cellulosae* when it was thought to be a parasite different from the adult taenia) takes place in 9 to 10 weeks. It is 8–15 by 5 by 10 mm in size, and resembles a fluid-filled bladder; it holds the invaginated scolex equipped with the suckers and hooks of the adult taenia. When a human consumes raw or undercooked pork that contains cysticerci, the larva is released from the surrounding tissue, the scolex is disinvaginated and attaches to the wall of the small intestine, usually in the jejunum, and begins to develop strobila. The first proglottids are expelled in the feces 62 to 72 days after infection. *T. solium* can survive in the human intestine for a long time; cases have been observed in which the cestode persisted for 25 years. Some authors have observed differences in the size of the hooks on the scolices of cysticerci found in humans, swine, cats, dogs, and baboons, and proposed the existence of different strains or subspecies. A multilobular cysticercus without a scolex has frequently been observed in human cysticercosis in Mexico; it has been designated *Cysticercus racemosus.* Most investigators are inclined to believe that it is a degenerative state of *T. solium* (see the chapter on Cysticercosis). The significance of *T. solium* for public health is that humans can become infected with the eggs of the taenia and develop cysticerci in their tissues.

T. saginata, or bovine taenia, is longer than *T. solium*; it is composed of 1,000 to 2,000 proglottids and is 4 to 10 m long. The gravid proglottids, which can contain more than 100,000 eggs, detach from the strobila one by one; they are motile and often exit actively through the anus. The eggs are either expelled from the proglottid or released when it disintegrates, contaminating the environment. Inside bovines, the viable eggs ingested by grazing cattle develop into cysticerci (still called *Cysticercus bovis)* in a manner similar to the eggs of *T. solium* in swine. Development takes 60 to 75 days. Cysticerci begin to degenerate in a few weeks, and after nine months, many of them are dead and calcified. Humans are infected by ingesting undercooked beef containing viable cysticerci. The adult taenia develops in the intestine in 10 to 12 weeks. Human cysticercosis caused by ingestion of *T. saginata* eggs either does not occur or is extremely rare (see the chapter on Cysticercosis). *T. saginata* eggs can survive several weeks or months in wastewater, bodies of water, or on grass, in moderate climatic conditions.

Geographic Distribution: *T. solium* and *T. saginata* are distributed worldwide. *T. solium* is much more common in developing countries, particularly in Latin America, eastern Europe, northern China, India, and eastern Africa. *T. saginata* is more universally distributed, particularly in eastern and western Africa (where both taenia coexist), North and South America, and Europe. *T. saginata* is approximately 10 times more prevalent than *T. solium. T. asiatica,* originally discovered in Taiwan, has since been identified in Ethiopia, Indonesia, Madagascar, the Republic of Korea, and Thailand (Fan *et al.,* 1990a; Fan *et al.,* 1990b).

Occurrence in Man: It was estimated in 1947 that nearly 39 million people in the world were infected by *T. saginata* and 2.5 million by *T. solium.* A 1973 estimate attributed 45 million cases to *T. saginata* and 3 million to *T. solium* (Strickland, 1991). Although the local prevalences of *T. asiatica* are known, there are no worldwide figures. Taeniases are not notifiable diseases, and the available information is based on isolated studies of specific sectors of the population, such as schoolchildren, recruits, and others. Also, since many studies of prevalence are based on the finding of eggs in feces, and the eggs of *T. solium, T. saginata,* and *T. asiatica* cannot be distinguished by conventional methods, the best-known prevalences do not establish differences among the species. A local report in Poland analyzed 736 cases of cestodiasis diagnosed in 1997: 634 were caused by *T. saginata,* 6 by *T. solium,* and 63 by *Taenia* sp. On a college campus in Chile, the 11 cases of taeniasis diagnosed at the species level between 1985 and 1994 were caused by *T. saginata.* In contrast, in Bali, Indonesia, one of every three cases of taeniasis was caused by *T. solium* and two were due to *T. saginata* (Sutisna *et al.,* 1999). *T. solium* parasites were identified in 98% of 56 cases of taeniasis in Guatemala (Allan *et al.,* 1996). The relative frequency of these species is strongly influenced by local customs. For example, *T. solium* is absent from Moslem and Jewish population groups that adhere to religious precepts prohibiting the consumption of pork.

In 216,275 fecal samples sent to state diagnostic laboratories in the US in 1987, 0.1% were found to contain *Taenia* sp. eggs (Kappus *et al.*, 1991). Based on these findings, any prevalence exceeding 1% in the general population should probably be considered very high. Hinz (1991) estimated that there were 900,000 infections in Germany, for a prevalence of 1.5%. Recent reports on high prevalence indicated a 12.4% infection rate in 1,008 people in a hamlet in Laos (Giboda *et al.*, 1991); 10.4% in 300 children in Sudan (Karrar and Rahim, 1995); 8.1% in the residents of 19 Ethiopian communities (Birrie *et al.*, 1994); and 2.9% in 171 adults in the general population of Thailand (Supanaranond *et al.*, 1990). The countries that historically have the highest prevalences of *T. saginata* (10% of the population) are Ethiopia, Kenya, and the Democratic Republic of the Congo. The endemic areas are the Caucasus region, the former Soviet republics in south and central Asia, and certain countries on the Mediterranean, such as Lebanon, Syria, and the former Yugoslavia. Up to 65% of the children were found to be infected in parts of the former Yugoslavia. South America, southwestern Asia, Europe, and Japan have moderate prevalences, while Australia, Canada, the US, and some countries in the western Pacific have low prevalences.

Infection by *T. solium* is endemic in southern Africa (especially among the Bantu), Latin America, and the non-Islamic countries of Southeast Asia. Little information is available on the prevalence of taeniasis in the Americas. Some studies recorded the following rates of infection by *T. saginata*: 0.6% in Argentina, 1%–2% in Brazil, 1.6% in Chile, 0.1% in Cuba, and 1.7% in Guatemala.

The prevalence of *T. asiatica* seems to be very high in the endemic areas. Fan (1997) reported a prevalence of 11% in the mountainous zones of Taiwan, 6% on Cheju Island in the Republic of Korea, and 21% on Samosir Island in Indonesia. But the natives of these areas engage in food and hygiene practices that greatly encourage the spread of parasites between man and swine (Depary and Kossman, 1991).

Occurrence in Animals: Animals are resistant to infection with the adult parasites. Animal cysticercosis is discussed in the chapter on Cysticercosis.

The Disease in Man: Taeniasis by *T. saginata* is often subclinical and is only revealed by fecal examination or when the infected person consults a physician after feeling the crawling movement of the proglottids in the anal region. In clinical cases, the most common symptomatology consists of abdominal pain, nausea, debility, weight loss, flatulence, and diarrhea or constipation. While a patient may have one or several of these symptoms, experience in Chile showed that only about a third of patients have any of these symptoms before becoming aware of the infection. The gravid proglottids of *T. saginata* sometimes travel to different organs (appendix, uterus, bile ducts, nasopharyngeal passages), causing disorders related to the site in which they settle. In rare cases, there may be intestinal obstruction and even perforation of the colon (Demiriz *et al.*, 1995). A high percentage of patients experience a decrease in gastric secretion. Individual reactions to the infection differ and may be influenced by psychogenic factors, since patients often notice symptoms only after they see the proglottids (Pawlowski, 1983).

Taeniasis caused by *T. solium* is more rarely clinically apparent than that caused by *T. saginata* and is usually benign and mild, possibly because its proglottids are less active and, therefore, less noticeable to the patient. In addition, complications such as appendicitis and cholangitis have not been recorded.

In a survey of 1,661 patients with *T. asiatica* in Taiwan, Fan *et al.* (1992) found that 78% had signs or symptoms. The most common signs were movement of proglottids (95% of patients), going on for years in some of them; anal pruritus in 77%; nausea in 46%; abdominal pain in 45%; dizziness in 42%; increased appetite in 42%; and headache in 26%.

Source of Infection and Mode of Transmission: In contrast to their role in other zoonotic infections, humans constitute an essential link in the epidemiology of taeniasis. Humans are the exclusive definitive host of the three species of *Taenia*; their feces contaminate cow pastures and areas where home-bred swine may eat. Taeniae can live for many years in the human small intestine, and can eliminate hundreds of thousands of eggs in a single day in the gravid proglottids. Consequently, the contamination can be extensive and intense. Sometimes, just one human carrier of *T. saginata* defecating in the grain silos or water reservoirs can infect several hundred cattle in a feedlot. Epizootic outbreaks of the cysticercosis caused by *T. saginata* have been described in Canada, the former Czechoslovakia, and the US. Survival of the eggs in pastures depends on the ambient temperature and humidity; in summer, *T. saginata* can survive for about two months in the environmental conditions found in Europe, while they may survive more than five months in winter. In the highlands of Kenya, eggs of *T. saginata* have been found to remain viable for up to a year. *T. solium* eggs seem to be a little less resistant to environmental factors.

In developing countries, where peasants on poor farms or large ranches often defecate in open fields, both swine and cattle have access to taenia eggs. The use of sewer water for irrigation or of contaminated water from rivers or other sources for watering animals contributes to the spread of cysticercosis. Another factor that has acted to raise the incidence of taeniasis in recent years is the increasing use of detergents that impede the natural destruction of the parasite's eggs in sewer systems. Taenia eggs can be carried several kilometers by river water, and they may be transported over long distances by gulls and other birds. An important role in the dissemination of taeniae eggs is also attributed to coprophagous insects. The cysticerci of *T. saginata* remain viable in live cattle for nine months, and in the tissues of the dead animal for two weeks; those of *T. solium* survive for several years in living swine, and nearly 60% remain viable if the carcass is stored at 4°C for 26 to 30 days (Fan *et al.*, 1998).

The distribution and prevalence rates of the human taeniases vary considerably in different geographic areas of the world. Several socioeconomic and cultural factors influence transmission. Taeniasis caused by *T. solium* is much more prevalent in the developing countries than in the industrialized ones. Taeniasis caused by *T. saginata* is prevalent in both developing and developed countries. It has been said that, while taeniasis caused by *T. solium* is especially prevalent in poor populations, taeniasis caused by *T. saginata* is "prevalent in wealthy nations because of their wealth and in the poor nations because of their poverty." Humans acquire *T. solium* taeniasis by eating raw or undercooked pork infected with cysticerci. The infection has almost disappeared from the more industrialized countries, where modern intensive swine-raising practices do not permit access to human feces. In developing countries, on the other hand, the breeding of small numbers of swine by households is still a common activity among impoverished rural inhabitants. Moreover, since this population group often does not have the benefit of drinking water and sewer systems, the swine have a much higher risk of infection by human feces. Finally, a high percentage of these swine are slaughtered at home for household or local consumption and, therefore, the animals are not subject to veterinary inspection.

In contrast, humans acquire *T. saginata* taeniasis by eating raw or undercooked beef infected with cysticerci. Human infection is closely related to the habit of eating dishes prepared with raw beef or beef cut into thick pieces that are not thoroughly cooked. The infection can also be contracted by tasting meat dishes during their preparation, before the meat is completely cooked. The risk of contracting the infection is five times greater in a family in which there is a carrier of *T. saginata*, which demonstrates the importance of the food handler in transmission of the disease. The risk is 14 times greater among workers involved in processing and marketing raw meat, probably due to their access to meat that is not subject to veterinary inspection or that is discarded during inspection. *T. saginata* taeniasis is widespread among the upper classes because beef costs more than pork and, therefore, is consumed more by the well-to-do, particularly in thick, undercooked portions (with the center still pink) or in sophisticated dishes intended to be eaten raw. However, as far as the poorer classes are concerned, the systems for supplying potable water, excreta removal, and veterinary inspection of slaughterhouses are often deficient, which facilitates the infection of cattle and, subsequently, of man. Man becomes infected with *T. asiatica* by eating the undercooked livers of infected swine.

There is some question about whether man can contract cysticercosis through regurgitation of distal portions of a *T. solium* from his own intestine, followed by activation of the eggs by his own gastric juices. While the majority of authors used to believe that the regurgitation of gravid proglottids from the jejunum or the ileum would be most unusual, the discovery of the oral expulsion of a *T. saginata* in a patient (Gupta *et al.*, 1997) requires another look at that opinion.

Diagnosis: *T. saginata* proglottids crawl the length of the intestine in order to exit, and *T. solium* proglottids adhere to the fecal matter. Thus, there is little opportunity for the eggs to be released in the intestine; parasite eggs are found in the feces of just one quarter of patients. Moreover, the various species of the genus *Taenia* cannot be distinguished by microscopic examination of the eggs. This is a major disadvantage because *T. solium* eggs pose a clear risk of cysticercosis to humans. For these reasons, diagnosis of human intestinal taeniasis is generally made by identifying gravid proglottids in the feces. In the case of infection by *T. saginata*, anal swabs should be used rather than direct examination of fecal samples. Proglottids are not eliminated on a daily basis, so the examination must be repeated if results are negative. Differential diagnosis between *T. saginata* and *T. solium* is based on the number of primary lateral branches of the uterus of the gravid proglottids, 16 to 30 in the former species and 7 to 12 in the latter. Differentiation of proglottids with 12 to 16 primary branches is unreliable. When the scolices are expelled (spontaneously or because of treatment), *T. saginata* can be identified by microscopy, since its scolex lacks hooks, but that of *T. solium* has them. Although *Taenia* spp. eggs are indistinguishable by conventional microscopy, techniques have been developed that differentiate the eggs of *T. solium* from those of *T. saginata* and other cestodes by the enzyme-linked immunosorbent assay (ELISA) (Montenegro *et al.*, 1996) and those of *T. saginata* with the polymerase chain reaction (Gottstein *et al.*, 1991). An ELISA that uses patients' feces to reveal *T. solium* coproantigens has also been developed (Allan *et al.*, 1996). This test is 2.5 times more sensitive than microscopic examination. A survey of 475 persons in a community endemic for *T. solium* in Mexico found no infection using parasitological methods but found 10 by looking for the coproantigen; 7 of these were confirmed by the subsequent discovery of proglottids (Rodríguez-Canul *et al.*, 1999).

Control: Human taeniases are not just a threat to public health, but also a factor in economic loss. According to estimates by Fan (1997), taenia infections resulted in an annual loss of US$ 11,327,423 in the mountainous areas of Taiwan, US$ 13,641,021 on Cheju Island in the Republic of Korea, and US$ 2,425,500 on Samosir Island in Indonesia. Almost all actions to control this zoonosis are based on appropriate health education of the at-risk population. Barriga (1997) proposes several control measures that consist of interrupting the epidemiological chain of the parasite at any of the following points of intervention:

1. The production of eggs and the consequent contamination of the environment. These are prevented by early diagnosis and effective treatment of infected persons, since man is the only definitive host. In the former Soviet Union, rates of *T. saginata* infection were reduced through health education of the public and the mass treatment of the population in endemic areas: between 1964 and 1972, the rate of infected bovines fell from 1.09% to 0.38%.

2. Dispersion of the eggs in the environment. This is prevented through an appropriate excreta disposal system, consisting not just of a traditional sewer system, but also well-built and utilized septic tanks and education of the population in their proper use. Unfortunately, the economic and cultural conditions of the rural populations in developing countries often preclude these actions. Also, traditional sewer systems can decrease the viability of taenia eggs up to approximately 8%, but the final solids can still contain significant numbers of viable eggs (Barbier *et al.*, 1990).

3. Ingestion of eggs by the natural intermediate host. This is avoided by preventing breeding swine and bovines access to food or drink contaminated with human feces. This is the rule on modern, large farms. However, poor peasants customarily breed a few swine for their own consumption or sale on the local market and, because of ignorance or lack of the means to implement hygienic breeding standards, the animals have easy access to places that have been contaminated with human feces, and they acquire cysticercosis.

4. Development of the cysticercus in the intermediate host. This can be prevented by treating the animals—which is too expensive, insufficiently effective, and not preventive of subsequent infections—or by vaccination. Studies of vaccination of the intermediate hosts of cestodiasis are very far advanced; in the case of bovine cysticercosis, there are just a few practical marketing problems to be resolved before its routine use can be initiated (Lightowlers, 1996). Attempts to vaccinate against porcine cysticercosis in Peru fared less well (Evans *et al.*, 1997).

5. The dissemination of cysticerci to the definitive host. This can be prevented by good veterinary inspection in slaughterhouses and educating the population against avoidance of inspection. Household slaughtering of swine and the consumption of pork that has not been subject to veterinary inspection is still very prevalent in eco-

nomically depressed agricultural communities and plays a large part in sustaining the human intestinal infection.

6. Personal human protection. This entails cooking pork and beef well to kill any cysticerci, and taking food hygiene measures such as washing food and washing the hands before eating to avoid ingesting *T. solium* eggs.

Bibliography

Allan, J.C., M. Velásquez-Tohom, R. Torres-Álvarez, P. Yurrita, J. García-Noval. Field trial of the coproantigen-based diagnosis of *Taenia solium* taeniasis by enzyme-linked immunosorbent assay. *Am J Trop Med Hyg* 54(4):352–356, 1996.

Barbier, D., D. Perrine, C. Duhamel, R. Doublet, P. Georges. Parasitic hazard with sewage sludge applied to land. *Appl Environ Microbiol* 56(5):1420–1422, 1990.

Barriga, O.O. *Veterinary Parasitology for Practitioners,* 2nd ed. Edina: Burgess International Group; 1997.

Birrie, H., B. Erko, S. Tedla. Intestinal helminthic infections in the southern Rift Valley of Ethiopia with special reference to schistosomiasis. *East Afr Med J* 71(7):447–452, 1994.

Demiriz, M., O. Gunhan, B. Celasun, E. Aydin, R. Finci. Colonic perforation caused by taeniasis. *Trop Geogr Med* 47(4):180–182, 1995.

Depary, A.A., M.L. Kosman. Taeniasis in Indonesia with special reference to Samosir Island, north Sumatra. *Southeast Asian J Trop Med Public Health* 22 Suppl:239–241, 1991.

Eom, K.S., H.J. Rim. Experimental human infection with *Asian Taenia saginata* metacestodes obtained from naturally infected Korean domestic pigs. *Kisaengchunghak Chapchi* 30(1):21–24, 1992.

Eom, K.S., H.J. Rim. Morphologic descriptions of *Taenia asiatica* sp. n. *Korean J Parasitol* 31(1):1–6, 1993.

Evans, C.A., A.E. González, R.H. Gilman, *et al.* Immunotherapy for porcine cysticercosis: Implications for prevention of human disease. Cysticercosis Working Group in Peru. *Am J Trop Med Hyg* 56(1):33–37, 1997.

Fall, E.H., S. Geerts, V. Kumar, T. Vervoort, R. De Deken, K.S. Eom. Failure of experimental infection of baboons (*Papio hamadryas*) with the eggs of Asian *Taenia*. *J Helminthol* 69(4):367–368, 1995.

Fan, P.C. Annual economic loss caused by *Taenia saginata asiatica* taeniasis in three endemic areas of East Asia. *Southeast Asian J Trop Med Public Health* 28 Suppl 1:217–221, 1997.

Fan, P.C., W.C. Chung, C.Y. Lin, C.C. Wu. Experimental infection of Thailand *Taenia* (Chiengmai strain) in domestic animals. *Int J Parasitol* 20(1):121–123, 1990a.

Fan, P.C., W.C. Chung, C.T. Lo, C.Y. Lin. The pig as an experimental host of Taenia saginata (Ethiopia and Madagascar strains). *Ann Trop Med Parasitol* 84(1):93–95, 1990b.

Fan, P.C., W.C. Chung, C.Y. Lin, C.H. Chan. Clinical manifestations of taeniasis in Taiwan aborigines. *J Helminthol* 66(2):118–123, 1992.

Fan, P.C., C.Y. Lin, C.C. Chen, W.C. Chung. Morphological description of *Taenia saginata* asiatica (Cyclophyllidea: Taeniidae) from man in Asia. *J Helminthol* 69(4):299–303, 1995.

Fan, P.C., Y.X. Ma, C.H. Kuo, W.C. Chung. Survival of *Taenia solium* cysticerci in carcasses of pigs kept at 4°C. *J Parasitol* 84(1):174–175, 1998.

Gemmell, M., Z. Matyas, Z. Pawlowski, *et al.*, eds. *Guidelines for Surveillance, Prevention and Control of Taeniasis/Cysticercosis.* Geneva: World Health Organization; 1983. (VPH/83.49).

Giboda, M., O. Ditrich, T. Scholz, T. Viengsay, S. Bouaphanh. Current status of food-borne parasitic zoonoses in Laos. *Southeast Asian J Trop Med Public Health* 22 Suppl:56–61, 1991.

Gottstein, B., P. Deplazes, I. Tanner, J.S. Skaggs. Diagnostic identification of *Taenia saginata* with the polymerase chain reaction. *Trans R Soc Trop Med Hyg* 85(2):248–249, 1991.

Gupta, R.L., V. Agrawal, S. Kumar, Monika. Oral expulsion of *Taenia saginata*. *Indian J Gastroenterol* 16(2):70–71, 1997.

Hinz, E. Current status of food-borne parasitic zoonoses in West Germany. *Southeast Asian J Trop Med Public Health* 22 Suppl:78–84, 1991.

Kappus, K.K., D.D. Juranek, J.M. Roberts. Results of testing for intestinal parasites by state diagnostic laboratories, United States, 1987. *Morb Mortal Wkly Rep CDC Surveill Summ* 40(4):25–45, 1991.

Karrar, Z.A., F.A. Rahim. Prevalence and risk factors of parasitic infections among under-five Sudanese children: A community based study. *East Afr Med J* 72(2):103–109, 1995.

Lightowlers, M.W. Vaccination against cestode parasites. *Int J Parasitol* 26(8-9):819–824, 1996.

Montenegro, T.C., E.A. Miranda, R. Gilman. Production of monoclonal antibodies for the identification of the eggs of *Taenia solium*. *Ann Trop Med Parasitol* 90(2):145–155, 1996.

Pawlowski, Z.S. Clinical expression of *Taenia saginata* infection in man. *In*: Prokopic, J.E., ed. *The First International Symposium of Human Taeniasis and Cattle Cysticercosis; 20-24 September 1982, Ceske Budejovice. Proceedings*. Prague: Academia; 1983.

Rodríguez-Canul, R., A. Fraser, J.C. Allan, *et al.* Epidemiological study of Taenia solium taeniasis/cysticercosis in a rural village in Yucatan state, Mexico. *Ann Trop Med Parasitol* 93(1):57–67, 1999.

Shulman, Y.S. Biology and taxonomy of *Taenia saginata* and *Taenia solium*. *In*: Lysenko, A., ed. Vol. 2: *Zoonoses Control*. Moscow: Centre of International Projects OKNT; 1982.

Strickland, G.T., ed. *Hunter's Tropical Medicine*, 7th ed. Philadelphia: Saunders; 1991.

Supanaranond, W., S. Migasena, P. Pitisuttitham, P. Suntharasamai. Health status of Thai volunteers in a cholera vaccine trial. *J Med Assoc Thai* 73(10):548–551, 1990.

Sutisna, I.P., A. Fraser, I.N. Kapti, *et al.* Community prevalence study of taeniasis and cysticercosis in Bali, Indonesia. *Trop Med Int Health* 4(4):288–294, 1999.

3. Acanthocephaliases and Nematodiases

ACANTHOCEPHALIASIS

ICD-10 B83.8 Other specified helminthiases

Synonym: Macracanthorhynchosis.

Etiology: The agents of this disease are the acanthocephalans, or thorn-headed helminths *Macracanthorhynchus hirudinaceus* (synonyms *Gigantorhynchus hirudinaceus, G. gigas, Echinorhynchus gigas*), *Moniliformis moniliformis, Acanthocephalus rauschi, A. bufonis (A. sinensis), Corynosoma strumosum,* and *Bolbosoma* sp. The first two are rare in man and the others are uncommon.

The definitive hosts of *M. hirudinaceus* are swine, wild boars, and, occasionally, bovines, rodents, dogs, monkeys, or man, in whose small intestine the parasite lives. The parasites are milky white or slightly pink, cylindrical, and somewhat flattened; females measure 35 cm or more in length by 4–10 mm in width, and males are about 10 cm long by 3–5 mm wide. On the surface, they resemble a wrinkled ascarid, but are easily distinguished from it because acanthocephalans have a retractile oral proboscis with five or six rows of curved spines. The eggs are ovoid and about 70–110 μm long; they are already embryonated when expelled with the feces of the definitive host. To continue their development, the eggs must be ingested by a beetle, usually a dung beetle of the family Scarabaeidae. Once inside these intermediate hosts, the eggs hatch in the midgut and the freed larvae penetrate the body cavity of the insect, where they continue their development and encyst. When a swine or another definitive host (peccary, squirrel, muskrat, or man) ingests a parasitized coleopteran, the larva sheds its cystic envelope and, after two to three months, reaches maturity and begins oviposition. A female can produce more than 250,000 eggs per day for approximately 10 months. The eggs are very resistant to environmental factors and can survive in the soil for several years.

Definitive hosts of *M. moniliformis* are several species of rats and other small rodents. Intermediate hosts are beetles and cockroaches. The vertebrate hosts of *Corynosoma strumosum* are the arctic fox (*Alopex lagopus*), dog, sea otter (*Enhydra lutris*), and several species of cetaceans and pinnipeds. The intermediate host is probably an amphipod crustacean (*Pontoporeia affinis*). Many species of fish serve as paratenic hosts. The intermediate hosts of *Acanthocephalus* are crustaceans. *Bolbosoma* is a parasite of cetaceans whose juvenile state has been found in fish.

Geographic Distribution and Occurrence: *M. hirudinaceus* is found in swine throughout much of the world; western Europe seems to be free of the infection. In some areas, the infection is common in swine and can reach high rates: in Belarus, 17% to 32% of the herds were found to be infected, and prevalence rates ranged from 0.9% to 5%, and occasionally up to 23% (Soulsby, 1982). Prevalence rates in China varied from 3% to 7.4% in one province, and from 50% to 60% in another (Leng *et al.*, 1983). Human infection was said to be common during the last century in the region of the Volga in the former Soviet Union, owing to the consumption of raw *Melolontha* beetles; however, other studies have not confirmed human cases (Leng *et al.*, 1983), with the exception of one case of a 5-year-old child recorded in 1958 (Faust *et al.*, 1974). Radomyos *et al.* (1989) reported on the ninth known human case in Thailand; isolated cases have also been described in Brazil, Bulgaria, the former Czechoslovakia, and Madagascar. Since 1970, human infection has necessitated emergency surgery on children in three provinces in northern China and one in southern China. A study of hospital records demonstrated that in Liaoning province, more than 200 surgical interventions were required for intestinal perforations, and that 115 cases of abdominal colic caused by macracanthorhynchosis were treated in another hospital (Leng *et al.*, 1983).

Isolated cases of human infection by *M. moniliformis* have been described in Israel, Italy, Indonesia (island of Java), and Sudan. In 1989, the first autochthonous case in the US was reported, in a 15-month-old child (Neafie and Marty, 1993). In Nigeria, a case of *M. moniliformis* was reported in a man (Ikeh *et al.*, 1992), and the infection was found to affect 39% of rats (*Rattus rattus*) (Mafiana *et al.*, 1997). A case of human infection by *Acanthocephalus bufonis* was described in Indonesia, one by *Corynosoma strumosum* in Alaska, US, and one by *A. rauschi,* also in Alaska (Schmidt, 1971). Prociv *et al.* (1990) reported two cases of unidentified acanthocephalans in two children from Australia.

The Disease in Man: The pathologic effect and symptomatology of the human infection have not been well studied. The case histories recorded in China, which are the most numerous, refer to extreme cases with acute abdominal colic and perforation of the intestine. The two most recent cases in children required resection of a part of the jejunum, which had multiple perforations (Leng *et al.*, 1983). In an experimental autoinfection by *M. moniliformis,* a researcher experienced acute gastrointestinal pain, diarrhea, somnolence, and general debility. The patient reported on by Ikeh *et al.* (1992) complained of weakness, occasional dizziness, and an intermittent burning sensation in the area of the navel. Other cases have been asymptomatic.

The Disease in Animals: *M. hirudinaceus* attaches with its proboscis to the wall of the swine's jejunum, duodenum, and ileum. The parasite produces an inflammatory reaction that can progress to necrosis and the formation of small, sometimes caseous nodules. Clinical manifestations depend on the intensity of infection, the degree of penetration of the parasite into the intestinal wall, and, especially, the presence of a secondary bacterial infection. The most severe cases are due to perforation of the intestine, leading to peritonitis and death. Generally, clinical symptoms are not apparent. In mink, which are accidental hosts, *C. strumosum* has caused bloody diarrhea and anemia.

Source of Infection and Mode of Transmission: The development of the parasite requires an intermediate host. Although swine and wild boars are the reservoirs and main hosts of *M. hirudinaceus*, the species specificity of the parasite is not strict and it can infect more than 12 different species of vertebrates, including man (De Giusti, 1971). Swine are infected by ingesting scarabaeid coleopterans, which serve as intermediate hosts. In China, besides these scarabaeids, members of the family Carambycidae were found infected with the larvae of the last immature stage of the acanthocephalus (cystacanth) (Leng *et al.,* 1983). Man becomes infected in a manner similar to swine, by accidental or deliberate ingestion of coleopterans. Most infections occur in children from rural areas, who catch beetles for play, and sometimes eat them lightly toasted but insufficiently cooked to kill the larvae. In southern China, some peasants believe that coleopterans are effective against nocturia and administer them to children for that reason.

Diagnosis: Diagnosis can be made by confirming the presence in the feces of thick-shelled eggs containing the first larval stage (acanthor). The eggs are easier to see after centrifugal concentration. The adult parasite can be examined after the patient is treated with piperazine citrate and expels it. In many cases, diagnosis is made after emergency surgery.

Control: Human infection can be prevented by avoiding the ingestion of coleopterans. To control the parasitosis in swine, the animals should be kept under hygienic conditions and provided with abundant food to discourage rooting and ingestion of coleopterans.

Bibliography

De Giusti, D.L. Acantocephala. *In:* Davis, J.W., R.C. Anderson. *Parasitic Diseases of Wild Mammals.* Ames: Iowa State University Press; 1971.

Faust, E.C, P.F. Russell, R.C. Jung. *Craig and Faust's Clinical Parasitology,* 8th ed. Philadelphia: Lea & Febiger; 1970.

Ikeh, E.I., J.C. Anosike, E. Okon. Acanthocephalan infection in man in northern Nigeria. *J Helminthol* 66(3):241–242, 1992.

Leng, Y.J., W.D. Huang, P.N. Liang. Human infection with *Macracanthorhynchus hirudinaceus* Travassos, 1916 in Guangdong Province, with notes on its prevalence in China. *Ann Trop Med Parasitol* 77(1):107–109, 1983.

Mafiana, C.F., M.B. Osho, S. Sam-Wobo. Gastrointestinal helminth parasites of the black rat (*Rattus rattus*) in Abeokuta, southwest Nigeria. *J Helminthol* 71(3):217–220, 1997.

Neafie, R.C., A.M. Marty. Unusual infections in humans. *Clin Microbiol Rev* 6(1):34–56, 1993.

Prociv, P., J. Walker, L.J. Crompton, S.G. Tristram. First record of human acanthocephalan infections in Australia. *Med J Aust* 152(4):215–216, 1990.

Radomyos, P., A. Chobchuanchom, A. Tungtrongchitr. Intestinal perforation due to *Macracanthorhynchus hirudinaceus* infection in Thailand. *Trop Med Parasitol* 40(4):476–477, 1989.

Soulsby, E.J.L. *Helminths, Arthropods and Protozoa of Domesticated Animals,* 7th ed. Philadelphia: Lea & Febiger; 1982.

Schmidt, G.D. Acanthocephalan infections of man, with two new records. *J Parasitol* 57(3):582–584, 1971.

ANGIOSTRONGYLIASIS

ICD-10 B81.3 Intestinal angiostrongyliasis;
B83.2 Angiostrongyliasis (*Parastrongylus cantonensis*)

Synonyms: Angiostrongylosis, eosinophilic meningitis, eosinophilic meningoencephalitis (*A. cantonensis*), abdominal angiostrongylosis (*A. costaricensis*).

Etiology: The agents of this disease are the metastrongylid nematodes *Angiostrongylus (Morerastrongylus) costaricensis*, *A. cantonensis*, and *A. malaysiensis*. Some authors prefer to place them in the genus *Parastrongylus*. The first of these nematodes was recognized as a parasite of man in Taiwan in 1944; the second was described in Costa Rica in 1971, although the human disease had been known since 1952; the third was identified in Japan in 1990 and was subsequently diagnosed in aborigines in Malaysia. The first species is responsible for abdominal angiostrongyliasis; the second for eosinophilic meningitis or meningoencephalitis; and the third, *A. malaysiensis*, has not been associated with any pathological picture. The definitive hosts of all three species are rodents; man is an accidental host. All three require mollusks as intermediate hosts.

A. costaricensis is a filiform nematode measuring 14–35 mm long by 0.3 mm in diameter which lives in the mesenteric arteries (and their arterioles) of the cecum of the cotton rat (*Sigmodon hispidus*). Some 12 other rat species have been found to be infected; coatis (*Nasua arica*), monkeys (*Saguinus mystax*), and dogs can be experimentally infected. The female lays eggs in those arteries; the eggs are then carried by the bloodstream and form emboli in the arterioles and capillaries of the intestinal wall. The eggs mature and form a first-stage larva which hatches, penetrates the intestinal wall to the lumen, and is carried with the fecal matter to the exterior, where it begins to appear around the twenty-fourth day of the prepatent period of the infection. In order to continue their development, the first-stage larvae have to actively penetrate the foot of a slug of the family Veronicellidae (particularly *Vaginulus plebeius*) or be ingested by it. In Brazil, four species of Veronicellidae slug were found to be infected: *Phyllocaulis variegatus*, *Bradybaena similaris*, *Belocaulus angustipes*, and *Phyllocaulis soleiformis* (Rambo *et al.*, 1997). In the slug, the larvae mature and change successively into second- and third-stage larvae in approximately 18 days. The third-stage larva, which is infective for the definitive host, is eliminated with the slug's mucous or slime, and contaminates the soil and plants around it (Mojon, 1994). When the definitive host ingests the infective larva in the free state or inside the mollusk, the larva migrates to the ileocecal region, penetrates the intestinal wall, and invades the lymphatic vessels. In this location the larvae undergo two molts before migrating to their final habitat: the mesenteric arteries of the cecal region. The parasite can complete the life cycle in man, an accidental host, reaching sexual maturity and producing eggs, but the eggs usually degenerate, causing a granulomatous reaction in the intestinal wall of the host.

A. cantonensis is a small, thin nematode, 17–25 mm long and 0.3 mm in diameter, that lives in the pulmonary arteries of rodents of the genera *Rattus* and *Bandicota*. The intermediate hosts are various species of land, amphibian, or aquatic gastropods, e.g., *Vaginulus, Laevicaulis, Achatina*, and *Bradybaena*. Five species of *Oncomelania* snails have been experimentally infected. The development cycle is similar to that of *A. costaricensis*. The definitive hosts can become infected by ingesting the infective third-stage larvae, either with infected mollusks or with plants or water contaminated with the larvae that abandon the mollusk. In addition, infection can occur as a result of consuming transfer hosts (paratenic hosts), such as crustaceans, fish, amphibians, and reptiles, which in turn have eaten infected mollusks or free larvae. When a definitive host ingests an infected mollusk or infective larvae, the larvae penetrate the intestine and are carried by the bloodstream to the brain, where they undergo two additional changes to become juvenile parasites 2 mm long. From the cerebral parenchyma, they migrate to the surface of the organ, where they remain for a time in the subarachnoid space and later migrate to the pulmonary arteries, where they reach sexual maturity and begin oviposition. The eggs hatch in the pulmonary arterioles or their branches, releasing the first-stage larva, which penetrates the pulmonary alveoli and migrates through the airways to the pharynx; there it is swallowed and is eliminated with the feces starting six weeks after infection. In man, who is an accidental host, the larvae and young adults of *A. cantonensis* generally die in the brain, meninges, or medulla oblongata. The nematode can occasionally be found in the eyes and, more rarely, the lungs. Snails or slugs, which are the intermediate hosts, become infected when they ingest the feces of infected rodents. The third-stage infective larva forms in the mollusk in 17 or 18 days and can remain there for some time or be expelled and contaminate the environment. A large number of paratenic or transport hosts, such as crustaceans, fish, amphibians, or reptiles, may become infected with these larvae and, in turn, infect rats or human beings.

A. *malaysiensis* is a nematode resembling *A. cantonensis;* it was isolated from *Rattus norvegicus* in Japan in 1990. This nematode showed biologic and isoenzymatic differences when compared to *A. cantonensis* (Sawabe and Makiya, 1995). Subsequently, the infection was diagnosed in 23% of 108 aborigines in Malaysia by enzyme-linked immunosorbent assay (ELISA) with monoclonal antibodies (Ambu et al., 1997). The adult parasite has been found in rats, and its larva infects the snail *Biomphalaria glabrata*, although not as easily as it infects *A. cantonensis*.

Geographic Distribution and Occurrence: Abdominal angiostrongyliasis caused by *A. costaricensis* is primarily a disease of the Americas. It has been identified in children in Costa Rica since 1952, and more than 130 human cases had been diagnosed when Morera and Cespedes described the parasite in 1971. Morera (1991) indicated that about 300 cases a year were diagnosed in Costa Rica alone. In 1992, two cases were discovered in children on the French island of Guadeloupe in the Caribbean (Juminer et al., 1993). Neafie and Marty (1993) described the first human case in the US. The first known epidemic occurred in 1994–1995 in Guatemala and affected 22 persons (Kramer et al., 1998). The human disease has also been confirmed in Brazil, El Salvador, and Honduras. Based on epidemiological studies, Graeff-Teixeira et al. (1997) found that the human prevalence in two endemic areas of southern Brazil was 30% and 66%, respectively. Suspected clinical cases have occurred in Nicaragua and Venezuela. With respect to the animal definitive hosts, 15% of *Rattus norvegicus* and 6% of *R. rattus* on the island of Guadeloupe were found to be infected (Juminer et al., 1993). In Panama, the adult parasite was found in five species of rodents belonging to three different families. Parasites were also found in several specimens of *Sigmodon hispidus* in the US state of Texas, *Oryzomys caliginosus* in Colombia, and slugs (*Vaginulus* spp.) in Guayaquil, Ecuador. It is highly probable that the parasitosis is much more widespread than is currently recognized. Morera (1991) mentions that a case was reported in Africa.

Human cases of angiostrongyliasis by *A. cantonensis* have occurred in Australia, Cambodia, the Philippines, Indonesia, Japan, Thailand, Taiwan, Viet Nam, and several Pacific islands. In 1992, 27 cases had been reported in Japan, the majority in the prefecture of Okinawa. The geographic distribution of *A. cantonensis* was once believed to be limited to Africa, Asia, Australia, and the Pacific islands. However, its presence has been confirmed in Cuba, where infected rats (*R. norvegicus*) and mollusks have been found (Aguiar *et al.*, 1981). Likewise, five human cases with meningoencephalitis have been attributed to *A. cantonensis* (Pascual *et al.*, 1981). It is believed that the parasite was introduced to the island some years ago by rats from a ship from Asia. A review published in a local journal in Japan in 1992 describes how *A. cantonensis* spread, after the Second World War, from South and Southeast Asia to the islands of the western Pacific and from there, east and south through Micronesia and Australia to Polynesia. Since 1950, cases have been identified in Indonesia (island of Sumatra), Philippines, Taiwan, and even Tahiti. Later, in the 1960s, there were cases in Cambodia, Thailand, Viet Nam, and even in the US state of Hawaii. It subsequently appeared in Australia, mainland China, India, and Japan (Okinawa). In the 1970s and 1980s, the parasite was found in rats in Cuba, Egypt, Puerto Rico, and the city of New Orleans, US; it has been found in man in the Côte d'Ivoire, Cuba, and the French island of Reunion. There seems to be an autochthonous focus in the city of New Orleans, Louisiana, US, since infections were found in a primate in a zoo and in rats (García and Bruckner, 1997). In a study carried out on rat species (*R. norvegicus, R. rattus,* and *R. exulans*) on the Hawaiian Islands, US, and the Society Islands, French Polynesia, the parasite was found in more than 40% of the specimens captured. In Egypt, 32.7% of 55 specimens of *R. norvegicus* harbored the parasite. In the province of Havana, Cuba, 12 of 20 captured *R. norvegicus* were infected (Aguiar *et al.*, 1981). The confirmed cases of eosinophilic meningitis caused by *A. cantonensis* number in the hundreds, and thousands have been diagnosed clinically.

A. malaysiensis has been found in rats in Japan (Sawabe and Makiya, 1995) and in aborigines in Malaysia (Ambu *et al.*, 1997).

The Disease in Man: The clinical manifestations of abdominal angiostrongyliasis caused by *A. costaricensis* are moderate but prolonged fever, abdominal pain on the right side, and, frequently, anorexia, diarrhea, and vomiting. Leukocytosis is characteristic (20,000 to 50,000 per mm^3), with marked eosinophilia (11% to 82%). Palpation sometimes reveals tumoral masses or abscesses. Rectal exploration is painful and a tumor can occasionally be palpated. Lesions are located primarily in the ileocecal region, the ascending colon, appendix, and regional ganglia. Granulomatous inflammation of the intestinal wall can cause partial or complete obstruction. Out of 116 children with intestinal eosinophilic granulomas studied from 1966 to 1975 in the National Children's Hospital in Costa Rica, 90 had surgery (appendectomy, ileocolonic resection, and hemicolectomy). Appendicitis was the preoperative diagnosis in 34 cases. All but two of the children survived and recovered. The highest prevalence (53%) was found in children 6 to 13 years old, and twice as many boys as girls were affected (Loría-Cortés and Lobo-Sanahuja, 1980). Ectopic localizations may occur, such as those found in the livers of Costa Rican patients with visceral larva migrans-like syndrome (Morera et al., 1982).

In Taiwan, the disease occurs mainly in children, but in other endemic areas it occurs in adults. A study of 82 children found that the incubation period was 13 days, shorter than the average of 16.5 days in adults; meningoencephalitis was the predominant clinical form in 30% of the children, as opposed to the 5% observed in adults in Thailand, and the most common symptom was fever (91.5% of patients), followed by vomiting and headache. Cranial nerves VI and VII showed alterations in 19.5% and 11% of the cases, respectively, and papilledema was found in 25% of the children but in just 12% of the adults (Hwang and Chen, 1991). The symptomatology of meningitis and eosinophilic meningoencephalitis was studied in 1968 and 1969 in 125 patients from southern Taiwan. Most patients had a mild or moderate symptomatology, and only a few suffered serious manifestations; four of the patients died and another three had permanent sequelae. Young specimens of A. cantonensis were found in the cerebrospinal fluid of eight patients, and the parasite was found during autopsy in another. In 78% of the patients, the disease had a sudden onset, with intense headache, vomiting, and moderate intermittent fever. More than 50% of the patients experienced coughing, anorexia, malaise, constipation, and somnolence, and less than half had stiffness in the neck. Pleocytosis in the cerebrospinal fluid was particularly pronounced in the second and third weeks of the disease. The percentage of eosinophils was generally high and was directly related to the number of leukocytes in the cerebrospinal fluid. Leukocytosis and eosinophilia in the blood were also high. Legrand and Angibaud (1998) found that the most common signs were moderate meningeal irritation, paresthesia, and abnormalities in cranial nerves II, III, IV, and VII. While there are no effective anthelminthic and the headaches and weakness can last a few weeks, as a general rule the patient recovers without sequelae.

Angiostrongyliasis caused by A. cantonensis is generally expressed as eosinophilic meningitis, but there have also been isolated outbreaks in which the spinal cord, spinal nerves, and brain were extensively affected. The reason for the different clinical pictures is not known, but the severe cases may be due to the higher number of parasites present (intensity of infection). Eosinophilic meningitis usually occurs after the ingestion of paratenic hosts or contaminated vegetables containing few larvae; the most serious forms of the disease are due to direct consumption of highly infected intermediate hosts (Kliks et al., 1982). In American Samoa, an outbreak of radiculomyeloencephalitis was described in 16 fishermen who had consumed raw or undercooked Achatina fulica (giant African snail), an intermediate host of A. cantonensis, considered a delicacy by many Asians. The incubation period was 1 to 6 days, and the disease lasted 10 weeks. In addition to eosinophilia in the spinal fluid and the blood, the disease was characterized by acute abdominal pain, generalized pruritus, and later by pain, weakness, and paresthesia in the legs, and dysfunction of the bladder (urinary retention or incontinence) and the intestine. Half of the patients suffered transitory hypertension or lethargy; three entered a coma and one died. Of the 12 hospitalized patients, 10 had to use wheelchairs (Kliks et al., 1982). Serologic surveys carried out in Australia, in human populations living in localities where the infection occurs in rats and those living in other places where it does not, indicate that many human infections are asymptomatic.

The Disease in Animals: In rodents, *A. costaricensis* lesions are located primarily in the cecum, with focal or diffuse edema of the subserosa, a reduction of mesenteric fat, and swelling of the regional ganglia. In highly parasitized animals, eggs and larvae may be found in various viscera of the body. No significant difference in weight between parasitized and nonparasitized animals has been confirmed.

Rats infected by *A. cantonensis* may have coughing, sneezing, dyspnea, and fibrosis in the lungs. However, the physical appearance of the animals does not reflect the degree of pathologic changes.

For both parasites, the prevalence of the infection is greater in adult than in young rodents, which suggests that rodents do not develop resistance to the infection.

Source of Infection and Mode of Transmission: Several species of rodents serve as definitive hosts of *A. costaricensis*. In a study carried out in Panama (Tesh *et al.*, 1973), the highest prevalence of the infection was found in the cotton rat (*S. hispidus*), which was also the most abundant rodent in the six localities studied. The cotton rat inhabits areas close to dwellings in both tropical and temperate zones, feeding on both plants and small vertebrate and invertebrate animals, including slugs. All these facts suggest that this rat is a prime reservoir and that it plays an important role in the epidemiology of the parasitosis. Rodents are infected by ingesting food or water contaminated with the infective larvae in the mollusk secretions (slime) or by eating the infected mollusks. Man may acquire the infection in the same way, for example, by eating poorly-washed vegetables containing small slugs or their secretions. A study in Guatemala showed that the consumption of mint leaves, alone or as a seasoning in traditional uncooked dishes, correlated directly with the presence of the infection in man (Kramer, 1998). It is believed that children can become infected while playing in areas where slugs are abundant by transferring mollusk secretions found on vegetation to their mouths. An increase in cases in children occurs in Costa Rica during the rainy season, when slugs are plentiful. Humidity is an important factor in the survival of both the first- and third-stage larvae, since they are susceptible to desiccation.

A. cantonensis has been found in a dozen species of the genus *Rattus* and in *Bandicota indica* and *Melomys littoralis*. These rodents, natural definitive hosts, are infected by consuming mollusks or paratenic hosts that harbor third-stage larvae. The infection rates of mollusks as intermediate hosts are usually high; both the prevalence and the number of larvae an individual mollusk can harbor vary according to the species. Man, who is an accidental host, is infected by consuming raw mollusks or paratenic hosts such as crustaceans or fish.

The ecology of angiostrongyliasis is closely related to the plant community in which the mollusks and rodents live. The frequency of the human parasitosis depends on the abundance of these hosts and the degree to which they are infected, and, also, in the case of *A. cantonensis,* frequency is connected with eating habits (consumption of raw mollusks, crustaceans, and fish).

Diagnosis: Diagnosis of the human infection caused by *A. costaricensis* can be made by examining biopsied or surgical specimens and confirming the presence of the parasites or their eggs. Graeff-Teixeira *et al.* (1991) established histopathological patterns for diagnosis. Also, an enzyme-linked immunosorbent assay (ELISA) was developed that demonstrated a sensitivity of 86% and a specificity of 83% when used with sera adsorbed with *Ascaris suum* antigens (Graeff-Teixeira *et al.*, 1997).

In endemic areas, meningitis or meningoencephalitis caused by *A. cantonensis* is suspected in the presence of the characteristic signs of eosinophilia in the blood and eosinophilic pleocytosis of the cerebrospinal fluid. In places such as Thailand, where infection of the central nervous system caused by *Gnathostoma spinigerum* has a high prevalence, the two diseases must be differentiated. Punyagupta *et al.* (1990) indicate that gnathostomiasis causes sharp pain in the nerve roots, signs of cerebral and spinal disease, and yellowish or bloody cerebrospinal fluid. Although most reports indicate that only in a few cases can the parasite be found in patients' cerebrospinal fluid or eyes, Hwang and Chen (1991) reported having recovered it by lumbar puncture in 41.5% of 84 pediatric cases. Serologic tests are useful for confirming the presumptive diagnosis (Legrand and Angibaud, 1998). Two varieties of ELISA have shown a specificity of 100%, but sensitivity of just 50% to 60% (Eamsobhana *et al.*, 1997).

Control: While human angiostrongyliasis is not very prevalent, except in a few areas of high endemicity, prophylaxis is important because there is no known therapeutic treatment for the infection. Theoretically, angiostrongyliasis could be controlled by reducing rodent and mollusk populations, though practical application seems doubtful. Preventive measures for individuals consist of thoroughly washing vegetables, and hands after garden or field work; not eating raw or undercooked mollusks and crustaceans; and not drinking water that may be unhygienic. Experiments have shown that incubation of infective *A. costaricensis* larvae for 12 hours at 5°C in 1.5% sodium hypochlorite kills all the larvae. Incubation in saturated sodium chloride or in commercial vinegar reduced the number of larvae but failed to prevent the infection in mice (Zanini and Graeff-Teixeira, 1995).

Bibliography

Aguiar, P.H., P. Morera, J. Pascual. First record of *Angiostrongylus cantonensis* in Cuba. *Am J Trop Med Hyg* 30(5):963–965, 1981.

Ambu, S., A.N. Rain, J.W. Mak, D. Maslah, S. Maidah. Detection of *Angiostrongylus malaysiensis* circulating antigen using monoclonal antibody-based enzyme-linked immunosorbent assay (MAb-ELISA). *Southeast Asian J Trop Med Public Health* 28 Suppl:143–147, 1997.

Eamsobhana, P., H.S. Yong, J.W. Mak, D. Wattanakulpanich. Detection of circulating antigens of *Parastrongylus cantonensis* in human sera by dot-blot ELISA and sandwich ELISA using monoclonal antibody. *Southeast Asian J Trop Med Public Health* 28(3):624–628, 1997.

García, L.S., D.A. Bruckner. *Diagnostic Medical Parasitology*, 3rd ed. Washington, D.C.: ASM Press; 1997.

Graeff-Teixeira, C., L. Camillo-Coura, H.L. Lenzi. Histopathological criteria for the diagnosis of abdominal angiostrongyliasis. *Parasitol Res* 77(7):606–611, 1991.

Graeff-Teixeira, C., A.A. Agostini, L. Camillo-Coura, M.F. Ferreira-da-Cruz. Seroepidemiology of abdominal angiostrongyliasis: The standardization of an immunoenzymatic assay and prevalence of antibodies in two localities in southern Brazil. *Trop Med Int Health* 2(3):254–260, 1997.

Hwang, K.P., E.R. Chen. Clinical studies on angiostrongyliasis cantonensis among children in Taiwan. *Southeast Asian J Trop Med Public Health* 22 Suppl:194–199, 1991.

Juminer, B., G. Borel, H. Mauleon, *et al.* L'infestation murine naturelle par *Angiostrongylus costaricensis* Morera et Cespedes, 1971 à la Guadeloupe. *Bull Soc Pathol Exot* 86(5 Pt 2):502–505, 1993.

Kliks, M.M., K. Kroenke, J.M. Hardman. Eosinophilic radiculomyeloencephalitis: An angiostrongyliasis outbreak in American Samoa related to ingestion of *Achatina fulica* snails. *Am J Trop Med Hyg* 31(6):1114–1122, 1982.

Kramer, M.H., G.J. Greer, J.F. Quiñonez, *et al.* First reported outbreak of abdominal angiostrongyliasis. *Clin Infect Dis* 26(2):365–372, 1998.

Legrand, G., G. Angibaud. La meningite à eosinophiles due à *Angiostrongylus cantonensis*. *Rev Neurol (Paris)* 154(3):236–242, 1998.

Loría-Cortés, R., J.F. Lobo-Sanahuja. Clinical abdominal angiostrongylosis. A study of 116 children with intestinal eosinophilic granuloma caused by *Angiostrongylus costaricensis*. *Am J Trop Med Hyg* 29(4):538–544, 1980.

Mojon, M. Angiostrongylose humaine à *Angiostrongylus costaricensis*. *Bull Acad Natl Med* 178(4):625–631, 1994.

Morera, P. Abdominal angiostrongyliasis. *In*: Strickland, G.T., ed. *Hunter's Tropical Medicine*, 7th ed. Philadelphia: Saunders; 1991.

Morera, P., F. Pérez, F. Mora. Visceral larva migrans-like syndrome caused by *Angiostrongylus costaricensis*. *Am J Trop Med Hyg* 31(1):67–70, 1982.

Neafie, R.C., A.M. Marty. Unusual infections in humans. *Clin Microbiol Rev* 6(1):34–56, 1993.

Pascual, J.E., R.P. Bouli, H. Aguiar. Eosinophilic meningoencephalitis in Cuba, caused by *Angiostrongylus cantonensis*. *Am J Trop Med Hyg* 30(5):960–962, 1981.

Punyagupta, S., T. Bunnag, P. Juttijudata. Eosinophilic meningitis in Thailand. Clinical and epidemiological characteristics of 162 patients with myeloencephalitis probably caused by *Gnathostoma spinigerum*. *J Neurol Sci* 96(2–3):241–256, 1990.

Rambo, P.R., A.A. Agostini, C. Graeff-Teixeira. Abdominal angiostrongylosis in southern Brazil—prevalence and parasitic burden in mollusc intermediate hosts from eighteen endemic foci. *Mem Inst Oswaldo Cruz* 92(1):9–14, 1997.

Sawabe, K., K. Makiya. Comparative infectivity and survival of first-stage larvae of *Angiostrongylus cantonensis* and *Angiostrongylus malaysiensis*. *J Parasitol* 81(2):228–233, 1995.

Tesh, R.B., L.J. Ackerman, W.H. Dietz, *et al. Angiostrongylus costaricensis* in Panama. Prevalence and pathologic finding in wild rodents infected with the parasite. *Am J Trop Med Hyg* 22(3):348–356, 1973.

Zanini, G.M., C. Graeff-Teixeira. Angiostrongilose abdominal: Profilaxia pela destruição das larvas infectantes em alimentos tratados com sal, vinagre ou hipoclorito de sodio. *Rev Soc Bras Med Trop* 28(4):389–392, 1995.

ANISAKIASIS

ICD-10 B81.0

Synonyms: Anisakiosis, anisakidosis, herring worm disease, cod worm disease.

Etiology: The agent of this parasitosis is the larval stage of nematodes of the genera *Anisakis, Pseudoterranova* (synonyms *Porrocaecum, Terranova, Phocanema*), or *Contracaecum*. These parasites belong to the order Ascaridida, family

Anisakidae, which some authors call "marine ascarids." The species mentioned most often in the literature as parasites of man are *Anisakis simplex* and *Pseudoterranova decipiens*. Before identification techniques were refined, the Japanese literature referred to the third-stage larva of *P. decipiens,* frequently found in man, as type A or type 1 Anisakidae larva.

The adult stage *Anisakis* and *Pseudoterranova* parasites lodge in the stomach or small intestine of piscivorous marine mammals such as dolphins, porpoises, whales, and seals; *Contracaecum* lodges in the digestive tract of fish, where it lays eggs which are expelled, unembryonated, in the feces of the definitive host. While floating in the water, the eggs form a second-stage larva and are ingested by a variety of small crustaceans that act as intermediate hosts, inside which the third-stage larva forms. Many fish ingest these parasitized crustaceans and act as transfer (paratenic) hosts; there the third-stage larvae accumulate and encyst, waiting for definitive hosts. These fish may be ingested by larger fish or by man, in which case the worm just transfers from one to the other, or by definitive hosts, in which case the worm matures, mates, and begins oviposition (Mehlhorn and Walldorf, 1988).

Man is an aberrant host in whom the larva ingested with raw fish or squid does not reach maturity. There are two exceptions in which juvenile *P. decipiens* were recovered from human hosts.

Geographic Distribution and Occurrence: Parasites of the genus *Anisakis* are found in most oceans and seas, but some species have a more restricted distribution. Human infection occurs in countries where marine fish are eaten raw, lightly salted, or smoked. From 1955, when human infection was described for the first time, to 1968, 160 cases occurred in the Netherlands. Since 1969, when freezing fish for 24 hours before marketing became mandatory, only a few cases have occurred. The country with the highest prevalence of human anisakiasis is Japan, where 487 cases occurred up to 1976. In both Japan and the Netherlands, the prevalence was found to be higher in men than in women. In Japan, the highest rate of infection is in the 20- to 50-year-old age group. In the Republic of South Korea, 107 cases were diagnosed between June 1989 and June 1992 in a parasitological laboratory in Seoul. Most of the cases were due to *A. simplex,* and the rest were due to *P. decipiens.* In France, about 80 cases had been described up to 1995, and isolated cases have been reported in Belgium, Denmark, England, and Germany. When 244 patients were examined in a hospital in Indonesia, 11% were found to have antibodies against *Anisakis* spp. (Uga *et al.*, 1996). Of 1,008 apparently healthy people examined for anisakiasis in Spain by enzyme-linked immunosorbent assay (ELISA), 47 showed titers 1.5 to 2 times higher than the controls, and 14 showed titers more than 2 times higher than the controls (García-Palacios *et al.*, 1996). Oliveira *et al.* (1999) identified seven clinical cases in three months in a Madrid hospital. In the Western Hemisphere, up to 1997, 23 cases had been recorded in North America, 16 of which occurred in the US (11 in the state of California and 5 in the state of Alaska) (Kliks, 1983), and 3 in Chile. Most of the cases in the US were due to *P. decipiens*, and the others were caused by *Anisakis* spp. The number of cases in the US increased during the 1990s; in 1991, four cases were described in the state of Hawaii, bringing the total number of cases for the Hawaiian Islands to seven.

Many species of fish have been found to be naturally infected. The prevalence of infection in fish can be very high. A study of Baltic herring found that up to 95% of the fish were infected at certain times of the year, with an average of 14 larvae each. In Peru, larvae of *Anisakis* spp. have been found in three species of marine fish caught close to the port of Callao: 48.6% of 222 specimens of jacks (*Trachurus murphyi*); 1.5% of 381 croakers (*Sciaena deliciosa*); 1.6% of 180 "cocos" (*Polyclemus peruanus*); and none of 250 "cojinobas" (*Seriolella violacea*). The highest rates of infection were found between December and March. In Chile, 27% of 311 jacks (*Trachurus murphyi*) harbored larvae of *Anisakis* spp.; likewise, infection by other Anisakidae has been confirmed in *Merluccius gayi* (hake), *Cilus montti* (corvina), and *Thyrsites atun* (sierra), all fish that are consumed regularly (Torres *et al.*, 1978). *P. decipiens* larvae have been found in cod caught in the Atlantic Ocean near the South Pole.

The Disease in Man: Anisakiasis can occur clinically in several forms (Ishikura *et al.*, 1993). The larvae may remain in the cavity of the stomach or intestine without penetrating the tissues, causing an infection that is often asymptomatic. In general, asymptomatic or mild cases are caused by *Pseudoterranova* spp. These infections are discovered when live larvae are expelled by means of coughing, vomiting, or defecating. In laboratory examinations of two cases recently infected by *Pseudoterranova* spp., only mild and transitory eosinophilia was found. In the invasive forms, the larvae penetrate the gastric or intestinal submucosa, causing edema, erosion, ulcers, and bleeding. In Japan, 56 *A. simplex* larvae were recovered from a woman (Kagei *et al.*, 1992). In the anatomicopathological examination of cases of invasive anisakiasis, ulcerations and hemorrhagic foci are found in the mucosa, and localized or diffuse tumors are found in the intestinal or stomach wall. An intense eosinophilic infiltration is observed in the histopathological sections, with edema, histiocytes, lymphocytes, neutrophils, plasmocytes, and sometimes, giant cells suggestive of an allergic reaction. Allergy symptoms have also been found in many patients suffering from anisakiasis caused by *A. simplex*, many with symptoms of acute urticaria (Mendizabal-Basagoiti, 1999), anaphylaxis, and, occasionally, gastric symptoms which are often attributed to fish or shellfish allergies (Moreno-Ancillo *et al.*, 1997). The considerable edema in the large gastric curvature observed by endoscopy and leukocytosis also suggest an allergic origin for the gastric pathology (Kakizoe *et al.*, 1995).

In gastric anisakiasis, the symptoms appear 12 to 24 hours after the consumption of raw fish, and consist of sudden epigastric pain, often with nausea and vomiting. Eosinophilia is present in about half of the patients, but not leukocytosis. The gastric form of the disease is seldom diagnosed correctly; it can become chronic, lasting more than a year. In Japanese patients, in whom gastric anisakiasis is more prevalent than intestinal anisakiasis, occult blood has been found in the gastric juice, as well as hypoacidity or anacidity. The clinical picture of gastric anisakiasis is similar to and has been confused with that of peptic ulcer, gastric tumor, acute gastritis, cholecystitis, and other gastrointestinal pathologies.

Intestinal anisakiasis has an incubation period of about seven days and manifests as severe pain in the lower abdomen, nausea, vomiting, fever, diarrhea, and occult blood in the feces. There is leukocytosis, but seldom eosinophilia (Smith and Wootten, 1978). Intestinal anisakiasis can be confused with appendicitis and peritonitis. Sometimes the parasites perforate the intestinal wall and lodge in the mesenteric veins and various organs. In these invasive forms, the larvae are found in eosinophilic granulomas, phlegmons, or abscesses. The clinical picture of mesenteric anisakiasis varies with the organ affected. There have been two reported cases of pulmonary infection with high fever, dyspnea, and pleural effusion after eating raw fish (Matsuoka et al., 1994).

In a clinicopathologic study of 92 cases in Japan, anisakiasis was localized in the stomach of 65% of patients and in the intestine (large or small) of 30%. In the Netherlands, intestinal anisakiasis was more prevalent than gastric anisakiasis. Most cases in the US were due to a transitory, noninvasive anisakiasis caused by larvae of *Pseudoterranova* spp. located in the lumen of the digestive tract. The main symptoms consisted of mild epigastric pain and nausea beginning when the infected fish was ingested and lasting up to 20 hours; in about 2 weeks, the parasite was expelled by coughing or vomiting or was found in the mouth (Kliks, 1983).

The Disease in Animals: The larvae of anisakids can cause pathologic changes in many species of marine fish. The parasitosis can affect various organs, and the number of larvae may reach several hundred per fish. The most commonly affected organ is the liver, and atrophy is the most frequent change. A cod parasitized by *Contracaecum* spp. weighs less than a normal fish, and if the number of larvae is large, the fat content of its liver may be significantly reduced. In young fish, *Contracaecum* can cause death when they invade the cardiac region. In addition to the liver, anisakid larvae can encapsulate in other organs, causing perforations of the stomach wall, visceral adhesions, and muscle damage. In spite of these observations by several researchers, the pathologic effects on fish are not clear (Smith and Wootten, 1978).

In marine mammals, the parasites are deeply embedded in tumors of the gastric mucosa. It can thus be assumed that parasitic invasion affects the health of these animals. Lesions are usually observed when the parasite burden is large, and especially when large numbers of nematodes are inserted in one spot of the gastric mucosa or submucosa. More than 500 parasites have been recovered from a sea lion. The parasites that are free in the lumen of the digestive tract do not cause any apparent pathology.

In 1993, the infection of cats' intestines with anisakid larvae was reported in Korea.

Source of Infection and Mode of Transmission: The main source of infection for man is marine fish, many species of which are highly parasitized. Human cases are caused by consuming raw, lightly salted, or smoked fish, whether or not it has been refrigerated. In the Netherlands, the occurrence of the disease is due to the habit of consuming raw or lightly salted herring ("green herring"). Although the habit persists, the incidence of human anisakiasis has been drastically reduced by the requirement that fish be frozen before it is sent to market. The highest incidence of the disease has been recorded in Japan, where various fish dishes are eaten raw or pickled in vinegar. In the US, at least two cases were caused by eating ceviche (a dish consisting of pieces of raw fish seasoned in lemon juice for 24 hours), and others by eating Japanese raw fish dishes. The conditions necessary for transmission to humans exist on the Pacific coast of Latin American countries. In Peru and Chile, anisakid larvae have been found in the stomach wall, intestinal wall, and mesentery, and on the surface of the gonads of several species of commercial marine fish. In addition, in Peru and other countries along the Pacific coast, ceviche is a very popular dish. According to Japanese parasitologists, anisakid larvae found in cephalopods such as cuttlefish and octopus are third-stage larvae and so would be infective for man (and for the natural definitive hosts) when the cephalopods are consumed raw or undercooked. Marine fish can become infected second intermediate hosts by eating invertebrates; they can also become paratenic hosts by ingesting the infective third-stage larvae of other fish.

Diagnosis: Direct diagnosis by examination of the parasite is the preferred method, but in 50% to 70% of gastric cases, the parasite can be visualized and recovered by endoscopy (Deardorff *et al.*, 1991). In colonic anisakiasis, it is difficult to see the parasite by endoscopy, but the lesions and X-rays are very useful for diagnosis. In fact, the parasites were visible on X-ray in four out of six cases (Matsumoto *et al.*, 1992). The presence of ascites, dilation of the small intestine, and edema of the Kerckring's folds found using sonography in patients with acute abdomen who have eaten fish or shellfish recently are indications of intestinal anisakiasis (Ido *et al.*, 1998). Serologic tests, particularly the enzyme-linked immunosorbent assay (ELISA) and Western blot, are very useful for clinical evaluation; but cross-reactions with *Ascaris* have been reported (Petithory *et al.*, 1991).

Control: Human infection can be prevented by not eating raw fish. Most species of anisakids that are dangerous for humans die when exposed to temperatures of –20°C for 24 hours or 60°C for one minute. Since these are the temperatures to which the larva must be exposed, and since there are a few species that are more resistant, it is recommended that the fish be cooked at 70°C or frozen to –20°C for 72 hours in order to have a margin of safety. The freezer unit of a good home refrigerator can generally achieve temperatures of –20°C. The requirement that fish be subjected to low temperatures before being sent to market has drastically decreased the infection in the Netherlands. Salting is also effective when concentrated salt solutions that reach all parts of the fish are used. Prohibiting the sale of fish that has not undergone these processes is the most effective measure for controlling anisakiasis in the community. It is also important to eviscerate fish immediately after they are caught to prevent the *Anisakis* larvae from passing from the intestine to the muscle. Apparently, salmon farming prevents their infection with anisakids; Deardorff and Kent (1989) found that all the wild salmon they caught in the state of Washington, US, were infected with *A. simplex,* but none of those bred in commercial pens had the parasite.

Bibliography

Deardorff, T.L., S.G. Kayes, T. Fukumura. Human anisakiasis transmitted by marine food products. *Hawaii Med J* 50(1):9–16, 1991.

Deardorff, T.L., M.L. Kent. Prevalence of larval *Anisakis simplex* in pen-reared and wild-caught salmon (Salmonidae) from Puget Sound, Washington. *J Wildl Dis* 25(3):416–419, 1989.

García-Palacios, L., M.L. González, M.I. Esteban, E. Mirabent, M.J. Perteguer, C. Cuéllar. Enzyme-linked immunosorbent assay, immunoblot analysis and RAST fluoroimmunoassay analysis of serum responses against crude larval antigens of *Anisakis simplex* in a Spanish random population. *J Helminthol* 70(4):281–289, 1996.

Ido, K., H. Yuasa, M. Ide, K. Kimura, K. Toshimitsu, T. Suzuki. Sonographic diagnosis of small intestinal anisakiasis. *J Clin Ultrasound* 26(3):125–130, 1998.

Ishikura, H., K. Kikuchi, K. Nagasawa, *et al.* Anisakidae and anisakidosis. *Prog Clin Parasitol* 3:43–102, 1993.

Kagei, N., H. Isogaki. A case of abdominal syndrome caused by the presence of a large number of *Anisakis larvae*. *Int J Parasitol* 22(2):251–253, 1992.

Kakizoe, S., H. Kakizoe, K. Kakizoe, *et al.* Endoscopic findings and clinical manifestation of gastric anisakiasis. *Am J Gastroenterol* 90(5):761–763, 1995.

Kliks, M.M. Anisakiasis in the western United States: Four new case reports from California. *Am J Trop Med Hyg* 32(3):526–532, 1983.

Matsumoto, T., M. Iida, Y. Kimura, K. Tanaka, T. Kitada, M. Fujishima. Anisakiasis of the colon: Radiologic and endoscopic features in six patients. *Radiology* 183(1):97–99, 1992.

Matsuoka, H., T. Nakama, H. Kisanuki, *et al.* A case report of serologically diagnosed pulmonary anisakiasis with pleural effusion and multiple lesions. *Am J Trop Med Hyg* 51(6):819–822, 1994.

McClelland, G. *Phocanema decipiens*: Pathology in seals. *Exp Parasitol* 49(3):405–419, 1980.

Mehlhorn, H., V. Walldorf. Life cycles. *In*: Mehlhorn, H., ed. *Parasitology in Focus: Facts and Trends*. Berlin: Springer-Verlag; 1988.

Mendizabal-Basagoiti, L. Hypersensibilité à l'*Anisakis simplex*: À propos de 36 cas. *Allerg Immunol (Paris)* 31(1):15–17, 1999.

Moreno-Ancillo, A., M.T. Caballero, R. Cabanas, *et al.* Allergic reactions to *Anisakis simplex* parasitizing seafood. *Ann Allergy Asthma Immunol* 79(3):246–250, 1997.

Oliveira, A., S. Sánchez Rancano, P. Conde Gacho, A. Moreno, A. Martínez, C. Comas. Anisakiasis gastrointestinal. Siete casos en tres meses. *Rev Esp Enferm Dig* 91:70–72, 1999.

Petithory, J.C., M. Rousseau, F. Siodlak. Données seroepidémiologiques sur l'anisakiase. Consequences prophylactiques pour les produits de la pêche. *Ann Gastroenterol Hepatol (Paris)* 27(6):285–287, 1991.

Smith, J.W., R. Wootten. Anisakis and anisakiasis. *Adv Parasitol* 16:93–163, 1978.

Torres, P., G. Pequeño, L. Figueroa. Nota preliminar sobre Anisakidae (Railliet and Henry, 1912, Skrjabin and Korokhin, 1945), en algunos peces de consumo habitual por la población humana de Valdivia (Chile). *Bol Chil Parasitol* 33(1):39–46, 1978.

Uga, S., K. Ono, N. Kataoka, H. Hasan. Seroepidemiology of five major zoonotic parasite infections in inhabitants of Sidoarjo, East Java, Indonesia. *Southeast Asian J Trop Med Public Health* 27(3):556–561, 1996.

ASCARIASIS

ICD-10 B77

Synonyms: Ascaridiasis, ascaridiosis.

Etiology: The agents of human ascariasis are the nematode of humans, *Ascaris lumbricoides*, and occasionally, the nematode of swine, *A. suum*. The two species are closely related and show only slight morphologic and physiologic differences (Barriga, 1982). Both species can occasionally infect the heterologous host and reach a certain degree of development inside it. The literature mentions that *A. lumbricoides* infects chimpanzees, gorillas, rhesus monkeys, and swine. Experimentally, it has been possible to infect suckling pigs with *A. lumbricoides,* and the nematodes have reached maturity and produced eggs. In addition to swine,

A. *suum* infects goats, bovines, sheep, and humans, but it rarely reaches maturity in the latter; in general, the nematode does not go beyond the larval stages in the lung and only rarely advances to the intestinal phase.

Ascarides are large nematodes: the female is 20–35 cm long and 3–6 mm in diameter; the males are smaller and have a curved distal portion. The life cycles of both seem to be similar. The eggs of *A. suum,* which are eliminated with the feces, contain just a single cell. Under ideal conditions of humidity, temperature, shade, and availability of oxygen, a third-stage infective larva develops within the egg in 15 to 20 days; under adverse conditions, this process can take much longer. Once a new host ingests the eggs with food or drinking water, the infective larvae emerge from the egg in the intestine and invade the mucosa of the cecum and colon in a few hours, remain there approximately 12 hours, and migrate to the liver via the portal circulation (Murrell *et al.,* 1997). The larvae are then carried in the bloodstream from the liver to the heart, and from there to the lungs. After a period of time, they break out of the pulmonary capillaries, enter the alveoli, and migrate through the bronchial tubes and trachea to the pharynx, from whence they are swallowed and carried to the intestine. In the intestine, they complete their maturation and develop into male and female adults. In man, the prepatent period of *A. lumbricoides*—from the onset of infection until the eggs appear in the feces—is 60 to 75 days; in swine, the prepatent period of *A. suum* is 50 to 60 days.

Geographic Distribution and Occurrence: Ascariasis is one of the most widespread parasitoses, and both *A. lumbricoides* and *A. suum* are found worldwide. It has been estimated that between 644 million and more than 1 billion persons are infected, 42 million of whom are in Central and South America. The estimated worldwide mortality due to ascariasis is 20,000 per year due to intestinal complications; annual morbidity is a million cases, mainly due to pulmonary disorders and malnutrition (Walsh and Warren, 1979). The parasitosis is most prevalent in rural areas, where contamination of the soil and contact between hands or food and larvae are more common, and in hot, humid areas, which favor maturation of the eggs. The highest rate of infection is found in children, probably because of their less hygienic habits, but also because an immune resistance is acquired along with the infection. Prevalence rates vary considerably according to differences in environmental sanitation, health education of the population, personal and food hygiene, type of soil and climate, and other factors.

A. suum is found wherever swine are raised. Studies carried out in slaughterhouses have shown that the prevalence rate is high, ranging from 20% to 70% or more. The highest rate is found in piglets 2 to 5 months old; it declines with age thereafter. Since swine have the same contact with the soil at any age, the difference is believed to represent some level of acquired immunity against the infection. It is not known to what extent *A. suum* is involved in human infection, but it is probably not very important. Suckling pigs have been infected experimentally with embryonated eggs of *A. lumbricoides,* resulting in a patent infection, with adult, egg-laying parasites. Cases caused by accidental ingestion of *A. suum* eggs have been seen in a laboratory worker and some students, and one case occurred in a child who ingested swine feces. Intestinal infection was verified in 7 of 17 volunteers after each one was administered 25 eggs of *A. suum* containing infective larvae. These facts indicate that human intestinal ascariasis by *A. suum* can occur, but is probably seldom recognized.

A World Health Organization (WHO) Expert Committee on the Control of Ascariasis said, "When infective eggs are ingested the larvae of *A. suum* unquestionably develop in the intestine, and migrate to the lungs in man as they do in many other mammals. It is a reasonable assumption that a significant proportion of respiratory illnesses observed in people having contact with pigs is caused by *A. suum* as well as by *A. lumbricoides*" (WHO, 1967). In developing countries where humans and swine are in close contact and personal and environmental hygiene are deficient, it could be anticipated that the larval phase of *A. suum* might participate together with *A. lumbricoides* in the pulmonary alterations caused by the parasite's migration, and that a small fraction of human intestinal ascariases might be due to the porcine parasite.

The Disease in Man and Animals: The course of the disease and the symptomatology are similar in both humans and swine. Children and suckling pigs are most affected. In the early age group, not only is the rate of infection higher, but parasite burden is larger. Two phases of the disease are distinguished: the initial phase, produced by migrating larvae, and the latter phase, caused by adult parasites.

Invasion of the liver of swine and turkeys by the ascarid larvae produces traumatic microfoci which become inflamed and heal with connective tissue. These microlesions are more serious and show allergic components in reinfections, but rarely result in clinical signs (Barriga, 1997). In man, there is generally no hepatic component in the migration, although it has been shown that the excreta and secretions of *A. lumbricoides* cause liver damage in hamsters (Mazumder *et al.*, 1992). The pulmonary phase is characterized by respiratory symptoms attributable to the damage produced by the larvae during pulmonary migration. In intense and repeated larval invasions, the symptomatology consists of fever, irregular and asthmatic breathing, and spasmodic coughing. Aberrant larvae located in the brain, eyes, and kidneys are rare, but can give rise to serious symptoms. Recently, studies conducted principally in Japan have confirmed several human cases of visceral larva migrans in patients with serologic reactivity against *A. suum*. These cases have been attributed to infections with the swine ascarides (Inatomi *et al.*, 1999). The same situation has occurred in France (Petithory *et al.*, 1994). Ascariasis caused by *A. lumbricoides* was once prevalent in Japan, but its incidence has been reduced to less than 0.01%. That notwithstanding, between 1994 and 1995, 14 human cases with high peripheral eosinophilia, elevated titers against *Ascaris,* and absence of *Ascaris* eggs in the feces were found. Most of the patients were asymptomatic, but laboratory tests showed liver dysfunction in seven and pulmonary infiltration in five. All lived in an area with many pig farms. Based on this evidence, the investigators believe that it was an epidemic of ascariasis by *A. suum* (Maruyama *et al.*, 1997). Japanese investigators also described an eosinophilic gastroenteritis caused by *A. suum* in man, similar to the one caused by *Ancylostoma caninum* and described by the Australians (Takeyama *et al.*, 1997).

In the intestinal phase with adult ascarides, the symptomatology also depends on the number of parasites. Mild infections are generally asymptomatic; but when the parasite burden is larger, there may be vague abdominal discomfort, colic, diarrhea, and vomiting. The most serious complications in children include intestinal obstruction by a large mass of parasites, obstruction of the pancreatic choledoch or duct, and complications resulting from the aberrant migration of adult parasites to various organs. Large numbers of ascarides in the intestines can cause diarrhea and stunted development in swine. Food conversion is affected and susceptibility to viral respiratory infections is increased in infected swine, but there are no other clinical manifestations (Barriga, 1997).

No information is available on the frequency and seriousness of the disease caused by the larval phase of *A. suum* in humans. Four students who ingested a large number of *A. suum* eggs with their food manifested, after 10 to 14 days, pulmonary infiltration, eosinophilia, asthmatiform symptoms, and an increase in circulating IgE, indicating the allergic nature of the disease. The adult larvae of *A. suum* remain in the human intestine a relatively short time—approximately 10 months—judging from the experimental infections induced in volunteers.

Source of Infection and Mode of Transmission: Humans are the reservoir of *A. lumbricoides,* as swine are for *A. suum.* The sources of infection include soil (geohelminthiasis), edible plants, or drinking water contaminated with fecal matter containing eggs of *Ascaris.* Transmission to man can occur directly from the soil or indirectly, by means of dust, water, vegetables, or objects to which the parasite's eggs have adhered. The infection is almost always acquired by ingestion, but there are unconfirmed reports that, in some areas, it may occur by inhalation of eggs. The main factor in maintaining human ascariasis is fecal contamination of the soil around dwellings, particularly in family gardens, and contamination of sources of water for drinking or irrigation. Clay soils are particularly suited to the survival of *Ascaris* eggs because they retain moisture. To have some idea of the degree of soil contamination possible, it should be borne in mind that a single female *Ascaris lumbricoides* can produce 200,000 or more eggs per day, and a female *A. suum* can produce 1 to 2 million. It is not uncommon to find 100 eggs per gram in a child's feces and 2,000 eggs per gram in swine feces. The higher rates of infection in preschool children are explained by their more frequent contact with soil and their lack of personal hygiene. The epidemiology of swine ascariasis is similar to that of human ascariasis, although the swine are in permanent and close contact with the soil.

Role of Animals in the Epidemiology of the Disease: The role played by swine in the epidemiology of human ascariasis is not well defined. It has been confirmed experimentally that cross-infections can occur between swine and humans or between humans and swine. However, the frequency of heterologous infections is unknown, given the difficulty of distinguishing between the two agents. In man, *A. suum* rarely achieves oviposition because it stays a relatively short time in the intestine. However, there is no doubt that intestinal infections by *A. suum* occur in humans, as illustrated by the case of a child in Great Britain who ingested dirt from a garden that had been fertilized with swine excreta. When the parasite was expelled, study showed it to be *A. suum* (Crewe and Smith, 1971). Later, a case of intestinal obstruction by multiple specimens of *A. suum* was described in a 9-year-old girl in Zimbabwe (Davies and Goldsmid, 1978).

An investigation into the role of swine in the epidemiology of *A. lumbricoides* ascariasis was carried out in a village in southwestern Nigeria where the inhabitants lived in close contact with swine. The study identified the intestinal infection caused by *A. lumbricoides* in both swine and the human population. However, an effort to experimentally infect pigs with eggs of *A. lumbricoides* was unsuccessful (Kofie and Dipeolu, 1983). Other studies have indicated that repeated exposure to small doses, as occurs in nature, is more effective than infection with a large number of eggs.

Occasionally, *A. lumbricoides* has been found in the intestine of nonhuman primates, and its larvae have been found in the lungs of several other species of animals. *A. suum* can infect cattle, sheep, and goats and can reach sexual maturity in these animals. However, in some described cases, doubt exists about the identity of the parasite. While *A. lumbricoides* and *A. suum* are distinguished by studying the denticles on the lips, which are different in the two species, it is now known that the shape of the denticles of the swine parasite changes over time.

Diagnosis: In the hepatic or pulmonary migration phase of the larvae, it is difficult or impossible to confirm the diagnosis by means of laboratory tests. Sometimes larvae can be found in the bronchial secretions of both humans and suckling pigs. Hepatic and pulmonary migrations produce antibodies that can be detected using various immunological tests. However, while cross-reactivity is rare with other superfamilies of nematodes, *Anisakis simplex, A. suum, A. lumbricoides,* and *Toxocara canis* share common somatic and excretory antigens (Kennedy *et al.*, 1988).

In the intestinal phase, the characteristic eggs are found in the feces.

Control: Human ascariasis is a public health problem, especially in areas with a low economic level, deficient environmental sanitation, and low standards of personal hygiene. In several industrialized countries, the prevalence rate of the parasitosis has been significantly reduced as a result of an improved standard of living, without the adoption of specific control measures. The principal measures that should be included in a control program consist of massive and periodic treatment of the human population to prevent environmental contamination, sanitary excreta disposal, provision of potable water, and health education for the purpose of instilling personal hygiene habits in the population. In some countries (Korea, Israel, and Japan), human ascariasis has been practically eradicated.

It is important to remember that ascaris eggs are extremely resistant to environmental factors. In experiments with *A. lumbricoides*, contamination of the soil with eggs has persisted for up to five years. Treatment of solid sewer waste in stabilization ponds is insufficient to kill the eggs of ascarides; Ayres *et al.* (1993) reported that up to 12% of *A. lumbricoides* eggs recovered from a pond were viable after 2.5 years of operation. Treatment of sewer waste with ammonium hydroxide at 30°C, or at 40°C without the alkali, destroys them, but a temperature of 22°C, with or without ammonium, has no lethal effect (Ghiglietti *et al.*, 1995). While it has not been employed, biological control of ascarides seems to be a possibility. Apart from the insects that eat the eggs, at least the fungus *Verticillium chlamydosporium* invades the eggs and kills the *A. lumbricoides* larvae (Lysek and Sterba, 1991).

Bibliography

Ayres, R.M., D.L. Lee, D.D. Mara, S.A. Silva. The accumulation, distribution and viability of human parasitic nematode eggs in the sludge of a primary facultative waste stabilization pond. *Trans R Soc Trop Med Hyg* 87(3):256–258, 1993.

Barriga, O.O. Ascariasis. *In*: Steele, J.H., section ed. Section B, Vol. 2: *CRC Handbook Series in Zoonoses*. Boca Raton: CRC Press; 1982.

Barriga, O.O. *Veterinary Parasitology for Practitioners*, 2nd ed. Edina: Burgess International Group; 1997.

Crewe, W., D.H. Smith. Human infection with pig *Ascaris (A. suum)*. *Ann Trop Med Parasitol* 65(1):85, 1971.

Davies, N.J., J.M. Goldsmid. Intestinal obstruction due to *Ascaris suum* infection. *Trans R Soc Trop Med Hyg* 72(1):107, 1978.

Galvin, T.J. Development of human and pig *Ascaris* in the pig and rabbit. *J Parasitol* 54(6):1085–1091, 1968.

Ghiglietti, R., P. Rossi, M. Ramsan, A. Colombi. Viability of *Ascaris suum, Ascaris lumbricoides* and *Trichuris muris* eggs to alkaline pH and different temperatures. *Parassitologia* 37(2–3):229–232, 1995.

Inatomi, Y., T. Murakami, M. Tokunaga, K. Ishiwata, Y. Nawa, M. Uchino. Encephalopathy caused by visceral larva migrans due to *Ascaris suum*. *J Neurol Sci* 164(2):195–199, 1999.

Kennedy, M.W., J. Tierney, P. Ye, *et al*. The secreted and somatic antigens of the third stage larva of *Anisakis simplex*, and antigenic relationship with *Ascaris suum, Ascaris lumbricoides,* and *Toxocara canis*. *Mol Biochem Parasitol* 31(1):35–46, 1988.

Kofie, B.A., O.O. Dipeolu. A study of human and porcine ascariasis in a rural area of southwest Nigeria. *Int J Zoonoses* 10(1):66–70, 1983.

Lysek, H., J. Sterba. Colonization of *Ascaris lumbricoides* eggs by the fungus *Verticillium chlamydosporium* Goddard. *Folia Parasitol* 38(3):255–259, 1991.

Maruyama, H., Y. Nawa, S. Noda, T. Mimori. An outbreak of ascariasis with marked eosinophilia in the southern part of Kyushu District, Japan, caused by infection with swine ascaris. *Southeast Asian J Trop Med Public Health* 28 Suppl 1:194–196, 1997.

Mazumder, D.N., A. Santra, G. Dutta, N. Ghosh, M.K. Chowdhury. Hepatic lesions caused by excretory and secretory products of *Ascaris lumbricoides* in golden hamster. *Indian J Gastroenterol* 11(3):117–120, 1992.

Murrell, K.D., L. Eriksen, P. Nansen, H.C. Slotved, T. Rasmussen. *Ascaris suum:* A revision of its early migratory path and implications for human ascariasis. *J Parasitol* 83(2):255–260, 1997.

Petithory, J.C., A. Beddok, M. Quedoc. [Ascaridiases zoonoses: Visceral larva migrans syndromes.] *Bull Acad Natl Med* 178(4):635–645, 1994.

Phills, J.A, A.J. Harrold, G.V. Whiteman, L. Perelmutter. Pulmonary infiltrates, asthma and eosinophilia due to *Ascaris suum* infestation in man. *N Engl J Med* 286(18):965–970, 1972.

Takeyama, Y., S. Kamimura, J. Suzumiya, *et al*. Case report: Eosinophilic colitis with high antibody titre against *Ascaris suum*. *J Gastroenterol Hepatol* 12(3):204–206, 1997.

Walsh, J.A., K.S. Warren. Selective primary health care. An interim strategy for disease control in developing countries. *N Engl J Med* 301(18):967–974, 1979.

World Health Organization (WHO). *Control of Ascariasis. Report of a WHO Expert Committee*. Geneva: WHO; 1967. (Technical Report Series 379).

BAYLISASCARIASIS

Etiology: The agents of this infection are larvae of *Baylisascaris procyonis*, an ascarid found in the small intestine of raccoons. Natural patent infections have been found in two dogs, and rats, squirrels, and opossums have developed some specimens of adult ascarids in experimental infections. Other species of *Baylisascaris* are found in skunks, badgers, sables, and bears; no human infections by these other species have been reported, although the larvae migrate in mice and experimental infections have been produced in mice and chickens with *B. transfuga*.

B. procyonis is a typical ascarid; the female measures about 23 cm and the male, about 12 cm. The females lay eggs in the small intestine; these are expelled with the feces and, in three to four weeks, develop into infective larvae. These eggs may be eaten by the raccoons themselves or by intermediate hosts such as rodents, rabbits, or birds. Larvae that seem to belong to *B. procyonis* have been found in 19 species of mammals—mainly rodents and lagomorphs—and in 13 species of birds. These appear to be intermediate rather than paratenic hosts (see below). Young raccoons can become infected by ingesting infective eggs, but adult raccoons become infected only by ingesting the parasites in intermediate hosts. In young raccoons, the larvae develop first in the intestinal mucosa and then in the lumen; the eggs start to appear in the feces 50 to 76 days after infection. In adult raccoons, the larvae develop in the intestinal lumen and the eggs start to appear 32 to 38 days after infection. There is no extra-intestinal migration; transmission through the uterus or milk has not been studied.

Geographic Distribution and Occurrence: The infection is presumed to occur in areas where raccoons live. The prevalence of the infection in these animals can be very high, particularly in the northern and northeastern parts of the US; the infection in young animals has been 92% and 94%, respectively, in these areas. Seventy-two percent of 1,425 raccoons studied in the state of Indiana, 82% of 310 raccoons in the state of Illinois, and 70% of 33 raccoons in the state of Texas were found to be infected (Kerr *et al.*, 1997). Prevalence of the infection is low in the western US and very low to nonexistent in the southeast.

The first human infection was reported in 1984 (Huff *et al.*, 1984). Up until 1989, there were just two confirmed and two suspected cases of cerebral baylisascariasis and two cases of ocular baylisascariasis. Between 1989 and 2000, there were reports of one case of subacute diffuse unilateral neuroretinitis (Goldberg *et al.*, 1993), one case of meningoencephalitis in a 13-month-old child (Cunningham *et al.*, 1994), and one cardiac case in a 10-year-old child (Boschetti *et al.*, 1995).

The Disease in Man: Man is an intermediate rather than paratenic host. The human infection seems to be identical to that found in laboratory animals, in which it has been shown that the *B. procyonis* larvae continue to migrate, and that they molt and grow from 300 to 1,900 μm until they develop into eosinophilic granulomas.

B. procyonis causes visceral, ocular, and cerebrospinal syndromes in man. The severity of the disease depends on the number, location, and activity of the larvae. A mild infection with a small number of larvae, which mostly encapsulate in the connective and muscular tissue, will probably not produce clinical manifestations. A more intense infection can cause the typical signs of visceral larva migrans: fever, leukocytosis, eosinophilia, hepatomegaly, and pneumonitis. Due to the size and motility of the larvae, any infection that causes symptoms of visceral larva migrans can probably also cause nervous symptoms. The symptoms appear two to four weeks after infection, and include lethargy, lack of muscular coordination, torticollis, ataxia, and nystagmus, which progress to stupor, coma, and death. Ocular cases occur when the larvae invade the eye; the symptoms include unilateral vision loss, photophobia, and retinitis. Tunnels have been observed in the retina at seven days postinfection in experiments in monkeys.

The Disease in Animals: Infected raccoons are asymptomatic. In endemic areas, adult animals harbor 12 to 14 parasites and young animals harbor 48 to 62. Severe infections in young animals produce intestinal obstruction. There have been cases of symptomatic systemic or fatal infection caused by *Baylisascaris* larvae in puppies (Rudmann *et al.*, 1996), a gibbon in a zoo (Ball *et al.*, 1998), and a newborn lamb (Anderson, 1999), and other cases have been reported in monkeys, rodents, lago-morphs, and birds.

Source of Infection and Mode of Transmission: The source of infection is infected raccoons, which can eliminate millions of eggs a day. The eggs can survive in the soil for months or years. Man is thought to become infected accidentally by ingesting food or water, or through hands contaminated with the feces of infected raccoons.

Diagnosis: The human infection is suspected when symptoms of visceral larva migrans are accompanied by signs of alteration of the central nervous system, high peripheral eosinophilia, eosinophilia of the cerebrospinal fluid, and a history of exposure to raccoons. There are immunological tests for baylisascariasis, in partic-ular, enzyme immunoassay and immunoelectrotransfer (Cunningham *et al.*, 1994). *Baylisascaris* is antigenically closer to *Ascaris* than to *Toxocara*. The four human cases reported since 1994 were positive for *Baylisascaris* and negative for *Toxocara*, but one was positive for *Ascaris*. In raccoons, diagnosis of the infection is made by a finding of eggs in the feces or parasites in the feces or vomit. The eggs are similar to those of *T. canis*, but smaller. *Baylisascaris* eggs measure 62–70 μm by 52–58 μm, while *T. canis* eggs measure 85–90 by 73–77 μm.

Control: According to the available information, human baylisascariasis is very rare, but its control is important because people tend to keep raccoons as pets and the disease has no treatment. Pet raccoons should be examined for the parasite's eggs. If the examinations are positive, they should be treated with a medication effective against ascarids. Also, it should be borne in mind that the eggs can appear in the feces up to two and a half months after infection. In areas where raccoons are present, chim-neys and other openings through which these animals can enter a dwelling should be sealed. If nests are found, the feces should be burned. Like those of the other ascarids, *Baylisascaris* eggs are highly resistant to external environmental factors and disinfec-tants. If an area needs to be decontaminated, it is best to treat it with fire. Dryness and sunlight will kill the eggs, but it is not known how long this takes.

Bibliography

Anderson, B.C. Congenital *Baylisascaris* sp. larval migrans in a newborn lamb. *J Parasitol* 85(1):128–129, 1999.

Ball, R.L., M. Dryden, S. Wilson, J. Veatch. Cerebrospinal nematodiasis in a white-handed gibbon (*Hylobates lar*) due to *Baylisascaris* sp. *J Zoo Wildl Med* 29(2):221–224, 1998.

Boschetti, A., J. Kasznica. Visceral larva migrans induced eosinophilic cardiac pseudotu-mor: A cause of sudden death in a child. *J Forensic Sci* 40(6):1097–1099, 1995.

Cunningham, C.K., K.R. Kazacos, J.A. McMillan, *et al.* Diagnosis and management of *Baylisascaris procyonis* infection in an infant with nonfatal meningoencephalitis. *Clin Infect Dis* 18(6):868–872, 1994.

Goldberg, M.A., K.R. Kazacos, W.M. Boyce, E. Ai, B. Katz. Diffuse unilateral subacute neuroretinitis. Morphometric, serologic, and epidemiologic support for *Baylisascaris* as a causative agent. *Ophthalmology* 100(11):1695–1701, 1993.

Huff, D.S., R.C. Neafie, M.J. Binder, G.A. De Leon, L.W. Brown, K.R. Kazacos. The first fatal *Baylisascaris* infection in humans: An infant with eosinophilic meningoencephalitis. *Pediatr Pathol* 2(3):345–352, 1984.

Kazacos, K.R., W.M. Boyce. *Baylisascaris* larva migrans. *J Am Vet Med Assoc* 195(7):894–903, 1989.

Kerr, C.L., S.E. Henke, D.B. Pence. *Baylisascariasis* in raccoons from southern coastal Texas. *J Wildl Dis* 33(3):653–655, 1997.

Rudmann, D.G., K.R. Kazacos, S.T. Storandt, D.L. Harris, E.B. Janovitz. *Baylisascaris procyonis* larva migrans in a puppy: A case report and update for the veterinarian. *J Am Anim Hosp Assoc* 32(1):73–76, 1996.

CAPILLARIASIS

ICD-10 B81.1 Intestinal capillariasis;
B83.8 Other specified intestinal helminthiases

Synonym: Capillariosis.

Etiology: The agents of intestinal, hepatic, and pulmonary capillariasis are the nematodes *Capillaria philippinensis, C. hepatica,* and *C. aerophila,* respectively. The three species have different development cycles.

C. philippinensis is a filiform nematode. The female measures 2.5–5 mm long, and the male 1.5–4 mm. Its anterior extremity lodges in the mucosa of the small intestine in humans, particularly in the jejunum. The females can produce either larvae or eggs. The eggs are barrel-shaped and have opercula at both ends, very similar to those of *Trichuris*; they are eliminated with the feces, and when they enter fresh or contaminated bodies of water, they embryonate in 10 to 14 days and are ingested by a fish, in whose intestine they form infective larvae in approximately three weeks. If a larva is eaten by an appropriate host (man or a bird), it continues to develop, reaches the adult stage in about two weeks, and begins to lay larvae. These larvae do not leave the host's intestine. They develop to maturity and lay eggs, which will begin the external infection cycle anew. However, some females continue laying eggs, which mature in the host intestine without leaving it. In most cases, there is an overlap of oviparous and larviparous females, and as a result there is a combination of eggs, larvae, and adults in the host's feces (Neva and Brown, 1994). Although man is the only known host, it is thought that piscivorous birds are the natural hosts and that man is merely an accidental host who becomes infected by eating infected fish, which are the intermediate hosts (Cross and Basaca-Sevilla, 1991). In addition, experimental infections have been produced, using fish larvae, in monkeys and gerbils.

C. hepatica is also a filiform nematode, but it is longer than *C. philippinensis*; the females measure 5–8 cm long, and the males about half that. This is a common parasite of rodents and, occasionally, many other mammals. It lodges in the hepatic parenchyma, where it lays eggs, which remain trapped in the organ but do not develop to the infective stage. In order for *C. hepatica* to continue its development, the infected rodent must be eaten by a carnivore, which digests and releases the eggs enclosed in the hepatic tissue and eliminates them with the feces into the external environment, where they disseminate. To become infective, the eggs require a one- to two-month incubation period under favorable conditions of temperature, shade, aeration, and moisture. When the infective eggs are again eaten by a rodent, the larvae are released in the intestine, enter the intestinal wall, and are carried through the bloodstream to the liver, where they mature in approximately a month. *C. hepatica* is a helminth that is transmitted via the soil; therefore, hepatic capillariasis is a geo-helminthiasis. In moist soils, the eggs can remain viable for many months.

C. aerophila is a filiform parasite some 2–3 cm long. Its anterior extremity lodges in the mucosa of the trachea and bronchi of foxes, dogs, coyotes, and more rarely, other wild animals or cats. Human infection is rare. The eggs enter through the air-ways, are carried by the cilia and by coughing to the pharynx, are swallowed, and are eliminated with the feces. They develop an infective larva in five to seven weeks. When an appropriate host, such as a fox or dog, ingests the eggs, the larvae are released into the intestine and migrate through the bloodstream to the lungs in 7 to 10 days. Around 40 days after infection they reach maturity and begin oviposition.

Geographic Distribution and Occurrence: Intestinal capillariasis caused by *C. philippinensis* was first recognized in 1963 on Luzon Island in the Philippines. During the next five years, more than 1,500 cases were reported, with a 6% fatality rate. However, the prevalence of the infection seems relatively low, as eggs of the parasite were found in the feces of less than 3% of the 4,000 inhabitants of the endemic area examined during the epidemic outbreak in 1967 (Banzón, 1982). Aside from the Philippines, the most affected country seems to be Thailand, where 17 reported cases were reviewed (Peng *et al.*, 1993). From 1989 to 2000, 41 cases were reported throughout the world: 3 in Egypt, 1 in the United Arab Emirates, 2 in Spain, 1 in Greece, 1 in India, 1 in Indonesia, 3 in the Republic of Korea, 20 in Thailand, and 9 in Taiwan. One of the cases diagnosed in Spain involved a citizen of Colombia (Dronda *et al.*, 1993).

C. hepatica is found on all continents among synanthropic and wild rodents, with a prevalence rate that ranges from 0.7% to more than 85%. In Marseilles, France, the par-asite was found in 44% of 82 rats (Davoust *et al.*, 1997), and in Thailand, in 8% of 76 rats (Namue and Wongsawad, 1997). Besides rodents, the parasite has occasionally been found in other species of domestic and wild mammals. Infection in man is very rare; up until 1985, 11 cases of hepatic infection had been confirmed in Europe (9 in the former Czechoslovakia and 2 in Italy) and 14 others in the rest of the world (among them, 1 in Brazil, 5 in the US, 1 in Mexico, and 3 in South Africa). From 1989 to 2000, 10 other cases were reported: 1 in Germany, 1 in Japan, 3 in Mexico, 1 in the Republic of Korea, 3 in Switzerland, and 1 in Yugoslavia. In 1997, the worldwide prevalence was estimated at some 30 cases (Davoust *et al.*, 1997).

C. aerophila has been identified in animals in North America, Europe, the former Soviet Union, Australia, Chile, and Uruguay. In most animals, the prevalence is under 5% and often below 1%. Prevalences as high as 38% have been reported. Up until 1977, there were only nine known cases of human infection: one in Iran, one in Morocco, and seven in the former Soviet Union (Aftandelians *et al.*, 1977).

The Disease in Man: Intestinal capillariasis caused by *C. philippinensis* is a serious and fatal disease if not treated in time. Most patients are 20–45 years of age, with males predominating. The disease begins with insignificant symptoms such as borborygmus and vague abdominal pains. Intermittent diarrhea, which becomes persistent as the disease progresses, begins in two or three weeks, along with marked weight loss and cachexia. Gastrointestinal function is seriously affected; in addition, malabsorption and the loss of large quantities of protein, fat, and minerals have been confirmed. Death occurs as a result of heart failure or an intercurrent infection a few weeks or months after the onset of symptoms (Cross, 1992).

Clinical cases of hepatic capillariasis are due to a massive invasion of the liver by *C. hepatica*, which reaches maturity and begins to produce eggs in that organ. The disease is serious and frequently fatal. A prominent sign is hepatomegaly; other very common symptoms are high morning fever, nausea, vomiting, diarrhea or constipation, abdominal distension, edema of the extremities, splenomegaly, and sometimes pneumonia. A large part of the symptomatology is due to secondary infections in weakened patients, most of them children. In a case in an adult from Nigeria, the most prominent pathological feature was severe hepatic fibrosis and functional disorders related thereto (Attah *et al.*, 1983). Laboratory examinations find hyperleukocytosis with eosinophilia and hypochromic anemia, with abnormal values in liver function tests. Autopsy reveals the presence of grayish-white nodules on the surface of the liver. Histologically, the principal lesions consist of necrotic foci and granulomas. The adult parasites and eggs are found in the necrotic masses. Subclinical human infections undoubtedly occur, as attested to by solitary hepatic granulomas found in nine individuals autopsied during a study in the former Czechoslovakia. In seven of the nine cases, only one parasite larva was found in the lesions (Slais, 1973).

Pulmonary capillariasis caused by *C. aerophila* causes asthmatiform symptoms with coughing, mucoid or sometimes blood-tinged expectoration, fever, dyspnea, and moderate eosinophilia. Biopsy reveals granulomatous lesions with cellular reaction to a foreign body (Aftandelians *et al.*, 1977).

The Disease in Animals: *C. philippinensis* has not been found in land animals, but fish-eating birds are believed to be the natural hosts, though it is not known whether it causes symptoms in them. Experimental infection in primates of the genus *Macaca* or in wild rats is asymptomatic. In gerbils, on the other hand, the infection is manifested by a symptomatology similar to that in man (Banzón, 1982).

C. hepatica infections in rodents cause damage proportional to the parasite burden: mild infections may be subclinical; intense infections can cause hepatitis, splenomegaly, ascites, and eosinophilia; and massive infections can eventually cause hepatic necrosis. Although hepatic capillariasis does not have a high mortality rate, it could contribute to the control of rodent populations (McCallum, 1993). The infection was also found in one dog (Brander *et al.*, 1990).

C. aerophila infections are most severe in foxes, particularly in young animals. Intense infections can cause rhinitis, tracheitis, and bronchitis, which may end in bronchopneumonia caused by a secondary bacterial infection. Massive infections are often fatal.

Source of Infection and Mode of Transmission: Man is the only known definitive host of *C. philippinensis*. There are epidemiological reasons to suspect that the definitive natural hosts are piscivorous birds and that the intermediate hosts are fish in clean or contaminated waters. The main source of infection for humans seems to be infected fish, and the manner of infection is the ingestion of undercooked fish. Contamination of bodies of water with the excreta of humans or the birds that serve as hosts ensures perpetuation of the cycle. Given that the infection can be transmitted experimentally from one gerbil to another, with the parasite at different intestinal stages of development, direct person-to-person transmission may also occur (Banzón, 1982).

The main reservoir of *C. hepatica* is rodents. The infection is transmitted by ingestion of embryonated eggs that have been released from the liver of rodents and disseminated through the external environment by carnivores. In the peridomestic environment, the disseminating agents can be cats and dogs that hunt rodents. The eggs can also be released by cannibalism among rodents or by death and decomposition of their cadavers. For man, the source of direct infection is the soil, and the source of indirect infection is contaminated hands, food, or water. There are more than 30 described cases of spurious infections due to the ingestion of raw liver of rodents or other mammals, such as squirrels, monkeys, and wild boars, infected with unembryonated eggs. In such cases, the eggs of the parasite pass through the human digestive tract and are eliminated with the feces without causing true infection.

The source of *C. aerophila* infection for man and animals is the soil, where the eggs deposited with the feces of animals continue their incubation and the larvae reach the infective stage. Larvae can remain viable inside the eggs for a year or more. Children probably acquire the infection by ingesting dirt or water and food contaminated with eggs.

Diagnosis: A diagnosis of intestinal capillariasis caused by *C. philippinensis* is suspected in endemic zones when prolonged diarrhea with borborygmus and abdominal pain is observed in individuals who eat raw fish. Coprologic examination confirms the diagnosis, though a series of them may be necessary.

A specific diagnosis of hepatic capillariasis is suspected from the presence of fever, hepatomegaly, and eosinophilia in a patient in an endemic area. Confirmation can be obtained only from liver biopsy and identification of the parasite or its eggs. The discovery of *C. hepatica* eggs in human feces does not signify infection, but rather the passage of eggs through the intestine after ingestion of the liver of an infected animal.

Diagnosis of pulmonary capillariasis can be obtained by confirmation of the presence of eosinophils or the typical eggs in the sputum, or by biopsy of pulmonary tissue in which larvae or aspirated eggs can be found.

Control: In endemic areas, intestinal capillariasis can be prevented by refraining from eating raw or undercooked fish. Patients should be treated with thiabendazole, both for therapeutic reasons and to decrease the dissemination of parasite eggs. Hygienic elimination of human excreta is very important.

Hepatic capillariasis is a geohelminthiasis in which the eggs develop to the infective stage in the soil; they then penetrate the host orally through contaminated food or water or, in the case of man, via contaminated hands that are brought to the mouth or handle food. Consequently, individual prevention consists of carefully washing suspected foods and avoiding eating them raw; boiling both water and suspected foods; and washing hands carefully before eating. Since the infection is common in young children, who often eat dirt, and in homes in which rats abound, supervision of children's hygiene and rodent control can be important.

To prevent pulmonary capillariasis in animals and personnel on fox breeding farms, the animals must be kept in clean, well-ventilated, and sunny facilities to promote the destruction of the eggs. Young animals, which are the most susceptible and have the largest parasite burden, must be separated from adults. Any infection must be treated as soon as possible to prevent contamination of the environment with the eggs. Individuals can avoid infection by following strict hygiene rules to prevent infections with geohelminths.

Bibliography

Aftandelians, R., F. Raafat, M. Taffazoli, P.C. Beaver. Pulmonary capillariasis in a child in Iran. *Am J Trop Med Hyg* 26(1):64–71, 1977.

Attah, E.B., S. Nagarajan, E.N. Obineche, S.C. Gera. Hepatic capillariasis. *Am J Clin Pathol* 79(1):127–130, 1983.

Banzón, T. Human intestinal capillariasis (*Capillaria philippinensis*). *In*: Schultz, M.O., section ed. Section B, Vol. 2: *CRC Handbook Series in Zoonoses*. Boca Raton: CRC Press; 1982.

Brander, P., T. Denzler, M. Henzi. *Capillaria hepatica* bei einem Hund und einem Igel. *Schweiz Arch Tierheilkd* 132(7):365–370, 1990.

Cross, J.H. Intestinal capillariasis. *Clin Microbiol Rev* 5(2):120–129, 1992.

Cross, J.H., V. Basaca-Sevilla. Capillariasis *philippinensis*: A fish-borne parasitic zoonosis. *Southeast Asian J Trop Med Public Health* 22 Suppl:153–157, 1991.

Davoust, B., M. Boni, D. Branquet, J. Ducos de Lahitte, G. Martet. Recherche de trois infestations parasitaires chez des rats capturés à Marseille: Évaluation du risque zoonosique. *Bull Acad Natl Med* 181(5):887–895, 1997.

Dronda, F., F. Chaves, A. Sanz, R. López-Vélez. Human intestinal capillariasis in an area of nonendemicity: Case report and review. *Clin Inf Dis* 17(15):909–912, 1993.

McCallum, H.I. Evaluation of a nematode (*Capillaria hepatica* Bancroft, 1893) as a control agent for populations of house mice (*Mus musculus domesticus* Schwartz and Schwartz, 1943). *Rev Sci Tech* 12(1):83–93, 1993.

Namue, C., C. Wongsawad. A survey of helminth infection in rats (*Rattus* spp.) from Chiang Mai Moat. *Southeast Asian J Trop Med Public Health* 28 Suppl 1:179–183, 1997.

Neva, F.A., H.W. Brown. *Basic Clinical Parasitology*, 6th ed. Norwalk: Appleton & Lange; 1994.

Peng, H.W., H.L. Chao, P.C. Fan. Imported *Opisthorchis viverrini* and parasite infections from Thai labourers in Taiwan. *J Helminthol* 67(2):102–106, 1993.

Slais, J. The finding and identification of solitary *Capillaria* hepatica (Bancroft, 1893) in man in Europe. *Folia Parasitol (Praha)* 20(2):149–161, 1973.

CUTANEOUS LARVA MIGRANS

ICD-10 B76.9 Hookworm disease, unspecified

Synonyms: Creeping verminous dermatitis, serpiginous eruption, larva currens (infection caused by the larvae of *Strongyloides* spp.).

Etiology: Cutaneous larva migrans is a clinical description more than an etiologic diagnosis. The principal etiologic agent is the infective larva of *Ancylostoma braziliense*, an ancylostomid of dogs, cats, and other carnivores. Experimental infections have been produced in human subjects with other animal ancylostomids, such as *A. caninum* of dogs, *Uncinaria stenocephala* of dogs and cats, and *Bunostomum phlebotomum* of cattle. Since cases of cutaneous larva migrans have been seen occasionally in areas where these latter parasites are prevalent, it is assumed that they can also infect man in nature. However, the larvae of *A. braziliense* produce much more hyaluronidase (the substance that makes it possible to break down intercellular cement and invade tissue) than do those of the other ancylostomids (Hotez *et al.*, 1992), which may explain the greater incidence of this species. Cutaneous infection caused by the larvae of *Strongyloides stercoralis*, which progresses more rapidly than that caused by the larvae of ancylostomids, is currently called "larva currens," but it is also known as cutaneous larva migrans. In addition, some authors extend the validity of this term to gnathostomiasis (Díaz-Camacho *et al.*, 1998). Also, a case of invasion of human skin by *Pelodera strongyloides*, a free-living soil nematode related to *S. stercoralis* (the third known case in the world), was reported as cutaneous larva migrans (Jones *et al.*, 1991). The name "cutaneous larva migrans" has even been applied to the larvae of some arthropods that can colonize human skin, such as *Gasterophylus* and *Hypoderma* (Cypess, 1982). In individuals who have suffered previous infections, the human ancylostomids *A. duodenale* and *Necator americanus* can cause a picture of cutaneous allergy similar to that of cutaneous larva migrans. Here consideration is given only to the canine ancylostomes, with particular focus on *A. braziliense*.

Man is an aberrant host, in which the infective larvae cannot complete their development cycle and become adults. *A. braziliense* is a small species of *Ancylostoma*; the female measures about 1 cm long by 0.37 mm wide. Its life cycle is similar to that of the other ancylostomes (see the chapter on Zoonotic Ancylostomiasis).

Geographic Distribution and Occurrence: *A. braziliense* occurs in tropical and subtropical areas; *A. caninum* and *B. phlebotomum*, in temperate climates; and *U. stenocephala*, in colder parts of temperate regions (Barriga, 1997). Human cutaneous larva migrans occurs more frequently in tropical and subtropical areas. The disease has been reported in Argentina, Australia, southern Brazil, the Caribbean islands, France, Germany, India, Israel, Mexico (especially along the Gulf Coast), the Philippines, South Africa, Spain, southeastern US, and Uruguay, among other places. The prevalence of human infection is unknown. The fact that cases appear only sporadically in the literature suggests that it is a relatively infrequent condition. Nevertheless, a hospital in Paris, France, recorded 269 cases in a two-year period (Caumes *et al.*, 1995), and a hospital in Munich, Germany, registered 98 cases in four years (Jelinek *et al.*, 1994), most of them in travelers who had acquired the infection outside the country.

Infections caused by *A. braziliense* and other ancylostomes in dogs and cats can reach high prevalence rates: Malgor *et al.* (1996) found *A. braziliense* in 49% and *A. caninum* in 96% of 80 dogs autopsied in Uruguay, while Saleh *et al.* (1988) found *Ancylostoma* sp. in 68% of dogs examined in the Netherlands Antilles.

The Disease in Man: The infective larva produces a pruriginous papule upon penetrating the skin. In the days that follow, the larva travels around in the germinal layer and produces sinuous tunnels, advancing a few millimeters to several centimeters a day and forming vesicles along the tunnels on the outer surface of the skin. The migration of the larvae and the corresponding tissue reaction cause intense pruritus, especially at night, and may keep the patient awake. Secondary bacterial infections are common because the pruritus induces the patient to scratch. The lesion, which can be single or multiple, is most often located on the lower extremities (73% of the cases) and less frequently on the trunk and upper extremities (7% of the cases), but it can occur on any part of the skin exposed to contaminated soil. Lesions on the palm of the hand or the sole of the foot are particularly painful. The larvae usually remain alive and travel in the skin for two to eight weeks, at the end of which the disease is cured spontaneously. However, there have been patients in whom the infection persisted for as long as 18 to 55 months (Richey *et al.*, 1996). In a few cases, the levels of IgE and peripheral eosinophilia are elevated (Jelinek *et al.*, 1994). In one-third of the cases, the larvae manage to invade the lungs. Some patients suffer a transitory pneumonitis with eosinophilia (Loeffler syndrome), and in such cases larvae may be found in the sputum. *Ancylostoma* larvae have also been found in the cornea. This finding confirms the hypothesis that the larvae of animal ancylostomids can sometimes produce visceral infections in man. When the cause of larva currens is *S. stercoralis*, the lesion is less clearly defined than in cutaneous larva migrans and is characterized by intense erythema as well as by its rapid progression and quick disappearance. Oral albendazole and ivermectin have given excellent therapeutic results.

The Disease in Animals: The disease caused by ancylostomes in carnivores is mainly intestinal and is manifested by diarrhea, anemia, and malabsorption. Invasion of the skin by the larvae of *B. phlebotomum* in cattle or *U. stenocephala* in dogs can cause an allergic dermatitis, especially in repeated infections, which is generally short lived. The lesions are limited to the interdigital spaces, and the most prominent signs are erythema, pruritus, and papules that disappear about five days after the initial infection. Occasionally, the reactions are quite severe, prompting self-mutilation.

Source of Infection and Mode of Transmission: The source of infection is infective ancylostomid larvae found in the soil. The larvae develop from eggs that are shed in the feces of infected dogs or cats and land in a favorable environment— i.e., with warm temperatures and high humidity and sheltered from direct sunlight. Moist and sandy soils are the most propitious for development of the larvae. In countries with a temperate climate, the human infections occur in summer, whereas in tropical climates, they occur during the rainy season. Man is infected by contact with contaminated soil. The groups most exposed to the infection are children who play in the sand; workers who have close contact with the soil, such as gardeners, farmers, construction workers, and miners; and people who spend time at the beach. A study of contamination of children's sandboxes showed that *Toxocara* species were much more prevalent than *Ancylostoma*, perhaps because *Toxocara* eggs are more resistant to environmental conditions (Barriga, 1997).

Diagnosis: Clinical diagnosis is based on the nature and symptomatology of the lesions—i.e., serpiginous inflammations and intense pruritus. Although clinical detection can be challenging, in a series of 269 patients presenting at a tropical disease unit, cutaneous larva migrans was the most frequent diagnosis (25%), compared with pyoderma (18%), pruritic arthropod-reactive dermatitis (10%), myiasis (9%), tungiasis (6%), and urticaria (5%) (Caumes *et al.*, 1995). Diagnosis can be confirmed by biopsy of the affected skin to confirm the presence of larvae, but this method is only about 25% efficient. It is also difficult to identify the parasite in histological section, and because of this difficulty, it has not been possible to determine the percentage of cases due to *A. braziliense* compared with other species. Differential diagnosis should take into account the other parasites mentioned at the beginning of this chapter.

Control: The principal control measures are regular treatment of dogs and cats and the elimination of stray animals to reduce contamination of the soil. Dogs and cats should not be allowed on beaches or in places where children play in the sand. Whenever possible, areas susceptible to contamination should be kept dry, clean, and free of vegetation. The larvae of *Ancylostoma* live for almost a month in moist and grassy soils, but only one or two days on terrain that is bare, dry, and in direct sunlight (Barriga, 1997). Since the infective larvae develop in about four to five days at optimum temperatures, the removal of canine feces twice a week also reduces contamination.

Bibliography

Barriga, O.O. *Veterinary Parasitology for Practitioners*, 2nd ed. Edina: Burgess International Group; 1997.

Caumes, E., J. Carriere, G. Guermonprez, F. Bricaire, M. Danis, M. Gentilini. Dermatoses associated with travel to tropical countries: A prospective study of the diagnosis and management of 269 patients presenting to a tropical disease unit. *Clin Infect Dis* 20(3):542–548, 1995.

Cypess, R.H. Cutaneous larva migrans. *In*: Steele, J.H., section ed. Section C, Vol. 2: *CRC Handbook Series in Zoonoses*. Boca Raton: CRC Press; 1982.

Díaz-Camacho, S.P., M. Zazueta Ramos, E. Ponce Torrecillas, *et al.* Clinical manifestations and immunodiagnosis of gnathostomiasis in Culiacán, Mexico. *Am J Trop Med Hyg* 59(6):908–915, 1998.

Hotez, P.J., S. Narasimhan, J. Haggerty, *et al.* Hyaluronidase from infective *Ancylostoma* hookworm larvae and its possible function as a virulence factor in tissue invasion and in cutaneous larva migrans. *Infect Immun* 60(3):1018–1023, 1992.

Jelinek, T., H. Maiwald, H.D. Nothdurft, T. Loscher. Cutaneous larva migrans in travelers: Synopsis of histories, symptoms, and treatment of 98 patients. *Clin Infect Dis* 19(6):1062–1066, 1994.

Jones, C.C., T. Rosen, C. Greenberg. Cutaneous larva migrans due to *Pelodera strongyloides*. *Cutis* 48(2):123–126, 1991.

Malgor, R., Y. Oku, R. Gallardo, I. Yarzabal. High prevalence of *Ancylostoma* spp. infection in dogs, associated with endemic focus of human cutaneous larva migrans, in Tacuarembó, Uruguay. *Parasite* 3(2):131–134, 1996.

Richey, T.K., R.H. Gentry, J.E. Fitzpatrick, A.M. Morgan. Persistent cutaneous larva migrans due to *Ancylostoma* species. *South Med J* 89(6):609–611, 1996.

Saleh, F.C., C.E. Kirkpatrick, O. De Haseth, J.B. Lok. Occurrence of some blood and intestinal parasites in dogs in Curaçao, Netherlands Antilles. *Trop Geogr Med* 40(4):318–321, 1988.

DIOCTOPHYMOSIS

ICD-10 B83.8 Other specified helminthiases

Synonym: Dioctophymiasis.

Etiology: *Dioctophyma* (*Dioctophyme*) *renale* is a large, blood-red nematode that in the adult stage lodges in the kidneys of minks, occasionally other mustelids, and at times, wild and domestic canids. In dogs, the adult female of the parasite can reach up to 1 m long and 5–12 mm wide and is therefore known as the "giant kidney worm." The male is much smaller. The size of the parasite depends on the host species; for example, in minks it is not more than a few centimeters long.

The definitive host eliminates the eggs of the parasite via the urine. The eggs develop in water and, depending on the temperature, form a first-stage larva in 15 to 102 days. The larval eggs must be ingested by the free-living aquatic oligochaete annelid *Lumbriculus variegatus*, in whose intestine they hatch quickly and then invade the coelomatic cavity. There, the larva undergoes two molts and becomes an infective, third-stage larva in 70 to 120 days or more. Several fish, such as *Ictalurus nebulosus* and *Esox lucius* in North America or *Idus* spp. in Europe, or frogs such as *Rana pipiens*, *R. clamitans*, and *R. septentrionalis*, can ingest the infected worm. In that case, the infective larva encysts in the mesentery or liver without continuing its development to the adult stage. These animals are paratenic or transport hosts. If a mink or other suitable host ingests an infected worm or paratenic host, the larva is released by digestion of the tissues, penetrates the mammal's stomach wall, molts in the submucosa, migrates to the liver, passes into the peritoneal cavity, and reaches the kidney. The juvenile nematodes, which are already several centimeters long, penetrate the renal pelvis, mature, and begin laying eggs five or six months after infection. In dogs, some specimens remain in the peritoneal cavity, near the kidney, but never really invade it (Barriga, 1982).

Geographic Distribution and Occurrence: With the possible exception of Africa and Oceania, the parasite is distributed worldwide and has been found in many species of carnivores. The most commonly reported form is canine dioctophymosis. In the Americas, the animal parasitosis has been described in Argentina, Brazil, Canada, Paraguay, Uruguay, and the US, and in other countries as well. Prevalences of between 18% and 48% have been found in minks, 2% in otters, and 1.5% in weasels. Although prevalences of 37% in dogs and 35% in jackals have occasionally been reported, in most cases the infection rate in dogs is under 1%. *D. renale* is, in fact, rarely discovered in veterinary practice; 60% of *D. renale* in dogs are not located in the liver and are therefore not patent and can go unnoticed. Until 1969, only 204 cases of canine dioctophymosis had been reported in the world literature. It is very infrequently reported in bovines, equines, and swine. These numbers, the fact that the parasite is almost always found in the kidney of minks, from which it can eliminate its eggs to the outside, and the fact that the parasite is found less than half the time in the kidney of dogs, indicate that mustelids, particularly minks, are the definitive natural hosts of the parasite. The infection is very rare in man. Until 1982, the literature described just 13 well-documented cases of infections in the human kidney (Barriga, 1982). There are also three human cases in which larvae of *D. renale* were found in ectopic locations (Gutiérrez *et al.,* 1989).

The Disease in Man and Animals: In humans and dogs, the nematode usually locates in just one kidney, most often the right one, and in most cases, only one parasite is found. As it grows, *Dioctophyma* destroys the renal parenchyma and, in extreme cases, leaves only the capsule of the organ. The most prominent symptoms include renal colic and hematuria or pyuria. In some cases, the parasite migrates to the ureter or urethra and blocks the flow of urine. In dogs, cases in which the parasite remains in the peritoneum are usually asymptomatic, though this localization can occasionally cause peritonitis. The healthy organ compensates for the loss of renal function and generally hypertrophies.

Source of Infection and Mode of Transmission: Minks seem to be the main reservoirs. The definitive wild hosts are infected when they ingest the infected intermediate hosts (worms) or the paratenic hosts (frogs or fish). Humans and, very probably, dogs are accidental hosts that almost always harbor only one parasite. Both are probably infected by eating undercooked fish or frogs. The rarity of human infection is explained by the fact that the larvae are located in the mesentery or liver of fish or frogs, organs that man generally does not consume.

Diagnosis: When the parasite infecting a human or dog is a female that is in contact with the urinary tract, the parasitosis can be diagnosed by observing its eggs in urinary sediment. Renal infections caused by a male parasite or located in the peritoneum can be diagnosed only by laparotomy or at autopsy.

Control: The infection can be prevented, both in humans and dogs, by avoiding the consumption of raw or undercooked frogs and fish.

Bibliography

Barriga, O.O. Dioctophymiasis. *In:* Schultz, M.O., section ed. Section C, Vol. 2: *CRC Handbook Series in Zoonoses.* Boca Raton: CRC Press; 1982.

Fyvie, A. *Dioctophyma renale. In:* Davis, J.W., R.C. Anderson, eds. *Parasitic Diseases of Wild Mammals.* Ames: Iowa State University Press; 1971.

Gutiérrez Y., M. Cohen, C.N. Machicao. Dioctophyme larva in the subcutaneous tissues of a woman in Ohio. *Am J Surg Pathol* 13(9):800–802, 1989.

DRACUNCULIASIS

ICD-10 B72

Synonyms: Dracontiasis, dracunculosis, guinea-worm disease.

Etiology: The agent of this infection is *Dracunculus medinensis*, one of the longest nematodes known, despite its variable size. The female measures 50–120 cm long and 1–2 mm wide, while the male is much smaller, measuring 12–29 mm long and 0.4 mm wide. The male is rarely seen in patients because it dies soon after copulation. In its adult stage, *D. medinensis* parasitizes man and a variety of domestic and wild animals, including monkeys, carnivores, cattle, and equines. The species *D. insignis*, found in North America, has a life cycle similar to that of *D. medinensis*, but it infects carnivores and rodents, especially those with semiaquatic habits such as raccoons, dogs, skunks, weasels, nutrias, and muskrats. The females of the two species are indistinguishable, but *D. insignis* has not been observed in human infections.

The first-stage larvae of *D. medinensis* are expelled through the skin by the gravid females. In order to continue its development, the larva must be ingested within one to three weeks by an intermediate host, which is a copepod microcrustacean of the genus *Cyclops*. About 15 different species of *Cyclops* are known to serve as intermediate hosts. Once the larva is ingested by an appropriate species of copepod, it will continue its development in the coelomic cavity of the intermediate host for three to six weeks, until it becomes an infective third-stage larva. When the copepod, acting as intermediate host, is ingested in turn by a definitive host, the larva is released in the intestine of the latter, traverses the intestinal wall, and, probably migrating through the lymphatic system, finds a site in deep subcutaneous or retroperitoneal conjunctive tissue, where it becomes embedded. The worms mature in about three to four months. They then copulate, after which the male dies and the female penetrates deeply into the tissue, remaining there for months until her uterus is filled with first-stage larvae. Ten to 14 months after the initial infection, the parasite migrates to the surface of the body, especially the legs, feet, ankles, knees, and wrists, and occasionally other parts, and positions its anterior end in close contact with the inner surface of the skin. There, it produces an irritation which at first forms a hard papule on the skin. The papule soon turns into a vesicle, and eventually, an ulcer. When this part of the skin is immersed in water, the parasite starts to have uterine contractions that rupture the vesicle (if it has not yet ulcerated), and releases about 500,000 first-stage larvae into the external environment. Subsequent contacts with water repeat the phenomenon, but the number of larvae released is smaller. In general, the females live for 12 to 18 months, although many of them die and are expelled spontaneously. Sometimes additional live larvae are extracted from patients.

Geographic Distribution and Occurrence: Dracunculiasis is restricted to tropical and subtropical regions of Africa and Asia, probably because the *D. medinensis* larva develops best at 25°C to 30°C and cannot grow at temperatures lower than 19°C (Muller, 1979). The infection is endemic in several regions of western and eastern Africa, as well as western India and Pakistan. In Africa, it is found within a triangle formed by Côte d'Ivoire, the border between Ethiopia and Kenya, and Mali. The countries most affected are Benin, Ghana, Nigeria, and Togo. In the past, there have been minor endemic foci in parts of Asia, such as Iran, Yemen, Saudi Arabia, and possibly Iraq, but these foci seem to have disappeared. In 1947, Stoll estimated that there were 43 million infections worldwide, but this figure would appear to be quite exaggerated. The World Health Organization (WHO) calculated the worldwide prevalence in 1976 at about 10 million. However, in 1978, only 26,980 cases were reported. This disease is obviously underregistered. A study carried out in Togo in 1977 found that less than 4% of the cases observed had been reported to the public health authorities (WHO, 1982). In Ghana and Nigeria, the countries with the highest prevalences of dracunculiasis, incidence of the infection in 1991 was down 33% relative to 1990 and 57% relative to 1989 (CDC, 1992). Although in 1992 there were still 3 million people infected and some 100 million at risk for the infection in India, Pakistan, and 17 African countries, these figures represented a dramatic improvement over the situation that existed a decade earlier (Hopkins and Ruiz-Tiben, 1992). In 2000, only 75,223 cases were reported to WHO, all of them from sub-Saharan Africa (WHO, 2003a).

In some endemic foci, a high proportion of the population is infected. In southern Togo, for example, in 1989 the prevalence of infection was estimated at 80% and the incidence at 50% (Petit et al., 1989). A study of 1,200 individuals in Nigerian villages revealed that 982 (82%) were infected (Okoye et al., 1995). In some villages of Ghana and southern India, 50% of the people have been found to be infected. The age group most affected was 20- to 40-year-olds, and reinfection was common (Johnson and Joshi, 1982).

In the Western Hemisphere, there have been foci in some parts of the Antilles, Brazil (Bahia), French Guiana, and Guyana, all of which have disappeared spontaneously. It is believed that the infection was brought from Africa along with the slave trade. In addition, there have been imported cases of dracunculiasis outside the known endemic areas. For example, since 1995 there have been two cases in the US, both of them imported from Sudan (CDC, 1998). In the eastern US, some sporadic cases of human dracunculiasis were attributed to *D. insignis* (WHO, 1979).

Dracunculus medinensis occurs naturally in monkeys, wild and domestic carnivores, cattle, and equines. In northern Argentina, four cases of *Dracunculus* infection were reported, but the species were not identified (Hoyos et al., 1995).

The Disease in Man: The prepatent period, from initial infection until emergence of the parasite in the skin, lasts about a year and does not produce any symptoms in the host. Indeed, the first sign of the infection is usually the papule or vesicle that appears prior to larviposition by the parasite, approximately a year after the initial infection. It may be that allergic symptomatology is absent during this period because the parasite covers itself with host proteins that hide it from the immune system (Bloch et al., 1999). Symptoms appear when the parasite initiates its final migration to the skin surface. Shortly before or at the same time the vesicle is formed, some of the following allergic manifestations begin to develop: urticaria, pruritus, dyspnea, vomiting, mild fever, and sometimes fainting. Once the vesicle is formed and before the parasite emerges, the patient feels a strong burning sensation, which he may try to alleviate by immersing the affected part in cold water. The symptoms disappear when the vesicle ruptures and the parasite emerges. The vesicle and subsequent ulcer usually appear on the skin of the feet, ankles, legs, knees, wrists, and, less often, the upper part of the body. The ulcer forms a scar about a month after the patient is rid of the parasite.

The most serious complications stem from secondary bacterial infections that gain entry through the open lesion and can propagate along the length of the tunnel excavated by the parasite. These infections often occur as a result of failed attempts to extract the parasite. If it ruptures in the process, larvae may remain trapped in the subcutaneous tissue and give rise to cellulitis and abscesses. Chronic ulcers, arthritis, and tendon contractions are other common sequelae. Although the parasite triggers antibody reactions, it does not appear to induce protective immunity (Bloch and Simonsen, 1998).

Even when there are no complications, many patients remain incapacitated for several weeks or months. According to a study conducted in the district of Ibadan, Nigeria, patients remained disabled for an average of 100 days. The degree of incapacity was related to the number of parasites and their localization: sites in the ankle and foot were the most serious (Kale, 1977). A study of 1,200 persons in Nigerian villages showed that 982 (82%) were infected. Of these, 206 (21%) were totally incapacitated; 193 (20%) were seriously incapacitated; 431 (44%), moderately incapacitated; and 152 (16%) were unaffected (Okoye et al., 1995).

The Disease in Animals: The course and clinical manifestations of dracunculiasis in animals are very similar to those seen in man. In dogs, there have been clinical cases of purulent fistulated skin nodules caused by *D. insignis* (Beyer et al., 1999).

Source of Infection and Mode of Transmission: The disease is found in rural areas and is directly linked to the lack of potable water in poor tropical and subtropical regions, an arid climate, or prolonged dry seasons. Transmission is more intense during the dry season, when lagoons, ponds, and other water bodies are at low levels and the density of infected copepods increases. In desert climates, however, transmission of the infection is more frequent during the rainy season. The main sources of infection for man are shallow lagoons, ponds, wells dug in dry river beds, cisterns, and wells that are accessed via steps and that people enter to obtain water. The infective element is the copepod harboring third-stage larva, which can only live in still water. Frogs and tadpoles are paratenic hosts for *D. insignis* (Eberhard and Brandt, 1995). It is not known if there are paratenic hosts for *D. medinensis*.

Infected humans contaminate the water with larvae escaping from their cutaneous parasitic ulcers, and the larvae, in turn, infect other humans when they drink water containing infected copepods. The infection is distinctly seasonal in nature because of two factors: a) climatic changes that affect the various sources of water, and b) the development cycle of the parasite itself (Muller, 1979). The transmission period peaks at different times depending on the particular endemic area and on ecological conditions. In the Sahel region of Africa, where annual precipitation is less than 75 cm^3, infection occurs during the rainy season and for a few months thereafter, until the lagoons dry up. On the other hand, in the desert foci of southern Iran, where rainwater is collected in large protected cisterns that are rarely empty, the incidence is higher during the dry season, when the density of copepods is greater. In each endemic area, one or two species of *Cyclops*—usually the largest and most carnivorous—serve as intermediate hosts. In an endemic region of Nigeria, it has been estimated that each inhabitant ingests some 75 infected copepods a year.

Man is undoubtedly the main definitive host and reservoir of the parasite. The role of animals in the epidemiology of human dracunculiasis is not yet clear and has been the subject of debate. Domestic animals, especially dogs, can be an additional reservoir of secondary importance in areas with high rates of human infection. Even though there are indications that these animals alone can maintain the infection in nature, the proportion of these hosts that may be infected by *D. medinensis* relative to other species of *Dracunculus* is still unknown. Indeed, *D. medinensis* occurs in some places where the human infection has not been recorded, such as Malaysia and Tanzania. In Kazakhstan, for example, after an endemic focus of human dracunculiasis was eradicated, a study found that 11.7% of 213 dogs examined were parasitized. However, the animal infection does not appear to have interfered with numerous successful campaigns to eradicate the human infection.

Diagnosis: Diagnosis presents no difficulties once the cephalic end of the parasite has emerged. If necessary, the infection can be confirmed by pouring a little cold water on the ulcer and then examining a drop of the exudate for the presence of first-stage larvae. Radiologic examination reveals dead and calcified parasites. Several immunologic tests have been used for diagnosing this parasite. The enzyme-linked immunosorbent assay (ELISA) used with the antigen of first-stage larvae to detect IgG4 antibodies was 83% sensitive and 97% specific. Moreover, it was possible to increase sensitivity to 97% by refining the antigen and measuring various types of antibody at the same time (Bloch and Simonsen, 1998). An attempt was made to diagnose the disease on the basis of parasite antigen in the bloodstream, but none could be found (Bloch *et al.*, 1998).

Control: In 1980, the US Centers for Disease Control initiated a global campaign to eradicate dracunculiasis, and WHO considers that it can be eradicated successfully (WHO, 2003b). The most important preventive measure is to provide populations with a regular supply of potable water. In Nigeria, the provision of piped water to a city of 30,000 inhabitants reduced incidence from 60% to 0% in the course of two years. When economic conditions in an area are inadequate to provide potable water, prevention consists of educating the population and identifying subterranean water sources. Individuals can boil or filter surface water, treat their drinking water to kill the intermediate hosts, and take precautions to avoid contaminating water sources.

Public health education is of the utmost importance in the control of dracunculiasis because patients in hyperendemic areas do not look upon the parasite as an agent of infection; they see it as a normal condition of the human body, and hence they do not associate it with the ingestion of contaminated water (Bierlich, 1995). Moreover, two-thirds of the population consider that boiling or filtering water is inconvenient and impractical (Ilegbodu *et al.*, 1991). Digging wells to extract subterranean water with hand pumps appears to be a very effective solution. When this approach was tried in Ghana's Upper Region, it protected between 88% and 96% of the population there (Hunter, 1997). Treatment of drinking water with temephos to kill the crustaceans that are intermediate hosts is simple and effective. Also, providing the population with nylon mesh strainers to filter out copepods has yielded excellent results (Kaul *et al.*, 1992). A study conducted in Pakistan showed that the filters were adequate to remove the copepods even after 12 to 15 months of use (Imtiaz *et al.*, 1990). Filters with 200-micron holes capture the large copepods, which are the ones that harbor *Dracunculus* larvae. Finally, in Tashkent and Samarkand,

Uzbekistan, the disease was eradicated more than half a century ago by the simple strategy of closing all the stepped wells and replacing them with curbed wells, so that people could no longer go inside and contaminate the water.

Bibliography

Beyer, T.A., R.D. Pinckney, A.J. Cooley. Massive *Dracunculus insignis* infection in a dog. *J Am Vet Med Assoc* 214:366–368, 1999.

Bierlich, B. Notions and treatment of guinea worm in northern Ghana. *Soc Sci Med* 41:501–509, 1995.

Bloch, P., P.E. Simonsen. Studies on immunodiagnosis of dracunculiasis. I. Detection of specific serum antibodies. *Acta Trop* 70:73–86, 1998.

Bloch, P., B.J. Vennervald, P.E. Simonsen. Studies on immunodiagnosis of dracunculiasis. II. Search for circulating antigens. *Acta Trop* 70:303–315, 1998.

Bloch, P., M. Lund, B.J. Vennervald, P.E. Simonsen. Human serum albumin and immunoglobulin on *Dracunculus medinensis*. *Acta Trop* 73:135–141, 1999.

Eberhard, M.L., F.H. Brandt. The role of tadpoles and frogs as paratenic hosts in the life cycle of *Dracunculus insignis* (Nematoda: Dracunculoidea). *J Parasitol* 81:792–793, 1995.

Hopkins, D.R., E. Ruiz-Tiben. Surveillance for dracunculiasis, 1981–1991. *MMWR CDC Surveill Summ* 41:1–13, 1992.

Hoyos, C.B., G.A. Jara, C.M. Monzon. Reporte de un caso de dracunculosis en un canino en la provincia de Formosa—Argentina. *Rev Inst Med Trop Sao Paulo* 37:273–275, 1995.

Hunter, J.M. Bore holes and the vanishing of guinea worm disease in Ghana's upper region. *Soc Sci Med* 45:71–89, 1997.

Ilegbodu, V.A., A.E. Ilegbodu, R.A. Wise, B.L. Christensen, O.O. Kale. Clinical manifestations, disability and use of folk medicine in *Dracunculus* infection in Nigeria. *J Trop Med Hyg* 94:35–41, 1991.

Imtiaz, R., J.D. Anderson, E.G. Long, J.J. Sullivan, B.L. Cline. Monofilament nylon filters for preventing dracunculiasis: Durability and copepod retention after long term field use in Pakistan. *Trop Med Parasitol* 41:251–253, 1990.

Johnson, S., V. Joshi. Dracontiasis in western Rajasthan, India. *Trans R Soc Trop Med Hyg* 76:36–40, 1982.

Kale, O.O. The clinico-epidemiological profile of guinea-worm in the Ibadan District of Nigeria. *Am J Trop Med Hyg* 26:208–214, 1977.

Kaul, S.M., R.S. Sharma, T. Verghese. Monitoring the efficacy of temephos application and use of fine mesh nylon strainers by examination of drinking water containers in guineaworm endemic villages. *J Commun Dis* 24:159–163, 1992.

Muller, R. Guinea-worm disease: Epidemiology, control, and treatment. *Bull World Health Organ* 57:683–689, 1979.

Okoye, S.N., C.O. Onwuliri, J.C. Anosike. A survey of predilection sites and degree of disability associated with guineaworm (*Dracunculus medinensis*). *Int J Parasitol* 25:1127–1129, 1995.

Petit, M.M., M. Deniau, C. Tourte-Schaefer, K. Amegbo. Étude epidémiologique longitudinale de la dracunculose dans le sud du Togo. *Bull Soc Pathol Exot Filiales* 82:520–530, 1989.

United States of America, Department of Health and Human Services, Centers for Disease Control and Prevention (CDC). Update: dracunculiasis eradication—Ghana and Nigeria, 1991. *MMWR Morb Mortal Wkly Rep* 41:397–399, 1992.

United States of America, Department of Health and Human Services, Centers for Disease Control and Prevention (CDC). Imported dracunculiasis—United States, 1995 and 1997. *MMWR Morb Mortal Wkly Rep* 47:209–211, 1998.

World Health Organization (WHO). *Parasitic Zoonoses. Report of a WHO Expert Committee, with the Participation of FAO.* Geneva: WHO; 1979. (Technical Report Series 637).

World Health Organization (WHO). Dracunculiasis surveillance. *Wkly Epidemiol Rec* 57:65–72, 1982.

World Health Organization (WHO). Dracunculiasis [web page]. Available at www.who.int/ctd/dracun/progress.htm. Accessed 11 March 2003. 2003a.

World Health Organization (WHO). Dracunculiasis Erradication [web page]. Available at www.who.int/ctd/dracun/index.html. Accessed 11 March 2003. 2003b.

ESOPHAGOSTOMIASIS AND TERNIDENSIASIS

ICD-10 B81.8 Other specified intestinal helminthiases

Synonyms: Helminthoma, helminthic abscesses, nodular worm infection.

Etiology: The agents of these diseases are strongylid nematodes of the species *Oesophagostomum bifurcum, O. stephanostomum, O. aculeatum (O. apiostomum),* and *Ternidens deminutus.* They live in the intestine of nonhuman primates and sometimes humans, causing the formation of nodules in the intestinal wall. The taxonomy of the esophagostomes in primates is still not fully understood. Levine (1980) has suggested that *O. bifurcum* is at least partially homologous with *O. stephanostomum, O. apiostomum,* and other species. Apparently most recent authors agree with this view, because *O. bifurcum* is the only human esophagostome mentioned in the literature since 1989.

The life cycles of the species of *Oesophagostomum* that occur in primates have not been fully elucidated, but it is assumed that they follow patterns similar to those of other species of the genus, which are common parasites of domestic animals. Adult females measure 8–13 mm long and live in the large intestine. The eggs are shed with feces, mature, and release a first-stage larva. In five to seven days at ambient temperature, the first-stage larva develops into a third-stage larva, which is encysted within the cuticle of the second-stage larva and is infective. Primates acquire the infection by ingesting third-stage larvae. In the stomach and small intestine of the host, the larva frees itself from its cuticular sheath, penetrates the intestinal mucosa, and transforms into the next stage. Growth of the fourth-stage larva in the mucosa, especially of the large intestine, produces nodules 1–3 mm in diameter, known as a "nodular worms." When the larva emerges from the intestinal lumen, it leaves an ulcer several millimeters in diameter, and the nodule fills with pus (Barriga, 1997). The larva continues to mature until it reaches the adult stage and mates. At 30 to 40 days after the initial infection, the female begins to lay eggs. However, most of the parasites found in man are immature or nongravid.

The females of *T. deminutus* measure 12–16 mm long and 0.6 mm wide. The parasite localizes mainly in the large intestine, but sometimes it has been found in the small intestine. Its life cycle is still not fully understood. From the time its eggs are shed in feces until it transforms into a third-stage larva in soil, its evolution is similar to that of the esophagostomes, but what happens to the parasite from that point on is not known. Attempts to infect human volunteers and baboons with third-stage larvae have failed. Consequently, some authors suspect that *T. deminutus* may require an intermediate host for its subsequent development, which would be unusual for this taxonomic group. The eggs of *Oesophagostomum* spp. and *T. deminutus* are indistinguishable from those of the ancylostomids.

Geographic Distribution and Occurrence: The esophagostomes that infect man are natural parasites of monkeys and apes. Human infection is accidental and relatively infrequent: as of 1989, about 70 cases had been reported, almost all of them in Africa (Ross *et al.*, 1989). There have also been cases of human esophagostomiasis attributed to various species in Brazil, Indonesia, and Nigeria, where it is said that 4% of a prison population was infected. The first human case in Malaysia was reported in 1992 (Karim and Yang, 1992). In West Africa, *O. bifurcum* is common in northern Ghana and Togo, where human prevalence can be as high as 59% in small isolated villages and the infection usually occurs in association with ancylostomids. The human infection begins to appear in children 3 to 5 years old, and prevalence stabilizes at the age of 10 (Krepel *et al.*, 1992). *Oesophagostomum* infection is common in nonhuman primates. Among imported monkeys in the US, the infection rate of *O. bifurcum* has been as high as 53%, and that of *O. apiostomum*, 70% (Flynn, 1973).

T. deminutus is found in nature among monkeys and apes of Africa, India, and Indonesia. It is infrequent in laboratory primates, but prevalence has been as high as 76% among monkeys in South Africa (Flynn, 1973). The human infection has been observed in the southern half of Africa in Malawi, Mauritius, Mozambique, Democratic Republic of Congo, Tanzania, South Africa, Uganda, Zambia, and Zimbabwe, as well as in Comoros (Goldsmid, 1982). In Zimbabwe, infection rates have been as high as 87%. A coprologic survey of 5,545 patients in a Zimbabwe hospital found that *T. deminutus* was the second most frequent parasite (3.75% versus 5.75% for ancylostomids), but the intensity of infection was almost always low.

The Disease in Man and Animals: Pages *et al.* (1988) reviewed 28 cases of intestinal pseudotumors caused by esophagostomes. The lesions consist of nodules in the intestinal wall, primarily the large intestine, each of which contains a larva surrounded by purulent or necrotic matter. These nodules can produce abscesses, fistulas, and tumors in the intestinal wall. Mild human infections caused by *Oesophagostomum* spp. go unnoticed. In clinical cases, the symptoms range from vague abdominal pain to intestinal obstruction associated with tumors. The disease can be mistaken for ameboma, carcinoma of the colon, appendicitis, or ileocecal tuberculosis. A subcutaneous nodule caused by one of these species has been reported in a human patient (Ross et al., 1989).

Heavily parasitized monkeys develop dysenteric diarrhea. Several authors think that *Oesophagostomum* spp. are important pathogenic agents in nonhuman primates that can sometimes cause fatal disease. However, the available descriptions are insufficient to determine whether the parasitosis was in fact the main cause of death.

The larvae of *T. deminutus* form nodules and even ulcers in the intestine. Despite the fact that the adult larvae ingest blood, the infections do not cause significant symptoms; many of them are asymptomatic, and the rest pass with only mild diarrhea and vague abdominal pain.

Source of Infection and Mode of Transmission: Nonhuman primates are the main reservoir of the infection. In esophagostomiasis, the source of infection is the soil, where the infective larvae are found. The infection is produced by the ingestion of larvae in food or water or from contaminated hands, and it occurs almost exclusively during the rainy season (Krepel *et al.*, 1995). Man is an accidental host in whom the parasite seldom reaches maturity and oviposition. The epidemiology of *T. deminutus* infection has not yet been clarified. Some investigators admit the possibility that, in addition to the cycle between monkeys and humans, there may be a person-to-person cycle as well, and they also suspect the intervention of an intermediate host (Goldsmid, 1982).

Diagnosis: Human esophagostomiasis is difficult to diagnose because the symptoms are not specific and, in most cases, the parasites do not reach maturity and do not lay eggs. In such cases, diagnosis is confirmed by histologic examination of biopsies or surgical material. When eggs are observed, they should be differentiated from other species. *T. deminutus* infection is diagnosed by examining eggs in feces. The eggs of ancylostomids, *T. deminutus, Oesophagostomum, Strongyloides,* and *Trichostrongylus* are very similar, and it is therefore necessary to culture them and study the third-stage larvae in order to differentiate the species. Goldsmid (1982) has published useful criteria for identifying the eggs and third-stage larvae of these species. It has been calculated that each female *O. bifurcum* lays an average of 33.7 eggs per gram of feces (Krepel and Polderman, 1992), but this figure is relatively unimportant because most of the damage produced by the esophagostomes results from the activity of larvae and not the adult parasites. Several immunologic tests have been tried for detecting esophagostomiasis, but most of them are not sufficiently specific. Nevertheless, up to 95% specificity has been attained with an enzyme-linked immunosorbent assay (ELISA) designed to detect IgG4 antibody (Polderman *et al.*, 1993). In addition, there are differences in rDNA between *O. bifurcum* and *Necator americanus,* which suggests that the two species could be differentiated using polymerase chain reaction (Romstad *et al.*, 1997).

Control: Esophagostomiasis, and probably ternidensiasis, are geohelminthiases in which the eggs reach the infective stage in soil and penetrate the host via the oral route through contaminated food, water, or hands. Therefore, protective measures for individuals consist of carefully washing or boiling suspicious foods, boiling water, and washing hands carefully before eating. The infections are not sufficiently frequent to justify community prevention campaigns.

Bibliography

Barriga, O.O. *Veterinary Parasitology for Practitioners,* 2nd ed. Edina: Burgess International Group; 1997.

Flynn, R.J. *Parasites of Laboratory Animals.* Ames: Iowa State University Press; 1973.

Goldsmid, J.M. Ternidens infection. In: Steele, J.H., section ed. Section C, Vol. 2: *CRC Handbook Series in Zoonoses.* Boca Raton: CRC Press; 1982.

Karim, N., C.O. Yang. Oesophagostomiasis in man: Report of the first Malaysian case with emphasis on its pathology. *Malays J Pathol* 14:19–24, 1992.

Krepel, H.P., A.M. Polderman. Egg production of *Oesophagostomum bifurcum,* a locally common parasite of humans in Togo. *Am J Trop Med Hyg* 46:469–472, 1992.

Krepel, H.P., S. Baeta, A.M. Polderman. Human *Oesophagostomum* infection in northern Togo and Ghana: Epidemiological aspects. *Ann Trop Med Parasitol* 86:289–300, 1992.

Krepel, H.P., S. Baeta, C. Kootstra, A.M. Polderman. Reinfection patterns of *Oesophagostomum bifurcum* after anthelmintic treatment. *Trop Geogr Med* 47:160–163, 1995.

Levine, N.D. *Nematode Parasites of Domestic Animals and of Man,* 2nd ed. Minneapolis: Burgess; 1980.

Pages, A., K. Kpodzro, S. Baeta, K. Akpo-Allavo. La "tumeur" de Dapaong. Helminthiase à Oesophagostome. *Ann Pathol* 8:332–335, 1988.

Polderman, A.M., H.P. Krepel, J.J. Verweij, S. Baeta, J.P. Rotmans. Serological diagnosis of *Oesophagostomum* infections. *Trans R Soc Trop Med Hyg* 87:433–435, 1993.

Romstad, A., R.B. Gasser, P. Nansen, A.M. Polderman, J.R. Monti, N.B. Chilton. Characterization of *Oesophagostomum bifurcum* and *Necator americanus* by PCR-RFLP of rDNA. *J Parasitol* 83:963–966, 1997.

Ross, R.A., D.I. Gibson, E.A. Harris. Cutaneous oesophagostomiasis in man. *J Helminthol* 63:261–265, 1989.

GNATHOSTOMIASIS

ICD-10 B83.1

Synonyms: Gnathostomosis, larva migrans caused by *Gnathostoma*, wandering swelling.

Etiology: The agents of this infection are larvae of *Gnathostoma spinigerum, G. hispidum, G. doloresi,* and *G. nipponicum. G. spinigerum* is a spiruriod nematode parasite of dogs and domestic and wild felines. It has been known since 1890 that it can infect man. *G. hispidum* is a parasite of swine and wild boars, and has been known as a parasite of humans since 1924. Only in 1989 was it recognized that *G. doloresi,* a parasite of swine and wild boars, also infects man (Nawa *et al.,* 1989). Around the same time, it was found that *G. nipponicum,* a parasite of weasels, can also occasionally infect man. The larvae of the various species are differentiated by the number of hooks on the head bulb (see below) and the structure of the intestinal canal section (Akahane *et al.,* 1998). For example, the infective larvae of *G. nipponicum* have three rows of hooks with an average of 34.5, 36.7, and 39.7 hooks in the first, second, and third rows, respectively.

G. spinigerum is a reddish worm that lives in the stomach wall of its definitive hosts. The cuticle forms a globose ring (the head bulb) behind the lips (characteristic of the genus), and it has eight transversal rows of small spines. The female parasite measures 2.5–5 cm, and the male, about half that. The eggs are eliminated with the feces of the definitive host; they hatch in water after one to three weeks of incubation and release a first-stage larva. This larva actively penetrates a copepod of the genus *Cyclops*, invades its hemocele and, in about 10 days, changes into a second-stage larva with a spiny head bulb. When an appropriate freshwater fish ingests the infected copepod, the larva continues its development; it passes from the fish's intestine to the musculature where, after a month, it transforms into a mature third-stage larva and encysts. This infective larva measures about 4 mm, has four rows of spines on the head bulb, and more than 200 rows on the body, and is coiled in a spiral inside a fibrous cyst about 1 mm in diameter. When one of these hosts eats another, infected, host, the larva transfers from the first to the second without developing, so the second host acts as a transport or paratenic host. Cats, dogs, and all other natural definitive hosts are infected by consuming fish or paratenic hosts that contain the infective larvae. In the stomach of the definitive hosts, the larvae are released from their cysts, penetrate the stomach wall, migrate to the liver, and from there, go to other organs and tissues (muscular and connective). Then, from the peritoneal cavity they again penetrate the stomach and lodge in the mucosa. After about six months, they mature into adults and begin oviposition.

Studies with *G. nipponicum* indicate that the larva which invades the copepod would be an early third-stage larva, which develops into the mature third-stage larva when it is ingested by a fish (Ando *et al.*, 1992). Experimental infection has shown that about 36 species of freshwater fish, amphibians, reptiles, crustaceans, birds, and rodents can serve as second intermediate hosts. In Thailand, certain freshwater fish, ducks, and chickens are particularly important as sources of infection for man. Many animal species, such as snakes, birds, and some mammals, can serve as transport hosts.

G. doloresi and *G. hispidum* parasitize the stomach mucosa of pigs and wild boars. The development cycle of *G. doloresi* also requires two intermediate hosts: the first are copepods and the second are salamanders and serpents. *G. hispidum* requires only one intermediate host: the larvae released by the eggs are ingested by *Cyclops* copepods and the infective larvae develop in their coelom in one or two weeks. Fish, frogs, and reptiles can serve as paratenic hosts. When the salamanders or snakes, in the case of *G. doloresi*, or the copepods, in the case of *G. hispidum*, are ingested by a pig, the larva develops into the adult stage in a manner similar to *G. spinigerum*.

G. nipponicum is a parasite of the esophageal mucosa of the weasel *Mustela sibirica itatsi*. This species also requires two intermediate hosts: the first are copepods and the second are fish and small snakes. Fish, salamanders, frogs, mice, and rats have been infected experimentally with immature larvae obtained from copepods, but small snakes, birds, or weasels have not. In other words, the infested species should be considered second intermediate hosts. However, it was possible to infect frogs, snakes, birds, and rats with mature larvae obtained from fish. Since the larvae do not develop into adults in these hosts, but remain in the larval state, they should be considered paratenic hosts. Weasels infected with mature larvae obtained from fish began to produce eggs 69 to 90 days after infection (Ando *et al.*, 1992).

Geographic Distribution and Occurrence: The most common gnathostomiasis is caused by *G. spinigerum*, which is endemic in the countries of Asia, especially China, Japan, and Thailand (Rusnak and Lucey, 1993). It is common in Thailand, which made it possible to carry out treatment studies with 98 patients in a Bangkok hospital in 1998. Gnathostomiasis caused by *G. spinigerum* seems to be an emerging disease in Latin America: the first two human cases there were recognized in Mexico in 1970, but 300 additional cases were identified between 1992 and 1995 in Culiacán, in northern Mexico (Díaz Camacho *et al.*, 1998), and between 1993 and 1997, there were 98 cases in Acapulco, in southern Mexico (Rojas-Molina *et al.*, 1999). Cases of human infection also have been described in Argentina and Ecuador (Ollague *et al.*, 1988). The highest concentration of human cases has been in Thailand and Japan, where hundreds of patients are reported every year. The human infection is infrequent or rare in China, India, Indochina, Indonesia, and Malaysia. Sporadic cases have also been registered in Australia, Israel, and the state of California, US. *G. spinigerum* in animals is much more widely distributed than in humans. In an endemic area in southern Japan, 35% of cats and 4% of dogs had *G. spinigerum* parasites, and 60% to 100% of freshwater fish (*Ophiocephalus argus*) contained larvae. In the markets of Thailand, larvae were found in 37% of fish, 80% of eels, and 90% of frogs.

G. hispidum has been found in humans in China, Korea, and Taiwan. Urban cases of gnathostomiasis in Japan are the result of *G. hispidum*, introduced by fish imported from China, Korea, or Taiwan. The infection is relatively common in pigs in Asia, Australia, and Europe. A study of 3,478 pigs carried out in China in 1991 found the infection in 15% of them. Of 38 species of animals that serve as intermediate or paratenic hosts, 23 are shared with *G. spinigerum*. *G. nipponicum* occurs in China, Japan, and Korea, due to imported fish. *G. doloresi* has been found in man only in southern Japan. The first case was reported in 1989, and 25 cases had been reported by 1997: 23 cutaneous, 1 pulmonary, and 1 colonic (Nawa *et al.*, 1997).

The Disease in Man: Man is an aberrant host in which the parasite only exceptionally reaches sexual maturity: the larva continuously migrates and does not become established in the human stomach. In most cases, a single larva is responsible for the clinical picture. The most common symptoms are localized, intermittent, and sometimes migratory swelling of the skin, often accompanied by pain, pruritis, and erythema. It can also affect the internal organs (Rusnak and Lucey, 1993). The first symptoms appear one or two days after the ingestion of raw fish or the meat of paratenic hosts, such as chickens and ducks. The symptoms include nausea, salivation, urticaria, pruritis, and stomach discomfort; mild leukocytosis and very marked eosinophilia are common. Later, the symptoms are due to the migration of the larva into the liver and other organs. The movements of the larva inside the abdominal or thoracic organs can cause acute pain of limited duration. The symptoms resemble cholecystitis, appendicitis, cystitis, or other diseases, depending on the organ affected by the larvae (internal or visceral gnathostomiasis). Approximately one month after the infective food is eaten, the larva locates in the subcutaneous tissue, usually of the abdomen, extremities, head, and chest. This is the beginning of the chronic phase, in which the organic symptoms abate or disappear and eosinophilia gradually decreases. The most prominent symptom is an intermittent subcutaneous edema that changes location each time the larva moves. The edema is pruriginous but not painful, and initially lasts a week or more; its duration then becomes progressively shorter. In older infections, the edemas recur at longer intervals. The larva can survive in the human body for a long time; and one case lasting 16 years has been recorded.

In its erratic migration, the larva can affect a variety of different organs and tissues. When it penetrates the skin, it can cause a clinical picture similar to that of cutaneous larva migrans (see the chapter on that disease). The most serious localizations, fortunately rare, are in the brain and eyes. In 300 cases of *G. spinigerum* in Mexico, the lesions occurred mostly on the face, neck, arms, and legs. There was just one ocular case, and 75% of the patients developed peripheral eosinophilia. Skin biopsies obtained from 35 patients showed larvae in just 12 of them. The infection in 93 individuals was identified by enzyme-linked immunosorbent assay (ELISA) with extracts of *G. doloresi* (Díaz Camacho *et al.*, 1998).

In a case of *G. doloresi* studied in Japan, the patient had epigastric pain three days after eating fish (*Oncorhynchus masou masou*) and developed a scaly rash on the trunk three days later. The rash spread and he sought medical attention 18 days after eating the fish. Biopsies were negative, but two days later blisters appeared on the lower abdomen, and a nematode was obtained from one of them. The next day he had swelling of the jaw that lasted for a week. All the lesions began to shrink on the 25th day and had disappeared by day 30 (Akahane *et al.*, 1998).

Punyagupta *et al.* (1990) believe that *G. spinigerum* is one of the main causes of meningitis and eosinophilic meningoencephalitis in Thailand and that it can be clinically distinguished from the similar disease caused by *Angiostrongylus cantonensis*, even though it is very difficult to recover the parasite for purposes of a definitive diagnosis. Intraocular gnathostomiasis is rare and should be differentiated from that caused by filariae or *Angiostrongylus*; up until 1994, just 12 cases had been found (Biswas *et al.*, 1994).

The Disease in Animals: *G. spinigerum* larvae can cause necrotic tunnels during their migration—before reaching the stomach—in the liver, pancreas, and other abdominal tissues of the natural definitive hosts (cats and dogs). In the adult stage, the parasite lodges in the stomach wall, where it produces intense inflammation, with the formation of cavities full of serosanguineous fluid that become fibrous cysts. These cavities develop fistules that are connected to the lumen of the stomach to discharge the parasite's eggs. When the fistules open onto the peritoneum, they can cause severe peritonitis (Barriga, 1997). *G. hispidum* and *G. doloresi* can cause similar damage to the abdominal organs and stomach ulcers in pigs. The disease is infrequent but, when it occurs, it manifests with anorexia and weight loss. *G. nipponicum* produces nodules in the esophagi of weasels that can interfere with swallowing.

Source of Infection and Mode of Transmission: The reservoirs of the parasite are cats, dogs, pigs, weasels, and several species of wild mammals that can act as paratenic hosts. The definitive hosts and humans become infected by consuming infected fish or paratenic hosts. The habit of eating fish or fowl raw or only seasoned with vinegar is the essential factor in the occurrence of the human disease and its endemicity in Japan and Thailand. The parasitosis in animals is much more widespread than the human infection, since it occurs even in places where people do not eat raw fish or fowl. In Japan, very high rates of infection were found in two species of fish, *Ophiocephalus argus* and *O. tadianus*; each fish can contain hundreds of larvae. In Thailand, besides several species of *Ophiocephalus*, sources of infection include catfish (*Clarias batrachus*), eels, frogs, freshwater snakes, chickens, and ducks (Daengsvang, 1982).

Diagnosis: In endemic areas, migratory and recurrent subcutaneous edemas accompanied by leukocytosis and high eosinophilia can be considered pathognomic. Since the parasites do not develop to the adult stage in man, eggs are not found in the feces. Specific diagnosis in man can be made by identifying the larva in surgically obtained specimens. The immunobiological tests include an intradermal reaction of questionable specificity. ELISA with *G. doloresi* antigens is widely used to identify infection by any species of *Gnathostoma*, despite the fact that it cross-reacts in patients with *Toxocara canis*, *Anisakis* sp., *Paragonimus westermani*, and *Fasciola* sp. The antigens obtained from infective larvae of *G. spinigerum* are more specific for the species (Anantaphruti, 1989). In patients with cerebral gnathostomiasis by *G. spinigerum*, attempts have been made to confirm the infection by looking for antigens, immune complexes, or antibodies in the cerebrospinal fluid; of 11 patients, just one had antigens and another had immune complexes, but nine had antibodies (Tuntipopipat *et al.*, 1989).

In dogs and cats, diagnosis can be made by detecting eggs in the feces, but it must be borne in mind that the eggs are sometimes few in number or are eliminated irregularly.

Control: In enzootic areas, the best way to prevent disease is by abstaining from eating raw or undercooked fish and fowl. According to García and Bruckner (1997), cooking or immersing raw meat in strong vinegar for five hours kills the larvae, but lemon juice or chilling at 4°C for a month does not kill them.

Bibliography

Akahane, H., M. Sano, M. Kobayashi. Three cases of human gnathostomiasis caused by *Gnathostoma hispidum*, with particular reference to the identification of parasitic larvae. *Southeast Asian J Trop Med Public Health* 29(3):611–614, 1998.

Akahane, H., K. Shibue, A. Shimizu, S. Toshitani. Human gnathostomiasis caused by *Gnathostoma doloresi*, with particular reference to the parasitological investigation of the causative agent. *Ann Trop Med Parasitol* 92(16):721–726, 1998.

Anantaphruti, M.T. ELISA for diagnosis of gnathostomiasis using antigens from *Gnathostoma doloresi* and *G. spinigerum*. *Southeast Asian J Trop Med Public Health* 20(2):297–304, 1989.

Ando, K., H. Tokura, H. Matsuoka, D. Taylor, Y. Chinzei. Life cycle of *Gnathostoma nipponicum* Yamaguti, 1941. *J Helminthol* 66(1):53–61, 1992.

Barriga, O.O. *Veterinary Parasitology for Practitioners*, 2nd ed. Edina: Burgess International Group; 1997.

Biswas, J., L. Gopal, T. Sharma, S.S. Badrinath. Intraocular *Gnathostoma spinigerum*. Clinicopathologic study of two cases with review of literature. *Retina* 14(5):438–444, 1994.

Daengsvang, S. Gnathostomiasis. *In*: Schultz, M.O., section ed. Section C, Vol. 2: *CRC Handbook Series in Zoonoses*. Boca Raton: CRC Press; 1982.

Díaz Camacho, S.P., M. Zazueta Ramos, E. Ponce Torrecillas, *et al.* Clinical manifestations and immunodiagnosis of gnathostomiasis in Culiacán, Mexico. *Am J Trop Med Hyg* 59(6):908–915, 1998.

García, L.S., Bruckner, D.A. *Diagnostic Medical Parasitology*, 3rd ed. Washington, D.C.: ASM Press; 1997.

Nawa, Y. Historical review and current status of gnathostomiasis in Asia. *Southeast Asian J Trop Med Public Health* 22 Suppl:217–219, 1991.

Nawa, Y., J. Imai, K. Ogata, K. Otsuka. The first record of a confirmed human case of *Gnathostoma doloresi* infection. *J Parasitol* 75(1):166–169, 1989.

Nawa, Y., H. Maruyama, K. Ogata. Current status of gnathostomiasis *dorolesi* in Miyazaki Prefecture, Japan. *Southeast Asian J Trop Med Public Health* 28 Suppl 1:11–13, 1997.

Ollague, W., E. Gómez, M. Briones. *Gnathostoma spinigerum* y su dinámica de transmisión al hombre. Primer reporte en Ecuador y América. *Med Cutan Ibero Lat Am* 16:291–294, 1988.

Punyagupta, S., T. Bunnag, P. Juttijudata. Eosinophilic meningitis in Thailand. Clinical and epidemiological characteristics of 162 patients with myeloencephalitis probably caused by *Gnathostoma spinigerum*. *J Neurol Sci* 96(2–3):241–256, 1990.

Rojas-Molina, N., S. Pedraza-Sánchez, B. Torres-Bibiano, H. Meza-Martínez, A. Escobar-Gutiérrez. Gnathostomosis, an emerging foodborne zoonotic disease in Acapulco, Mexico. *Emerg Infect Dis* 5(2):264–266, 1999.

Rusnak, J.M., D.R. Lucey. Clinical gnathostomiasis: Case report and review of the English-language literature. *Clin Infect Dis* 16(1):33–50, 1993.

Tuntipopipat, S., R. Chawengkiattikul, R. Witoonpanich, S. Chiemchanya, S. Sirisinha. Antigens, antibodies and immune complexes in cerebrospinal fluid of patients with cerebral gnathostomiasis. *Southeast Asian J Trop Med Public Health* 20(3):439–446, 1989.

GONGYLONEMIASIS

ICD-10 B83.8 Other specified helminthiases

Synonym: Gongylonematosis.

Etiology: The agent of this disease is *Gongylonema pulchrum*, a spiruroid nematode of the family Thelaziidae, whose main hosts are ruminants, swine, and wild boars. It is also found in horses, carnivores, monkeys, rodents, and other animals (Cappucci *et al.*, 1982). Moreover, it has been found in macaques in Japan and squirrels (*Sciurus niger*) in the state of Florida, US (Coyner *et al.*, 1996).

The adult parasite lives in the esophageal mucosa and submucosa of the definitive hosts, but can also be found in the rumen and oral cavity. It is filiform and its size varies according to the host. In ruminants, the male can reach approximately 62 mm in length and 0.15–0.3 mm in diameter, and the females, up to 145 mm by 0.2–0.5 mm. The parasite is smaller in humans and swine.

The females of *G. pulchrum* lay embryonated eggs in the esophagus or rumen of the definitive host. The eggs are eliminated to the exterior with the feces, and must be ingested by an intermediate host for the life cycle to continue. These hosts are several species of coprophilic beetles of the genera *Aphodius, Blaps, Ontophagus,* and others. Experimental infection of the cockroach *Blatella germanica* was also possible. The egg hatches in the insect's intestine, and the larva penetrates its hemocele where, in about a month, it develops into the third (infective) stage and encysts. Ruminants acquire the parasitosis upon ingesting the small beetles with grass or other infested food, and swine become infected by coprophagia. The migration route of the larva in the definitive host is not well known, but experimental infections in guinea pigs provide evidence that the larva frees itself from the coleopteran in the stomach and migrates through the stomach wall to the esophagus, where it matures in about two months and reinitiates the cycle with oviposition.

Geographic Distribution and Occurrence: Human infection by *G. pulchrum* is rare: just 46 cases were recorded between 1864 and 1982, 2 more were reported by 1994, and an additional 2 by the year 2000. Of these, one was in the US (Eberhard and Busillo, 1999) and the other was in Germany, but originated in Hungary (Jelinek and Loscher, 1994). The human infection has been diagnosed in China, Bulgaria, Germany (in a Greek immigrant), Hungary, Italy, Morocco, New Zealand, the former Soviet Union, Sri Lanka, Turkey, the US, and the former Yugoslavia.

G. pulchrum is widely distributed geographically in animals. It has been found in Asia, the US, Europe, and the Russian Federation. The prevalence of the infection in domestic ruminants varies with the area. In surveys carried out in the US, the parasite was found in 5.9% of 1,518 pigs, with a range of 0% to 21% depending on geographic origin; in 10% of 29 bovines in the state of Georgia; and in 5% of 20 bovines in the state of Florida. In slaughterhouses in Ukraine, the parasite was found in 32% to 94% of adult cattle, 39% to 95% of sheep, and 0% to 37% of swine. In a slaughterhouse in Teheran, Iran, *G. pulchrum* was found in the esophagi of 49.7% of the cattle examined.

The Disease in Man: The lesions caused by the parasite are mainly irritative, due to its movement through the mucosa and submucosa; parasites have been found actively moving in the submucosa of lips, gums, hard palate, soft palate, and tonsils. Pharyngitis and stomatitis have sometimes been confirmed. Two cases described in China included bloody sialorrhea and eroded and bleeding patches on the esophageal mucosa.

The Disease in Animals: In ruminants, *G. pulchrum* is found mainly in the mucosa and submucosa of the esophagus, but the mature parasite can move in different directions and invade the pharynx, oral cavity, and rumen. In swine, it is found in the stratified squamous epithelium of the tongue mucosa. According to observations in Iran, there were no lesions that would indicate that the infection produced a pathologic condition. Histologic examination of swine tongues in the US revealed a mild and chronic inflammatory process. On the other hand, in the former Soviet Union, lesions, sometimes important, of the esophagi of infected bovines have been found, with hyperemia, edema, and deformations of the organ. Likewise, the infection is blamed for occlusions of the esophagus due to a reflex reaction caused by irritation of the nerve receptors.

Source of Infection and Mode of Transmission: Ruminants and other animals become infected by ingesting coleopterans containing third-stage larvae. Man is an accidental host who does not play any role in the maintenance of the parasite in nature and probably is infected by the same mechanism. Salads and raw vegetables are thought to be the vehicles by means of which man ingests the small beetles. It has also been suggested that the species of *Aphodius,* because of its size (4–6 mm) and capacity for flight, could be accidentally inhaled and then swallowed.

The maintenance of the parasite in nature is assured by its broad diffusion and prevalence among herbivores, swine, and other animals (definitive hosts), and the large number of susceptible species of beetles (intermediate hosts). In Ukraine, 60% to 90% of the beetles were found to be infected. The highest rates corresponded to several species of *Aphodius* and *Geotrupes*; the number of larvae ranged between 1 and 193.

Diagnosis: Most of the human cases were diagnosed because the patient felt something moving in the submucosa of the oral cavity or observed the parasite emerging from the mouth. Specific diagnosis is done by extracting the parasite and identifying it under the microscope.

Diagnosis in live animals is rarely achieved. The eggs are not always found by fecal examination, even when flotation or sedimentation methods are used. The parasites can be detected by postmortem examination of the esophagus (ruminants) or the tongue (swine).

Control: Because of the rarity and mildness of human infection, special control measures are not justified. Individual protection can be obtained by observing the rules of personal, food, and environmental hygiene. With a few exceptions, helminthologists agree that *G. pulchrum* does not cause major damage to animals. Moreover, it would not be feasible to adopt measures aimed at protecting animals at pasture from ingestion of beetles.

Bibliography

Cappucci, D.T., J.K. Augsburg, P.C. Klinck. Gongylonemiasis. *In*: Steele, J.H., section ed. Section C, Vol. 2: *CRC Handbook Series in Zoonoses*. Boca Raton: CRC Press; 1982.

Coyner, D.F., J.B. Wooding, D.J. Forrester. A comparison of parasitic helminths and arthropods from two subspecies of fox squirrels (*Sciurus niger*) in Florida. *J Wildl Dis* 3(3)2:492–497, 1996.

Eberhard, M.L., C. Busillo. Human *Gongylonema* infection in a resident of New York City. *Am J Trop Med Hyg* 61(1):51–52, 1999.

Jelinek, T., T. Loscher. Human infection with *Gongylonema pulchrum*: A case report. *Trop Med Parasitol* 45(4):329–330, 1994.

LAGOCHILASCARIASIS

ICD-10 B83.9 Helminthiasis, unspecified

Etiology: The vector of this disease is *Lagochilascaris minor*, a small ascarid. The female measures 6–20 mm long by 0.20–0.80 mm wide; the male is smaller. It has been identified in man, but parasites that seem to belong to the same species have been found in wild carnivores and in the agouti. Eggs, larvae, and adults of the ascarid are continually found in the abscesses produced by the parasite in man, suggesting ongoing reproduction in the lesion (Moraes *et al.,* 1983). While the parasite's natural life cycle is not known, laboratory mice have been infected with larvae from eggs obtained from human beings; infections have been produced with adult parasites in cats infected by those mice. In mice, the larvae encysted in the muscular and subcutaneous tissue. In cats, the larvae were released in the stomach and migrated through the esophagus, pharynx, trachea, otorhinopharynx, and cervical lymph nodes, to mature into adults in any of these organs 9 to 20 days after infection (Campos *et al.*, 1992).

Geographic Distribution and Occurrence: The disease occurs in Latin America and the Caribbean. It is very rare: only 19 human cases were known up to 1982 (7 in Brazil, 1 in Costa Rica, 5 in Suriname, 5 in Trinidad and Tobago, and 1 in Venezuela) (Volcan *et al.*, 1982; Moraes *et al.*, 1983). Between 1982 and 2000, 7 more cases were described (1 in Bolivia, 5 in Brazil, and 1 in Mexico).

The Disease in Man: The disease begins with a tumor in the neck, mastoid apophysis, tonsils, maxillae, or paranasal sinuses. Eventually, it opens to the surface of the skin, releasing pus, in which adult parasites, larvae, and eggs are intermittently found. Fistulas form, and may open in the nasopharynx, in which case purulent material and parasites are eliminated through the nose and mouth. The process is chronic and may last for years. The case of a girl in Mexico began with a hard, lobulate tumor in the neck, measuring 3 cm by 5 cm, with a purulent central pustule that contained parasites and that had been developing for six months. Neither repeated treatment with thiabenzadole nor surgical removal improved the picture (Vargas-Ocampo and Alvarado-Alemán, 1997). Three Brazilian patients had fistulous abscesses in the area of the neck and ear, and a mastoid process containing parasites; two of them had central nervous system involvement. Treatment with anthelmintics and surgical removal of the abscesses produced temporary improvement, but there were relapses in two of the cases (Veloso *et al.*, 1992). Treatment with ivermectin, a veterinary anthelmintic, was successful in the other case (Bento *et al.*, 1993).

The Disease in Animals: Just two cases have been described, both in Brazil, of fistulated abscesses in cats (Amato and Pimentel-Neto, 1990). The parasite has also been discovered in the trachea of a bush dog (*Speothos venaticus*) (Volcan and Medrano, 1991).

Source of Infection and Mode of Transmission: The natural reservoir is unknown. The rarity of the human infection would indicate that man is an accidental host and is unable by himself to maintain the parasite in nature. It is not known how humans become infected. In a review of the genus *Lagochilascaris*, the possibility was suggested that man is infected by ingesting embryonated eggs (possibly eliminated by another animal species), and that the third-stage larva ascends to the trachea, but rather than being swallowed, as occurs with the larva of *Ascaris lumbricoides*, it would become established in the retropharyngeal region. The findings of Campos *et al.* (1992) provide some support for this theory.

Diagnosis: Specific diagnosis is made by identifying the parasite found in lesions. The eggs are also characteristic and resemble those of *Toxocara cati* or *A. lumbricoides*. In a case described in Venezuela, eggs of *L. minor* were found in the feces of the patient (an occurrence that had not been observed before) and were at first confused with *A. lumbricoides* (Volcan *et al.*, 1982).

Control: Lack of knowledge about the transmission cycle of this parasite to man prevents determination of effective control measures.

Bibliography

Amato, J.F., L. Grisi, M. Pimentel-Neto. Two cases of fistulated abscesses caused by *Lagochilascaris major* in the domestic cat. *Mem Inst Oswaldo Cruz* 85(4):471–473, 1990.

Bento, R.F., C. do C. Mazza, E.F. Motti, Y.T. Chan, J.R. Guimaraes, A. Miniti. Human lagochilascariasis treated successfully with ivermectin: A case report. *Rev Inst Med Trop Sao Paulo* 35(4):373–375, 1993.

Campos, D.M., L.G. Freire Filha, M.A. Vieira, J.M. Paco, M.A. Maia. Experimental life cycle of *Lagochilascaris minor* Leiper, 1909. *Rev Inst Med Trop Sao Paulo* 34(4):277–287, 1992.

Moraes, M.A., M.V. Arnaud, P.E. de Lima. Novos casos de infecção humana por *Lagochilascaris minor* Leiper, 1909, encontrados no estado do Para, Brasil. *Rev Inst Med Trop Sao Paulo* 25(3):139–146, 1983.

Vargas-Ocampo, F., F.J. Alvarado-Alemán. Infestation from *Lagochilascaris minor* in Mexico. *Int J Dermatol* 36(6):56–58, 1997.

Veloso, M.G., M.C. Faria, J.D. de Freitas, M.A. Moraes, D.F. Gorini, J.L. de Mendonca. Lagoquilascariase humana. Sobre tres casos encontrados no Distrito Federal, Brasil. *Rev Inst Med Trop Sao Paulo* 34:587–591, 1992.

Volcan, G.S., C.E. Medrano. Infección natural de *Speothos venaticus* (Carnivora: Canidae) por estadios adultos de *Lagochilascaris* sp. *Rev Inst Med Trop Sao Paulo* 33(6):451–458, 1991.

MAMMOMONOGAMIASIS

ICD-10 B83.3 Syngamiasis

Synonym: Syngamosis.

Etiology: The agents of this disease are the nematodes *Mammomonogamus (Syngamus) laryngeus* and *M. nasicola* of the family Syngamidae. The former is a parasite of the laryngotracheal region, and the latter is a parasite of the nasal fossae of bovines, bubalines, and occasionally sheep, goats, and deer. Some helminthologists consider *M. nasicola* and *M. laryngeus* to be homologous.

The nematodes are red; the female measures about 10 mm by 0.5 mm and the male measures 3 mm by 0.3 mm. Since they remain in permanent union and the female has the vulva near the anterior end, they look like the letter Y. The development cycle of syngamids in mammals is not well known; it is believed to be similar to that of the fowl parasite *Syngamus trachea*. The eggs deposited by the parasite in the tracheal mucus are swallowed and eliminated with the feces. In the external environment, the infective larvae (third stage) can develop within or outside of the egg. Herbivores are infected by ingesting the infective larva, inside or outside of the egg, when they consume contaminated fodder or water. The infection can also probably be produced by ingestion of paratenic hosts, such as earthworms, snails, and several types of arthropods, as happens with avian *S. trachea*. In a herbivore's digestive tract, the larvae are released from their protective membranes, cross the intestinal wall to the mesenteric veins, and migrate to their final localization (tracheolaryngeal or nasal), where the two sexes couple and remain in permanent union. The cycle is reinitiated with oviposition.

Geographic Distribution and Occurrence: *M. laryngeus* is found in ruminants in tropical America and in the Philippines, India, Malaysia, and Viet Nam. *M. nasicola* occurs in Africa, Brazil, the Caribbean, and the eastern region of the former Soviet Union.

In a slaughterhouse in the state of São Paulo, Brazil, 27 (45%) of 60 slaughtered cows were found to be infected (Santos and Fukuda, 1977), as were 18 (37.5%) of 48 young bulls in the state of Rio de Janeiro (Freire and Biachin, 1979). In Honduras, only 2.8% of 70 bovines examined were parasitized (Secretariat of Natural Resources of Honduras, 1980). In the Philippines, 23% of 597 bovines were parasitized with *M. laryngeus* (Van Aken *et al.*, 1996).

Human infection is rare. Only 79 cases had been reported up to 1988 (Cunnac *et al.*, 1988)—51 of them in inhabitants of or visitors to Martinique (Mornex *et al.*, 1980)—and about 100 up to 1995 (5 of them in North America) (Nosanchuk *et al.*, 1995). Nine more cases were reported between 1988 and 2000. With the exception of three cases in Asia—one each in the Philippines, Thailand (Pipitgool *et al.*, 1992), and Korea (Kim *et al.*, 1998)—all the cases occurred in the Caribbean and Brazil.

The Disease in Man and Animals: In man, the symptomatology consists of tracheolaryngeal irritation with persistent cough but without fever. Some patients experience hemoptysis. A case was reported (Birrel, 1977) in an Australian woman who lived in Guyana for 10 months; she had respiratory symptoms consisting of a chronic cough and hemoptysis, and experienced loss of weight. In April 1977, she was admitted to Brisbane Hospital, Queensland, Australia, where bronchoscopy revealed larvae of a parasite that was identified as *M. laryngeus*. Extraction of the parasite resulted in disappearance of the symptoms. A similar case was described in the US (Gardiner and Schantz, 1983).

The animal infection is rarely symptomatic, and large numbers of *M. laryngeus* are required to produce an afebrile laryngitis or tracheitis. No symptoms have been observed in nasal infections caused by *M. nasicola*.

Source of Infection and Mode of Transmission: The reservoirs of *M. laryngeus* and *M. nasicola* are ruminants. Man is infected only accidentally. The sources of infection for man are probably raw plant foods and water contaminated with eggs or free larvae of the parasite. The sources of infection for ruminants are soil, pasture, and water. It is thought that the exogenous development of these parasites is similar to that of *Syngamus trachea* of fowl. In this parasite, the paratenic hosts are very important, since the third stage infective larva encysts in the coelom and can survive a year or more.

Diagnosis: The eggs of the parasite can be observed in feces and, more rarely, in sputum. Coughing fits may expel these parasites, which are easy to identify. Animal mammomonogamiasis is most often found on autopsy. Diagnosis in humans is usually effected by bronchoscopy and detection of the parasite.

Control: Prevention consists of observing the rules of food hygiene: wash raw food very well, boil suspicious drinking water, and wash hands well before eating.

Bibliography

Cunnac, M., J.F. Magnaval, D. Cayarci, P. Leophonte. À propos de 3 cas de syngamose humaine en Guadeloupe. *Rev Pneumol Clin* 44:140–142, 1988.

Freire, N.M.S., I. Biachin. Prevalência de *Mammomonogamus laryngeus* (Raillet, 1899) em bovinos no Rio de Janeiro. *Arq Esc Vet UEMG (Minas Gerais)* 31:23–24, 1979.

Gardiner, C.H., P.M. Schantz. *Mammomonogamus* infection in a human. Report of a case. *Am J Trop Med Hyg* 32(5):995–997, 1983.

Honduras, Secretaría de Recursos Naturales. *Muestreo patológico de Honduras.* Tegucigalpa: Secretaría de Recursos Naturales; 1980.

Kim, H.Y., S.M. Lee, J.E. Joo, M.J. Na, M.H. Ahn, D.Y. Min. Human syngamosis: The first case in Korea. *Thorax* 53:717–718, 1998.

Macko, J.K., V. Birova, R. Flores. Deliberations on the problems of *Mammomonogamus* species (Nametoda, Syngamidae) in ruminants. *Folia Parasit (Praha)* 28(1):43–49, 1981.

Mornex, J.F., J. Magdeleine, J. de Thore. La syngamose humaine *(Mammomonogamus nasicola)* cause de toux chronique en Martinique. 37 observations recentes. *Nouv Presse Med* 9(47):3628, 1980.

Nosanchuk, J.S., S.E. Wade, M. Landolf. Case report of and description of parasite in *Mammomonogamus laryngeus* (human syngamosis) infection. *J Clin Microbiol* 33(4):998–1000, 1995.

Pipitgool, V., K. Chaisiri, P. Visetsupakarn, V. Srigan, W. Maleewong. *Mammonogamus (Syngamus) laryngeus* infection: A first case report in Thailand. *Southeast Asian J Trop Med Public Health* 23(2):336–337, 1992.

Santos, I.F., R.F. Fukuda. Ocorrência de *Syngamus laryngeus* em bovinos do Município de Novo Horizonte. *S P Científica (S Paulo)* 5:391–393, 1977.

Van Aken, D., J.T. Lagapa, A.P. Dargantes, J. Vercruysse. *Mammomonogamus laryngeus* (Railliet, 1899) infections in cattle in Mindanao, Philippines. *Vet Parasitol* 64(4):329, 1996.

MICRONEMIASIS

ICD-10 B83.8 Other specified helminthiases

Etiology: *Micronema deletrix*, a very small, free-living nematode with a rhabditiform esophagus. The female measures barely 250–445 μm in length. It was originally described as *Halicephalobus gingivalis* by Stefanski in 1954. Anderson *et al.* (1998) reviewed the taxonomy of *M. deletrix* and concluded that both parasites were the same; consequently, *M. deletrix* is a synonym for *H. gingivalis*, although the latter name has priority. Other authors, such as Teifke *et al.* (1998), call it *H. deletrix*. We will use the name *Micronema deletrix* because it is the most widely known by health professionals.

The parasite lives as a saprophyte in soil rich in decomposing organic matter. All developmental stages of the nematode are found in that natural environment: eggs, larvae, and the female and male adult forms (Shadduck *et al.,* 1979). *M. deletrix* is a facultative parasite of man and equines. Eggs, larvae, and mature females, but not males, have been found in animal tissue; therefore, it has been deduced that the parasitic females are parthenogenic, like *Strongyloides stercoralis*. It has been suggested that it may be erroneous to attribute all the cases of infection to *M. deletrix* without having more information on the different species of the genus *Micronema* (Gardiner *et al.*, 1981). At least one case of granulomatous verminous mastitis in a mare, which could have been confused with micronemiasis, was due to another free-living nematode of the genus *Cephalobus* (Greiner *et al.*, 1991).

Geographic Distribution and Occurrence: The distribution of the nematode in its natural habitat has been studied very little; presumably it is distributed worldwide. Only three human cases are known, and all of them were fatal: one in Canada (Hoogstraten and Young, 1975) and two in the US (Shadduck *et al.*, 1979; Gardiner *et al.*, 1981). No cases were described between 1988 and 2000.

Cases of micronemiasis in equines have been diagnosed in North America, Europe, and in Egypt. Its occurrence is rare: only 7 cases were reported up to 1985, and 12 more were reported between 1988 and 2000 (2 in Germany, 1 in Canada, 8 in the US, and 1 in Great Britain). However, the infection may occur more frequently in equines and go undiagnosed. For example, a study carried out in Egypt found *M. deletrix* in 2 of 28 dead equines that had shown symptoms of encephalitis (Ferris *et al.*, 1972).

The Disease in Man and Animals: The three known human cases died after manifesting symptoms of meningoencephalitis. In two patients, the lesions and nematodes were limited to the brain; in the third, micronemes were also found in the liver and heart.

The disease in equines can take several forms, depending on the localization of the parasites. Chorioretinitis, gingivitis, rhinitis, sinusitis, encephalomyelitis, pneumonitis, nephritis, osteoarthritis, and osteomyelitis have been described. A nasal tumor was described in one horse, and in another, granulomas in the maxillae and the respective sinuses. In this last case, up to 87,500 parasites per gram of granulomatous mass were extracted. In two cases, other organs were affected in addition to the brain (Alstad *et al.*, 1979). In the forms that affect the central nervous system, the symptomatology is similar to that of viral encephalitides, with lethargy, ataxia, incoordination, lateral or sternal decubitus, and kicking; these often end in death.

In both humans and equines, the lesions consist of numerous foci of granulomatosis or encephalomalacia when they occur in the brain, especially in areas adjacent to the larger blood vessels. The nematodes are found in the walls of the vessels and the perivascular spaces, and are abundant in the lesions (Shadduck *et al.*, 1979).

Source of Infection and Mode of Transmission: The source of infection is soil rich in humus and decomposing organic matter, which is the natural habitat of *M. deletrix*. Neither the mode of transmission nor the route of penetration of the nematode into the animal body is known. In the case of a Canadian child, the nematode probably entered through the multiple lacerations the child received in an accident that became contaminated with equine feces. In another case, it is suspected that the nematode penetrated through decubitus ulcers. In equines, the cases of gingivitis may have been acquired by ingestion of the parasite; the nasal and pneumonic forms may have been acquired by inhalation, and the rest of the systemic cases may have been acquired by penetration of the parasite through pre-existing wounds.

Diagnosis: Diagnosis can be made by biopsy and histopathologic examination of the affected tissues and identification of the nematode. In all of the human cases and several of the equine cases, diagnosis was made postmortem.

Control: Because of the rareness of the disease, special control measures are not justified.

Bibliography

Alstad, A.D., I.E. Berg, C. Samuel. Disseminated *Micronema deletrix* infection in the horse. *J Am Vet Med Assoc* 174(3):264–266, 1979.

Anderson, R.C., K.E. Linder, A.S. Peregrine. *Halicephalobus gingivalis* (Stefanski, 1954) from a fatal infection in a horse in Ontario, Canada with comments on the validity of *H. deletrix* and a review of the genus. *Parasite* 5(3):255–261, 1998.

Ferris, D.H., N.D. Levine, P.D. Beamer. *Micronema deletrix* in equine brain. *Am J Vet Res* 33(1):33–38, 1972.

Gardiner, C.H., D.S. Koh, T.A. Cardella. *Micronema* in man: Third fatal infection. *Am J Trop Med Hyg* 30(3):586–589, 1981.

Greiner, E.C., M.B. Mays, G.C. Smart, Jr., S.E. Weisbrode. Verminous mastitis in a mare caused by a free-living nematode. *J Parasitol* 77(2):320–322, 1991.

Hoogstraten, J., W.G. Young. Meningo-encephalomyelitis due to the saprophagous nematode, *Micronema deletrix*. *Canad J Neurol Sci* 2(2):121–126, 1975.

Shadduck, J.A., J. Ubelaker, V.Q. Telford. *Micronema deletrix* meningoencephalitis in an adult man. *Am J Clin Pathol* 72(4):640–643, 1979.

Teifke, J.P., E. Schmidt, C.M. Traenckner, C. Bauer. *Halicephalobus* (Syn. *Micronema*) *deletrix* als Ursache einer granulomatosen Gingivitis und Osteomyelitis bei einem Pferd. *Tierarztl Prax Ausg G Grosstiere Nutztiere* 26(3):157–161, 1998.

STRONGYLOIDIASIS

ICD-10 B78

Synonym: Strongyloidosis.

Etiology: The agents of this disease are the nematodes *Strongyloides stercoralis* and *S. fuelleborni*. Although man can be infected experimentally with the swine parasite *S. ransomi*, this latter infection does not appear to occur in humans spontaneously in nature. A prominent characteristic of these nematodes is that free-living generations alternate with parasitic ones.

The adult female of *S. stercoralis* is filariform, measures about 2.2 mm in length and 50 microns in diameter, and lives in the mucosa of the duodenum and jejunum of man, other primates, and dogs. Cats have been infected experimentally. Reproduction is parthenogenetic; males are never observed during the parasitic phase of the nematode's life cycle. Oviposition takes place in the epithelium or even in the submucosa. The eggs are transformed into first-stage larvae with a rhabditiform esophagus and migrate to the intestinal lumen. These larvae are shed with feces and may follow either of two courses of development: a direct (homogonic) cycle, or an indirect (heterogonic) cycle. In the direct cycle, the larva undergoes two successive molts and is transformed into a third-stage larva with a filariform esophagus, which is the infective element for the host. In the indirect cycle, the rhabditiform larvae undergo four successive molts, and within two to five days they turn into free-living adult males and females. Like all free-living adult nematodes, these adults have a rhabditiform esophagus. The males and females mate, and the fertilized females lay eggs in the soil. The eggs develop in a few hours and turn into first-stage free-living rhabditiform larvae. The larvae undergo a second stage, and finally they develop into third-stage filariform larvae, which are infective for the host. Hence the indirect (heterogonic) cycle introduces a generation of free-living worms between the generations of parasitic worms. There is evidence that the free-living parasites give rise to only one generation of free-living larvae and that the next generation is always parasitic. The parthenogenetic female apparently produces three types of eggs: haploid, which generate free-living males; diploid, which generate free-living females; and triploid, which generate female parasites. Although all eggs develop to the point of becoming first-stage larvae, only those that can tolerate the prevailing environmental conditions continue to evolve. Adverse conditions (acid or wet soils, temperatures under 20°C or over 37°C, shortage of food) inhibit development of the larvae that will turn into free-living worms, but they favor the formation of infective larvae. Favorable conditions, on the other hand, inhibit development of the infective larvae but stimulate development of the free-living cycle (Barriga, 1997).

The filariform larvae produced by either cycle penetrate the skin of the host with the assistance of enzymes and travel via the bloodstream and lymphatic system to the heart and the lungs, where they settle within 24 hours after the initial infection. Once there, they rupture the capillaries and pulmonary alveoli, crawl through the respiratory tract to the pharynx, are swallowed, and reach the intestine, where they are transformed into parthenogenetic females. The larvae of this generation appear in the feces of man between two and four weeks after the initial infection, and in dogs, after 8 to 16 days.

In dogs, three other routes of infection have been observed: oral, transmammary, and uterine. In all three instances, the larvae settle in the intestine, where they mature into adults, and do not migrate to the lungs. The only difference occurs when the ingested larvae gain entry via blood vessels in the oral mucosa instead of being swallowed. In this case, they follow the same migration pattern as in transcutaneous penetration.

In man, there are two forms of superinfection (acquisition of a new infection on top of a previous one): hyperinfection and autoinfection. In hyperinfection, the rhabditiform larvae turn into infective filariform larvae in the upper part of the intestine; penetrate the mucosa in the lower part of the ileum or the colon; migrate to the lungs, trachea, and esophagus; and, finally, are carried by the bloodstream back to the intestine, where they mature. In autoinfection, some of the filariform larvae shed with the feces remain in the perianal or perineal region long enough to repenetrate the skin of the same host. In both cases, the ultimate effect is that, unlike any other nematodes of man, *S. stercoralis* is capable of reproducing itself in the host without having to abandon it, and thus causes prolonged, very intense infections. It is not known if these forms of superinfection occur in dogs, but persistent strongyloidiases have been observed that could have been the result of self-infection. Nearly one-third of experimentally exposed dogs are unable to eliminate the infection spontaneously, which is somewhat similar to the situation in man. Persistence of the chronic infection in man is illustrated by the fact that 30% of the US veterans who were prisoners of war in Southeast Asia were still infected 35 years later (Grove and Northern, 1982).

Although the canine nematode *S. stercoralis* is similar to the *S. stercoralis* that infects man in terms of both morphology and physiology, animals vary in their susceptibility to different biotypes and geographic strains. Trials by several researchers have shown that dogs were susceptible to human strains of *S. stercoralis* coming from one region of the world but not from another (Grove and Northern, 1982). However, studies elsewhere have made it possible to document molecular differences between the human and canine strains of *S. stercoralis*, and hence it is possible that the two strains are really different species or subspecies.

S. fuelleborni inhabits the intestine of man and nonhuman primates in Africa and Asia. Its development cycle is similar to that of *S. stercoralis*, except that the eggs hatch in the external environment rather than in the intestine. Hence eggs, rather than larvae, appear in fresh feces. Other animal species of *Strongyloides* can also infect man, but they remain as larval forms in the skin and cause symptoms similar to those of cutaneous larva migrans (WHO, 1979).

Geographic Distribution and Occurrence: *S. stercoralis* occurs worldwide, but it is more common in tropical and subtropical climates than in temperate regions. Not much is known about the prevalence of the infection. In 1947, it was estimated that nearly 34 million people throughout the world were parasitized, distributed as follows: 21 million in Asia, 8.6 million in Africa, 4 million in tropical regions of the Americas, 400,000 in North America, and 100,000 in the Pacific islands. A subsequent estimate in 2000 increased the number of human infections throughout the world to 200 million (Marquardt *et al.*, 2000). The infection has been observed in Mexico, all the countries of Central America, and parts of South America. Between 1965 and 1985, the following rates were cited: Argentina, 7.6%; Colombia, 16%; French Guiana, 23.6%; Panama, 20%; and Uruguay, 4.3%. In Iquitos, Peru, the rate was 60%; in Brazil, prevalence ranged from 4% to 58% depending on the area of the country; and in Chile, there have been only occasional cases in man or dogs. In Brazil, in an indigenous group of the Amazon region, the prevalence was 5.6% in 126 individuals in 1992 and subsequently dropped to 0% in 174 subjects from the same locality in 1995. Other studies in Brazil showed a prevalence of less than 1% in 264 food handlers in the state of Minas Gerais; 10.8% in 37,621 parasitologic examinations performed at a São Paulo hospital in 1993; 10.4% in 222 individuals from São Paulo in 1995 and 11.3% in 432 persons from the same locality in 1997; 5.8% in 485 persons from Pernambuco; and 15.2% in 99 AIDS patients in Rio de Janeiro. In Argentina during 1989–1999, the prevalence rate was 2% in 207 children from Corrientes and 83.3% in 36 children hospitalized in Salta. In Peru, the rate was 16% in 110 children and 2.4% in 1,511 hospitalized patients. During that same period, the infection was found in 20% of 241 Sudanese refugees and in 33% of 275 children in southern Sudan; 4% of 70 children in Kenya; 6.4% of 800 children in Guinea; 2.2% of 137 children in the Lao People's Democratic Republic; 10.1% of

2,008 inhabitants and 25.1% of 2,462 people from two communities in Nigeria; and 0.4% of 216,275 coprologic examinations performed by state laboratories in the US. The infection rate can reach as high as 85% in poor socioeconomic groups living in warm, humid regions of the tropics and in institutions such as hospitals for the mentally ill, where there are frequent opportunities for fecal contamination. On the other hand, in hot, semiarid areas the infection rate rarely exceeds 3%.

Strongyloidiasis in dogs appears to be distributed worldwide, but its prevalence is moderate. It was found in 6.3% of dogs and 4.8% of cats in Malaysia; in 2% and 1.5% of dogs in Canada and the US, respectively; and in only 2 of 646 dogs examined in Australia.

S. fuelleborni is a common parasite of nonhuman primates in Africa and Asia. It is frequently found in these animals both in the wild and in colonies. At a primate center in California, US, the parasite was detected in 50% of the imported monkeys and 75% of those born in captivity (Flynn, 1973). In man, it is more prevalent than *S. stercoralis* in the humid jungle regions of Central Africa—for example, Cameroon, Ethiopia, and the Central African Republic. Human *S. fuelleborni* infection is also prevalent in the African savannah. For example, Hira and Patel (1977) found that 9.9% of the strongyloidiasis cases in Zambia were caused by *S. fuelleborni*. In a study conducted in a small town in the Democratic Republic of Congo, the prevalence was 34% in 76 children examined and 48% in 185 individuals from the general population (Brown and Girardeau, 1977). In a jungle area of southern Cameroon, *S. fuelleborni* was found 31% of 154 Pygmies examined, while the rate for *S. stercoralis* was only 1%. In another area, the infection rates were 7% and 2%, respectively, for the two species.

The Disease in Man: In a high proportion of human patients, *S. stercoralis* infection can be of very long duration. The evidence suggests that, even though host immunity inhibits the development and pathogenicity of larvae, it does not terminate the infection. These hypobiotic larvae can remain in the patient's tissues for years as an asymptomatic and overlooked infection, until a breakdown of immunity enables them to resume their development and become pathogenic once again. Mild infections are usually well tolerated in immunocompetent individuals and produce no symptoms at all, or at most only vague and variable intestinal complaints. However, in persons with large parasite burdens or lowered immunity, the clinical picture can be cutaneous, pulmonary, or digestive, depending on the localization of the parasite, and the seriousness of the infection can range from mild to fatal (Liu and Weller, 1993).

The cutaneous symptoms that develop when the larva penetrates the skin may be the only manifestation of the infection apart from peripheral eosinophilia. The first sign is a small erythematous papule at the invasion site, which may be associated with intense pruritus, urticaria, and petechiae in patients who have been sensitized by previous exposure. After that, a linear, serpiginous, urticarial inflammation appears, known as *larva currens*, which is virtually pathognomonic of the infection; a similar lesion can be caused by the larvae of nonhuman ancylostomids such as *Ancylostoma braziliense* and *A. caninum* (Chabasse *et al.*, 1995). Some patients experience periodic urticaria, maculopapular exanthema, and pruritus, coinciding with attacks of diarrhea and the reappearance of larvae in feces. Skin lesions can be caused by other species of *Strongyloides* in addition to *S. stercoralis*. Based on experimental infections in a volunteer, it is suspected that cases of dermatitis with serpiginous eruptions among hunters in swampy areas of Louisiana, US, were caused by *S. procyonis*, a parasite of raccoons, or *S. myopotami*, of otters.

During the larvae's pulmonary migration phase, symptoms may range from an irritating cough to full-blown pneumonitis or bronchopneumonia, sometimes with eosinophilic pleural effusion (Emad, 1999). A review of patients with severe pulmonary manifestations revealed that most of them had had some risk factor for strongyloidiasis, such as corticosteroid use, age over 65 years, chronic pulmonary disease, use of antihistamines, or some chronic debilitating disease. Almost all the patients were experiencing cough, dyspnea, panting, and hemoptysis; in addition, 90% had pulmonary infiltrates, 75% had peripheral eosinophilia, 60% were suffering from secondary infections, 45% had adult respiratory distress syndrome, 15% had bacterial lung abscesses, and 30% of the patients died (Woodring *et al.*, 1996). In most cases, the bronchopulmonary manifestations are discrete and disappear within a few days. The serious pulmonary symptoms are usually associated with autoinfection.

Intestinal symptoms are predominant in the clinical picture. The intestine of parasitized individuals shows villous atrophy and cryptal hyperplasia (Coutinho *et al.*, 1996). Depending on the severity of the lesions caused by the parasites in the intestinal mucosa, the symptoms may correspond to an edematous catarrhal enteritis with thickening of the intestinal wall or an ulcerative enteritis. Among the other symptoms, epigastric pain, diarrhea, dyspepsia, nausea, and vomiting are common. Both abdominal pain and diarrhea occur intermittently. Leukocytosis and peripheral eosinophilia are common. Although 50% or more of infected individuals do not present symptoms, it should be kept in mind that asymptomatics can suddenly develop serious clinical disease if their immune resistance is lowered. This aggravation of a preexisting infection may come from a rapid rise in the parasite burden due to an endogenous hyperinfection triggered by the renewed development of hypobiotic larvae following the breakdown of immunity. A disruption of this kind in the equilibrium of the host-parasite relationship can occur in individuals weakened by concurrent illnesses, malnutrition, treatment with immunosuppressive drugs, or immunodeficiency diseases.

Several fatal cases of strongyloidiases have occurred in patients treated with corticosteroid or cytotoxic drugs. Most of these patients did not have symptoms of the infection and were not shedding larvae until the treatment was initiated. The clinical picture consists of ulcerative enteritis with abdominal pain, intense diarrhea, vomiting, malabsorption, dehydration, hypoproteinemia, and hypokalemia, and it can sometimes lead to death. In immunocompromised individuals such as patients with AIDS, strongyloidiasis becomes a disseminated infection, often with hyperinfection, which can affect any organ and be very serious. In most of these cases, the predominant symptoms are respiratory and pulmonary (Celedón *et al.*, 1994) and may include asthma, cavitation, opacities, consolidation, and infiltrates. Often, secondary bacterial infections can develop, such as bacteremia, peritonitis, meningitis, endocarditis, and abscesses at various sites. It is believed that the filariform larvae spread bacteria from the intestine to different parts of the body (Ramos *et al.*, 1984). There have also been reports of purulent meningitis (Foucan *et al.*, 1997) and nephrotic syndrome (Wong *et al.*, 1998) caused by the parasitosis. In addition, cases have been described of strongyloidiasis transmitted through an organ transplant obtained from a donor with a hypobiotic infection. The parasite does not seem to affect the organ recipient as long as he or she is receiving cyclosporin but can appear when the drug is suspended, perhaps because cyclosporin also has an inhibitory effect on the nematode (Palau and Pankey, 1997).

The pathogenicity of *S. fuelleborni* has been studied very little. Because simultaneous parasitoses occur so frequently in the tropics, it is difficult to link a particular symptom to a specific parasite. The most common complaints associated with this agent are abdominal pain and occasional diarrhea, as was observed in patients in Zambia and also in an experimentally infected volunteer (Hira and Patel, 1977). In general, infections caused by *S. fuelleborni* are not sufficiently intense to cause illness, and no superinfections have been reported.

The Disease in Animals: In dogs, the age of the host is an important factor. Clinical manifestations of *S. stercoralis* infection are seen only in young animals. Dogs and cats that have gotten rid of the parasite, either spontaneously or with treatment, are resistant to reinfection for more than six months. Unlike the human infection, which generally lasts for a long time if left untreated, the parasitosis in animals is of limited duration. The infection can be subclinical or symptomatic. In symptomatic cases, the first signs to appear in puppies are loss of appetite, purulent conjunctivitis, cough, and sometimes bronchopneumonia. The larval penetration phase can produce violent pruritus, erythema, and alopecia. The intestinal phase begins a week to 10 days later, with diarrhea, abdominal pain, and vomiting. Serious cases may include dehydration, emaciation, bloody diarrhea, and anemia, and they can even lead to death. In experimental infections, it has been observed that strongyloidiasis can become chronic in some adult dogs, but in veterinary practice the disease is limited to puppies.

In nonhuman primates infected with *S. fuelleborni*, the predominant symptom is diarrhea, which can vary from mild and benign to intense and hemorrhagic. In massive infections, the disease can be severe in weakened or very young animals.

Source of Infection and Mode of Transmission: Man is the principal reservoir of *S. stercoralis*. For both man and animals, the main source of infection is feces that contaminate the soil. The parasite usually enters by the cutaneous—rarely the oral—route, when the host comes in contact with third-stage or filariform larvae. Warm, moist soil is propitious for exogenic development of the heterogonic (indirect) cycle, which produces the free-living nematodes, because it allows for rapid multiplication of the infective larvae. For this reason, the infection is more common in tropical than in subtropical regions.

The role of dogs and cats in the epidemiology of strongyloidiasis has not yet been fully clarified. The susceptibility of dogs to certain biotypes or geographic strains would suggest that, at least in some parts of the world, these animals may contribute to human infection by contaminating the soil. However, the literature has recorded only one case (Georgi and Sprinkle, 1974) in which the source of human infection was attributed to canine feces. It is difficult to determine the frequency of human-animal cross-infections because there are no characteristics that distinguish the adults or larvae of *S. stercoralis* in man from those that occur in animals, but there are molecular differences, as mentioned earlier, that would suggest the human and canine parasites are different species or subspecies.

The reservoirs of *S. fuelleborni* are African and Asian simians. The source of infection is primate feces (nonhuman and human). Originally, the infection was zoonotic (from nonhuman to human primates), but there is growing evidence that *S. fuelleborni* in various parts of Africa is transmitted from human to human. Studies carried out in Zambia have confirmed that the parasitosis occurs among populations in periurban and urban areas, settings in which nonhuman primates are not usually found, and also in very young children (34% of 76 infants under 200 days old) (Hira and Patel, 1980; Brown and Girardeau, 1977). In such cases, it is undoubtedly man who maintains the cycle in nature. Likewise, the high prevalence of infection in some communities, such as the Pygmies, would suggest that the parasite has a tendency to adapt to the human species.

Other animal species of *Strongyloides* rarely succeed in completing their life cycle in man. In a volunteer experimentally infected with infective *S. procyonis* larvae from raccoons, very few specimens reached maturity and oviposition. Most animal species of *Strongyloides* are capable of invading human skin and causing transitory dermatitis.

Role of Animals in the Epidemiology of the Disease: Strongyloidiasis caused by *S. stercoralis* is a common disease and apparently intercommunicable between man and dogs. It has been thought that, in some areas, the infection can be transmitted from one species to another by means of contaminated soil, but the evidence of transmission from dog to man and vice versa is scant and circumstantial.

Strongyloidiasis caused by *S. fuelleborni* is an infection of both zoonotic and interhuman transmission. Dermatitis in man caused by other species of *Stongyloides* is zoonotic.

Diagnosis: Laboratory confirmation of the infection consists of finding rhabditiform *S. stercoralis* larvae or *S. fuelleborni* eggs in host feces. With strongyloidiasis, there are various means of improving the results of the coprologic examination. De Kaminsky (1993) studied 427 fecal samples to compare direct smear, the modified Baermann technique, and agar-plate culture: the smear revealed 9 infections; the Baermann technique, 42; and the culture, 70. However, the smear is the most economical; the Baermann technique was 4 times more expensive, and the culture, 15 times more costly. The larvae or eggs can be shed intermittently, and the tests should be repeated on three different days. Duodenal aspiration varies in its effectiveness, and this method is best used as a complement to the coprologic examination. Larvae can occasionally be observed in sputum. An enzyme-linked immunosorbent assay (ELISA) has been introduced which has presented some problems of cross-reactivity with other nematodes. However, adsorption of problem sera with *Onchocerca gutturosa* extract and the use of selected antigens has made it possible to achieve 94% to 97% specificity and 100% sensitivity (Lindo *et al.*, 1994). The conventional ELISA test is only 13% sensitive in immunodeficient patients, but it improves to 100% with the use of biotinylated conjugates or avidin-peroxidase (Abdul-Fattah *et al.*, 1995). Also, indirect immunofluorescence reaction has been reported to produce 92% to 94% sensitivity and 94% to 97% specificity (Costa-Cruz *et al.*, 1997).

Control: The most important community control measure is reduction of the source of infection through the sanitary disposal of human feces. It is important to treat all infected persons, even if they are asymptomatic, in order to reduce the possibility of contaminating the environment. As with ancylostomiasis, wearing shoes provides good protection in endemic areas because it prevents larvae from penetrating the skin of the foot. Since strongyloidiasis can be acquired by the oral route, good personal hygiene habits, such as washing one's hands before eating, are also important.

Prior to the initiation of any immunosuppressive treatment, it is recommended that the patient be tested for *S. stercoralis*. In the event that the results are positive, this infection should be treated first to prevent the possibility of hyperinfection.

Although the importance of domestic pets in transmission of the infection to man has not been determined, it is recommended to take basic precautions, such as treating infected dogs or cats.

Bibliography

Abdul-Fattah, M.M., M.E. Nasr, S.M. Yousef, M.I. Ibraheem, S.E. Abdul-Wahhab, H.M. Soliman. Efficacy of ELISA in diagnosis of strongyloidiasis among the immune-compromised patients. *J Egypt Soc Parasitol* 25:491–498, 1995.

Barriga, O.O. *Veterinary Parasitology for Practitioners*, 2nd ed. Edina: Burgess International Group; 1997.

Brown, R.C., M.H. Girardeau. Transmammary passage of *Strongyloides* sp. larvae in the human host. *Am J Trop Med Hyg* 26:215–219, 1977.

Celedón, J.C., U. Mathur-Wagh, J. Fox, R. García, P.M. Wiest. Systemic strongyloidiasis in patients infected with the human immunodeficiency virus. A report of 3 cases and review of the literature. *Medicine (Baltimore)* 73:256–263, 1994.

Chabasse, D., C. Le Clec'h, L. de Gentile, J.L. Verret. Le larbish. *Sante* 5:341–345, 1995.

Costa-Cruz, J.M., C.B. Bullamah, M.R. Gonçalves-Pires, D.M. Campos, M.A. Vieira. Cryo-microtome sections of coproculture larvae of *Strongyloides stercoralis* and *Strongyloides ratti* as antigen sources for the immunodiagnosis of human strongyloidiasis. *Rev Inst Med Trop Sao Paulo* 39:313–317, 1997.

Coutinho, H.B., T.I. Robalinho, V.B. Coutinho, *et al.* Immunocytochemistry of mucosal changes in patients infected with the intestinal nematode *Strongyloides stercoralis*. *J Clin Pathol* 49:717–720, 1996.

de Kaminsky, R.G. Evaluation of three methods for laboratory diagnosis of *Strongyloides stercoralis* infection. *J Parasitol* 79:277–280, 1993.

Emad, A. Exudative eosinophilic pleural effusion due to *Strongyloides stercoralis* in a diabetic man. *South Med J* 92:58–60, 1999.

Flynn, R.J. *Parasites of Laboratory Animals*. Ames: Iowa State University Press; 1973.

Foucan, L., I. Genevier, I. Lamaury, M. Strobel. Meningite purulente aseptique chez deux patients co-infectés par HTLV-1 et *Strongyloides stercoralis*. *Med Trop (Mars)* 57:262–264, 1997.

Georgi, J.R., C.L. Sprinkle. A case of human strongyloidiasis apparently contracted from asymptomatic colony dogs. *Am J Trop Med Hyg* 23:899–901, 1974.

Grove, D.I., C. Northern. Infection and immunity in dogs infected with a human strain of *Strongyloides stercoralis*. *Trans R Soc Trop Med Hyg* 76:833–838, 1982.

Hira, P.R., B.G. Patel. *Strongyloides fuelleborni* infections in man in Zambia. *Am J Trop Med Hyg* 26:640–643, 1977.

Hira, P.R., B.G. Patel. Human strongyloidiasis due to the primate species *Strongyloides fuelleborni*. *Trop Geogr Med* 32:23–29, 1980.

Lindo, J.F., D.J. Conway, N.S. Atkins, A.E. Bianco, R.D. Robinson, D.A. Bundy. Prospective evaluation of enzyme-linked immunosorbent assay and immunoblot methods for the diagnosis of endemic *Strongyloides stercoralis* infection. *Am J Trop Med Hyg* 51:175–179, 1994.

Liu, L.X., P.F. Weller. Strongyloidiasis and other intestinal nematode infections. *Infect Dis Clin North Am* 7:655–682, 1993.

Marquardt, W.C., R.S. Demaree, Jr., R.B. Grieve, eds. *Parasitology and Vector Biology*, 2nd ed. San Diego: Academic Press; 2000.

Palau, L.A., G.A. Pankey. *Strongyloides* hyperinfection in a renal transplant recipient receiving cyclosporine: Possible *Strongyloides stercoralis* transmission by kidney transplant. *Am J Trop Med Hyg* 57:413–415, 1997.

Ramachandran, S., A.A. Gam, F.A. Neva. Molecular differences between several species of *Strongyloides* and comparison of selected isolates of *S. stercoralis* using a polymerase chain reaction-linked restriction fragment length polymorphism approach. *Am J Trop Med Hyg* 56:61–65, 1997.

Ramos, M.C., R.J. Pedro, L.J. Silva, M.L. Branchinni, F.L. Gonçales Jr. Estrongiloidiase maciça. A propósito de quatro casos. *Rev Inst Med Trop Sao Paulo* 26:218–221, 1984.

Wong, T.Y., C.C. Szeto, F.F. Lai, C.K. Mak, P.K. Li. Nephrotic syndrome in strongyloidiasis: Remission after eradication with anthelmintic agents. *Nephron* 79:333–336, 1998.

Woodring, J.H., H. Halfhill II, R. Berger, J.C. Reed, N. Moser. Clinical and imaging features of pulmonary strongyloidiasis. *South Med J* 89:10–19, 1996.

World Health Organization (WHO). *Parasitic Zoonoses. Report of a WHO Expert Committee, with the Participation of FAO*. Geneva: WHO; 1979. (Technical Report Series 637).

THELAZIASIS

ICD-10 B83.8 Other specified helminthiases

Synonyms: Conjunctival spirurosis, thelaziosis, eyeworm.

Etiology: The agents of this disease are *Thelazia callipaeda, T. californiensis,* and *T. rhodesii.* These parasites are nematodes of the superfamily Thelazioidea whose adult stage lodges in the conjunctival sac and conjunctiva of domestic and wild mammals and, occasionally, of man. The other species of the genus *Thelazia* have not been found in humans; the correct identification is doubtful in the only human case attributed to *T. rhodesii.*

T. callipaeda is a parasite of dogs and other canids. The female measures 7 mm to 17 mm and the male measures 7 mm to 11.5 mm. The female lays embryonated eggs in the conjunctival sac, and the first-stage larvae are released and deposited on the conjunctiva. To continue their development, *Thelazia* spp. require a fly as an intermediate host. The flies, by sucking conjunctival secretions, ingest the larvae (or the eggs containing them). These larvae develop inside the insect for several weeks, until they become infective third-stage larvae. The infective larvae migrate to the proboscis of the fly and infect new conjunctiva when the arthropods resume sucking conjunctival secretions. In 2 to 6 weeks, the third-stage larva matures into an adult and begins to produce eggs. The intermediate host of *T. callipaeda* is not well known. In the Russian Far East, larvae of the parasite have been found in the fly *Phortina variegata,* and it is believed that this species could be the vector. The intermediate host of *T. californiensis* is the fly *Fannia thelaziae*, a member of the *F.*

benjamini complex (Weinmann, 1982). The intermediate hosts of *T. rhodesii* are various species of *Musca* (*M. autumnalis*, *M. convexifrons*, *M. larvipara*), *Morellia simplex,* and *Stomoxys calcitrans.*

Geographic Distribution and Occurrence: *T. callipaeda* is found in dogs and wild canids in the Far East. Up until 1985, more than 20 human cases had been reported in China, Korea, Japan, India, Thailand, and the eastern region of the former Soviet Union. Up until 2000, 9 more cases were reported: 1 in China; 4 in Korea, bringing that country to a total of 24 cases (Hong *et al.*, 1995); 1 of an undetermined species in India; 1 in Indonesia; 1 in Thailand; and 1 in Taiwan.

T. californiensis occurs in the western US, where it parasitizes the black-tailed jackrabbit (*Lepus californicus*), deer, coyotes, foxes, raccoons, bears, dogs, and less frequently, cats and sheep. Up until 1985, approximately 10 human cases had been reported, and 3 more had been reported by 2000. All the cases occurred in California, US, or in neighboring states.

T. rhodesii parasitizes bovines, goats, sheep, bubalines, and deer in North Africa, Europe, and the Middle East. One human case was described in Spain, but the identification of the etiologic agent has been questioned (Weinmann, 1982).

The Disease in Man and Animals: In man, *Thelazia* sp. lodge in the conjunctival sac, where they cause irritation, lacrimation, conjunctivitis, and sometimes, corneal scarring and opacity (Cheung *et al.*, 1998; Doezie *et al.*, 1996). Some infections manifested only as a bothersome sensation of a foreign body in the affected eye.

In animals, the parasite is found under the nictitating membrane. The symptomatology is similar to that of human thelaziasis. Conjunctivitis is often aggravated by pruritis, which causes the animal to rub against various objects. Corneal lesions are more common in animals than in humans, but it has not been well established whether they are due to the parasites or to other, concurrent causes. The intensity of symptoms is quite variable and may depend on the species of *Thelazia* affecting the animal; *T. rhodesii* is considered to be the most pathogenic, but it may not be infective for humans.

Source of Infection and Mode of Transmission: The reservoirs are several species of domestic and wild mammals. In a village in Thailand, where one human case caused by *T. callipaeda* occurred, five of seven dogs examined were infected. The infection is transmitted from one animal to another or from animal to man by various species of flies. Some species of *Thelazia* are very particular about their intermediate hosts and the first-stage larva develops only in certain species. This particularity largely determines the geographic distribution of both *T. californiensis* and *T. callipaeda.* The predilection of the different vectors for feeding on particular animal species is important in the epidemiology and is a factor that limits the number of human cases. Transmission is seasonal and occurs when vector flies are abundant.

Diagnosis: After a local anesthetic is administered, the parasites are seen as white threads in the conjunctiva or conjunctival sac, and are extracted with ophthalmic forceps and identified.

Control: Special prevention measures are not justified because human infection is so rare.

Bibliography

Bhaibulaya, M., S. Prasertsilpa, S. Vajrasthira. *Thelazia callipaeda* (Raillet and Henry, 1910), in man and dog in Thailand. *Am J Trop Med Hyg* 19(3):476–479, 1970.

Cheung, W.K., H.J. Lu, C.H. Liang, M.L. Peng, H.H. Lee. Conjunctivitis caused by *Thelazia callipaeda* infestation in a woman. *J Formos Med Assoc* 97(6):425–427, 1998.

Doezie, A.M., R.W. Lucius, W. Aldeen, D.V. Hale, D.R. Smith, N. Mamalis. *Thelazia californiensis* conjunctival infestation. *Ophthalmic Surg Lasers* 27(8):716–719, 1996.

Hong, S.T., Y.K. Park, S.K. Lee, *et al.* Two human cases of *Thelazia callipaeda* infection in Korea. *Korean J Parasitol* 33(2):139–144, 1995.

Smith, T.A., M.I. Knudsen. Eye worms of the genus *Thelazia* in man, with a selected bibliography. *Calif Vect News* 17:85–94, 1970.

Weinmann, C.J. Thelaziasis. *In*: Steele, J.H., section ed. Section C, Vol. 2: *CRC Handbook Series in Zoonoses*. Boca Raton: CRC Press; 1982.

TRICHINOSIS

ICD-10 B75 Trichinellosis

Synonyms: Trichiniasis, trichinelliasis.

Etiology: The agents of this disease are nematodes of the genus *Trichinella*, particularly *T. spiralis*. This species is a small nematode of the intestine of predatory mammals and the muscles of mammals preyed upon by other animals. In the intestine, the adults measure 1–3 mm; in the muscles, the larvae measure less than 1 mm. *T. spiralis* was described by Owen in 1835 and was thought to be a single species until, in 1972, Soviet researchers determined that there were several species. The taxonomic category, species, subspecies, strains, or varieties of the new entities were debated for a long time. After the detailed review by Pozio *et al.* (1992), most authors seem to have accepted their categorization as comparatively new species. Differentiation of those species by polymerase chain reaction restriction fragment length polymorphism (Wu *et al.*, 1999) supports this opinion. Bessonov (1998) holds the opposite opinion, but his writings are less widely read, being in Russian. Apart from three phenotypes of *T. spiralis* of uncertain taxonomic category, the generally accepted species (Barriga, 1997) are *T. spiralis*, *T. nativa*, *T. nelsoni*, *T. pseudospiralis*, and *T. britovi*. Most of our knowledge about the parasite, the infection, and the disease results from studies of the classic species, *T. spiralis*.

T. spiralis is adapted to temperate zones where swine are raised; it is found in domestic, peridomestic, and wild epidemiological cycles. It is highly infective to mice, rats, guinea pigs, rabbits, and swine, and moderately infective to hamsters. It does not infect birds. The species is highly pathogenic to mice and rats and moderately pathogenic to humans. In the muscle, the larva does not survive more than 10 or 20 days at −15°C.

T. nativa is adapted to the northern circumpolar regions, above the 40th parallel, where it circulates among wild carnivores, such as bears and foxes, and their prey. The species is highly infective to mice and slightly infective to rats, hamsters, guinea pigs, rabbits, and swine. It does not infect birds. The larva survives in the muscle for more than 12 months at temperatures of –15°C.

T. *nelsoni* is adapted to the tropical and semitropical areas of Africa, Asia, and Europe, and areas near the Mediterranean Sea; it circulates among carnivores such as foxes, panthers, leopards, lions, hyenas, and wild boar. The species is slightly infective to mice, rats, hamsters, and swine, moderately pathogenic to mice, slightly pathogenic to rats, and less pathogenic than T. *spiralis* to humans. It does not infect birds. The larva survives in the muscle for 6 or more months at –12°C or –17°C and is resistant to high temperatures.

T. *pseudospiralis* is distributed in North America, India, and the former Soviet Union; it is thought to circulate among predators of birds and their prey. The species is highly infective to hamsters, slightly infective to rats, and less pathogenic than T. *spiralis* to monkeys and, presumably, to humans. Unlike the other species, it does not encyst, and it infects birds. The larva in the muscle dies in three days at –12°C or –17°C.

T. *britovi* is adapted to the temperate and subarctic regions of Eurasia; it circulates among wild carnivores, mainly foxes, but also wolves and mustelids, and their prey, the wild boar. The species is slightly infective to mice, rats, and swine, less pathogenic than T. *spiralis* to humans, and less resistant to freezing than T. *nativa*.

When a carnivore or omnivore ingests meat with infective first-stage *Trichinella* larvae, the larvae are released in the small intestine, penetrate the mucosa, go through four rapid molts, return to the lumen, and mature into adults in just two days. The adult parasites mate, the female invades the intestinal mucosa again, and begins to release live larvae on the fifth day of infection, with the highest number being released on the ninth day. The period of larviposition and the number of larvae produced are limited by the immune response of the host. In a primary infection, larviposition lasts 10 to 20 days in mice and rats, and about 6 weeks in man; each female produces between 200 and 1,700 larvae. The larvae are disseminated through the organism by the circulatory system and, in a few hours, penetrate the striated muscle fibers, where they coil up and grow for the next 10 days. The parasite prefers the most active muscle groups, especially the jaw, lingual, ocular, back, and lumbar muscles, and the pillars of the diaphragm. The larva quickly takes control of the muscle cell's function and converts it to a nurse cell which satisfies the metabolic needs of the parasite. The larvae that penetrate tissues other than the striated muscles do not continue to develop. The larva becomes infective for the next host approximately 16 days after invading the muscle. At around day 10, a collagen cyst formed by the host starts to surround the larva. The cyst is completely formed in about three months, is shaped like a lemon measuring approximately 1 mm, and, in most cases, contains a single larva. The cysts generally begin to calcify at around six months, but the parasites can live inside them for up to three years or more. Ingestion of those infected muscles by another host reinitiates the cycle. It is worthy of note that the same host acts first as the definitive host and then as the intermediate host.

Geographic Distribution: T. *spiralis* is widely distributed in the temperate countries. Steele (1982) undertook a detailed review of its distribution up until approximately 1980. Its presence has not been confirmed in Australia or in several tropical or semitropical countries in Africa, Latin America, and Asia. However, it should be borne in mind that research has been limited for the most part to the domestic cycle in swine, rats, and man. Thus, the possibility exists that the infection may occur in wild or synanthropic animals without human cases having been reported. For information on the geographic distribution of the other species, see Etiology. In several countries there is more than one species. For example, *T. spiralis* and *T. britovi* have been found in China and Spain; *T. spiralis* and *T. nelsoni* in France; and *T. spiralis*, *T. britovi*, and *T. nativa* in Estonia. *T. spiralis* is found in domestic or peridomestic environments, and the other species in wild environments (Pozio *et al.*, 1998).

Occurrence in Man: There is a great difference between the real prevalence of trichinosis and that diagnosed or reported. During the time when approximately 2% of the US population was infected, there were less than two hundred known clinical cases. This may be due to the fact that trichinosis is easy to confuse with influenza, which results in many erroneous diagnoses.

In the Americas, the disease has occurred in Argentina, Canada, Chile, Mexico, the US, Uruguay, and Venezuela. In some other countries or territories, isolated cases have been recorded, but it is not clear whether they were autochthonous or imported cases. Few outbreaks of trichinosis have been recorded in Canada. In 1974, 1975, and 1976, there were 49, 3, and 31 clinical cases, respectively. Examination of the diaphragms of persons who died from other causes revealed percentages of infection ranging from 1.5% in Toronto to 4%–6% in British Columbia. Infection among indigenous peoples is frequent in northern Canada, but clinical cases are sporadic or affect only small groups. In that region the source of infection is wild mammals, both terrestrial and marine, and the etiologic agent is probably *T. nativa*. While the parasite is virtually nonexistent in swine, and human cases originating in swine have not occurred for nearly 20 years, cases still occur because of the consumption of wild boar. The 1993 outbreak in Ontario affected 24 people (Greenbloom *et al.*, 1997). In the US, 1,428 cases were recorded in the 10 years from 1972 to 1981, for an annual average of 143 cases, 7 deaths, and a fatality rate of 0.49%. Distribution of the disease was unequal: of the 188 cases that occurred in 1981, 81.3% originated in five northeastern states and Alaska. The rate per million inhabitants was 0.8 for the whole country, 36.7 for Rhode Island, and 33.9 for Alaska (CDC, 1982).

The reduction in the incidence and intensity of the disease is noteworthy: in the period 1947–1956, an average of 358 cases were recorded each year, with 84 deaths and a fatality rate of 2.3%; between 1984 and 1988, just 44 cases per year were recorded on average. The reduction is due essentially to the decline of the infection in swine, but the importance of the infection from game animals has increased: Dworkin *et al.* (1996) reported on an epidemic of 15 cases in Idaho caused by cougar meat infected with *T. nativa*. While the rates are low, the infection still exists in swine in the US and can affect humans who eat the raw pork: 90 refugees from Southeast Asia were infected in Iowa in 1990 by eating raw sausages prepared with store-bought pork (McAuley *et al.*, 1992). The real prevalence of the infection has also declined, as confirmed by autopsies. Between 1936 and 1941, an estimated 12% of the population was infected, while in 1970 the adjusted rate of infection was 2.2%. In 1940, 7.3% of inhabitants had live trichinae in their diaphragms—suggesting relatively recent infection—while in 1970, the rate was 0.7%. In Mexico, studies carried out between 1939 and 1953 discovered trichinae in 4% to 15% of autopsies; a study in 1972–1973 found the larvae in 4.2% of cadavers. In 1975, just three cases were diagnosed in the country. However, in Zacatecas, there were 17 outbreaks with a total of 108 cases between 1978 and 1983 (Fragoso et al., 1984).

Outbreaks of trichinosis occur periodically in Argentina and Chile, which are the only South American countries where the disease is important from the public health standpoint. In 1976, the rate per 100,000 population was 0.1 for Argentina and 0.5 for Chile. In 1982, in Santiago, Chile, a 2.8% rate of infection was found in the cadavers of people who died in accidents or by other violent means. The percentage is similar to that reported in studies carried out in 1966–1967 and 1972; however, in 1982, all the larvae were calcified and the prevalence shifted to older age groups, which could be interpreted as a decrease in new infections. The epidemic reported in Argentina in 1991 affected 18 people in southern Buenos Aires (Venturiello et al., 1993), and the epidemic reported in Chile in 1992 affected 36 people in the southern part of that country (Zamorano et al., 1994).

The morbidity rate has also declined in Europe. For example, in Poland, where previously more than 500 cases occurred per year, the incidence has diminished notably and no major outbreaks were reported in the last years of the twentieth century. In the former Soviet Union, the endemic area with the highest prevalence is found in Belarus, where 90% of all cases have occurred. The sporadic cases recorded in the northern and central Asian regions of the former Soviet Union resulted from the consumption of wild animal meat. An outbreak in Italy in 1975, which affected 89 people who ate horse meat imported from eastern Europe, was attributed to T. nelsoni. A similar outbreak occurred in France (Bellani et al., 1978). Later, an outbreak of trichinosis was discovered in Paris, France, with more than 250 human cases caused by the consumption of raw or undercooked horse meat imported from the US (Ancelle and Dupouy-Camet, 1985). In 1993, there was another outbreak in France, affecting 554 people, attributed to the consumption of horse meat (Dupouy-Camet et al., 1994). Infection caused by horse meat is surprising because strictly herbivorous animals such as horses would not have the opportunity to become infected. It has been hypothesized that these animals may have inadvertently eaten infected rodents with their fodder, or that the horses became infected by eating necrophagous insects in their pasture. Trichina larvae have been proven to survive five to eight days in the intestines of these insects and, since they multiply in the host's intestine, a few larvae ingested in this manner could cause a significant infection in a horse (Barriga, 1997).

In Asia, human trichinosis was not considered important until the 1960s and 1970s. In Thailand, the first outbreak occurred in 1962 in the northern part of the country, and from then until 1973, 975 cases and 58 deaths were recorded. The first outbreak in Japan occurred in 1974, and a total of three outbreaks had been reported by 1991: the first affected 15 people in 1974; the second affected 12 people in 1980; and the third affected 60 people in 1981. All the infections were due to consumption of bear meat (Yamaguchi, 1991). A domestic cycle does not seem to exist in that country. In Lebanon, an epidemic probably affected more than 1,000 people in 1982, and another affected 44 people in 1995 (Haim et al., 1997). Two epidemics reported in China occurred in an endemic area in the center of the country: one affected 54 people in the 1980s and the other affected 291 in the period 1995–1996 (Cui et al., 1997). In China, larvae have been found in swine, dog, sheep, and bear meat.

The situation in Africa is peculiar. In countries of northern Africa bordering on the

Mediterranean, some outbreaks of human trichinosis were known in Algeria and in Egypt among Copts and tourists, but it was believed that the disease did not exist south of the Sahara. The first outbreak in Kenya, due to *T. nelsoni*, was diagnosed in 1959. The investigation demonstrated that the human infection originated as a result of consumption of meat from a bush pig (*Potamochoerus porcus*). Later research discovered that the infection is widely distributed in the wild fauna of Africa, including warthogs (*Phacochoerus aethiopicus*), hyenas, jackals, and some felids.

The infection is frequent in the Arctic regions and is mainly due to the consumption of bear meat. Cases linked to walrus meat were first described in Greenland and then in the northern part of Alaska. The species that circulates at these latitudes is *T. nativa*, which is characterized by greater resistance to freezing temperatures.

Human cases are unknown in Australia. The Hawaiian Islands are the only endemic area in the Pacific; a survey conducted in 1964 found the parasite in 7.4% of cadavers autopsied. In New Zealand, the first human case was diagnosed in 1964, and the first human infection attributed to *T. pseudospiralis* was identified in 1994; the species of the parasite was confirmed by molecular biology techniques (Andrews *et al.*, 1995). In 1994–1995, an epidemic in Thailand caused by raw meat from an infected wild pig affected 59 people and caused one death (Jongwutiwes *et al.*, 1998).

In general, human trichinosis is still widespread in many parts of the world, but morbidity rates are low and declining.

Occurrence in Animals: *T. spiralis* has a wide range of hosts among domestic and wild animals. The infection has been confirmed in 150 species of mammals, from primates to marsupials, including cetaceans and pinnipeds. Of special interest among domestic animals are swine, whose meat and by-products are the main source of infection for man. The infection rate in swine depends on how they are managed and, in particular, how they are fed. There is a marked difference in the rates of infection in grain-fed swine and those fed raw waste from either the home or from slaughterhouses. In the US, in 1950, the prevalence of trichinosis in swine fed waste was 11%, while it was only 0.63% in those fed grain. When mandatory cooking of waste intended for swine food was established in order to prevent viral infections, the prevalence decreased rapidly to 2.2% between 1954 and 1959, to 0.5% in the 1970s, and to even lower rates later on, when less than 1% of swine in the US were fed waste. The source of the infection is not clear, especially because, on several occasions, the role of rats was discounted. In a serologic examination of 4,078 swine on 156 farms in the region of New England and the state of New Jersey, US, 15 positive swine were found on 10 farms, for an individual prevalence of 0.37% and a herd prevalence of 6.4%. The most important risk factors were access of swine to live wildlife and wildlife carcasses on the farm. However, since there was no association between the infection and the consumption of scraps of human food, the recycling of infected pork is no longer an important factor in that area (Gamble *et al.*, 1999).

In many European countries, the parasitosis is no longer found in swine; the highest frequency is 0.1%, usually on small farms. In 1976 in Germany, only one infected pig was found out of 32 million examined by trichinoscopy (observation of larvae by pressing a muscle sample between two slides and viewing it under a microscope). In the Netherlands, not a single infected pig was discovered by trichinoscopic examination between 1926 and 1962. However, use of the digestion method (digestion of muscle samples and observation of larvae in the sediment) demonstrated that some pigs had very low intensity infections, with 0.025 larvae per gram of meat (Ruitenberg *et al.*, 1983).

In Brazil, Colombia, Ecuador, Paraguay, and Venezuela, the parasite has not been found by trichinoscopic examination. In Argentina and Chile, trichinoscopy records indicate a general frequency of 0.14% and 0.33%, respectively. Of course, the prevalence is much higher in selected samples, such as pigs that roam around garbage dumps or pigs from small farms that are fed kitchen waste, and it is these animals that frequently give rise to epidemic outbreaks in South America.

Dogs and cats have ample opportunity to become infected both in the domestic cycle, with raw meat provided by their owners, and in the wild cycle, through the hunting of omnivorous rodents. For this reason, the prevalence in these animals is generally higher than in pigs. Studies of street dogs in Santiago, Chile (Letonja and Ernst, 1974) found rates ranging from 1.2% to 4%, while 72% of 36 dogs captured in 1955 in the municipal slaughterhouse were infected. In a later study in Valdivia Province, in southern Chile, 30 urban dogs and 30 rural dogs were examined, and 6.6% and 16.6%, respectively, were found to be infected (Oberg *et al.*, 1979). In Mexico City, 3.3% of 150 dogs examined had trichinellosis, while in Maracay, Venezuela, all 600 animals examined were free of infection. Infection rates of 45% to 60% have been found in dogs in Alaska, Greenland, and Siberia. The parasite was discovered in 7 of 12 cats examined in San Luis, Argentina; in 2% of 50 cats in Santiago, Chile; and in 25% of 300 cats studied in Mexico. By contrast, in Maracay, Venezuela, none of the 120 cats examined gave a positive result. In the US, Europe, and the former Soviet Union, the infection in dogs and cats is relatively frequent, with prevalence rates higher than those in pigs.

Rats also participate in the synanthropic or peridomestic cycle. In the US, rural rats are not infected, but a high rate of infection has been found among rats living in garbage dumps (5.3% of 1,268). In the former Soviet Union, 1.6% of 8,037 rats were found to be infected. High rates of infection have been found in Lebanon (36% in a survey in 1952) and in British Columbia, Canada (25% in 1951). Studies in Costa Rica, Ecuador, Panama, Puerto Rico, and Venezuela, and more recently in Santos and São Paulo, Brazil (Paim and Cortes, 1979), yielded negative results. Almost all of these studies employed trichinoscopy, which is not very sensitive for detection of the parasite, so very low levels of infection cannot be discounted. Numerous surveys have been done in Chile, where an important role in the epizootiology is attributed to rats. Of rats captured in garbage dumps in Santiago and Antofagasta, 8% and 28.6%, respectively, were found to be infected. Surveys conducted in 1951 and 1967 in the municipal slaughterhouse of Santiago revealed infection rates in *Rattus norvegicus* of 10% and 25%, respectively. A high rate of infection (86%) was also found in rats captured in 1983 in several sectors of the city of Concepción. In the epidemiologic investigation of an outbreak that affected 60 persons, 12.3% of swine and 30.7% of *R. norvegicus* were found to be infected.

The main reservoirs of trichina in nature, however, seem to be the wild carnivores. The fox (*Vulpes vulpes*) is important in Europe because of its abundance and high infection rates. Trichinosis is also frequent among Old World badgers (*Meles meles*), wolves (*Canis lupus*), lynxes (*Felis lynx*) and wild boar (*Sus scrofa*). In the state of Alaska and other areas of the Arctic and Subarctic, high rates of infection have been found in the polar bear (*Thalarctos maritimus*), with an average of 45% parasitized, as well as in other ursids, Arctic and red foxes, and several species of mustelids. Among marine mammals, the infection has been confirmed in walruses (*Odobenus rosmarus*), with a prevalence of 0.6% to 9%, and low rates have been found in other pinnipeds and cetaceans. In the US, the parasite was discovered in 5% of minks and 6.4% of foxes in Iowa. Low-intensity infection was found in wild rodents (*Microtus pennsylvanicus*, *Sigmodon hispidus*, and others) in Virginia (Holliman and Meade, 1980). There is enough evidence to assume that the wild cycle of trichinosis is self-sustainable. However, on at least one occasion, it seems that a coyote became infected through infected swine (Minchella *et al.*, 1989).

In sub-Saharan Africa, only the wild cycle is known. The parasite is widely distributed among wild carnivores. The infection has been confirmed in hyenas, jackals, leopards, lions, servals (*Felis serval*), and wild pigs. Hyenas (*Crocuta crocuta* and *Hyaena hyaena*) seem to be the main reservoirs; 10 of 23 *C. crocuta* tested were positive.

Except in Argentina and Chile, studies have not been done on the wild fauna of Latin America. In central Chile, 2,063 wild animals were examined, of which 301 were carnivores (usually very parasitized) and 1,762 were rodents (generally not very parasitized), and the infection was not found in any of them. Out of 20 animals examined in Argentina, a fox (*Pseudalopex gracilis*), an armadillo (*Chaetophractus villosus*), and a rodent (*Graomis griseoflavus)* were found to be infected.

The Disease in Man: Only a small proportion of infections—those that are intense—are manifested clinically. It is thought that man needs 10 to 100 parasites per gram of muscle in order to show symptoms. Many sporadic cases pass unnoticed or are confused with other diseases.

In classic trichinosis caused by *T. spiralis*, the incubation period lasts about 10 days, but can vary greatly—from 1 to 43 days—and seems to be directly related to the number of larvae ingested. Three phases of the disease are described: intestinal, larval migration, and convalescence. The intestinal phase is uncommon and occurs in about 15% of patients; it is expressed as a nonspecific gastroenteritis, with anorexia, nausea, vomiting, abdominal pain, and diarrhea.

Seven to 11 days after ingestion of the infective food, the signs of the larval migration phase begin, with fever, myalgias (which may be pronounced and in diverse locations), edema of the upper eyelids (a very common and prominent sign), cephalalgia, sweating, and chills. In a small proportion of patients with severe disease there may be urticaria or scarlatiniform eruptions, and respiratory and neurologic symptoms. The vast majority of patients have leukocytosis and eosinophilia. In 95.9% of 47 Chilean patients, eosinophilia with values above 6% was found. The disease lasts about 10 days in moderate infections, but may persist a month or more in massive infections. In the convalescent phase, muscular pains can sometimes persist for several months. In cases of infection caused by *T. spiralis* in Italy, Pozio *et al.* (1993) found eosinophilia in 100% of the patients, specific IgG antibodies in 100%, high levels of creatine phosphokinase in 90%, fever in 60%, myalgia in 50%, diarrhea in 40%, and antibodies against the newborn larva in 30%. In epidemic outbreaks, mortality is usually under 1%.

In a study of 150 patients suffering from trichinosis due to *T. nelsoni* in an outbreak in Italy, myalgia was found in 88%, myositis in 62%, muscular weakness in

60%, and arthralgia in 20%. The degree of myositis was directly related to the degree of hypereosinophilia, and the muscle damage observed microscopically was often related to eosinophilic infiltration of the muscle. The arthralgia was closely related to the myalgias/myositis. There was no relationship between the clinical manifestations and the IgG or IgE antibodies. There was no vascularitis or involvement of the nervous system or heart. *T. nelsoni* seems to mainly affect the muscular system, with a favorable prognosis (Ferraccioli *et al.*, 1988).

In *T. britovi* infections, Italian authors have observed that the patients present milder gastrointestinal symptoms, lower levels of creatine phosphokinase, and less persistence of specific IgG antibodies in comparison with patients suffering from classic *T. spiralis* (Pozio *et al.*, 1993).

In an outbreak caused by *T. pseudospiralis* in Thailand, the most striking clinical manifestations were muscular swelling, myalgia, and asthenia of more than four months' duration (Jongwutiwes *et al.*, 1998).

The Disease in Animals: Trichinosis does not cause clinical manifestations in animals at the level of infection found in nature. However, massive experimental infections cause illness or death in rats, dogs, cats, and swine; the infected animals exhibit peripheral eosinophilia, fever, anorexia, emaciation, and muscle pain.

Source of Infection and Mode of Transmission: Trichinosis in nature is an infection of wild animals. The parasite circulates between predatory carnivores and omnivorous or necrophagous animals. The former become infected by hunting and consuming the latter, and the latter become infected by eating the carcasses of the former. From the epidemiological standpoint, the parasite's resistance to putrefaction is important; live, often infective, larvae have been found in badly decayed flesh for up to four months, which facilitates the infection of carrion eaters. A domestic, peridomestic, or synanthropic cycle derives from this wild cycle when synanthropic animals such as rats, dogs, cats, and swine become infected by eating infected wild animals and carry the infection to the domestic environment. In an extensive study, Gamble *et al.* (1999) found that the risk factors for the infection in swine are access to live wildlife or wildlife carcasses on the farm. The consumption of garbage did not constitute a risk for infection. In places where modern technology is applied to swine breeding, such as Japan and Switzerland, the wild cycle can exist without extending to the domestic environment (Gotstein *et al.*, 1997; Yamaguchi, 1991). There is some evidence that the infection can also extend from the domestic to the wild environment: Minchella *et al.* (1989) found a coyote infected with swine trichinae.

It is assumed that, once in the domestic environment, the parasite circulates among pigs, dogs, cats, and rats. The parasite is transmitted from pig to pig mainly by the ingestion of food scraps containing raw pork. The incidence of trichinosis in swine fed raw waste from kitchens, restaurants, or slaughterhouses is 20 times higher than that in grain-fed swine. Another source of infection for swine may be dead infected animals, including rats, but also dogs, cats, or wild animals, which are sometimes found in garbage dumps. One theory is that the consumption of infected rats explains the swine infections which, in turn, cause outbreaks of the infection in man. While it is true that an association between high rates of infection in rats and swine has sometimes been found, there is also solid research that casts doubt on this association (Campbell, 1983). It has also been shown that the pig can acquire the infection from another pig by coprophagia, since some trichina larvae are eliminated in the feces of swine that ingest infected meat for up to five days after ingestion, and they can infect another swine that eats them. Infection of swine by chewing the tails of other (infected) swine has also been described. These last two transmission mechanisms are of little practical importance.

Dogs and cats probably become infected when they eat scraps of infected raw pork provided by their owners or by hunting infected rats or ingesting infected dead domestic, peridomestic, or wild animals. Sled dogs in the Arctic are infected by eating wild animal meat fed to them by man or by consuming carrion they find in their habitat. This explains the extremely high rates (50% or more) found among dogs in that region. In turn, dog and cat carcasses transmit the infection to other carrion eaters, rats, and swine.

Rats become infected by eating infected domestic or wild animals and by cannibalism. The role of the rat in the epidemiology of trichinosis, considered central for a long time, has not been objectively proven. In the opinion of most modern investigators, its epidemiological role seems to be secondary.

Man is an accidental host in whom the parasite finds a dead end, except in unusual circumstances, such as in eastern Africa, where some tribes abandon the dead or dying to the hyenas. The human infection occurs mainly as a result of consuming raw or undercooked pork or pork by-products, but also as a result of eating wild game. It is estimated that the meat of a single parasitized pig weighing 100 kg can be a potential source of infection for 360 persons. Since pork is frequently added to beef in the manufacture of sausage, the potential risk is even greater. In Argentina and Chile, outbreaks most commonly occur in rural areas, with the source of infection being a pig killed by its owner and thus not subjected to veterinary inspection. The sources of infection are almost always pigs fed waste from kitchens, restaurants, or local slaughterhouses and, in small towns, animals kept at garbage dumps. However, even pigs inspected in slaughterhouses can give rise to infections, albeit probably mild infections, since trichinoscopy cannot detect low-level parasitoses (fewer than 1–3 larvae per gram of muscle). The US is one of the few developed countries in which trichinosis is still a public health problem, although on a much smaller scale than it used to be. Of 947 human cases for which the source of infection could be ascertained, 79.1% were attributable to pork products, 6% were due to ground beef (probably contaminated with pork), and 13.9% were linked to wild animal meat, especially bear. In Alaska, half the cases were due to bear meat and the other half to walrus meat. In Japan, all the cases were due to the consumption of wild animals. In contrast to the epidemiological pattern in Latin America, where the infection often results from slaughter of animals and preparation of sausages at home, 81% of the tainted pork products in the US were acquired in supermarkets, butcher shops, or similar outlets. Products acquired directly from farms caused only 13.8% of the cases recorded between 1975 and 1981 (Schantz, 1983). This is due to the fact that inspection for *Trichinella* is mandatory in slaughterhouses in most of the Latin American countries where the parasite occurs, but not in the US.

In man, as in animals, the frequency of the infection and its intensity increase with age, as a result of longer opportunity for infection and reinfection. In the US, between 1966 and 1970, the average intensity for people who died under the age of 45 was 2.4 trichinae per gram of diaphragm material, while the same study found that for older persons, it was 12.2 per gram (Zimmermann and Zinter, 1971).

Religion and ethnic origin have a great influence on the prevalence of the infection. The prevalence of trichinosis is very low among Muslims, Jews, and Seventh Day Adventists, whose religious beliefs prohibit the consumption of pork. In the Middle East, the disease occurs in Lebanon, where the Christian population is large, but is very rare in the predominantly Muslim countries. On the other hand, prevalence rates in the US are higher in some ethnic groups, such as Italians, Germans, and Poles, because of their preference for pork products processed at a temperature insufficient to destroy the larvae. In the former Soviet Union, the habit of consuming raw salt pork (which contains muscle fibers) explains why this product is one of the main sources of infection.

Food preservation technology and the peculiarities of the different variants of *Trichinella* also influence the occurrence and prevalence of trichinellosis. The reduction in the incidence and intensity of human infection observed in the US in the last decades of the twentieth century is due in large part to the generalized practice of freezing pork products, both commercially and at home. Freezing is an effective means of killing the *T. spiralis* larvae found in pork or pork products. Regulations in Canada and the US establish that pork products less than 15 cm thick must be frozen at −15°C for 20 days or −30°C for six days. These temperatures are sufficient to kill the *T. spiralis* larvae, but not the *T. nativa* larvae, which are found in terrestrial and marine mammals of the Arctic region. For example, viable larvae have been found in bear meat frozen at an ambient temperature of −32°C for several weeks, and in walrus meat kept in a home freezer at −12°C for a month.

Most outbreaks in Argentina and Chile occur in winter or early spring when home slaughter of pigs is more frequent. Neighbors usually participate in sausage-making and eat the recently made products at community meals.

In some parts of the world, such as the Arctic and Subarctic and eastern Africa, the meat of wild animals constitutes the main source of human infection. In Africa, three outbreaks are known to have been caused by consumption of bush pig (*Potamochoerus porcus*) meat. Although the immediate source of human infection was the meat of wild swine, the main reservoirs seem to be wild canids, especially hyenas. Outbreaks in the Arctic region generally affect only a few persons. Nevertheless, an epidemic was recorded in Greenland in 1947 that caused 300 cases and 33 deaths. The origin of that epidemic was not discovered, but in a later outbreak, the source of infection was found to be walrus meat. Two more outbreaks were subsequently described in Alaska due to the consumption of walrus meat (Margolis *et al.*, 1979). The relative rarity of clinical cases at those latitudes is explained by the low intensity of the parasitosis in wild animals. Outside the Arctic region, cases of human trichinosis whose source of infection was bear meat have occurred. Between 1967 and 1981, 5% of the human cases in the US resulted from the ingestion of such meat (Schantz, 1983). In several European countries, infection due to bear or wild boar meat is playing an increasing role in the epidemiology of the disease, and outbreaks of this nature have been described in the former Czechoslovakia and the former Soviet Union (Ruitenberg *et al.*, 1983). There were also 58 cases of trichinosis in China due to consumption of bear meat (Wang and Luo, 1981) and 87 in Japan (Yamaguchi, 1991).

Role of Animals in the Epidemiology of the Disease: Trichinosis is an infection

of wild and domestic animals that is accidentally transmitted to man by the ingestion of raw or undercooked meat or meat products. It is a food-originated zoonosis.

Diagnosis: The clinical diagnosis of trichinosis is difficult due to its nonspecific
symptomatology and its similarity to common infectious diseases such as influenza.
Individual or sporadic cases are often confused with other diseases, but the diagnosis can be supported by the epidemiological circumstances (such as the recent consumption of pork or bear meat and the concurrent occurrence of other, similar cases)
and with confirmation of peripheral eosinophilia, increased enzymes that indicate
muscle damage, and increased erythrosedimentation. Specific diagnosis can be
made by muscle biopsy and observation of the larvae. This technique is rarely used
in man because it is painful and of limited utility. It is justified only for ruling out
collagen diseases with which trichinosis may be confused.

Very precise immunobiologic and molecular biology tests are available (Ko,
1997). The preferred tests for diagnosis of the human infection, because of their sensitivity and specificity, are indirect immunofluorescence, enzyme-linked
immunosorbent assay (ELISA), immunoelectrotransfer, and polymerase chain reaction. Some authors still recommend the use of undefined mixtures as antigens
(Sandoval *et al.*, 1995), but there is strong evidence that the antigen used is crucial
to the sensitivity and specificity of the tests and how early they will detect the disease (Homan *et al.*, 1992). Consequently, modern authors prefer to use well-defined
antigens. Ben *et al.* (1997) compared indirect immunofluorescence with the enzymatic immunohistochemical technique and found a high correlation between them;
the latter showed sensitivity of 100% and specificity of 93%. ELISA is considered
to be sensitive and versatile because it detects different classes of immunoglobulins.
In a study during an outbreak caused by bear meat in which 58 persons were
affected (92% confirmed by muscle biopsy), ELISA detected IgG specific antibodies in 100% of the cases in the first month of the disease and IgM antibodies in 86%
of the cases. In a high percentage of cases, these antibodies persisted up to 11
months after the study. It was also possible to detect IgA antibodies, which were presumed to have been of intestinal origin, in 62% of the patients in the first month of
the disease; their detection is important, since patients can be treated with
anthelmintics at that stage. The indirect immunofluorescence test was somewhat
less sensitive (95%), but became negative faster (van Knapen *et al.*, 1982). A problem with immunobiologic reactions is that they take about three weeks to appear and
last months or years. This hinders early diagnosis and the ability to distinguish current infections from long-standing ones. To resolve these problems, ELISA techniques have been designed to detect the parasite antigens, rather than the antibodies,
in the patient's blood. In experimentally infected rats, the antigen is found starting
on the fourth day of infection and, in a third of human patients, at the end of the third
week of infection (Dzbenski *et al.*, 1994). In these patients, the sensitivity was 100%
and the specificity was 96.8%; there were cross reactions with capillariasis, gnathostomiasis, opisthorchiasis, and strongyloidiasis (Mahannop *et al.*, 1995). As with
other diseases, two blood samples should be taken two weeks apart to observe the
change in the antibody titers, which can indicate an active infection.

To diagnose the infection in animals, direct methods are used, such as
trichinoscopy and artificial digestion; immunobiologic methods such as indirect
immunofluorescence, ELISA, and Western blot; and molecular biology techniques

such as PCR and random amplified polymorphic DNA analysis (RAPD). Unlike the human infection, in which early diagnosis is needed, only a sensitive diagnosis is needed in swine because the larvae do not become infective until after the 16th day of infection. Trichinoscopy is used in the veterinary inspection of pork in slaughter-houses and meat-packing facilities in many countries. It is a rapid process, but it is not very sensitive and does not reveal light infections. In Sweden in 1961 and in Germany in 1967, epidemic outbreaks involving several hundred cases occurred fol-lowing consumption of pork and pork products that had passed trichinoscopic exam-ination. Some experts estimate that trichinoscopy can detect the infection only when there are three or more larvae per gram of muscle; according to others, the figure is 10 or more larvae per gram. The artificial digestion method is much more efficient and cheaper, but it is slow and does not lend itself to the rhythm of hog processing in large slaughterhouses and industrial packing plants. Its sensitivity is primarily attributed to the use of a sample that is 50 to 100 times larger than that used in trichinoscopy. A practical modification of this method has been proposed, which consists of mixing samples of the diaphragmatic pillars of 20 to 25 hogs from the same source. If trichinae are found in the composite sample, a 50–100 g sample of diaphragm muscle tissue from each individual pig is examined. Venturiello et al. (1998) compared trichinoscopy, artificial digestion, indirect immunofluorescence, and ELISA in 116 swine and found that the direct parasitology techniques were much less sensitive than the indirect techniques, and that ELISA was less sensitive than immunofluorescence when the intensity of the infection was low. ELISA has been automated for use in slaughterhouses, with substantial savings of resources and time. One of the drawbacks of this test was the high proportion of false positives (about 15%). This drawback has been surmounted by the use of purified antigens (Gamble and Graham, 1984). RAPD has shown a sensitivity of 100% and a speci-ficity of 88% to 100% for detection of a single larva of the parasite (Pozio et al., 1999).

Control: The purpose of a control program should be to reduce and eventually eradicate the infection in swine, whose meat is the main source of human infection. The requirement that kitchen or slaughterhouse waste intended for pigs be heat-treated (100°C), introduced as part of the campaign to eradicate vesicular exanthema in swine and hog cholera, has proven beneficial in controlling trichinosis in the US. However, compliance with this regulation is very difficult to ensure, and, therefore, the results are not always satisfactory.

The trichinosis problem in some Latin American countries centers on the small rural farms raising a few pigs fed with household or restaurant scraps. These farms are very difficult to supervise, and pigs are slaughtered by the farmers without vet-erinary inspection. Continuous education of the population could at least partially remedy the situation. Another source of human infection is swine kept in town or village garbage dumps. In these cases, municipal and health authorities should pro-hibit this practice.

Trichinoscopy, which is practiced in slaughterhouses in Argentina, Chile, and other countries, has been shown to be effective in protecting the population. Although its sensitivity and cost leave much to be desired, when correctly executed, it protects the consumer against massive infections. The digestion method is much more efficient and cheaper in large slaughterhouses, but is costly for small plants in developing countries. Hopes are founded on implementing automated immunologic or molecular biology tests.

At the individual level, humans can avoid the infection by abstaining from eating pork or pork products of dubious origin, without veterinary inspection. Pork or pork products that have not been inspected can be submitted to several processes to destroy the trichinae. Cooking at 57°C is more than sufficient to inactivate the parasites. This temperature turns the raw pork, which is pink and semi-translucent, whitish and opaque. Special care should be taken with rib roasts, pork chops, and pork sausages, which are not always sufficiently cooked, particularly close to the bone. The use of microwave ovens is not recommended because they heat unevenly and they may leave live parasites in portions of the meat. Trichinae are also destroyed by freezing the meat at –15°C for 20 days or at –30°C for 6 days, as long as the piece is not thicker than 15 cm. Smoking, salting, or drying of pork are not sure methods of killing larvae. The meat of wild animals should be cooked; this is the only sure method of destroying the larvae in the Arctic.

Bibliography

Andrews, J.R., C. Bandi, E. Pozio, M.A. Gómez Morales, R. Ainsworth, D. Abernethy. Identification of *Trichinella pseudospiralis* from a human case using random amplified polymorphic DNA. *Am J Trop Med Hyg* 53(2):185–188, 1995.

Barriga, O.O. *Veterinary Parasitology for Practitioners*, 2nd ed. Edina: Burgess International Group; 1997.

Bellani, L., A. Mantovani, S. Pampilione. Observations on an outbreak of human trichinellosis in Northern Italy. *In*: Kim, C.W., Z.S. Pawlowski, eds. *Trichinellosis. Proceedings of the Fourth International Conference on Trichinellosis, August 26–28, 1976, Poznan, Poland.* Hanover, New Hampshire: University Press of New England; 1978.

Ben, G.J., S.L. Malmassari, G.G. Núñez, S.N. Costantino, S.M. Venturiello. Evaluation of an enzymatic immunohistochemical technique in human trichinellosis. *J Helminthol* 71:299–303, 1997.

Bessonov, A.S. [The taxonomic position of nematodes in the genus *Trichinella* Railliet, 1895]. *Med Parazitol (Mosk)* Jan–Mar(1):3–6, 1998.

Campbell, W.C. Epidemiology. I. Modes of transmission. *In*: Campbell, W.C., ed. *Trichinella and Trichinosis.* New York: Plenum Press; 1983.

Cui, J., Z.Q. Wang, F. Wu, X.X. Jin. Epidemiological and clinical studies on an outbreak of trichinosis in central China. *Ann Trop Med Parasitol* 91(5):481–488, 1997.

Dupouy-Camet, J., C. Soule, T. Ancelle. Recent news on trichinellosis: Another outbreak due to horsemeat consumption in France in 1993. *Parasite* 1(2):99–103, 1994.

Dworkin, M.S., H.R. Gamble, D.S. Zarlenga, P.O. Tennican. Outbreak of trichinellosis associated with eating cougar jerky. *J Infect Dis* 174(3):663–666, 1996.

Dzbenski, T.H., E. Bitkowska, W. Plonka. Detection of a circulating parasitic antigen in acute infections with *Trichinella spiralis*: Diagnostic significance of findings. *Zentralbl Bakteriol* 281(4):519–525, 1994.

Ferraccioli, G.F., M. Mercadanti, F. Salaffi, F. Bruschi, M. Melissari, E. Pozio. Prospective rheumatological study of muscle and joint symptoms during *Trichinella nelsoni* infection. *Q J Med* 69(260):973–984, 1988.

Fragoso, R., P. Tavizón, H. Villacaña. Universidad Autónoma de Zacatecas, 1984. (Personal communication).

Gamble, H.R., C.E. Graham. Monoclonal antibody-purified antigen for immunodiagnosis of trichinosis. *Am J Vet Res* 45(1):67–74, 1984.

Gamble, H.R., R.C. Brady, L.L. Bulaga, et al. Prevalence and risk association for Trichinella infection in domestic pigs in the northeastern United States. Vet Parasitol 82(1):59–69, 1999.

Gottstein, B., E. Pozio, B. Connolly, H.R. Gamble, J. Eckert, H.P. Jakob. Epidemiological investigation of trichinellosis in Switzerland. Vet Parasitol 72(2):201–207, 1997.

Greenbloom, S.L., P. Martin-Smith, S. Isaacs, et al. Outbreak of trichinosis in Ontario secondary to the ingestion of wild boar meat. Can J Public Health 88:52–56, 1997.

Haim, M., M. Efrat, M. Wilson, P.M. Schantz, D. Cohen, J. Shemer. An outbreak of Trichinella spiralis infection in southern Lebanon. Epidemiol Infect 119(3):357–362, 1997.

Holliman, R.B., B.J. Meade. Native trichinosis in wild rodents in Henrico County, Virginia. J Wildl Dis 16(2):205–207, 1980.

Homan, W.L., A.C. Derksen, F. van Knapen. Identification of diagnostic antigens from Trichinella spiralis. Parasitol Res 78(2):112–119, 1992.

Jongwutiwes, S., N. Chantachum, P. Kraivichian, et al. First outbreak of human trichinellosis caused by Trichinella pseudospiralis. Clin Infect Dis 26(1):111–115, 1998.

Ko, R.C. A brief update on the diagnosis of trichinellosis. Southeast Asian J Trop Med Public Health 28 Suppl 1:91–98, 1997.

Letonja, T., S. Ernst. Triquinosis en perros de Santiago, Chile. Bol Chil Parasitol 29(1–2):51, 1974.

Mahannop, P., P. Setasuban, N. Morakote, P. Tapchaisri, W. Chaicumpa. Immunodiagnosis of human trichinellosis and identification of specific antigen for Trichinella spiralis. Int J Parasitol 25(1):87–94, 1995.

Margolis, H.S., J.P. Middaugh, R.D. Burgess. Arctic trichinosis: Two Alaskan outbreaks from walrus meat. J Infect Dis 139(1):102–105, 1979.

McAuley, J.B., M.K. Michelson, A.W. Hightower, S. Engeran, L.A. Wintermeyer, P.M. Schantz. A trichinosis outbreak among Southeast Asian refugees. Am J Epidemiol 135(12):1404–1410, 1992.

Minchella, D.J., B.A. Branstetter, K.R. Kazacos. Molecular characterization of sylvatic isolates of Trichinella spiralis. J Parasitol 75(3):388–392, 1989.

Oberg, C., S. Ernst, P. Linfati, P. Martin. Triquinosis en perros de la comuna de Máfil, Provincia de Valdivia, Chile. Bol Chil Parasit 34(1–2):46–47, 1979.

Pozio, E., G. La Rosa, K.D. Murrell, J.R. Lichtenfels. Taxonomic revision of the genus Trichinella. J Parasitol 78(4):654–659, 1992.

Pozio, E., P. Varese, M.A. Morales, G.P. Croppo, D. Pelliccia, F. Bruschi. Comparison of human trichinellosis caused by Trichinella spiralis and by Trichinella britovi. Am J Trop Med Hyg 48(4):568–575, 1993.

Pozio, E., I. Miller, T. Jarvis, C.M. Kapel, G. La Rosa. Distribution of sylvatic species of Trichinella in Estonia according to climate zones. J Parasitol 84(1):193–195, 1998.

Pozio, E., C.M. Kapel, H.R. Gamble. Specificity and sensitivity of random amplified polymorphic DNA analysis for the identification of single larvae of Trichinella after experimental infection of pigs. Parasitol Res 85(6):504–506, 1999.

Ruitenberg, E.J., F. van Knapen, A. Elgersma. Incidence and control of Trichinella spiralis throughout the world. Food Technology 37:98–100, 1983.

Sandoval, L., P. Salinas, E. Rugiero, M.C. Contreras. Valor diagnóstico de la ELISA IgG para triquinosis, usando antígeno de Melcher. Bol Chil Parasitol 50(3–4):92–96, 1995.

Schantz, P.M. Trichinosis in the United States, 1947–1981. Food Technology 37:83–86, 1983.

Steele, J.H. Trichinosis. In: Steele, J.H., section ed. Section C, Vol. 2: CRC Handbook Series in Zoonoses. Boca Raton: CRC Press; 1982.

Steele, J.H., P. Arámbulo III. Trichinosis. A world problem with extensive sylvatic reservoirs. Int J Zoonoses 2(2):55–75, 1975.

United States of America, Department of Health and Human Services, Centers for Disease Control and Prevention (CDC). Trichinosis surveillance annual summary 1981. *MMWR Morb Mortal Wkly Rep CDC Surveill Summ*, 1982.

van Knapen, F., J.H. Franchimont, A.R. Verdonk, J. Stumpf, K. Undeutsch. Detection of specific immunoglobulins (IgG, IgM, IgA, IgE) and total IgE levels in human trichinosis by means of the enzyme-linked immunosorbent assay (ELISA). *Am J Trop Med Hyg* 31(5):973–976, 1982.

Venturiello, S.M., R.A. Caminoa, R. Veneroni, *et al.* Aspectos serológicos, clínicos y epidemiológicos de un brote de triquinosis en Azul, Provincia de Buenos Aires. *Medicina (B Aires)* 53(1):1–5, 1993.

Venturiello, S.M., G.J. Ben, S.N. Costantino, *et al.* Diagnosis of porcine trichinellosis: Parasitological and immunoserological tests in pigs from endemic areas of Argentina. *Vet Parasitol* 74(2–4):215–228, 1998.

Wu, Z., I. Nagano, E. Pozio, Y. Takahashi. Polymerase chain reaction-restriction fragment length polymorphism (PCR-RFLP) for the identification of *Trichinella* isolates. *Parasitology* 118 (Pt 2):211–218, 1999.

Yamaguchi, T. Present status of trichinellosis in Japan. *Southeast Asian J Trop Med Public Health* 22 Suppl:295–301, 1991.

Zamorano, C.G., M.C. Contreras, A. Espinoza, *et al.* Brote de triquinosis en la Comuna de Purranque, Región X, Chile, octubre-noviembre, 1992. *Bol Chil Parasitol* 49(1–2):38–42, 1994.

Zimmermann, W.J., D.E. Zinter. Trichiniasis in the US population, 1966–1970. Prevalence and epidemiologic factors. *Health Serv Rep* 88:606–623, 1971.

TRICHOSTRONGYLIASIS

ICD-10 B81.2

Synonyms: Trichostrongylosis, trichostrongylidosis.

Etiology: The agents are several species of the genus *Trichostrongylus* (nematode) that inhabit the small intestine and stomach of sheep, goats, and bovines, and sometimes infect other domestic and wild animals or man. The following have been identified in humans: *T. axei, T. colubriformis, T. orientalis, T. skrjabini, T. vitrinus, T. probolurus, T. capricola, T. brevis, T. affinis,* and *T. calcaratus.* The species are difficult to differentiate, and human case histories often indicate only the genus and not the species. Other trichostrongylids have occasionally been found in humans. Among these are three cases caused by *Haemonchus contortus* in Australia, one in Brazil, and one in Iran; two cases caused by *Ostertagia ostertagi* in Iran and one in Azerbaijan; and one case caused by *O. circumcincta,* also in Azerbaijan.

Trichostrongylids are short parasites, measuring 1 cm or less in length, and are as slender as an eyelash, and therefore, difficult to see. The mouth is a simple orifice and the males have a well-developed copulatory sac. The development cycle is direct. The eggs of the parasite are eliminated with the feces of the host, and, under favorable conditions of temperature, humidity, shade, and aeration, they release the first-stage larva in one or two days. This is a free-living worm that makes its home in the soil and feeds on organic waste or small organisms; it quickly molts into a second-stage larva, which is also free-living; then it molts into a third-stage larva, which is infective to the host. The infective larva can develop in just a week; when ingested by a host, it matures into the adult stage in close contact with the intestinal or gastric mucosa, mates, and begins to produce eggs during the fourth week of infection.

Geographic Distribution and Occurrence: Trichostrongylids are very common parasites of domestic ruminants and their distribution is worldwide. Human trichostrongyliasis occurs sporadically. In general, the prevalence is very low, but where people live in close contact with ruminants and food hygiene conditions are inadequate—as in nomadic communities—high rates of infection can occur. Human prevalence rates found in Iran were 7.5% in the northern part of the country and 69% to 85% in Isfahan. In southern Sudan, 2.5% of 275 children were found to be infected (Magambo et al., 1998). In 1993, a 1% rate of infection with *Trichostrongylus* sp. was found in 99 Thai workers in Israel. In southern Ethiopia, 19 communities were studied, and 0.3% of those examined were found to be infected (Birrie et al., 1994). In a total of 52,552 stool samples examined in a hospital in Seoul, Republic of Korea, 0.1% were found to contain *T. orientalis* eggs (Lee et al., 1994). In Australia, 5 cases were found out of 46,000 coprologic examinations (Boreham et al., 1995).

Endemic areas are dispersed; in particular, they cover southern Asia from the Mediterranean to the Pacific, and the Asian areas of the former Soviet Union, where nomadic tribes are still found. In some localities in Iraq, up to 25% of the population has been found to be infected. The infection is very common in some areas of Korea and Japan, as well as in parts of Africa, such as the Democratic Republic of the Congo and Zimbabwe.

Human infection has also been described in Germany, Australia, and Hungary. In the Americas, the infection has been confirmed in Brazil, Chile, Peru, the US, and Uruguay. In Brazil, 75 cases of infection by *Trichostrongylus* spp. were found in 46,951 persons examined. In Chile, 45 cases were diagnosed between 1938 and 1967, and 17 cases were found among 3,712 persons examined in the province of Valdivia between 1966 and 1971.

The Disease in Man: The parasites lodge in the duodenum and jejunum. Infections are usually asymptomatic or mild and are discovered in coprologic examinations carried out to diagnose other parasitoses. In acute infections, with several hundred parasites, there may be transitory eosinophilia and digestive disorders, such as diarrhea, abdominal pain, and weight loss; sometimes, slight anemia is observed. The infection can last several years if left untreated. The clinical picture in man has not been studied very much and is difficult to define, since other species of parasites are generally found in an individual infected with trichostrongylids.

The Disease in Animals: The different species of *Trichostrongylus*, together with gastrointestinal parasites of other genera, constitute the etiologic complex of parasitic or verminous gastroenteritis of ruminants, an important disease in terms of its economic impact, because it causes major losses in meat, milk, and wool production, and occasionally causes death (Barriga, 1997).

In ruminants, trichostrongylids cause accelerated reproduction of the cells of the intestinal epithelium, which alters the structure of the epithelium and permits the filtration of plasma proteins to the lumen (Hoste *et al.*, 1995). This does not seem to occur in man, probably because of the small number of parasites he harbors. In animals, peripheral eosinophilia is also uncommon.

Source of Infection and Mode of Transmission: The reservoirs of trichostrongylids are domestic and wild ruminants. However, *T. orientalis* is a parasite of man and only occasionally of sheep. This species occurs in Asia and is transmitted between humans, especially in areas where human fecal matter is used as fertilizer in agriculture. *T. orientalis* is the predominant species in human infections. *T. brevis* is another human species that has been described in Japan. The species of animal origin produce rather sporadic cases in man, although areas of high prevalence are known. The number of species of *Trichostrongylus* that infect man varies in different areas. In Isfahan, Iran, seven different species have been found in the rural inhabitants of the region.

The source of infection is the soil where infected ruminants deposit the eggs when they defecate. Man and animals are infected orally by consuming contaminated food or water. Man acquires the infection mainly by consuming raw vegetables. The rains that wash the feces of infected ruminants out of the soil and carry them to bodies of water can contaminate sources of drinking water. A lack of food hygiene, and close contact with ruminants, which is common among rural populations at a low socioeconomic level in endemic areas, facilitate transmission. The use of manure as fertilizer or fuel can also facilitate transmission.

Diagnosis: The infection can go unnoticed because patients are asymptomatic; sometimes they present only peripheral eosinophilia or mild gastrointestinal disturbances (Boreham *et al.*, 1995). Diagnosis often occurs accidentally while looking for another parasite. Parasitological confirmation is established by identifying the eggs in the feces. The eggs of *Trichostrongylus* are quite similar to those of six or seven other genera, including ancylostomids found in man. Therefore, it may be necessary to cultivate the eggs to produce third-stage larvae and study their morphology in order to determine the genus. In the case of human ancylostomids, the eggs are much smaller than those of *Trichostrongylus* (56–75 µm by 36–45 µm versus 73–95 µm by 40–50 µm).

Parasitic gastroenteritis in ruminants can be diagnosed by finding and counting the eggs in the feces, but autopsy is more effective for determining the number and species of infective parasites.

Control: Preventive measures for the human infection consist of improved food, environmental, and personal hygiene. In endemic areas, it is prudent to avoid eating vegetables or other raw foods that could be contaminated with the larvae of the parasite and to boil suspicious drinking water.

In animals, control measures are directed toward keeping both pasture contamination and animal infections at low levels. To achieve this objective, the animals must be kept well nourished. Anthelmintics should be administered at the appropriate times of the year to prevent the accumulation of parasites in animals and pastures.

Bibliography

Barriga, O.O. *Veterinary Parasitology for Practitioners*, 2nd ed. Edina: Burgess International Group; 1997.

Birrie, H., B. Erko, S. Tedla. Intestinal helminthic infections in the southern Rift Valley of Ethiopia with special reference to schistosomiasis. *East Afr Med J* 71(7):447–452, 1994.

Boreham, R.E., M.J. McCowan, A.E. Ryan, A.M. Allworth, J.M. Robson. Human trichostrongyliasis in Queensland. *Pathology* 27(2):182–185, 1995.

Ghadirian, E., F. Arfaa. First report of human infection with *Haemonchus contortus, Ostertagia ostergagi,* and *Marshallagia marshalli* (Family Trichostrongylidae) in Iran. *J Parasitol* 59(6):1144–1145, 1973.

Ghadirian, E., F. Arfaa, A. Sadighian. Human infection with *Trichostrongylus capricola* in Iran. *Am J Trop Med Hyg* 23(5):1002–1003, 1974.

Hoste, H., J.L. Nano, S. Mallet, F. Huby, S. Fournel, P. Rampal. Stimulation of HT29-D4 cell growth by excretory/secretory products of the parasite nematode *Trichostrongylus colubriformis*. *Epithelial Cell Biol* 4(2):87–92, 1995.

Lee, S.K., B.M. Shin, N.S. Chung, J.Y. Chai, S.H. Lee. [Second report on intestinal parasites among the patients of Seoul Paik Hospital (1984–1992)]. *Korean J Parasitol* 32(1):27–33, 1994.

Magambo, J.K., E. Zeyhle, T.M. Wachira. Prevalence of intestinal parasites among children in southern Sudan. *East Afr Med J* 75(5):288–290, 1998.

Tongston, M.S., S.L. Eduardo. Trichostrongylidiosis. *In*: Steele, J.H., section ed. Section C, Vol. 2: *CRC Handbook Series in Zoonoses*. Boca Raton: CRC Press; 1982.

TRICHURIASIS OF ANIMAL ORIGIN

ICD-10 B79 Trichuriasis

Synonyms: Trichocephaliasis, trichocephalosis.

Etiology: The agent of trichuriasis is *Trichuris vulpis* of canids and, secondarily, *T. suis* of swine. *Trichuris trichiura* is a species that parasitizes man and that has been found in chimpanzees, monkeys, and lemurs. However, there is no proof that its transmission is zoonotic, except in unusual circumstances. Despite the fact that the name *Trichuris* means "tail as thin as a hair," the thin portion of the parasite's body is actually the head. For this reason, various authors prefer the term *Trichocephalus*, which is morphologically correct. While it should be noted that the name *Trichuris* has priority, some authors incorrectly use *Trichocephalus* as the taxonomic denomination.

T. vulpis lives in the cecum and in neighboring portions of the large intestine of domestic and wild canids. It measures 4.5 cm to 7.5 cm long, and the posterior two fifths are much thicker than the anterior portion. This is typical of the genus and is the reason the English literature refers to it as whipworm. The male has a very long spicule, 8 mm to 11 mm, with a sheath that is also very long. The females produce eggs which, as in all species of *Trichuris*, resemble lemons: they are oval, thick-shelled, and have two polar plugs; they measure 72–90 μm by 32–40 μm.

T. suis lives in the cecum and in neighboring portions of the large intestine of domestic pigs and wild boars. It measures 30 cm to 50 cm in length; the male's spicules measure 2–2.3 mm and the female's eggs measure 50–56 µm by 21–25 µm.

T. trichiura lives in the cecum and in neighboring portions of the large intestine of humans and some lower primates. The worms, spicules, and eggs are the same size as those of *T. suis* (Barriga, 1997). These parasites must belong to different species because *T. suis* has six chromosomes and *T. trichiura* has just four, and its ability to infect heterologous hosts is deficient. That notwithstanding, the authors who compared the two species insist that they cannot be differentiated on morphological bases (Barriga, 1982).

The development cycle is similar in all species of *Trichuris*: the female lays eggs that are eliminated to the exterior with the feces. Under favorable conditions of humidity, temperature, shade, and aeration, in two weeks or more the zygote develops inside the egg into the infective first-stage larva. When the host ingests those eggs, the larvae are released in the small intestine, lodge in the crypts for about 10 to 14 days, return to the lumen, and move to the large intestine, where they mature and begin oviposition in about three months. The prepatent period of *T. vulpis* is 70 to 90 days in dogs; that of *T. suis* is 41 to 45 days in swine; and that of *T. trichiura* is 1 to 3 months in humans. *T. vulpis* lives approximately 16 months in dogs, and *T. suis*, approximately 4 to 5 months in swine.

Geographic Distribution and Occurrence: The two zoonotic species and *T. trichiura* occur all over the world and, in general, their distribution is similar to that of the ascarids transmitted through the soil, such as *Toxascaris leonina* (dogs and cats), *Ascaris suum* (swine), and *A. lumbricoides* (man). This is because *Trichuris* spp. and *Ascaris* spp. need very similar environmental conditions in order for their infective larvae to develop, and the mechanisms of transmission to the host are almost identical. Both are highly prevalent in warm, humid climates, less prevalent in moderate humidity or temperatures, and scarce or nonexistent in arid and hot or very cold climates.

T. vulpis is very common in dogs. The prevalence of the infection in dogs brought to veterinary clinics is generally between 10% and 20%, and in stray dogs, approximately 40%. For example, in the state of New Jersey, US, 38% of 2,737 dogs examined were infected; in New York, the prevalence was 31%, and in Detroit, 52%. The first case of human infection caused by *T. vulpis* was reported in 1956; Barriga (1982) compiled 40 more reports, 34 of which were from Viet Nam, by 1980. By 2000, 8 more cases were reported: 1 in an autopsy in the US (Kenney and Yermakov, 1980), 5 in a survey in India (Singh *et al.*, 1993), and 2 clinical cases involving children in India (Mirdha *et al.*, 1998). It is interesting that three cases prior to 1980 were found on fecal examination of 1,710 patients in the state of New York; the 34 cases in Viet Nam were found in 276 individuals examined, and the 5 cases reported by Singh *et al.* (1993) were found in 83 individuals studied. In these examples, the prevalences were 0.2%, 12.3%, and 6%, respectively. However, it must be taken into consideration that most diagnoses of *T. vulpis* in humans were made by measuring eggs in the feces, which might not be completely reliable. Moreover, only a particularly discerning technician would note that the eggs he or she is observing are larger than usual, so many cases of human infection caused by *T. vulpis* may go undetected.

In general, *T. suis* is common in swine, with prevalences of 2% to 5% in adult animals and 15% to 40% in suckling pigs. In 1938 and 1940, unsuccessful attempts were made to infect humans experimentally with swine parasites. In the 1970s, two human volunteers were infected, and later an accidental infection in a laboratory worker was studied. The three subjects passed a few eggs of low fertility in 11 to 84 days (Barriga, 1982). While these studies documented the possibility of human infection with swine parasites, their practical importance is not known. Moreover, experiments involving the infection of swine with *T. trichiura* failed to produce patent infections.

The Disease in Man and Animals: Trichuriasis is very similar in humans and canines. The infection is much more common than the disease and much more prevalent in young individuals. In infections with a large number of parasites, there may be abdominal pain and distension as well as diarrhea, which is sometimes bloody. In very heavy infections in children (hundreds or thousands of parasites), there can be strong tenesmus and rectal prolapse. Massive parasitoses occur mainly in tropical regions, in children 2 to 5 years old who are usually malnourished and often infected by other intestinal parasites and microorganisms. Geophagy and anemia are common signs among these children. Most cases of human infection with zoonotic *Trichuris* have been asymptomatic or the patients have complained only of vague intestinal disturbances and moderate diarrhea.

Source of Infection and Mode of Transmission: The reservoirs of zoonotic species of *Trichuris* are dogs and other wild canids and, possibly, the swine. The sources of infection are soil or water contaminated with eggs of the parasite. The mode of transmission is, as in other geohelminthiases, the ingestion of eggs in the food or water, or hands contaminated with infective eggs. As indicated earlier, *Trichuris* eggs have the same climatic requirements as *Ascaris* eggs and, therefore, occur in the same regions. However, *Trichuris* eggs are considerably more sensitive to climatic conditions. With constant temperatures of 22°C, the infective larva forms in 54 days; with temperatures fluctuating between 6°C and 24°C, the process takes 210 days. It is also less resistant to drought, heat, and chemical disinfectants. Even in a moist environment, few eggs survive more than two weeks. Soil contamination studies carried out in Switzerland showed that 16% of samples of dog feces had *Toxocara canis* eggs, but fewer than 1% had *T. vulpis* eggs (Tost *et al.*, 1998). In Nigeria, it was found that 10% to 20% of soil samples from playgrounds were contaminated with *Ascaris lumbricoides* eggs, 8% with *T. canis,* and 4% with *T. vulpis* (Umeche, 1989).

Therefore, infection by *Trichuris* occurs more often when there is a constant source of environmental contamination, such as infected small children who defecate on the ground. The role of dogs or swine does not seem to be important in human trichuriasis.

Diagnosis: Diagnosis is based on confirmation of the presence in the feces of the typical eggs. The eggs of *T. vulpis* (72–90 µm by 32–40 µm) can be distinguished from those of *T. suis* (50–56 µm by 21–25 µm) or *T. trichiura* by their size, although the reliability of this characteristic is not known. The eggs of *T. suis* are indistinguishable from those of *T. trichiura*. The females of these species can be distinguished by the size of the eggs inside them. *T. vulpis* males can be distinguished from *T. suis* or *T. trichiura* males by the size of the spicules.

Control: As with all geohelminthiases, prevention of human trichuriasis requires improvement of environmental hygiene through the adequate disposal of excreta to avoid contamination of the soil, personal hygiene, the washing of raw food and of hands, and the boiling or filtering of suspicious water. For obvious reasons, the adequate disposal of excreta is difficult in the case of zoonotic diseases and, while the infected animals can be treated to prevent them from contaminating the environment, zoonotic trichuriasis is so rare that mass methods of control are not justified except under highly unusual circumstances.

Bibliography

Barriga, O.O. Trichuriasis. *In*: Steele, J.H., section ed. Section C, Vol. 2: *CRC Handbook Series in Zoonoses*. Boca Raton: CRC Press; 1982.

Barriga, O.O. *Veterinary Parasitology for Practitioners,* 2nd ed. Edina: Burgess International Group; 1997.

Kenney, M., V. Yermakov. Infection of man with *Trichuris vulpis*, the whipworm of dogs. *Am J Trop Med Hyg* 29(6):1205–1208, 1980.

Mirdha, B.R., Y.G. Singh, J.C. Samantray, B. Mishra. *Trichuris vulpis* infection in slum children. *Indian J Gastroenterol* 17(4):154, 1998.

Singh, S., J.C. Samantaray, N. Singh, G.B. Das, I.C. Verma. *Trichuris vulpis* infection in an Indian tribal population. *J Parasitol* 79(3):457–458, 1993.

Tost, F., A. Hellmann, G. Ockert. *Toxocara canis*-Infektion. Umweltparasitologische und epidemiologische Untersuchungen. *Ophthalmologe* 95(7):486–489, 1998.

Umeche, N. Helminth ova in soil from children's playgrounds in Calabar, Nigeria. *Centr Afr J Med* 35(7):432–434, 1989.

World Health Organization (WHO). *Intestinal Protozoan and Helminthic Infections. Report of a WHO Scientific Group*. Geneva: WHO; 1981. (Technical Report Series 666).

VISCERAL LARVA MIGRANS AND TOXOCARIASIS

ICD-10 B83.0 Visceral larva migrans

Synonym: Larval granulomatosis.

Etiology: Visceral larva migrans refers to the presence of parasite larvae that travel in the systemic tissues of man but not in the skin. The use of the qualifier "visceral" should be discontinued because it corresponds to only one of the four clinical forms of the disease. There are several helminths whose larvae can cause this condition: for example, species of *Baylisascaris, Gnathostoma, Gongynolema, Lagochilascaris, Dirofilaria*, and *Angiostrongylus*. However, the term visceral larva migrans is usually reserved for extraintestinal visceral infections caused by nematodes of the genus *Toxocara*, especially *Toxocara canis*, and to a lesser extent, *T. cati* (*T. mystax*), which will be covered in this chapter.

T. canis is an ascarid which, in its adult stage, lives in the small intestine of dogs and several wild canids. The female measures 9–18 cm long and the male, 4–10 cm. One of the characteristics of the genus is that the males have a caudal terminal appendage, which is digitiform. The eggs contain a zygote and they are shed in the host feces. These eggs are very resistant to environmental conditions, and they can remain viable for several years in moist, shaded soils when temperatures are cool. Under favorable environmental conditions of humidity, temperature, shade, and aeration, a third-stage infective larva forms inside the egg in about 10 days at 24°C and 90% relative humidity, or in about 15 days at 19°C (Araujo, 1972; Maung, 1978). When a puppy under 4 or 5 weeks old ingests eggs containing infective larvae, the parasites emerge in the intestine, pass through the intestinal wall, and enter the bloodstream, which carries them to the liver and then to the lungs. There they rupture capillaries and pulmonary alveoli and migrate through bronchioles, bronchi, and the trachea to the pharynx, where they are swallowed. Once again the parasite reaches the intestine, and this time it develops into the adult stage. The first eggs begin to appear in feces between four to five weeks after the initial infection. The average lifespan of *T. canis* in the intestine is about four months, and most of the parasites are expelled six months after the onset of infection (Schantz and Glickman, 1983).

In puppies older than 5 weeks, the ingested larvae initiate the migration described above, but increasingly larger proportions go into hypobiosis in different systemic tissues, and they do not reach the airway or the intestine. In those 3 months of age and older, almost none of the parasites reach the intestine; some settle in the liver, others in the hepatic parenchyma, and the rest bypass the lungs and lodge in muscle, the kidneys, etc. (Barriga, 1997). This migration that bypasses the lungs is referred to as somatic migration. Since the larvae lapse into hypobiosis within a few days, they become very resistant to anthelmintics (Carrillo and Barriga, 1987). In gravid females, the parasites remain resistant until the final third of pregnancy. In addition to the age factor, the ultimate destination of the larvae (whether by tracheal or somatic migration) is determined by the infective dose. Dubey (1978) demonstrated experimentally that puppies infected orally with 10,000 eggs did not exhibit patent parasitosis—with the elimination of eggs in their feces—but did do so when they received 1,000 eggs. Patent infection was observed in 3 of 6 adult dogs that were infected with 100 eggs. It may be speculated that a large parasite burden stimulates immunologic mechanisms that prevent maturation of the parasite (Barriga, 1998). When bitches harboring hypobiotic larvae reach the final third of their pregnancy (starting at approximately day 42), the larvae reactivate and resume their migration, many of them traveling to the liver of the fetuses and, after the birth of the pups, migrating to the trachea and appearing in their feces when the animals are about 21 days old.

Almost all puppies born of infected mothers are infected, which indicates that transplacental infection is a highly important mode of transmission for the parasite. Other reactivated larvae pass into the intestine of the mother and mature. Starting at day 25 postpartum, the adult parasites lay eggs for three and a half months. One-third to half of all bitches shed eggs after they deliver a litter. Finally, some of the larvae in their bloodstream also pass to their pups through their milk for up to five weeks (Barriga, 1991).

When man and other noncanid hosts, such as rodents, swine, and lambs, ingest infective eggs, the larvae are released into the intestine, where they initiate somatic migration and remain in the tissues as hypobiotic larvae. These species can act as paratenic, or transport, hosts.

T. cati is a somewhat smaller ascarid than *T. canis*. Its natural hosts are cats and wild felids. Although the life cycle of *T. cati* is similar to that of *T. canis*, there are a few important differences: the cat develops patent infection with eggs ingested at any age; it does not experience prenatal infection; and transmammary infection appears to be common. Eberhard and Alfano (1998) reported the presence of adult or subadult *T. cati* in the intestine of four children who did not have symptoms or antibodies corresponding to the infection. The authors consider it more likely that the children became infected from ingesting subadult parasites passed on by cats than that they ingested infective eggs. The role of *T. cati* in the production of human larva migrans is still being debated (see below).

Geographic Distribution and Occurrence: *T. canis* and *T. cati* are found in dogs and cats throughout the world. Data collected by Barriga (1988) from around the world indicate that the infection is present in 99.4% of all newborn pups, about 40% of dogs of both sexes under 6 months of age, and 20% of males and 5% of females over 6 months old. In studies of apparently healthy humans using the enzyme-linked immunosorbent assay (ELISA), 6.7% of 1,150 sera in the US, 4.7% of 358 sera in Canada, and 3.6% of 1,321 sera in Great Britain had antibodies to the parasite. In 1981 alone, 675 cases of ocular toxocariasis were diagnosed in the US. The clinical disease has been diagnosed in 48 different countries, and more than 1,900 human cases were reviewed by Ehrhard and Kernbaum (1979). Of 780 well-documented cases, 56% were in children under 4 years old. Most of the clinical cases have been reported in industrialized countries because they have better diagnostic facilities, but the data collected by Barriga (1988) indicate that the infection is actually more prevalent in the developing countries.

Intestinal infection with adult parasites is very rare in man. Two cases have been attributed to *T. canis* and a somewhat larger number due to *T. cati* have been described, but the accuracy of these diagnoses has been questioned in several reports.

The Disease in Man: Toxocariasis is caused by the presence of *T. canis* or *T. cati* larvae in various human tissues. These larvae produce small tunnels of traumatic, inflammatory, and necrotic lesions in the course of their migration, followed by a granulomatous reaction with an abundance of eosinophils, and sometimes abscesses, once the larvae settle in a particular site. Toxocariasis is basically an allergic disorder. Originally two forms were described (visceral and ocular), but later four clinical forms were recognized: visceral (perhaps better referred to as systemic), ocular, neurological, and covert.

The visceral, or systemic, form occurs when most of the larvae are lodged in the liver or lungs, the first organs they travel through in the course of their migration. Clinical manifestations depend on the number of larvae and their anatomic localization. Usually, the infections are mild and asymptomatic, with the exception of persistent eosinophilia. In symptomatic cases, the seriousness of the clinical picture varies, but cases with mild symptomatology are predominant. The most notable sign is chronic eosinophilia. Eosinophils can represent more than 50% of the total leukocyte count. Hepatomegaly and pneumonitis with hypergammaglobulinemia are common during the early stages of the disease. In the cases reviewed by Ehrhard and Kernbaum (1979), 56% of the patients were under 3 years old and 18% were adults. The most frequent manifestations in children were hepatomegaly (79%), respiratory signs (72%), and fever (69%); in adults, the most common signs were fever (71%), asthenia (63%), and digestive symptoms (60%). Reinfections often affect the liver and lungs at the same time, weakening the patient considerably. Older children and adolescents frequently have fever, coughing spells, nausea, vomiting, and dyspnea during the first week, and the symptoms may recur for several months. The disease can be more severe in younger children, with asthmatic attacks, high fever, anorexia, arthralgia, myalgia, nausea, vomiting, hepatomegaly, lymphadenopathy, and sometimes urticaria and angioneurotic edema. Four of eight patients with systemic toxoplasmosis studied by Rugiero et al. (1995) had cardiac symptoms, three had pulmonary symptoms, and two were affected in various organs, while all of them had eosinophilia (35% to 90%) and seven had leukocytosis (14.5 to 160 million per mL). All were positive in the ELISA test, with titers ranging from 64 to 1,000. The cardiac cases responded only moderately to treatment; the patients suffered frequent decompensation, and one of them died. Eosinophilia has been known to last for up to 20 years, which suggests how long the larvae can survive.

The ocular form occurs in older children and sometimes adults. It is seldom preceded by or concurrent with the visceral form. The presence of larvae in the eye can cause progressive loss of vision and sudden blindness. Strabismus is common. The infection is unilateral and generally without systemic symptoms or eosinophilia. The single granulomatous lesion is located near the optic disc and the macula retinae. Endophthalmias caused by *Toxocara* larvae have often been mistaken for retinoblastomas, resulting in enucleation of the affected eyeball. Apart from the fact that the migrating larvae induce a granulomatous response in the host, the mechanism by which they cause damage is still not understood. It has been found that in visceral and optical cases the symptoms correlate with the presence of antigen-antibody complexes and with levels of IgE, suggesting that the pathogenic mechanism includes type I and III hypersensitivities (Obwaller et al., 1998). Eosinophils have also been mentioned as possible agents of pulmonary damage.

The neurological form occurs when the larvae settle in the central nervous system. There, they can give rise to meningoencephalitis (Barra et al., 1996) or other neurological manifestations. This form appears to be more common than was once believed: when irritability and minor behavioral disorders are excluded, one-fourth of 233 patients reviewed by Ehrhard and Kernbaum (1979) exhibited neurological symptoms, consisting mainly of convulsions and motor deficiencies, and 15 cases of encephalitis or meningitis were reported, some of them fatal. Several authors have found a correlation between this infection and epileptic symptoms, although others have not been able to verify such a connection.

The covert form is considered more common than any of the other forms. It is described as a disorder found in patients with positive serology for *Toxocara* and a few systemic or localized symptoms, mainly abdominal pain, which do not correspond to the syndrome of the visceral, ocular, or neurological form of the disease. One-fourth of these patients did not have peripheral eosinophilia, and in some cases, the symptoms lasted for months or even years (Nathwani et al., 1992).

Regardless of the form of the disease, fatal cases of visceral larva migrans are rare.

The Disease in Animals: Adult dogs and cats with larva migrans do not appear to suffer. Both species can maintain a large number of larvae in their tissues. Otherwise, uterine and lacteal transmission of *T. canis* and lacteal transmission of *T. cati* would not be possible. However, veterinarians in small animal practice do not see clinical signs attributable to the larvae of these nematodes. Intestinal infection with adult parasites can cause symptoms in puppies and kittens a few weeks old, especially digestive disorders, diarrhea, vomiting, flatulence, and loss of vitality. Puppies infected prenatally with a large number of parasites can die at the age of 2 or 3 weeks. Sudden death is often due to obstruction and rupture of the small intestine and consequent peritonitis. Prenatally infected puppies sometimes exhibit signs of pneumonia immediately after birth because their lungs have been invaded by a large number of larvae passed on by the mother. Intestinal infections with few parasites tend to be asymptomatic, as is often the case in adult animals as well. Dogs and cats that survive the critical period of infection recover fully and expel the parasites from their intestine during the first six months of life.

Source of Infection and Mode of Transmission: The reservoir of larva migrans for man is infected dogs. The source of infection is soil contaminated with infective eggs, and the mechanism of transmission is the ingestion of these eggs in contaminated food or water, or via contaminated hands.

For a long time, there was speculation about whether the feline *T. cati* is equally dangerous for man. Using the Western blot technique, Petihory *et al.* (1994) found that twice as many patients responded to *T. canis* antigen as they did to *T. cati*, and other authors have published similar results. In Iceland, however, the virtual elimination of dogs (but not cats) nearly eradicated the visceral form of larva migrans, suggesting that the parasite of cats plays an insignificant role as an etiologic agent.

A mild *T. canis* infection produces 10,000 eggs per gram of feces, and a dog sheds an average of 136 grams of feces daily; hence every mildly infected dog contaminates the environment with nearly 1.4 million *T. canis* eggs in a single day (Barriga, 1988). The eggs of *T. canis* are highly resistant to physical and chemical factors in the environment. Since the eggs can survive for years in a place that is cool, humid, and shady, once the environment is contaminated it remains so for a long time. On the other hand, since the eggs take 10 days to become infective, direct contact with dogs is less significant than contact with soil contaminated with their feces. The dog itself becomes a risk when it picks up infective eggs in the environment (Overgaauw, 1997). A review of reports from around the world as of 1986 regarding contamination of the soil with *T. canis* eggs revealed that usually 2% to 25% of the samples were contaminated, and in some places, the percentages were much higher (Barriga 1988). In Japan, Shimizu (1993) found that 68% of 144 puppies were infected and that 87.5% of the soil samples from parks and children's playgrounds were contaminated. Cases of human infection usually occur individually, but small outbreaks of up to seven people have been described (Bratt and Tikasingh, 1992).

Dogs are infected by transplacental and transmammary transmission, by ingestion of paratenic hosts, or by ingestion of infective eggs. The transplacental route is the most important: five experiments with a total of 669 newborn puppies found that 99.4% were born with the infection (Barriga, 1988). Cats can be infected by transmammary transmission, by ingestion of paratenic hosts, or by ingestion of infective eggs.

Since children have more contact with the soil and tend to be more lax about personal hygiene, they are more exposed and have the highest rates of prevalence. Moreover, geophagy is not uncommon in children and plays an important role in transmission of the infection. Adults can acquire the infection if they do not follow the basic rules of personal hygiene: dirty hands are almost always the vehicle for the parasite's eggs.

Diagnosis: Human larval toxocariasis is suspected mainly when there is leukocytosis, persistent eosinophilia, hypergammaglobulinemia, and hepatomegaly. Other factors to be considered in the diagnosis are age under 4 years and a history of geophagy or exposure to soil contaminated with canine feces. In the case of ocular toxocariasis, the diagnosis is confirmed by ophthalmoscopic examination, and by histopathologic examination of the eyeball if it has been enucleated. Histopathology is also used with biopsies of the liver. Identification of the larvae in tissue is a painstaking procedure that requires serial sections from the pathologic specimen. Even with an organ as small as the eyeball, it is sometimes necessary to study more than 100 sections before finding any larvae. In several extraocular cases, definitive diagnosis was obtained by laparotomy and resection of a visible granuloma on the surface of the liver. Differential diagnosis between ocular larva migrans and retinoblastoma is especially important. In the case of ocular larva migrans, examination of the aqueous humor usually reveals numerous eosinophils.

The difficulty of basing the diagnosis on clinical signs and the uncertainty of the diagnosis has stimulated the development of immunobiologic tests. In particular, ELISA has been used with larval excretory-secretory antigen and sera adsorbed with extracts of *Ascaris lumbricoides* to eliminate cross-reacting antibodies. It is estimated that this test is 78% sensitive and 92% specific in the visceral form and 73% sensitive and 95% specific in the ocular form (Schantz and Glickman, 1983). A modified ELISA test to show *T. canis* antigen in circulating blood was positive in 68% of 28 acute patients, 10% of 10 patients with inactive infection, and 28% of 7 with ocular infection; at the same time, however, 25% of patients with schistosomiasis or filariasis had false positive reactions (Gillespie *et al.*, 1993). Since larva migrans does not cause pathology in animals, no immunologic tests have been developed for diagnosis, although the tests used for human infection should serve the purpose. Diagnosis of intestinal infection with adult parasites is made by observing the parasite's eggs in feces.

Control: The primary control measure consists of deworming dogs and cats. Since a high proportion of dogs are born infected, newborn pups are especially important in prophylaxis (Barriga, 1991). It is recommended to treat 2-week-old puppies with any anthelmintic that is effective against ascarids and repeat the medication at 4, 6, and 8 weeks of age (Barriga, 1991). This measure eliminates the parasites before they have time to pass on eggs and contaminate the environment. The mothers should be treated at the same time.

Although most adult *T. canis* larvae are eliminated spontaneously from the intestine when dogs reach puberty (about 8 to 10 months of age), between 5% and 30% of adult dogs are infected with the parasite. Therefore, adult dogs should be treated twice a year, or else examined regularly for eggs in feces and treated if they are infected. Although hypobiotic larvae in the bitch are resistant to anthelmintics, treatment can kill the parasites when they renew their migration before they are passed on to the fetuses. For this purpose, the mother should be given a daily dose of 50 mg/kg of fenbendazole, or 0.3 mg/kg from day 40 of pregnancy to day 14 postpartum (Barriga, 1997).

Since even the best treatment has not been shown to be more than 50% effective (Barriga, 1991), other complementary measures should be used at the same time. One of these is to reduce the population of stray dogs and require all other dogs to have a socially responsible owner. Dogs should not be allowed to run free in public parks, especially where there are sandboxes for children. Owners can walk their dogs on a leash and pick up their feces in a plastic bag; the feces should then be burned or disposed of in the trash at home. Flushing the feces down the toilet is not as effective because some *T. canis* eggs can be resistant to wastewater treatment. Finally, the most important measure is to educate the public about the transmission of toxocariasis and the importance of washing hands and raw food before eating.

Bibliography

Araujo, P. Observações pertinentes as primeiras ecdises de larvas de *Ascaris lumbricoides*, *A. suum* e *Toxocara canis*. *Rev Inst Med Trop Sao Paulo* 14(2):83–90, 1972.

Barra, L.A., W.F. dos Santos, P.P. Chieffi, *et al*. Larva migrans visceral: forma mista de apresentação em adulto. Aspectos clínicos e laboratoriais. *Rev Soc Bras Med Trop* 29(4):373–376, 1996.

Barriga, O.O. A critical look at the importance, prevalence, and control of toxocariasis, and the possibilities of immunological control. *Vet Parasitol* 29(2–3):195–234, 1988.

Barriga, O.O. Rational control of canine toxocariasis by the veterinary practitioner. *J Am Vet Med Assoc* 198(2):216–221, 1991.

Barriga, O.O. *Veterinary Parasitology for Practitioners*, 2nd ed. Edina: Burgess International Group; 1997.

Barriga, O.O. La inmunobiología de las larvas migratorias de nematodos (con énfasis en *Toxocara* spp.). *Parasitol al Día* 22(número especial):44–54, 1998.

Bratt, D.E., E.S. Tikasingh. Visceral larva migrans in seven members of one family in Trinidad. *Trop Geogr Med* 44(1–2):109–112, 1992.

Carrillo, M., O.O. Barriga. Anthelmintic effect of levamisole hydrochloride or ivermectin on tissue toxocariasis of mice. *Am J Vet Res* 48(2):281–283, 1987.

Dubey, J.P. Patent *Toxocara canis* infection in ascarid-naive dogs. *J Parasitol* 64(6):1021–1023, 1978.

Ehrhard, T., S. Kernbaum. *Toxocara canis* et toxocarose humaine. *Bull Inst Pasteur* 77:225–227, 1979.

Eberhard, M.L., E. Alfano. Adult *Toxocara cati* infections in U.S. children: Report of four cases. *Am J Trop Med Hyg* 59(3):404–406, 1998.

Gillespie, S.H., D. Bidwell, A. Voller, B.D. Robertson, R.M. Maizels. Diagnosis of human toxocariasis by antigen capture enzyme linked immunosorbent assay. *J Clin Pathol* 46(6):551–554, 1993.

Kayes, S.G. Human toxocariasis and the visceral larva migrans syndrome: Correlative immunopathology. *Chem Immunol* 66:99–124, 1997.

Maung, M. The ocurrence of the second moult of *Ascaris lumbricoides* and *Ascaris suum*. *Int J Parasitol* 8(5):371–378, 1978.

Nathwani, D., R.B. Laing, P.F. Currie. Covert toxocariasis—a cause of recurrent abdominal pain in childhood. *Br J Clin Pract* 46(4):271, 1992.

Obwaller, A., E. Jensen-Jarolim, H. Auer, A. Huber, D. Kraft, H. Aspock. *Toxocara* infestations in humans: Symptomatic course of toxocarosis correlates significantly with levels of IgE/anti-IgE immune complexes. *Parasite Immunol* 20(7):311–317, 1998.

Overgaauw, P.A. Aspects of *Toxocara* epidemiology: Human toxocarosis. *Crit Rev Microbiol* 23(3):215–231, 1997.

Petithory, J.C., A. Beddok, M. Quedoc. Zoonoses d'origine ascaridienne: les syndromes de Larva migrans visceral. *Bull Acad Natl Med* 178(4):635–645, 1994.

Rugiero, E., M.E. Cabrera, G. Ducach, I. Noemi, A. Viovy. Toxocariasis sistémica en el paciente adulto. *Rev Med Chil* 123(5):612–616, 1995.

Schantz, P.M., L.T. Glickman. Ascáridos de perros y gatos: un problema de salud pública y de medicina veterinaria. *Bol Oficina Sanit Panam* 94(6):571–586, 1983.

Schottler, G. Studie zum Vorkommen von Wurmeiern—insbesondere von Eiern des Hundespulwurmes (Larva migrans visceralis-Syndrom) im Strandsand von Warnemunde 1997. *Gesundheitswesen* 60(12):766–767, 1998.

Shimizu, T. Prevalence of *Toxocara* eggs in sandpits in Tokushima city and its outskirts. *J Vet Med Sci* 55(5):807–811, 1993.

ZOONOTIC ANCYLOSTOMIASIS

ICD-10 B76.0 Ancylostomiasis; B76.8 Other hookworm diseases

Synonyms: Ankylostomiasis, hookworm disease, necatoriasis, uncinariasis.

Etiology: The agents of these diseases are the nematodes *Ancylostoma caninum* (of dogs) and *A. ceylanicum* (of cats). Up until 1982, just six cases of human infection caused by *A. caninum*, which affected the intestine, had been reported (Barriga, 1982). However, based on reports from Australia in the 1990s, it is now known that the parasitosis is common in that region. Human intestinal infection with *A. ceylanicum* has been described, but it is uncommon. In the 1950s, several cases of human intestinal infection due to *A. braziliense* were reported before the difference between *A. braziliense* and *A. ceylanicum* was understood. Since that difference became widely accepted, just one case has been reported (in Portugal in 1970). It is likely, therefore, that the previous reports confused the two species. However, *A. braziliense* seems to be a common agent of cutaneous larva migrans (Cypess, 1982), which is discussed in the respective chapter.

A. malayanum in Argentina and Brazil, *A. japonica* in Japan, *Necator suillis* in Malaysia, and *N. argentinus* in Trinidad and Brazil were once reported as causing infection in the human intestine (Barriga, 1982). Since these species have not been confirmed, their identity is questionable and they will not be addressed here. *Ancylostoma duodenale* and *Necator americanus* are exclusively human parasites, although the former infects dogs and cats under experimental conditions (el-Naggar *et al.*, 1994); *N. americanus* infects hamsters (Rose and Behnke, 1990) and mice (Wilkinson *et al.*, 1990). The nematode *A. duodenale* was identified in 83% of 1,000 swine in Nigeria, but only by examination of the eggs (Salifu *et al.*, 1990). The oldest literature mentions that *A. duodenale* is occasionally found in Old and New World monkeys, swine, and domestic and wild felids; *N. americanus* has been found in Old and New World monkeys, rhinoceri, an African rodent, domestic carnivores, and a rabbit (Barriga, 1982). Albonico and Savioli (1997) believe that there are probably 1.3 billion people infected with ancylostomes worldwide, and that perhaps 96 million have symptoms.

The life cycles of *A. caninum* and *A. ceylanicum* are essentially identical; therefore, only the former will be described here. The adult parasites are grayish-white to reddish-white, although they may also be dark red. They measure from 11–20 mm in length and 0.3–0.6 mm in diameter (the females are larger) and have three pairs of teeth on the ventral rim of the buccal capsule. The morphology of the bursa copulatrix in males is an aid to identification. They live in the small intestine of the host, and each female lays some 16,000 eggs per day, which are eliminated to the exterior with the fecal matter. Under favorable environmental conditions (humidity above 90%, temperature between 23°C and 30°C, shade, availability of oxygen, and absence of predators), embryogeny is rapid, and the first-stage larva, which has a rhabditiform esophagus, can hatch from the egg in 24 to 48 hours. These larvae are not resistant to low temperatures or a dry environment. In the course of a week, the larva undergoes two molts and develops into a third-stage larva, which is infective for the host. In this stage, the larva has a filiform esophagus, is encysted in the cuticular envelope of the second-stage larva, does not feed, and can survive in the soil for approximately three weeks.

Hosts can become infected through the skin or orally, in the latter case by ingestion of milk from infected mothers or consumption of paratenic hosts. Both methods occur in the case of *A. caninum,* for which dogs are natural hosts. Transmission of this species through the placenta is considered an exceptional situation (Barriga, 1997). When the infection route is through the skin, the infective larvae lodge in the host, attracted by the temperature and chemical substances (Ashton *et al.*, 1999), penetrate the skin by means of mechanical and enzymatic phenomena, probably with the aid of a hyaluronidase (Hotez *et al.*, 1994), and are carried by the bloodstream to the lungs. Once there, they pass through the capillary and alveolar walls and advance up the tracheobronchial tree to the pharynx, molt into the fourth stage 44 to 48 hours after infection, and are swallowed. The larvae develop into juvenile nematodes in the small intestine prior to the sixth day of infection. Subsequently, they reach maturity and the females begin to lay eggs 14 days after infection. In infections via the oral route, a few larvae may penetrate the digestive mucosa and follow a systemic cycle similar to that of the transcutaneous infection, but most penetrate the gastric or intestinal mucosa and mature there without leaving the gastrointestinal tract. The discovery of adult ancylostomes in human infants suggests the possibility of either transplacental or transmammary transmission. The persistence of infective ancylostome larvae for days or months in rodents, rabbits, or chickens as transport hosts suggests that transmission in man can occur through paratenic hosts.

A. ceylanicum is smaller than *A. caninum* and has just two pairs of teeth. The natural hosts of *A. caninum* are dogs and other wild canids; the natural hosts of *A. ceylanicum* are cats and other wild felids.

Geographic Distribution and Occurrence: The human intestinal infection is very rare almost everywhere in the world. The literature mentions just six cases up to 1982 (Barriga, 1982). However, an epidemic of 93 human cases was reported in northeastern Australia in 1990, with an eosinophilic enteritis that seemed to be caused by this parasite (Prociv and Croese, 1990). Six years of research confirmed *A. caninum* as the culprit, and a few cases were found in other parts of Australia (Prociv and Croese, 1996). There seems to be no reason why the infection cannot be found in other parts of the world, especially since *A. caninum* is very common in dogs, with prevalences of 20% to 60%. Of 80 stray dogs autopsied in Uruguay, 99% were infected with *A. caninum* and 49% were infected with *A. braziliense* (Malgor *et al.*, 1996).

The geographic distribution of *A. ceylanicum* is difficult to determine because of the long-standing confusion with *A. braziliense*. The locations reported since 1967, when the difference from *A. braziliense* was already well known, include eastern Asia, Brazil, the Philippines, Guyana, India, Indonesia (Sumatra), Japan, Liberia, Madagascar, Malaysia, Sri Lanka, Suriname, Thailand, Taiwan, and Zimbabwe. Between 1968 and 1982, 1 human case in Japan and 1 in the Philippines were reported; *A. ceylanicum* was reported in 5 of 140 people examined in Taiwan, 7 of 45 people in Thailand, 2 of 15 soldiers returning to the Netherlands from Suriname, and 16 of 183 ancylostomiasis patients in India (Barriga, 1982). *A. ceylanicum* infection occurs sporadically and, in general, with few specimens: 29 infected individuals had an average of 2.6 specimens of *A. ceylanicum*, with a maximum of 23 specimens. For the most part, the patients are also infected with a large number of human ancylostomes: a study of 16 ancylostomiasis patients found a ratio of 1:25:54 for *A. ceylanicum*, *A. duodenale*, and *N. americanus*.

In India, Japan, Malaysia, and Taiwan, high rates of infection due to *A. ceylanicum* were found in dogs and cats. In Suriname, *A. ceylanicum* was found in 80% of 102 dogs and in 60% of 50 stray cats that were autopsied. In South Africa, autopsies of 1,502 cats found 41% with *Ancylostoma tubaeforme*, 25% with *A. braziliense*, 3.3% with *A. caninum*, and 1.4% with *A. ceylanicum* (Baker *et al.*, 1989).

The Disease in Man: The most important signs of nonzoonotic ancylostomiasis are anemia caused by an anticoagulant peptide which inhibits the coagulation factor Xa (Cappello *et al.*, 1995) and atrophy of the intestinal villi. These signs are not seen in the zoonotic ancylostomiases because of the limited number of parasites in man. Human infection with *A. caninum* is probably asymptomatic in a large proportion of cases, but it causes eosinophilic enteritis in some. The most common clinical manifestation is abdominal pain, sometimes very intense, with or without eosinophilia. In no case has more than one parasite been found, always juvenile larvae, so the infections did not become patent. The lesions associated with the infection are focal or diffuse eosinophilic inflammation, probably caused by reaction to the parasite's antigens, and aphthous ulcers of the terminal ileum, cecum, or colon, visible on endoscopy. These lesions were found in 5% of patients in northeastern Australia. The clinical manifestations and pathology of this infection are similar to those of anisakiasis (Prociv and Croese, 1996).

In the few confirmed cases of intense infection by *A. ceylanicum*, the symptomatology was similar to that caused by human ancylostomes, and anemia was the main sign. Eight volunteers who received 50 to 150 *A. ceylanicum* larvae via the percutaneous route developed papules at the inoculation site; 15 to 20 days later they complained of epigastric discomfort, headache, fatigue, and eosinophilia. The prepatent period lasted three to five weeks. The early symptoms described were similar to those observed in volunteers who received the human ancylostome *N. americanus* or *A. duodenale* (Wijers *et al.*, 1966).

The Disease in Animals: Animal ancylostomiasis can manifest itself clinically on the skin due to the entry of the parasites, in the lungs due to the migration of the larvae, or in the intestine due to the activity of the adults. The intensity of the infection depends on several factors, such as the number of parasites, nutritional state of the animal, age, or previous infections by these nematodes. Young animals are the most affected. Entry of larvae through the skin in a first infection causes microscopic wounds that heal quickly. Subsequent infections can cause allergic inflammation with extensive pruritus, which can lead to further tissue damage due to scratching and rubbing. The signs are more acute in infection by *Uncinaria stenocephala* than *A. caninum*. In general, migration of the larvae in the respiratory system is asymptomatic. Extensive infections can cause petechiae and foci of traumatic inflammation, and the subsequent infections can cause more intense allergic inflammations, but these rarely have clinical manifestations. In intense infections, enteritis (sometimes with hemorrhagic diarrhea), atrophy of the intestinal villi, and deficiencies in intestinal absorption are frequent. Loss of blood caused by suction and the subsequent bleeding, associated with malnutrition caused by diarrhea and malabsorption, leads to hypochromic microcytic anemia. Eosinophilia, generally 10% to 15%, is lower than in human patients. Mild infections are generally asymptomatic.

It has been confirmed that some *A. caninum* larvae can remain hypobiotic in female dogs and, in gravid animals, become active again toward the end of pregnancy and be passed on to the newborn puppies in the mother's milk (Barriga, 1997).

Source of Infection and Mode of Transmission: There is epidemiological evidence that human infection with *A. caninum* is acquired from infected dogs (Croese *et al.*, 1994). The sources of infection for humans are soil and vegetables contaminated with the feces of infected dogs or cats. Soils that retain moisture are the most favorable for the larvae because they prevent desiccation. While the larvae do not develop at temperatures below 12°C, temperatures close to that favor the survival of infective larvae because they do not accelerate the consumption of food reserves. While human ancylostomiasis can be acquired through the transcutaneous or digestive route, infection with *A. caninum* in its normal host occurs more efficiently by the oral route, and there is some evidence that infection of man by *A. ceylanicum* is also more efficient by the oral route.

Diagnosis: As was shown in Australia, infection by *A. caninum* cannot be diagnosed by the presence of eggs in the feces because the nematode does not reach sexual maturity in man. The observation of aphthous ulcers of the terminal ileum, cecum, or colon, associated with the clinical manifestations, can be an aid to diagnosis. The parasite itself is observed in just 10% to 15% of endoscopies. Enzyme-linked immunosorbent assays (ELISA) with secretory and excretory products of the parasite have revealed specific IgG and IgE antibodies. The Western blot technique with a 68 kDa antigen appears to be more sensitive and specific, even though a similar antigen seems to be present in human ancylostomes (Prociv and Croese, 1996).

Infection with *A. ceylanicum* can be confirmed by discovery of the eggs in fecal matter, but it is not possible to distinguish them from the eggs of *A. duodenale*, with which it is frequently associated. Counting the number of eggs (Stoll or Kato-Katz method) indicates the intensity of the infection: less than 2,000 eggs per gram of feces in man corresponds to less than 50 parasites and a subclinical infection; 5,000 eggs per gram of feces are found in infections with clinical significance; and more than 11,000 eggs per gram are found in cases of frank anemia. However, it is not known whether these figures are valid for *A. ceylanicum*. For specific diagnosis, the patient should be given an anthelmintic (bephenium hydroxynaphthoate, pyrantel pamoate, mebendazole, or thiabendazole), and the expelled parasites identified.

Control: Zoonotic human ancylostomiasis is so infrequent as compared to the nonzoonotic variety that specific control measures are not justified, unless they also help reduce human infection with ancylostomes or other, more prevalent parasites. Since both zoonotic ancylostomes are prevalent in areas in which the nonzoonotic infection also occurs, the recommendations to avoid walking barefoot in areas that may be contaminated with ancylostomes, boil untreated water, avoid eating suspicious foods, and wash the hands before eating can help prevent both types of infection. Seventy years of research have brought about important advances in the development of vaccines against ancylostomiasis (Hotez *et al*., 1996), but it is not known whether a single vaccine can protect against all species of ancylostomes. Mechanical vectors may play a role in ancylostome infection: a study in Nigeria of 5,000 domestic flies found 2.6% to have *Ancylostoma caninum* eggs and 6.2% to have *A. caninum* larvae on their external surface and their digestive system (Umeche and Mandah, 1989). Health education regarding the role of pets in human infection would be the most effective method of controlling this and other zoonoses.

Bibliography

Albonico, M., L. Savioli. Hookworm infection and disease: Advances for control. *Ann Ist Super Sanita* 33(4):567–579, 1997.

Ashton, F.T., J. Li, G.A. Schad. Chemo- and thermosensory neurons: Structure and function in animal parasitic nematodes. *Vet Parasitol* 84(3–4):297–316, 1999.

Baker, M.K., L. Lange, A. Verster, S. van der Plaat. A survey of helminths in domestic cats in the Pretoria area of Transvaal, Republic of South Africa. Part 1: The prevalence and comparison of burdens of helminths in adult and juvenile cats. *J S Afr Vet Assoc* 60(3):139–142, 1989.

Barriga, O.O. Ancylostomiasis. *In*: Schultz, M.O., section ed. Section C, Vol. 2: *CRC Handbook Series in Zoonoses*. Boca Raton: CRC Press; 1982.

Barriga, O.O. *Veterinary Parasitology for Practitioners*, 2nd ed. Edina: Burgess International Group; 1997.

Cappello, M., G.P. Vlasuk, P.W. Bergum, S. Huang, P.J. Hotez. *Ancylostoma caninum* anticoagulant peptide: A hookworm-derived inhibitor of human coagulation factor Xa. *Proc Natl Acad Sci USA* 92(13):6152–6156, 1995.

Croese, J., A. Loukas, J. Opdebeeck, S. Fairley, P. Prociv. Human enteric infection with canine hookworms. *Ann Intern Med* 120(5):369–374, 1994.

Cypess, R.H. Cutaneous larva migrans. *In*: Schultz, M.O., section ed. Section C, Vol. 2: *CRC Handbook Series in Zoonoses*. Boca Raton: CRC Press; 1982.

el-Naggar, H.M., A.M. el-Shazly, M. el-Mahdy. Immune response in dogs infected with *Ancylostoma duodenale*. *J Egypt Soc Parasitol* 24(1):77–83, 1994.

Harvey, J.B., J.M. Roberts, P.M. Schantz. Survey of veterinarians' recommendations for treatment and control of intestinal parasites in dogs: Public health implications. *J Am Vet Med Assoc* 199(6):702–707, 1991.

Hotez, P., M. Cappello, J. Hawdon, C. Beckers, J. Sakanari. Hyaluronidases of the gastrointestinal invasive nematodes *Ancylostoma caninum* and *Anisakis simplex*: Possible functions in the pathogenesis of human zoonoses. *J Infect Dis* 170(4):918–926, 1994.

Hotez, P.J., J.M. Hawdon, M. Cappello, *et al.* Molecular approaches to vaccinating against hookworm disease. *Pediatr Res* 40(4):515–521, 1996.

Malgor, R., Y. Oku, R. Gallardo, I. Yarzabal. High prevalence of *Ancylostoma* spp. infection in dogs, associated with endemic focus of human cutaneous larva migrans, in Tacuarembó, Uruguay. *Parasite* 3(2):131–134, 1996.

Prociv, P., J. Croese. Human eosinophilic enteritis caused by dog hookworm *Ancylostoma caninum*. *Lancet* 335(8701):1299–1302, 1990.

Prociv, P., J. Croese. Human enteric infection with *Ancylostoma caninum*: Hookworms reappraised in the light of a "new" zoonosis. *Acta Trop* 62(1):23–44, 1996.

Rose, R.A., J.M. Behnke. *Necator americanus* in the DSN hamster: Density-dependent expulsion of adult worms during primary infection. *Parasitology* 100 Pt 3:469–478, 1990.

Salifu, D.A., T.B. Manga, I.O. Onyali. A survey of gastrointestinal parasites in pigs of the Plateau and Rivers States, Nigeria. *Rev Elev Med Vet Pays Trop* 43(2):193–196, 1990.

Umeche, N., L.E. Mandah. *Musca domestica* as a carrier of intestinal helminths in Calabar, Nigeria. *East Afr Med J* 66(5):349–352, 1989.

Wijers, D.J.B., A.M. Smith. Early symptoms after experimental infection of *Ancylostoma braziliense* var. *ceylanicum*. *Trop Geogr Med* 18:48–52, 1966.

Wilkinson, M.J., C. Wells, J.M. Behnke. *Necator americanus* in the mouse: Histopathological changes associated with the passage of larvae through the lungs of mice exposed to primary and secondary infection. *Parasitol Res* 76(5):386–392, 1990.

World Health Organization (WHO). *Intestinal Protozoan and Helminthic Infections. Report of a WHO Scientific Group.* Geneva: WHO; 1981. (Technical Report Series 666.)

ZOONOTIC FILARIASES

ICD-10 B74.1 Filariasis due to Brugia malayi; B74.8 Other filariases

Etiology: The agents of these infections are the zoonotic filariae *Brugia malayi* (subperiodic form), possibly *B. pahangi* and *B. leporis, Dirofilaria immitis, D. (Nochtiella) tenuis, D. (Nochtiella) repens, Loaina* sp., *Meningonema* sp., *Onchocerca* sp., and several species of unidentified animal filariae, including some that manifest themselves in man and that have been identified only as *Microfilaria semiclarum* and *M. bolivarensis* (Beaver *et al.*, 1984; Orihel and Eberhard, 1998).

The subperiodic form of *B. malayi* infects man as well as monkeys, cats, and dogs in the Orient. While *B. pahangi* infects the same animals as subperiodic *B. malayi* and has been experimentally transmitted to man (Nutman, 1991), its presence in man has not been reported under natural conditions. Eberhard *et al.* (1991) found a *Brugia* microfilaria similar to that of *B. leporis* in 60% of the rabbits on the island of Nantucket, in the state of Massachusetts, US. The authors believe that this microfilaria could be the agent of the 21 cases of human brugiasis reported in the northeastern US. Two years earlier, Orihel and Beaver (1989) had described nine cases of human brugiasis, eight acquired in the US and one in Brazil, and reclassified as brugiasis three other cases whose etiologic agents had been identified as "similar to" *Dirofilaria, Dipetalonema,* or *Brugia. D. immitis* is a filaria of the heart and great vessels of dogs, wild canids, and, less frequently, cats. It has also been described in almost 30 other wild species, mainly carnivores, mustelids, and primates (Barriga, 1982). On rare occasions, the dead parasites are found in the lungs of man. The subgenus *Nochtiella* is a dirofilaria of the subcutaneous tissue; it is characterized by fine transversal striations and prominent longitudinal ridges along the cuticulae. *D. tenuis* is a filaria of the subcutaneous tissue in raccoons and man; it is found in the southern US. *D. repens* is a filaria of the subcutaneous tissue of dogs and cats in Africa, Asia, and Europe; it is also found occasionally in man. *Onchocerca* (possibly *O. cervicalis* in horses or *O. gutturosa* in cattle) is a filaria that has been found just six times anywhere in the world in the form of subcutaneous nodules; on the seventh occasion, it was found embedded in the cornea (Burr *et al.*, 1998). *Loaina* is a filaria that has been found at least once in the human eye (Beaver, 1989). *Meningonema* (possibly *M. peruzzii*) is a filaria of the nervous system of *Cercopithecus* monkeys; it has been found in man in Cameroon and may also occur in Zimbabwe (Boussinesq *et al.*, 1995).

Animals do not participate to a significant extent in the epidemiology of human filariases caused by *Wuchereria bancrofti*, *B. malayi* (periodic form), *B. timori*, *Onchocerca volvulus*, *Loa loa*, *Mansonella ozzardi*, *Tetrapetalonema (Dipetalonema) perstans*, or *T. (Dipetalonema) streptocerca*, which are all considered to be parasites specific to humans (Dissanaike, 1979). Some findings in animals are so limited that zoonotic classification is not practicable. *O. volvulus* has only been found in one gorilla in the Democratic Republic of the Congo and in one spider monkey (*Ateles geoffroyi*) in Mexico (Dissanaike, 1979). The mandrill worm, similar to *L. loa* in man, is considered a different subspecies, *L. loa papionis*, which is transmitted by a different vector, *Chrysops*. Parasites similar to *M. ozzardi* have been observed in neotropical monkeys, but there is no certainty that this is the same species that infects man (Dissanaike, 1979). Also, *T. perstans* and *T. streptocerca* have been found in anthropoid monkeys, but there is not enough information available about their biology to determine their epidemiological importance (WHO, 1979).

One of the prominent features in the biology and epidemiology of filariae is that their life cycle requires an arthropod host. The adult parasites are long, thin nematodes that live in the host's tissues or body cavities. The females are viviparous, incubating their eggs *in utero* and releasing embryos called microfilariae, which live in the blood or lymph, or, sometimes, in the skin. The presence or absence of a sheath (the stretched shell of the egg) around the microfilariae is an important factor in diagnosis. The microfilariae are ingested by an arthropod during feeding and continue their development into a third-stage larva inside the host; then they migrate to the invertebrate host's mouthparts. When the arthropod feeds again, it releases the infective larvae, which enter the body of a vertebrate host and continue their development, reaching sexual maturity and producing microfilariae.

The microfilariae of some species appear in the blood with a marked nocturnal or diurnal periodicity. Those that do not display this phenomenon to a high degree are called subperiodic. *B. malayi* has a nocturnal periodic form in which the microfilariae disappear or are very rare during the day, and a subperiodic form with maximum filaremia during the night, but with filariae also present during the day. *D. repens* is of diurnal periodicity, while *D. immitis* has a nocturnal subperiodicity, with filaremia 5 to 10 times greater in the afternoon or at night than in the morning or at midday. This phenomenon, which is interpreted as an adaptation of the filariae to the feeding habits of the vectors, is important in the epidemiology and diagnosis.

Geographic Distribution and Occurrence: Periodic *B. malayi* is the cause of most of the human cases of brugiasis *malayi* that occur in Southeast Asia, China, Korea, and India, but it is a parasite exclusive to man that is transmitted only experimentally to cats and monkeys. The subperiodic form is limited to wooded and swampy regions of Indonesia, peninsular Malaysia, Thailand, southern Viet Nam, and three foci in the Philippines. Transmission occurs between jungle animals and man by means of mosquitoes, primarily those of the genus *Mansonia*. The parasite has been found in several species of nonhuman primates, domestic cats, wild felids, and pangolins (*Manis javanica*). *B. pahangi*, whose microfilariae are not easily distinguished from those of *B. malayi*, is a parasite of dogs, cats, wild felids, and less frequently, primates. Experimentally, the infection was transmitted from cat to man, but it is not known if the human infection occurs naturally, given the difficulty in distinguishing the two species. Its vectors are *Armigeres subalbatus* and *Mansonia* spp. mosquitoes; its area of distribution in Malaysia coincides with that of *B. malayi*. In the US, up until the year 2000, 22 cases of human infection by *Brugia* spp. of animal origin were described, but it was not possible to determine the species of filariae. *B. beaveri*, of raccoons, and *B. leporis*, of rabbits, are found in that country. Judging by their geographic distribution, the human cases could be due to *B. leporis* (Eberhard *et al.*, 1991). Two cases of a human infection by a zoonotic *Brugia* of unknown species have been described in Colombia (Kozek *et al.*, 1984).

D. immitis is widespread among dogs throughout the world, although the prevalence varies greatly in different areas. In the endemic areas, the prevalence is generally 40% to 70% in dogs and 1% to 4% in cats. Up until 1982, just 44 human cases had been reported (Barriga, 1982), but then Rodrigues-Silva *et al.* (1995) mentioned 229, and Echeverri *et al.* (1999), 150. Of the cases reported between 1995 and 2000, 10 were in Japan, 6 in Germany, 4 in the US, 3 in Italy, and 1 each in Argentina, Brazil, Puerto Rico, and Thailand. Some 87 cases had been reported in the US by 1992 (Asimacopoulos *et al.*, 1992), and 5 more were reported by 2000. The human infection was rare in Japan, with just 2 cases reported up to 1968, but an additional 118 cases had been reported by 1995 (Makiya, 1997) and 10 more by the year 2000. Subcutaneous human dirofilariasis is usually due to *D. tenuis*, a parasite of raccoons *(Procyon lotor)*, in the US, and to *D. repens*, a parasite of dogs and felids, in other countries. Many cases of human subcutaneous dirofilariasis have been diagnosed in numerous countries of Africa, the Americas (Argentina, Brazil, Canada, and the US), Asia, and Europe. The greatest numbers of cases have been recorded in Italy, Sri Lanka, and the former Soviet Union (Dissanaike, 1979).

D. repens occurs in Africa, Asia, and Europe. In Europe, it is known to exist in France, Greece, Italy, Spain, and the former Yugoslavia. In the endemic areas, the prevalence in dogs generally ranges from 5% to 20%. Up to 1995, 397 cases of human infection by *D. repens* had been reported worldwide. The highest number of cases, 168, occurred in Italy (Pampiglione *et al.*, 1995). There were just 4 human cases in Spain up to 1998. There were about 60 cases in France up to 1996, but only about 30 were well documented (Marty, 1997). While a prevalence rate of 1.4% for *D. repens* was found in 5,000 dogs (Marty, 1997), in some populations of military dogs the prevalence exceeded 20% (Chauve, 1997). In Greece, 20 human cases were recognized up to 1990, but 20 more cases were identified by 1997 (12 unpublished); 4 cases were ocular and the rest were subcutaneous. There has been just one known human case of *D. repens* in Japan (Makiya, 1997).

Four species are recognized in dogs: *D. repens*, *D. immitis*, *D. reconditum*, and *D. grassii*. The overall prevalence rate is 12% to 37% (Vakalis and Himonas, 1997). The infection is common in Sri Lanka: up until 1997, there were 70 human cases, and the prevalence in dogs was 30% to 60% (Dissanaike *et al.*, 1997).

The few cases of zoonotic onchocerciasis reported have been diagnosed in Canada, the US, Japan, Switzerland, and the former Soviet Union (Burr *et al.*, 1998). Human cases of cutaneous or ocular infection by filariae "similar to *Dipetalonema*" have been diagnosed in Costa Rica (one case) and in the US (four cases: three in Oregon and one in Alabama) (Beaver *et al.*, 1984).

The Disease in Man: The main symptomatology of filariases due to *B. malayi*, both periodic and subperiodic (zoonotic), consists of lymphadenopathies, lymphangitis, and high eosinophilia. Attacks of lymphadenopathy lasting several days occur at irregular intervals, with fever, malaise, cephalalgia, nausea, swelling of one leg, and sterile abscesses. In advanced cases, elephantiasis of the lower extremities may occur due to obstruction of the lymphatic circulation. Elephantiasis of the scrotum, such as is seen in Bancroft's filariasis *(Wuchereria bancrofti)*, is rare in brugiasis. Many infections among the natives of endemic regions occur asymptomatically in spite of the presence of filaremia. In the cases of human infection by *Brugia* spp. of animal origin in the US, the parasite was unexpectedly found in infarcted ganglia in patients who had no other symptomatology related to this infection (Gutiérrez and Petras, 1982). The two Colombian cases were also characterized by lymphadenopathy (Kozek *et al.*, 1984).

The dirofilariae that infect man (*D. immitis*, *D. repens*, and *D. tenuis*) often cause pulmonary or cutaneous symptoms. *D. immitis* is transmitted by a variety of mosquitoes. In man, it appears that the parasite begins its cycle from the subcutaneous tissue, reaches the heart and dies, and is carried in the bloodstream to the lung, where it forms a thrombus. The parasites are usually found dead, forming a 1–4 cm nodule in the lung. In general, the parasite is a juvenile specimen; mature females have been found on a few occasions, and parasitemia was observed only in the case of a girl who received immunosuppressant therapy (Barriga, 1982). The X-ray image is known as a coin lesion (Echeverri *et al.*, 1999). In 39 patients, 22 (56%) were asymptomatic and the infection was discovered during routine examination (Flieder and Moran, 1999). However, the parasite is often removed unnecessarily when it is suspected that it is a neoplasm (Rodrigues-Silva *et al.*, 1995). In the symptomatic cases, cough and thoracic pain lasting a month or more have been reported, along with occasional hemoptysis, fever, malaise, chills, and myalgia. X-rays show the coin lesion, and eosinophilia is rarely confirmed.

Subcutaneous dirofilariasis and, frequently, subconjunctival dirofilariasis is due to *D. tenuis* in the US and *D. repens* in Africa, Asia, Europe, and South America. Other, unidentified species of animal dirofilariae may also be involved. Up until 1995, 397 cases of human dirofilariasis by *D. repens* had been reported worldwide. Italy had the highest number of cases (168). The lesion is generally a subcutaneous nodule or submucosal swelling which may or may not be nodular. The nodules and swelling may or may not be painful, and some are migratory. The most frequent localizations are the head, chest wall, upper extremities, and, occasionally, under the conjunctiva. Sometimes it is internal, mainly in the lung (Pampiglione *et al.*, 1995). In general, a single parasite is responsible for the lesion, and on some occasions, it has been retrieved alive. In a few cases, microfilariae have been observed in the uterus of the parasite, and in just one case, in the patient's blood (Marty, 1997). The lesion is inflammatory, with accompanying histiocytes, plasmocytes, lymphocytes, and abundant eosinophils. Blood eosinophilia is unusual (Marty, 1997).

D. tenuis seems to have a greater affinity for subconjunctival localization. It was originally identified as *D. conjunctivae* because of the frequency with which it affected the eyelids. Periorbital dirofilariasis caused by *D. tenuis* is suspected in the presence of migratory swelling in patients who have lived or traveled in the southeastern US. The infection must be differentiated from sarcoidosis, ruptured dermoid cyst, infectious abscesses, neoplasms, and idiopathic pseudotumors (Kersten *et al.*, 1994). Some 56 cases of human intraocular filariasis in which the parasite was a specimen of a variety of species, predominantly nonzoonotic worms such as *L. loa* and *W. bancrofti*, have been described (Beaver, 1989). In Oregon, US, there were three cases with actively motile filariae in the anterior chamber of the eye. The causal agent was classified as *Dipetalonema* spp., with morphology similar to that of *D. arbuta* of porcupines (*Erethizon dorsatum*) or *D. sprenti* of beavers (*Castor canadensis*).

The cases of zoonotic onchocerciasis in North America were manifested as fibrotic nodules on the wrist tendon and, in one case, the nodule was embedded in the cornea (Burr *et al.*, 1998).

The Disease in Animals: Dogs and cats do not seem to suffer symptoms of infection due to subperiodic *B. malayi* or *B. pahangi*, but in the laboratory, both species—especially *B. pahangi*—can cause changes in the lymphatic circulation, with edema in the hind legs of infected animals. Dogs develop lymphangitis with fibrotic lymphadenopathy similar to that of man (Snowden and Hammerberg, 1989). The infection in domestic carnivores is probably underdiagnosed.

D. immitis lives in the pulmonary artery of dogs and, secondarily, in the right ventricle; it almost always forms a mass that includes numerous parasites. When the number of parasites is small, the infection may be asymptomatic. In cases of more intense or protracted infections, the living or dead filariae cause stenosis of the pulmonary vessels, obstructing the flow of blood. Over time, this causes failure of the right ventricle (Barriga, 1997). The most prominent signs are chronic cough, loss of vitality, and, in serious forms, right cardiac insufficiency. Chronic passive congestion can develop in several organs and produce ascites; thromboses caused by dead parasites can lead to pulmonary infarctions, resulting in sudden death. The acute hepatic syndrome consists of obstruction of the vena cava inferior by a large number of adult parasites that matured simultaneously, with consequent acute congestion of the liver and kidneys, hemoglobinuria, and death in 24 to 72 hours.

D. tenuis and *D. repens* do not cause illness in the animal; they may occasionally cause pruritis and eczema, leading to hair loss and scab formation.

Source of Infection and Mode of Transmission: The reservoirs of subperiodic brugiasis, which occurs in the wooded and swampy regions of Southeast Asia, are monkeys, cats, and wild carnivores. High rates of infection have been found in the monkeys *Presbytis obscurus* and *Macaca irus*. The relative importance of wild and domestic animals as reservoirs is unknown, but it is likely that the latter serve more frequently as a source of infection for man (Denham and McGreevy, 1977). The infection is transmitted by mosquitoes of the genus *Mansonia* from animal to animal, from animal to human, and from human to human. The maximum concentration of microfilariae in the blood occurs at night to coincide with the nocturnal feeding habits of the vectors. Although *Mansonia* mosquitoes usually feed outside houses, they have also been found inside them, as is demonstrated by the fact that the infection occurs in children. In other zoonotic human infections by *Brugia* spp., *Onchocerca* spp., and *Dipetalonema* spp. (or similar species), the source of infection is wild animals of undetermined species. The main reservoir of *D. immitis* is the dog, and the disease is transmitted by a variety of mosquitoes; man is infected only accidentally. The reservoir of *D. repens* is the dog, and that of *D. tenuis* is the raccoon. Man is an accidental host of zoonotic filariae (with the exception of subperiodic *B. malayi*) and does not play any role in the epidemiology.

Role of Animals in the Epidemiology of the Disease: Of the large number of filariae species that exist in nature, only eight have fully adapted to man, and their transmission is exclusively or mainly person to person (see Etiology). The other species of filariae are parasites of animals, affecting man only occasionally and thus not constituting a public health problem. One exception is subperiodic *Brugia malayi*, which is an important pathogen for man.

Diagnosis: Of all the filariases presented in this section, only subperiodic *B. malayi* infection can be diagnosed in man when microfilariae are detected in the patient's blood; the others are not evident in man. The most common techniques are the blood smear stained with Giemsa stain, the Knott concentration, and Millipore filter concentration. Since microfilaremia takes many months to appear after infection, ganglion biopsy can be useful for early diagnosis.

In man, diagnosis of pulmonary or subcutaneous dirofilariasis is made by morphologic examination of parasites obtained through biopsy or surgery. In dogs and cats, diagnosis is made by identifying microfilariae in the blood, using a smear, the modified Knott method, or Millipore filters. In the case of *D. immitis*, a blood sample should preferably be obtained during the nocturnal hours, when the microfilaremia reaches its maximum level. Microfilaremia by *D. immitis* appears in dogs six months after infection; microfilaremia is not detectable (occult dirofilariasis) in approximately 15% of dogs infected by *D. immitis*. It is also necessary to differentiate the microfilariae of *D. immitis* from those of *D. repens* and *Dipetalonema reconditum*. *D. reconditum* is a nonpathogenic filaria of dogs, but its microfilariae can be confused with those of *D. immitis*. This need has been the impetus for the development of indirect diagnostic tests. The detection of an antigen of female *D. immitis* in the bloodstream of infected dogs by enzyme-linked immunosorbent assay (ELISA) makes a very sensitive and specific diagnosis possible. In man, it has been found that both *D. immitis* and *D. repens* cause the formation of antibodies and that both parasites have specific antigens. Consequently, it is possible to differentiate the respective infections serologically (Simon *et al.*, 1997). The polymerase chain reaction has also been used successfully to differentiate infections caused by *D. immitis* and *D. repens* (Favia *et al.*, 1997). However, the polymerase chain reaction and the Western blot technique seem to be more sensitive than ELISA in detecting infections by *D. repens* (Cancrini *et al.*, 1999).

Control: Human filariasis is combated by controlling the vector arthropods, mainly with insecticides. Mass therapeutic treatment of human communities has also been successfully used to decrease the source of infection for the vectors. Control of subperiodic brugiasis is more difficult because of the ecologic characteristics of the endemic area and because of the abundance of wildlife reservoirs. In India and Sri Lanka, population levels of the intermediate host and vector of subperiodic *B. malayi* (*Mansonia* mosquitoes) were reduced by eliminating several species of floating aquatic plants to which the mosquito larvae attached. In highly enzootic areas, *D. immitis* infection in dogs can be prevented by periodic administration of an appropriate oral anthelmintic to kill the infective larvae when they are introduced by the mosquito. The drug should not be given to dogs with microfilaremia, as it can destroy the microfilariae and produce anaphylactic shock in sensitized animals. While this preventive treatment is not used against *D. repens* because the infection in dogs is asymptomatic, it could be used to decrease the reservoir of vectors in areas of high human endemicity. The other human zoonotic filariases are very rare, so individual protective measures against vectors are sufficient.

Bibliography

Asimacopoulos, P.J., A. Katras, B. Christie. Pulmonary dirofilariasis. The largest single-hospital experience. *Chest* 102(3):851–855, 1992.

Barriga, O.O. Dirofilariasis. *In*: Steele, J.H., section ed. Section C, Vol. 2: *CRC Handbook Series in Zoonoses*. Boca Raton: CRC Press; 1982:93–109.

Barriga, O.O. *Veterinary Parasitology for Practitioners*, 2nd ed. Edina: Burgess International Group; 1997.

Beaver, P.C. Intraocular filariasis: A brief review. *Am J Trop Med Hyg* 40(1):40–45, 1989.

Beaver, P.C., R. Brenes, G. Vargas Solano. Zoonotic filaria in a subcutaneous artery of a child in Costa Rica. *Am J Trop Med Hyg* 33(4):583–585, 1984.

Boussinesq, M., O. Bain, A.G. Chabaud, N. Gardon-Wendel, J. Kamgno, J.P. Chippaux. A new zoonosis of the cerebrospinal fluid of man probably caused by *Meningonema peruzzii*, a filaria of the central nervous system of Cercopithecidae. *Parasite* 2(2):173–176, 1995.

Burr, W.E., Jr., M.F. Brown, M.L. Eberhard. Zoonotic *Onchocerca* (Nematoda: Filarioidea) in the cornea of a Colorado resident. *Ophthalmology* 105(8):1494–1497, 1998.

Cancrini, G., G. Prieto, G. Favia, *et al.* Serological assays on eight cases of human dirofilariasis identified by morphology and DNA diagnostics. *Ann Trop Med Parasitol* 93(2):147–152, 1999.

Chauve, C.M. Importance in France of the infestation by *Dirofilaria (Nochtiella) repens* in dogs. *Parassitologia* 39(4):393–395, 1997.

Dissanaike, A.S. Zoonotic aspects of filarial infections in man. *Bull World Health Organ* 57(3):349–357, 1979.

Dissanaike, A.S., W. Abeyewickreme, M.D. Wijesundera, M.V. Weerasooriya, M.M. Ismail. Human dirofilariasis caused by *Dirofilaria (Nochtiella) repens* in Sri Lanka. *Parassitologia* 39(4):375–382, 1997.

Eberhard, M.L., S.R. Telford III, A. Spielman. A *Brugia* species infecting rabbits in the northeastern United States. *J Parasitol* 77(5):796–798, 1991.

Echeverri, A., R.F. Long, W. Check, C.M. Burnett. Pulmonary dirofilariasis. *Ann Thorac Surg* 67(1):201–202, 1999.

Favia, G., A. Lanfrancotti, A. della Torre, G. Cancrini, M. Coluzzi. Advances in the identification of *Dirofilaria repens* and *Dirofilaria immitis* by a PCR-based approach. *Parassitologia* 39(4):401–402, 1997.

Flieder, D.B., C.A. Moran. Pulmonary dirofilariasis: A clinicopathologic study of 41 lesions in 39 patients. *Hum Pathol* 30(3):251–256, 1999.

Gutiérrez, Y., R.E. Petras. *Brugia* infection in northern Ohio. *Am J Trop Med Hyg* 31(6):1128–1130, 1982.

Kersten, R.C., A.J. Locastro, M.L. Eberhard, A.G. Spaulding, D.R. Kulwin. Periorbital dirofilariasis. *Ophthal Plast Reconstr Surg* 10(4):293–296, 1994.

Kozek, W.J., M.A. Reyes, J. Ehrman, F. Garrido, M. Nieto. Enzootic *Brugia* infection in a two-year old Colombian girl. *Am J Trop Med Hyg* 33(1):65–69, 1984.

Makiya, K. Recent increase of human infections with dog heart worm *Dirofilaria immitis* in Japan. *Parassitologia* 39(4):387–388, 1997.

Marty, P. Human dirofilariasis due to *Dirofilaria repens* in France. A review of reported cases. *Parassitologia* 39(4):383–386, 1997.

Nutman, T.B. Experimental infection of humans with filariae. *Rev Infect Dis* 13(5):1018–1022, 1991.

Orihel, T.C., P.C. Beaver. Zoonotic *Brugia* infections in North and South America. *Am J Trop Med Hyg* 40(6):638–647, 1989.

Orihel, T.C., M.L. Eberhard. Zoonotic filariasis. *Clin Microbiol Rev* 11(2):366–381, 1998.

Pampiglione, S., G. Canestri Trotti, F. Rivasi. Human dirofilariasis due to *Dirofilaria (Nochtiella) repens*: A review of world literature. *Parassitologia* 37(2–3):149–193, 1995.

Rodrigues-Silva, R., H. Moura, G. Dreyer, L. Rey. Human pulmonary dirofilariasis: A review. *Rev Inst Med Trop Sao Paulo* 37(6):523–530, 1995.

Simon, F., G. Prieto, A. Muro, G. Cancrini, M. Cordero, C. Genchi. Human humoral immune response to *Dirofilaria* species. *Parassitologia* 39(4):397–400, 1997.

Snowden, K.F., B. Hammerberg. The lymphatic pathology of chronic *Brugia pahangi* infection in the dog. *Trans R Soc Trop Med Hyg* 83(5):670–678, 1989.

Vakalis, N.C., C.A. Himonas. Human and canine dirofilariasis in Greece. *Parassitologia* 39(4):389–391, 1997.

World Health Organization (WHO). *Parasitic Zoonoses. Report of a WHO Expert Committee, with the Participation of FAO.* Geneva: WHO; 1979. (Technical Report Series 637).

Section C

ARTHROPODS

DERMATITIS CAUSED BY MITES OF ANIMAL ORIGIN

ICD-10 B88.0 Other ascariasis

Etiology: In addition to the mite that causes sarcoptic scabies, or mange (see the chapter on Zoonotic Scabies) and ticks (see the chapter on Tick Infestations), there are other acarid parasites that can infest the skin of man and cause a temporary dermatitis, although they are incapable of becoming established on this aberrant host. These parasites belong to the families Cheyletiellidae, Dermanyssidae, and Macronyssidae.

In the family Cheyletiellidae, only the genus *Cheyletiella* is of importance for present purposes. The members of this genus are obligate ectoparasites of lagomorphs, dogs, cats, wild animals, and, occasionally, man. The species transmissible to man are *C. parasitovorax*, a parasite of rabbits; *C. yasguri*, associated with dogs; and *C. blakei*, found on cats. The mites of this genus are grayish white and measure approximately 0.4 mm by 0.3 mm. Each palp has a claw directed toward the mouth, and at the end of the legs is a double row of hairs instead of suckers. The entire life cycle takes place on the host and is completed in about 35 days. The female attaches her eggs (0.2 mm by 0.1 mm) to the animal's hair about 2 mm or 3 mm from the skin. The hexapod larvae develop within the egg and then go through two nymphal stages before becoming adults. They are superficial parasites of the skin and fur and do not dig galleries into the host. They feed on keratinized skin cells and occasionally suck lymph. Off the host, the adult female and the eggs can survive up to 10 days in a cool place, but the larvae, nymphs, and adult males are less resistant and die in about 2 days in the open environment. Because of their appearance and the way they move, they are popularly referred to as "walking dandruff."

The family Dermanyssidae includes hematophagous ectoparasitic mites of birds and mammals. They measure approximately 0.8–1.0 mm in length and are grayish white when fasting and reddish when engorged. The zoonotic species are *Dermanyssus gallinae*, a parasite of chickens, turkeys, pigeons, canaries, and wild fowl, and *Liponyssoides* (*Allodermanyssus*) *sanguineus*, found on small rodents. *D. gallinae* live in hens' nests and nearby cracks, where the female lays her eggs. At night, they come out of their hiding places and feed on the birds. The females initiate oviposition 12 to 24 hours after feeding. The eggs can hatch in two to three days, releasing a six-legged larva that goes through two nymphal stages before becoming an adult. Under favorable environmental conditions, the entire life cycle can be completed in a week. The adults can live up to 34 weeks without feeding, and hence their spontaneous elimination is difficult. *L. sanguineus* has a similar cycle in rodents, but it takes 18 to 23 days, and the female can survive up to 51 days without feeding.

The family Macronyssidae includes hematophagous ectoparasites of birds, mammals, and reptiles. The potentially zoonotic species are *Ornithonyssus bacoti*, which parasitizes rodents and small marsupials, and *O. bursa* and *O. sylviarum*, found on birds. The genus *Ornithonyssus* has undergone several name changes, and its species are sometimes considered to belong to the genera *Liponyssus* or *Bdellonyssus*. *O. bacoti* lays its eggs in the burrows or nests of rodents, and in the case of laboratory animals such as mice, rats, and hamsters, in the cracks and corners of the cages. Under ideal conditions, the parasite can complete its life cycle in only 11 to 16 days, going from egg to larva and then through two nymphal stages, the adult stage, and finally, oviposition. Hence, it can generate large populations in a short time. *O. bursa* infests chickens, turkeys, pigeons, sparrows, and other fowl. It lives mostly in the birds' nests, where it goes through its life cycle, but it spends more time on fowl than do *D. gallinae*, and less time than *O. sylviarum*. It does not survive more than 10 days in the absence of an avian host. Unlike the other species, *O. sylviarum* is for the most part a permanent ectoparasite which lays its eggs, develops, and spends most of its life on its host. It can complete its life cycle in only seven days and survive for three to four weeks off the host.

Geographic Distribution and Occurrence: Mites of the genus *Cheyletiella* and the species *Dermanyssus gallinae* are distributed worldwide. *Liponyssoides sanguineus* is found in northern Africa, Asia, Europe, and the US. *Ornithonyssus bacoti* is found throughout the world, especially in association with the black rat, *Rattus rattus*. It appears to be common in the Russian Federation because the local literature reports that 36 foci were identified and eradicated in Moscow between 1990 and 1991. *O. bursa* is found mainly in tropical and subtropical regions, and *O. sylviarum*, in temperate regions of the northern hemisphere and also in Australia and New Zealand. The prevalence in man is difficult to determine accurately because these infestations occur only in special circumstances that enable the arthropod to transfer from its usual host to man.

C. yasguri has been found in dog kennels and, occasionally, in veterinary practices. Many cases of *C. blakei* infestations on cats have been detected because their owners were also affected and had sought medical care (Paradis, 1998). Sometimes the infestation is discovered in a coprologic examination, as happened in a laboratory in the US when very large eggs (0.23 mm by 0.11 mm) were found in the feces of a cat. This finding prompted examination of another 41 cats from the same supplier, and 10 of them were found to be infested; at the same time, 28 cats from two other suppliers were negative (McKeevar and Allen, 1979). *C. parasitovorax*, found on rabbits, can invade laboratory colonies and affect a large number of animals. *D. gallinae* is rarely present in modern establishments where fowl are raised in cages; the species is more commonly seen on rural poultry farms and rustic hen houses that afford suitable hiding places for the arthropod. Human homes can be invaded by mites from nearby hen houses or pigeon cotes, especially when the birds leave their nests and the mites have to look for a new source of food. In Rotterdam, Netherlands, 23 individuals from 8 families were found to be infested. *L. sanguineus* is an abundant parasite of mice (*Mus musculus*), but when it needs food, it can readily feed on other rodents or man. *O. bacoti* is frequent wherever the black rat exists in large numbers, and it can be quite common in poorly maintained laboratory rodent colonies. It tends to invade human dwellings when campaigns to eliminate rats have not included treatment to suppress the arthropods. Like *D. gallinae*, *O. bursa* is not often seen on modern farms, which do not provide suitable hiding places. Humans experience only a passing infestation because the mite cannot survive more than 10 days without feeding on its natural host. *O. sylviarum* is more common, even on modern farms, because it lives mainly on the fowl and does not need nests or cracks to hide in.

The Disease in Man: Human infestation with *Cheyletiella* spp. results from close contact with infested animals. The disease consists of an unspecific papular, pruriginous dermatitis on the arms, thorax, waist, and thighs. In man, the infestation is transitory and disappears spontaneously once the reservoir animals in the household—the source of infestation and reinfestation—are treated. The bite of *D. gallinae* is painful, and the infestation usually causes a papular, pruriginous urticaria, although sometimes the only manifestation is persistent pruritus. *L. sanguineus* infestation is similar, but this mite can also transmit *Rickettsia akari*, the agent of vesicular rickettsiosis in man. *O. bacoti* causes a similar condition, with painful bites and sometimes allergic dermatitis. *O. sylviarum* attacks man in the absence of its natural hosts, and it can sometimes cause immediate irritation, followed by erythema, edema, and pruritus. The other avian mite, *O. bursa*, frequently attacks man as well, causing a mild skin irritation. In the laboratory, several of these mites have been infected with organisms that are pathogenic for man, but none except *R. akari* is known to transmit pathogens to man in nature.

The Disease in Animals: The symptoms of animal infestation with *Cheyletiella* spp. are variable. In dogs, an exfoliative and a crusted form have been described. In the former, there is abundant formation of dandruff on the back, which is more noticeable in the fur than as a scaly condition of the skin. There is pruritus to varying degrees, alopecia, and inflammation, which is mainly the result of scratching. In the crusted form, the noticeable manifestation is multiple circular areas of alopecia on the back and sides of the trunk, crusted with no inflammation underneath, which bear a resemblance to tinea. In cats, the infection is often asymptomatic, and when it is manifested, it usually assumes a crusted form very similar to tinea, except that it appears on the trunk and neck instead of the face and paws.

D. gallinae does not appear to cause dermal lesions that can be detected, but in birds it produces anemia and irritation. When the infestation is very intense, it can cause lowered egg production and even an interruption in oviposition, and blood loss can be so severe that the birds die of anemia. In Australia, *D. gallinae* is a vector of *Borrelia anserina*, the agent of fowl spirochetosis. *L. sanguineus* is likely to cause irritation, anemia, and debility in mice. It is the vector of *R. akari*, the agent of human vesicular rickettsiosis, for which the reservoirs are mice and rats. An intense infestation of *O. bursa* in chickens, and even more so, of *O. sylviarum*, gives the plumage a dirty appearance because of the presence of mites, their eggs, and their excrement. A large concentration of mites around the cloaca can cause the skin to crack and form scabs. *O. bacoti* infestation in laboratory rodents can result in debility, anemia, reduced reproduction, and even death (Flynn, 1973).

Source of Infestation and Mode of Transmission: Man is an accidental host. These mites do not colonize permanently in the human skin and, in fact, they stay there for only a short time. Man becomes infested with *Cheyletiella* spp. as a result of close contact with cats, dogs, or rabbits carrying the mites. The infestation usually results from handling infested animals, but it can also be acquired indirectly because the females can survive off the animal's body for about 10 days. It has been pointed out that this latter mode of transmission could occur when infested cats are allowed to sleep on people's beds. *Cheyletiella* females have been found stuck to fleas and louse flies (Hippoboscidae), and it is believed that this may also be a transmission mechanism in certain hosts. *D. gallinae* and the other avian mites can also cause human infestation as a result of contact with infested birds. *D. sylviarum* is found abundantly on birds' eggs, and the handling of them can often cause infestation. Both avian mites and those of rodents may invade human habitations simply because of the proximity of the animals' nests on roofs, between floors, underneath the dwelling, or in the vicinity. The situation becomes worse when the birds leave their nests or the rodents are eliminated, leaving the arthropods to search for new sources of food.

Diagnosis: In the absence of the parasite itself or epidemiologic background, diagnosis of the infestation in man is very difficult because the condition can be mistaken for pediculosis, scabies, or a flea infestation (Engel *et al.*, 1998). For a definitive diagnosis, it is necessary to find the arthropod that caused the lesion. This is important because, even though human dermatitis due to zoonotic mites does not require treatment, it is often recurrent if the source of infestation is not eliminated. Dermatologists recommend that zoonotic mites be taken into account in the differential diagnosis of any cutaneous eruption of unexplained etiology (Blankenship, 1990).

Mites of the genus *Cheyletiella* are too small to be seen by the naked eye, but they can be detected on animals by microscopic examination of impressions, comb residue, or skin scrapings, or by coprologic examination, since they are often ingested. Impressions are made using strips of transparent cellophane tape: the tape is pressed against the animal's skin to capture dandruff and any mites that may be present, and it is then examined under a microscope. Dandruff and mites may be collected by combing or superficial scraping and then studied microscopically. These methods are not as effective in man because the skin has no fur, frequent bathing dislodges the mites (Miller, 1983), and their numbers are limited since they do not reproduce on the human skin. *D. gallinae* and other avian and rodent mites can be seen with the naked eye as a red dot on the skin when they are feeding, or as rapidly running dots in the cracks where they hide. To determine whether they are present in a dwelling, the dust in the home can be vacuumed up, especially in the areas where pets sleep or where birds might enter from outdoors, and examined by flotation: the mites will rise to the surface because they have numerous hairs that trap the air and allow them to float easily in water. Taxonomic differentiation of the species is easy as long as sufficient clues are present.

Control: To prevent human infestation with *Cheyletiella*, pets such as dogs, cats, and rabbits that are suspected of being infested should be treated with appropriate acaricides. In cases of intense infestation, it is necessary to vacuum and apply powdered acaricides in the areas they frequent; however, a veterinarian should be consulted because many of these compounds can be toxic for both man and the pets. To avoid infestations with avian or rodent mites, contact with these animals should be avoided. Repellants should be used on visits to rural areas, or else clothing should protect the body and leave no openings by which the mites could enter. When homes are infested with unwanted birds or rodents, these animals and their nests should be eliminated, and insecticides or acaricides should be applied as part of the treatment to destroy any surviving arthropods.

Bibliography

Blankenship, M.L. Mite dermatitis other than scabies. *Dermatol Clin* 8(2):265–275, 1990.

Engel, P.M., J. Welzel, M. Maass, U. Schrammi, H.H. Wolff. Tropical rat mite dermatitis: Case report and review. *Clin Infect Dis* 27:1465–1469, 1998.

Flynn, R.J. *Parasites of Laboratory Animals*. Ames: Iowa State University Press; 1973.

McKeevar, P.J., S.K. Allen. Dermatitis associated with *Cheyletiella* infestation in cats. *J Am Vet Med Assoc* 174(7):718–720, 1979.

Miller, W.H. *Cheyletiella* infestation. *In*: Parish, L.C., W.B. Nutting, R.M. Schwartzman, eds. *Cutaneous Infestations of Man and Animal*. New York: Praeger; 1983.

Paradis, M. Mite dermatitis caused by *Cheyletiella blakei*. *J Am Acad Dermatol* 38(6 Pt 1):1014–1015, 1998.

Pecheur, M., H. Wissocq. Un cas de gale due à *Cheyletiella parasitovorax* chez un chat. *Ann Med Vet* 125:191–192, 1981.

MYIASES

ICD-10 B87 Myiasis

Myiases are conditions caused by the infestation of animal tissues or open cavities by dipteran larvae. The flies that produce myiases are classified as: a) obligate or specific parasites, when the larvae require a host in order to develop; b) facultative or semispecific parasites, when the larvae normally develop in dead tissue (human or animal remains) or decomposing animal or vegetal matter but can also develop in necrotic tissue of live animals (these flies are usually secondary invaders, attracted by fetid odors of purulent or contaminated wounds); and c) accidental parasites, when the larvae normally develop in excrement, decomposing organic matter, or food, and the flies only accidentally invade wounds, the gastrointestinal system, or the urinary tract of live animals or humans. Numerous species of flies can cause myiases, but only the most important ones will be covered in this chapter, namely: *Cochliomyia hominivorax*, *Chrysomya bezziana*, *Cordylobia anthropophaga*, *Dermatobia hominis*, *Cuterebra* spp., *Gasterophilus* spp., *Hypoderma* spp., *Oestrus ovis*, *Rhinoestrus purpureus*, and *Wohlfahrtia* spp. In addition, reference will be made to some of the semispecific and accidental parasites that cause myiases.

1. Myiasis Caused by Larvae of *Cochliomyia hominivorax*

Synonym: Screwworm.

Cochliomyia hominivorax (synonyms *Cochliomyia americana* or *Callitroga americana*), of the family Calliphoridae, is a bluish green fly with three dark bands on its back that measures about 10–15 mm in length. It is found almost exclusively in the Americas. In 1988, a focus of myiasis appeared in Libya, but the fly was eliminated in May 1991 thanks to an eradication program based on an approach similar to the sterile insect technique used in the US (Barriga, 1997). *C. macellaria*, a species which is morphologically very similar, is not a parasite. Differentiation of these two species used to be a problem, but now they can be distinguished rapidly using low-cost molecular biology techniques (Taylor *et al.*, 1996).

The larva of this fly (screwworm) is an obligate parasite that can invade the tissues of any warm-blooded animal. It is one of the main agents of myiasis over an area ranging from the southern US to northern Argentina. This species and *Dermatobia hominis* appear to be the principal obligate agents of myiases in Latin America. *C. hominivorax* causes the largest number and most serious cases of human myiases in the Americas. Animal myiases cause heavy economic losses in terms of cattle, sheep, goats, and equines. Prior to an eradication campaign in southern and southeastern US, annual losses in that country due to animal myiases were estimated at between US$ 50 million and US$ 100 million.

The females of *C. hominivorax* mate only once, and they deposit packets of 12 to 400 eggs, overlapped like roof tiles, on the skin of the host. A single female can produce up to 4,000 eggs. The larvae emerge after 11 to 21 hours, penetrate any preexisting wound, and begin to feed on the surrounding tissue. Between four and eight days later, they fall to the ground, bury themselves about 2 cm deep, and turn into pupae. The adult flies emerge a little less than a week afterwards if the weather is warm and humid, or longer if the climate is cooler. The flies mate within three or four days, and in a few more days, the females begin to lay eggs. In summer the entire development cycle can be completed in just over three weeks, so that several generations of flies can be born in a single season. Adult flies live for about two weeks and feed on plant juices. Females can travel about 50 km from their birthplace under their own power, and they are also carried considerable distances by automobiles on which they alight. These facts suggest that eradication programs based on the sterile insect technique need to cover extensive areas in order to achieve a lasting effect.

In the temperate zones, myiases occur in the hot season, from the end of spring to the beginning of autumn, whereas in the tropical zones, they occur all year long and are more frequent in summer (Amarante *et al.*, 1992). The larvae, which are screw-shaped and measure about 12 mm in length, destroy the tissue in which they lodge and become covered by exudate from the wound. The profuse reddish brown exudate from the wound stains the skin, fur, or wool, and attracts other flies of both the same and other species, which deposit more eggs or larvae. The larvae of *C. hominivorax* can invade and produce myiases in all types of accidental wounds regardless of their size, surgical incisions (from castration, dehorning, docking, or other procedures), shearing cuts, umbilical wounds, and even skin abrasions and tick bites. It has been demonstrated that the larvae can penetrate the intact skin of rabbits and guinea pigs. Secondary bacterial infections are common in wounds invaded by the larvae of *C. hominivorax* and aggravate the clinical picture, both by their own action and by the attraction of other flies that are semispecific parasites, which in turn deposit eggs and larvae in the lesion. Larval invasions are not limited to tegumentary wounds; they can also occur in open cavities of the body such as the nostrils, mouth, eye socket, outer ear, and vagina.

The clinical manifestations are severe pain in the affected region and intense pruritus obliging the animal or person to scratch. If the animals are not treated, continuous tissue destruction produces pain and restlessness, which interferes with grazing and leads to weight loss. Sometimes prostration and death ensue, and when the flies are very abundant, the fatality rate can be as high as 20%. The most serious clinical pictures are usually seen in sheep, goats, and equines, which often develop secondary infections.

Human myiases occur in rural populations, especially in areas and at the times when there is an abundance of *C. hominivorax*, which depend mainly on domestic animal hosts in order to reproduce. When myiases are abundant in animals, many cases can occur in man. Human myiasis is clinically similar to that of animals. In addition to the invasion of wounds and ulcers (varicose ulcers of the legs), myiasis also occurs in a furuncular form characterized by a nonmigratory cutaneous nodule. Most of the myiases seen in natural cavities are also due to the larvae of *C. hominivorax*. Invasion of the nasal fossae (rhinomyiasis) is most frequent, and it usually occurs as a complication of ozena. The larvae of *C. hominivorax* often destroy the cartilage and palatine vault, and they can penetrate the nasal sinuses and even the cranial cavity. The ocular form can destroy the eye (Chodosh and Clarridge, 1992).

To prevent this myiasis, care should be taken to keep domestic animals from giving birth during the season when the flies are abundant. The navel of animals born during the hot season should be treated with fly repellents. In addition, castrations, dehorning, docking, branding, and other interventions that leave tegumentary lesions should be avoided during this season. All accidental wounds, whether affected by myiasis or not, should be cleaned and properly treated as soon as possible and covered with an effective repellent or insecticide.

Regional eradication programs based on the sterile insect technique have yielded good results. The technique consists of releasing large numbers of artificially bred males sterilized with gamma rays, which are intended to compete with fertile males in the natural population and mate with the females. Since the females mate only once, they do not become fertilized if they copulate with the sterile males. The first pilot program was initiated in Curacao in 1954 and was successful in eradicating the infestation. The island remained free of the fly until 1975, but then, in the first nine months of that year, there were 261 cases of myiasis, including 14 in humans. The animals most affected were dogs, with 179 cases. The southeastern US was freed of *C. hominivorax* in 1959, as were Puerto Rico and the Virgin Islands in 1974. On the other hand, despite application of this measure, the southwestern US continued to remain infested, especially because of the steady introduction of fertile males from the Mexican side of the border. For this reason, a joint initiative was undertaken with Mexico in 1972 to establish a barrier of sterile males across the isthmus of Tehuantepec. This program has led to eradication of the screwworm in the US and Mexico, and it is expected to extend its impact southward. In 1991, *C. hominivorax* was declared eradicated in Mexico, and campaigns were intensified or initiated in Central America. In 1988, the technique proved to be effective in Africa, when the fly that had appeared in Libya was eradicated (Krafsur and Lindquist, 1996).

The sterile insect campaign is not a universal panacea, and it is very expensive: for example, in the US-Mexico border campaign, some 200 million sterile males were released each week. The campaign must be kept up continuously to prevent the introduction of fertile males or the reproduction of residual local males; otherwise, the epizootic often reappears. The technique only works with species that can be bred in the laboratory in massive numbers and are still able to mate despite sterilization, and it is only effective when the density of fertile males is low (Reichard, 1999). For this reason, an additional measure has been introduced whereby insecticide-saturated bait is distributed to reduce the natural population of *C. hominivorax* before releasing the sterile males.

2. Myiasis Caused by Larvae of *Chrysomya bezziana*

The fly *Chrysomya bezziana* is a species similar to *C. hominivorax* and produces similar lesions. It is found in the tropical regions of Africa, Asia (India, Indonesia, Philippines, Taiwan), the Pacific islands, and Papua New Guinea. Moreover, climatic simulation studies indicate that it could possibly spread to Australia and the Americas (Sutherst *et al.*, 1989). The animals most often attacked are cattle, but it also infests sheep, goats, buffalo, equines, swine, and dogs. The human myiasis is more frequent in India and other parts of Asia than in Africa. Like *C. hominivorax,* this fly deposits its eggs near wounds, ulcers, and natural openings (genitals, nose, labial commissure, eyes). The lesions produced on the face can be deforming, and they are fetid and frequently subject to secondary infections. Invasion of the eye is uncommon, but when it occurs, it can destroy the eyeball in two days (Sachdev *et al.*, 1990).

3. Furuncular Myiasis Caused by Larvae of *Cordylobia anthropophaga*

Cordylobia anthropophaga ("tumbu fly" or "mango fly") is another fly belonging to the family Calliphoridae. It is found in sub-Saharan Africa, and a few human cases were reported in Saudi Arabia which were believed to have been autochthonous (Omar and Abdalla, 1992). Imported cases have been seen in persons and dogs from Europe and the US who visited Africa (Jelinek *et al.*, 1995). The larvae mature in about one week and abandon the host in order to pupate for three to four weeks and give birth to the adult fly. The dog is the domestic animal most affected, but this fly can infest many other domestic and wild species. *Cordylobia rodhaini*, a species of African fly that attacks man less often, produces more intense and more severe infestations. A case was reported in which 150 *C. rodhaini* larvae were recovered from a single individual. Its main hosts are the antelope and the giant rat (Soulsby, 1982).

4. Furuncular Myiasis Caused by Larvae of *Dermatobia hominis*

Synonyms: Torsalo (Central America), moyocuil (Mexico), berne (Brazil), mucha (Colombia), mirunta (Peru), ura (Argentina, Paraguay, and Uruguay).

Dermatobia hominis is a large fly, about 12–18 mm long, which belongs to the family Cuterebridae. It has an opaque, dark blue, hairy thorax that contrasts with its bright blue abdomen. *D. hominis* is widely distributed in tropical America, from Mexico to Paraguay and northeastern Argentina. Several dozen imported cases have been described in Canada and the US (Sampson *et al.*, 2001). It attacks a wide variety of mammals, both domestic and wild, as well as several avian species, and causes heavy economic losses, especially in the case of cattle.

The fly lives in moist forest and underbrush. Its life cycle begins when the female lays its eggs on the abdomen of a hematophagous insect (any of some 50 zoophilic species), which it captures in flight. This nonparasitic transport relationship is known as phoresy. From 15 to 20 eggs are deposited in this manner, and the incubation period lasts 7 to 10 days. When the insect transporting the incubated eggs comes into contact with an animal, the larvae hatch, penetrate its skin (often via the lesion created by the bite of the carrier insect, but they can also penetrate healthy skin), and a few minutes later reach subcutaneous tissue, where they produce a furuncular lesion with an orifice on the top through which to breathe. This outlet to the exterior facilitates the development of secondary infections. The larvae do not migrate; they live in the animal for a period of 4 to 18 weeks, at the end of which they abandon their furuncles early in the morning and fall to the ground in order to pupate. The pupae remain in the ground for 28 to 77 days before developing into adult flies. They mate 24 hours after emerging, and the female lives only 1 to 9 days, during which it does not eat because it has only a vestigial mouth. As a rule, each lesion contains a single larva, but there may be several furuncles, depending on the number of larvae deposited. In cattle, the preferred sites are the forequarters and the back. In man, the lesions are found most often on exposed parts of the body, such as the scalp, legs, arms, hands, face, and neck. Besides causing myiasis in the skin, the larvae of *D. hominis* can invade the eyelids, eye sockets, and mouth. Such cavity myiases are seen primarily in children.

Cattle and dogs can be afflicted by large numbers of parasitic furuncles. Often, these nodules are invaded by the larvae of other flies or bacteria, giving rise to abscesses. The hides of heavily parasitized animals lose much of their value. It has been estimated that Brazil loses about US$ 200 million a year from lowered meat, milk, and hide production as a result of this myiasis.

In man, pain in the affected areas is intermittent; it is especially intense in furuncular myiasis of the scalp. In some regions, human myiases caused by *D. hominis* can be quite common. In Brazil, for example, 41.3% of 363 people living on a eucalyptus plantation had parasitic nodules. In Venezuela, 104 cases of myiasis caused by this fly have been described. In Panama, several palpebral cases were reported, as well as one cerebral case in which larvae on the scalp penetrated through the fontanelle of a child. The number of larvae invading a given person is variable.

The primary objective of a control program should be to prevent myiases in domestic animals by applying insecticides or repellents. In the event of an infestation, care should be taken to keep the larvae from falling to the ground, where they can then transform into pupae. Larvae on animals can be destroyed by systemic insecticides. However, since the flies cover a large range of territory, a control program needs to cover an extensive area in order to be effective. The success of a program also entails the collaboration of cattlemen and control of animal movement. Use of the sterile insect technique to control and eradicate the fly has been tested in large-scale breeding studies, but this approach has a disadvantage in the case of *Dermatobia* because, unlike *C. hominivorax*, the female mates several times in the course of her life.

5. Furuncular Myiasis Caused by the Larvae of *Cuterebra* spp.

Flies of the genus *Cuterebra* resemble bees and measure 20 mm or longer. Their larvae are obligate parasites of rodents and lagomorphs in North America.

The adult females deposit eggs on vegetation in the habitat of their hosts. The larvae are born at intervals, invade the host via natural cavities or penetrate intact skin, and apparently travel extensively throughout the body. They finally appear as third-stage larvae under the skin, where they form subcutaneous furunculoid nodules. Approximately one month after the initial infestation, these nodules rupture, and the larvae fall to the ground and begin to pupate.

The larvae of *Cuterebra* spp. cause subcutaneous cysts in rodents and lagomorphs. *C. emasculator* often parasitizes the scrotum of mice and chipmunks, destroying their testicles. In addition to their natural hosts, the larvae of *Cuterebra* spp. occasionally invade humans, cats, dogs, and domestic rabbits. In cats, the larvae may be found in subcutaneous pruriginous lesions, frequently in the nape of the neck or the submandibular region. In addition, there have been serious or fatal cases in which the parasite was found in the eyeball or surrounding tissue, trachea, or central nervous system of cats (Glass *et al.*, 1998).

In 1989, Baird *et al.* (1989) reviewed 54 human cases in the US, plus an additional 8 cases that had been reported as of mid-2001. Most of these cases involved second- or third-stage larvae that had formed furuncular lesions in the neck, chest, or back, and they occurred at the end of summer or in early autumn. It is unusual to recover first-stage larvae; when this happens, the parasite is found in the vitreous humor or the upper respiratory tract, and the lesions appear at the end of spring or in early summer. The same pattern has been reported in cats. The times of the year when the first-, second-, and third-stage larvae of *Cuterebra* appear would suggest that the parasite migrates through the lungs and the head before maturing in subcutaneous tissue.

6. Furuncular Myiasis Caused by Larvae of *Hypoderma* spp.

This myiasis is caused by the larvae of two fly species, *Hypoderma lineatum* and *H. bovis*, which belong to the family Oestridae. Both are parasites of cattle and are found in the Northern Hemisphere (Canada, the US, Europe, and certain parts of Asia and northern Africa). Parasitized cattle have occasionally been introduced in Australia, South Africa, and several South American countries, but the species did not become permanently established.

The flies resemble bees. In cattle, they lay their eggs on hairs on the lower part of the body, preferentially the feet. *H. lineatum* deposits a row of eggs, and *H. bovis* lays isolated eggs. The larvae are born after two to six days and invade the subcutaneous connective tissue, from which they migrate to the rest of the body. The first-stage larvae of *H. bovis* migrate along the nerves and settle in the epidural fat of the spinal canal. The larvae of *H. lineatum* settle in the submucosa of the esophagus. In both cases, the larvae remain for a while in their respective sites, and then in winter (January and February), they finally migrate to the subcutaneous tissue of the dorsolumbar region, where they arrive as second-stage larvae and mature into third-stage larvae within 10 to 11 weeks. During this time, they form cysts about 3 cm in diameter, with a pore through which to breathe. The larvae spend about 10 months of their 11- to 12-month development cycle inside the animal's body. In their final stage, the larvae emerge through the hole in the cyst, fall to the ground, and pupate. The pupal stage lasts from one to three months, depending on climatic conditions. Once the adult flies emerge, they mate very quickly and begin to lay eggs. The adult flies live only eight days at most.

The animals most affected are calves. Adult animals suffer less, since some resistance is acquired with age. The number of furuncles on a given animal can range from one to hundreds. Secondary infection usually leads to the formation of abscesses. The migration of *H. bovis* larvae in the epidural fat along the spinal canal can produce inflammation and necrosis of the adipose tissue of the periosteum, as well as neurologic alterations. The larvae of *H. lineatum*, in turn, can produce inflammation of the tissue underlying the esophageal mucosa and stenosis of the esophageal tract. An abundance of adult flies causes restlessness in cattle and can provoke stampedes and interfere with their feeding. In some regions, the larvae of *Hypoderma* take a heavy economic toll. Annual losses attributable to this myiasis in cattle have been estimated at US\$ 35 million in France, US\$ 192 million in the US (in 1956), and UK£ 13 million in Great Britain (Soulsby, 1982). These losses are due to delayed growth, lowered milk and meat production, and damage to the hides.

Man is an accidental and aberrant host of the larvae of *H. bovis*, *H. lineatum*, and, less often, *H. diana* (whose larvae parasitize European deer). Development of the parasite in humans is usually arrested in the first larval stage and rarely reaches the third, or mature, stage. A serologic study of more than 100 cases in France led to the conclusion that the species that most frequently affects man is *H. bovis* (Doby and Deunff, 1982). The myiasis it causes is subcutaneous and only occasionally conjunctival or palpebral-conjunctival. Endophthalmias are rare. The cutaneous forms can be manifested as a serpiginous myiasis, similar to cutaneous larva migrans, or as a subcutaneous myiasis with moving furuncles that appear and disappear. The parasitosis can cause pruritus, restlessness, pain, and stomach upset. Children are affected more frequently than adults. The cutaneous myiasis associated with *Hypoderma* spp. would appear to be less common in humans than those caused by other species; Jelinek *et al.* (1995) found only 1 case in a series of 13 myiases reviewed. Authors have described several cases of eosinophilic syndrome with fever and muscle pain, as well as respiratory, muscular, cardiac, dermal, or neurologic symptoms, in patients who turned out to have myiasis caused by *H. lineatum*. In several of these cases, the diagnosis was made when furuncular lesions appeared, usually in the scalp, and the symptoms disappeared spontaneously after they were excised (Navajar *et al.*, 1998; Starr *et al.*, 2000). In addition, two cases of cerebral *H. bovis* invasion were observed in human patients (Kalelioglu *et al.*, 1989). It is possible that the human parasitosis is more common than has been believed in the past, but that it goes unnoticed.

The use of insecticides or repellents in animals at risk can be successful if they are applied at the appropriate time of year, since the season for adult infestation is relatively brief. Most of the development of *Hypoderma* takes place inside the animal (10 months to a year), and hence the larval phase is a good point at which to attack the fly. Control consists of treating cattle with larvicides at the beginning of autumn to prevent the larvae from completing their development cycle and becoming established under the skin. Treatment at this point interrupts the life cycle of the fly and at the same time avoids damage to the hide. To prevent neurological damage to the animals, the larvicide should not be applied in late autumn, when *H. bovis* larvae have reached the spinal canal. In animals being raised for food, the application of insecticides should take into account the time lapse required between administration of the insecticide and use of the meat or milk. Also, delayed treatment can be given in the spring when the subcutaneous larvae are first noticed; in this case, topical insecticides are used, reaching the larvae through the furuncular orifices.

Several European countries—Cyprus, Denmark, Germany (Bavaria), the Netherlands, and Sweden—have succeeded in eradicating the infestation. Promising results have also been obtained in Ireland, where the infestation rate has been reduced to very low levels.

7. Myiasis Caused by Larvae of *Oestrus ovis* and *Rhinoestrus purpureus*

The adult fly of *Oestrus ovis* is gray and measures 10–12 mm in length. It is larviparous and deposits its larvae in the nostrils of sheep, goats, and, occasionally, man. Its distribution is worldwide, and it is found wherever sheep are raised. *Rhinoestrus purpureus* is similar to *O. ovis* in its morphology and development cycle. The larval forms are obligate parasites of equines—in whose nostrils and larynx they develop—found in Africa, Asia, and Europe.

The first-stage larvae enter the nasal fossae, where they feed on mucus and desquamated cells, and they then move on to the frontal or maxillary sinuses, where they mature. After 2 to 10 months, the mature larvae return to the nasal fossae, where they are expelled by sneezing, fall to the ground, and pupate for four to five weeks. The fly that emerges from the pupa lives for 2 to 28 days. The adult flies are annoying to the animals, and when they are very abundant, they cause the animals to become restless. The larvae cause chronic rhinitis and sinusitis. The morbidity rate in a flock may be very high, but mortality is nil. The most prominent symptom is a mucopurulent nasal discharge. Breathing is sometimes difficult because of swelling of the nasal mucosae. The pathology of this condition has been attributed to the mechanical effect of the size of the larvae and the irritation caused by their spines on the mucosae of the nose, pharynx, and sinuses. Some findings indicate that hypersensitivity, probably IgE-mediated, plays an important role. The examination of human cases, however, has not demonstrated the presence of hypersensitivity in man (Dorchies, 1997).

Human cases of myiasis caused by *O. ovis* have been described in several countries of the world, including Chile, Ecuador, Uruguay, and the US. The parasitosis occurs most often in sheep herders and is also seen in urban dwellers who keep sheep in residential areas (Dar *et al.,* 1980). Man is an accidental and aberrant host, but apparently not an uncommon one. The form for which people most often seek treatment is invasion of the conjunctiva, evidenced by lacrimation and the sensation of a foreign body in the eye. Of 112 sheep herders interviewed in Italy, 80% stated that they had had the infestation at some time, and 54% reported that more than one site had been infected at the same time. The sites where larvae were found most frequently were the larynx (77 times), the conjunctiva (56 times), and the nasal fossae (32 times). They were also found in the ears (1 time). The most common sign was pain, sometimes accompanied by fever and general malaise (Pampiglione *et al.,* 1997). In Benghazi, Libya, 80 cases of external ocular myiasis were diagnosed over a two-year period, representing an estimated incidence of 10 per 100,000 population (Dar *et al.,* 1980). In a case in Thailand, eight larvae were recovered from the palpebral conjunctiva (Nacapunchai *et al.,* 1998). Human oestriasis is usually a benign condition that lasts only a few days because the larvae cannot develop beyond the first stage in man. Serious cases, with destruction of the eye and perforation of the orbital walls, are rare. In Africa, cases of oral and nasal myiases have been described in which the larvae have entered the nasal fossae and frontal sinuses, causing localized pain, frontal cephalalgia, and insomnia over a period of 3 to 10 days. There have also been reports of invasion of the outer ear (otomyiasis). *R. purpureus* appears to be an uncommon parasite, having been described only once in burros (Zayed, 1992) and once in man (Rastegaev, 1980).

Treatment with modern systemic insecticides is effective against all the larval phases, and, if it is applied annually, it can greatly reduce the populations of these flies at livestock-raising establishments.

8. Myiasis Caused by Larvae of *Gasterophilus* spp.

The three most important species of this genus are *Gasterophilus intestinalis*, *G. nasalis*, and *G. haemorrhoidalis*, which are widely distributed on all continents. The species *G. inermis*, *G. pecorum*, and *G. nigricornis* are found only in the Old World. The normal hosts of these flies are horses and other equines, in which the larvae lodge in the stomach. Larval infestation rates are high in equines in many parts of the world. *G. intestinalis*, which is the most common, deposits its eggs primarily on the lower part of the animals' forelegs; *G. nasalis*, on the submaxillary region; and *G. haemorrhoidalis*, on the lip hairs. The first-stage larvae hatch in two to seven days and are carried to the mouth when the animal licks itself, or they can travel there on their own. From there they invade the oral or lingual mucosa, where they develop for three to four weeks until they become second-stage larvae. They are then swallowed, travel to the lumen, and attach themselves to the mucosa of the stomach, where they remain for 8 to 10 months. It has been estimated that fewer than 1% of the larvae lodge in the glandular portion of the stomach. Finally, when they mature, these larvae are shed in the animal's feces, pupate in the ground for about one month, and give rise to adult flies, which reinitiate the cycle. The adult flies live for only a few days, but since the flies do not all emerge from the pupal stage at the same time, populations of *Gasterophilus* spp. can be present from mid-spring until mid-summer.

Little is known about the effect of stomach infestation by *Gasterophilus* larvae on the health of equines. According to some observations, it can cause anorexia and mild colic. Ulceration of the nonglandular portion of the stomach was the most frequent lesion. Abscesses, rupture of the stomach, and peritonitis can occasionally occur (Soulsby, 1982).

Adult flies frighten and disturb the animals.

Human infestation is apparently rare; only a single case was reported during the period from 1989 to 2001 (Royce *et al.*, 1999). The larvae rarely develop beyond the first stage, and only exceptionally do they reach the stomach. The common clinical form is a dermal affliction similar to cutaneous larva migrans, with superficial serpiginous tunnels within the tegument that look like red stripes on the surface of the skin. The lesion is characterized by intense itching. The species that most often attacks man is *G. intestinalis*, and the lesions are almost always located on the extremities. The persons most affected are those who are in close contact with equines.

Since the larvae remain for a long time in the horse's stomach, this stage poses a good point of attack for interrupting the life cycle and reducing the population of *Gasterophilus* spp., but it is difficult to determine the optimum time to administer treatment. For example, in Kentucky, US, it has been found that the second-stage larvae of *G. intestinalis* continue to arrive in the stomach until April, while the third-stage larvae abandon the host to pupate starting in August. Accordingly, the best time for treatment is May, June, or July (the end of spring and beginning of summer) because two generations can be eliminated at once. However, the third-stage larvae of *G. nasalis* become detached between March and August, while the new second-stage larvae reach the stomach in July. In this case, the treatment needs to be applied in February (winter) to eliminate the previous generation and in August (summer) to eliminate the new generation.

9. Furuncular Myiasis Caused by Larvae of *Wohlfahrtia* spp.

Specific myiases are also caused by the larvae of *Wohlfahrtia vigil* and *W. magnifica*, flies belonging to the family Sarcophagidae. Both species are larviparous.

W. vigil is found in Canada and the US, where its larvae parasitize rodents, lagomorphs, foxes, mink, dogs, and other carnivores, and occasionally man. The adult flies feed on plant nectar. The larvae are deposited in packets, either on the animals or in their vicinity, and they then penetrate intact skin and produce a furuncular lesion. The larvae mature in 7 to 9 days, abandon the animal, and pupate for 10 to 12 days. When the adults emerge 11 to 17 days later, the females lay their eggs, and thus the cycle is completed. *W. vigil* is a pest of mink and fox farms in Canada and northern US. Newborn and young animals are the most vulnerable. In rodents, this fly can cause severe tissue destruction. In humans, the infestation is found only in children who spend time outdoors, in whom it causes small subcutaneous abscesses, irritability, fever, and dehydration.

W. magnifica is found in China, the African and European areas of the Mediterranean, the Middle East, and the Russian Federation. The fly is attracted by skin wounds, where it deposits its larvae, but it also does so in natural orifices of humans, sheep, bovine cattle, and other domestic animals, including fowl (especially geese). The myiasis caused by *W. magnifica* is an important disease of sheep in the southern part of the Russian Federation. Human infestation does not appear to be frequent; during the 1990s, only five cases were reported. The following sites were involved: the eye (one case), vulva (in an elderly woman), orotracheal region (in an elderly intubated man), ear (one case), and scalp (in a child) (Ciftcioglu *et al.*, 1997; Delir *et al.*, 1999; Iori *et al.*, 1999).

Facultative or Semispecific Myiases

A large variety of dipterans can be facultative parasites of animal and human tissue. These flies, which normally lay their eggs or larvae on decomposing meat or animal or human remains, can sometimes invade the necrotic tissue of wounds in live animals. The larvae of these dipterans do not penetrate healthy skin and rarely invade recent wounds that have been kept clean. Their medical importance lies in the fact that the larvae of some species do not always restrict themselves to feeding on necrotic tissue but can occasionally penetrate deeply and damage healthy tissue. One such species is *Lucilia* (*Phaenicia*) *sericata*, whose larvae do not usually cause serious damage but can sometimes destroy healthy tissue surrounding wounds and can also invade the human nasal fossae in large numbers.

Most of the dipterans that cause semispecific myiases in man belong to the families Sarcophagidae (*Sarcophaga* and *Parasarcophaga*) and Calliphoridae (*Lucilia*, *Phormia*, and *Paraphormia*). The larvae of the latter are agents of "calliphorine myiasis" ("blowfly" or "fleece-fly strike" in Australia), which can cause heavy economic losses in sheep in certain areas. The most susceptible breed is the merino, and the highest incidence rates are in Australia, Great Britain, and South Africa. In hot, humid summers, when the population of calliphorine flies is at its peak, this myiasis often affects the development of sheep and causes losses in both wool and meat production. Invasions by the larvae of these flies can also lead to high mortality. In Australia, the most important flies are *Lucilia cuprina*, *L. sericata*, and several species of the genus *Calliphora*, while in Canada and the US, the prominent species are *Phormia regina* and *Protophormia terraenovae*. The most common site of larval invasion is the ano-vulvar or ano-preputial region, where the skin often becomes excoriated from soft feces and urine, the smell of which attracts the flies. Any accidental or surgical wound can be the site of calliphorine myiasis. According to some authors, a lesion is not required in order for invasion to occur; during hot summers with abundant rain followed by sunshine, the matted wool can become rotten and attract swarms of flies. When the density of calliphorine flies is low, their larvae breed in carcasses or garbage containing scraps of meat. The situation changes when climatic conditions favor a rapid increase in the fly population, at which point the larvae also invade contaminated wounds and damp, dirty wool. The development cycle of these flies can be completed in a few weeks, and, under highly favorable conditions, within a single week. As a result, many generations of flies are born in the course of one season. In areas where calliphorine flies are a problem for sheep, all wounds should be treated immediately and the animals should be protected with larvicides or repellents.

According to reports published in different parts of the world between 1989 and 2001, the most common larvae that produce facultative human myiases belong to the genera *Lucilia*, *Sarcophaga*, *Parasarcophaga*, *Phormia*, and *Paraphormia*. *Lucilia* larvae appear to be the most frequent: of 14 human myiases reported over approximately two years in Brisbane, Australia, 10 were caused by *L. cuprina* and 2 by *Parasarcophaga crassipalpis*, while 2 were unidentified (Lukin, 1989). These myiases, because of their nature, affect wounded, bedridden, or otherwise debilitated people who are unable to take care of themselves. There have been a number of reports of nosocomial infestations caused by *L. sericata*: in the former Czechoslovakia, one case in the tumor of a dying 87-year-old woman, and two cases in the mouth and nose of patients with multiple traumas (Daniel *et al.*, 1994); in Korea, one case in the nasopharyngeal tube of a paraplegic patient; in Israel, one case in an extreme premature newborn; and in Spain, one case in the cutaneous orifice of an osteoplastic tibial extension (Mateos *et al.*, 1990). Cases have also been reported in apparently healthy individuals, such as a cattle-rancher in Korea who had five larvae in the auditory canal which did not appear to be bothering him, and an urban case acquired in Spain.

The larvae of *Sarcophaga* also appear to be a frequent cause of facultative human myiases. Two nosocomial infestations were described in Spain: one in a 77-year-old woman with radionecrotic wounds and another in an 87-year-old man with dementia (Merino *et al.*, 2000). One infestation was reported in Japan, with nine larvae in the eye of a debilitated patient. Also, in Spain, one case of vulvar myiasis in an 86-

year-old woman living in a home for the elderly was reported. In India, 64 cases of myiases in the nasal cavity, hands, and toes of leprosy patients were reported, from whom the larvae of *Sarcophaga haemorrhoidalis*, *Chrysomya bezziana*, *Callitroga americana*, and *Musca domestica* were recovered (Husain *et al.*, 1993). Also in India, a case of cutaneous myiasis with *Sarcophaga* sp. and *Chrysomya bezziana* larvae was observed in a drug addict. In Japan, two cases of intestinal myiases caused by *S. peregrina* were reported: one was in an 8-month-old girl with hemorrhagic mucous feces, and the other was asymptomatic. In Morocco, a case of intestinal myiasis caused by *S. haemorrhoidalis* in a 15-year-old girl produced abdominal pain, hematemesis, and vomiting of the larvae (Abkari *et al.*, 1999). In Israel, larvae from the same fly were found in the auditory canal of four children, resulting in pain, pruritus, and secretions. A case of *Parasarcophaga argyrostoma* larvae in the gangrenous toe of an elderly man was described in England, and in Japan, an intestinal myiasis caused by *Parasarcophaga crassipalpis* was reported. *Phormia regina* was identified in a case in Pennsylvania and another in Florida, US.

In ancient times, the larvae of *L. sericata*, *L. illustris*, or *P. regina* were used to get rid of necrotic tissue in wounds. The technique is still being applied successfully using sterilized *L. sericata* larvae with infected wounds that are resistant to antibiotics and difficult to treat with surgery (Fleischman *et al.*, 1999). In forensic medicine, the larvae of *Phormia regina*, *L. sericata*, *Eucalliphora latifrons*, *Lucilia illustris*, *Calliphora vicina*, and other flies found on cadavers help to determine the time elapsed since death. Since the identification of some of these larvae is difficult, polymerase chain reaction techniques have been developed for this purpose (Vincent *et al.*, 2000).

Accidental Myiases

Accidental myiases are caused by numerous species of flies that normally lay their eggs or larvae on decomposing organic matter and accidentally deposit them on the food or wounds of humans or animals, giving rise to intestinal or cutaneous myiases. Most eggs or larvae ingested in this way are destroyed in the digestive tract, but some of them survive and continue their larval development. The larvae of *Musca domestica*, *Fannia canicularis*, *F. scalaris*, and *Muscina stabulans*, as well as several species of Calliphoridae and Sarcophagidae, can produce intestinal myiases.

Often, the ingested larvae are eliminated in feces without causing any damage or symptoms. In other cases, however, there can be abdominal pain and nausea, and, in very intense infestations, damage to the intestinal mucosa and bloody diarrhea. Myiases have been described in the urinary tract (cystomyiasis), but they are rare. In India, Gupta *et al.* (1983) reported that a bedridden hospital patient had developed a case of urethral myiasis (associated with necrosis of part of the glans) from the larvae of a domestic fly. Cases of urogenital myiasis have also been seen in other parts of the world. These infestations have occurred mainly in immobilized elderly patients suffering from incontinence. In rural areas, there have been cases caused by the larvae of *Fannia* spp., which are frequently found in the vicinity of latrines. In some cases of urogenital myiasis, the larvae do not go beyond the first stage—in other words, they cannot feed or develop ("pseudomyiasis"). In other cases, however, second- and third-stage larvae have been found in the bladder. A urinary myiasis caused by *Fannia canicularis* was identified in France. Finally, two cases of cutaneous myiasis caused by *Musca domestica* were described in England, as was a third case, attributed to the same species, in a leprosy patient in India.

Role of Animals in the Epidemiology of the Disease: Animals play an essential role in the epidemiology of the flies that cause obligate myiases; without their animal hosts, the flies could not exist. Man is only an accidental host of these larvae, and in some myiases, such as those caused by *O. ovis* and *Gasterophilus* spp., an aberrant host in which the larvae cannot complete their development. The obligate myiases occur in humans when there is a high incidence of animal myiases, typically in the spring or summer. The victims are usually people who live in rural areas where both the flies and the natural hosts of their larvae are abundant. With the facultative myiases, the role of animals is much less significant—indeed, debatable: it could be argued that most of the flies that produce facultative myiases normally develop in the feces of domestic animals, so that the humans living in the proximity of domestic animals increase their risk of becoming infested with facultative myiases.

Control: Human obligate myiases are controlled by eliminating or reducing infestations in the animal reservoirs. The primary means of achieving this goal is preventive treatment of the animals at risk with insecticides or repellents to keep them from becoming infested, or, once they are infested, curative treatment with insecticides to eliminate the larvae before they abandon the host and begin to pupate. With both animals and humans in areas where myiases are common, any wound should be treated as soon as possible and watched closely until it forms a scar. Particular care should be taken with bedridden patients who have wounds and cannot protect themselves from flies. To prevent the disease in man, both personal and environmental hygiene should be observed, including steps to eliminate the breeding sites of flies.

Bibliography

Abkari, A., Z. Jouhadi, A. Hamdani, N. Mikou, N. Guessous, H.H. Khalifa. La myiase gastro-intestinale. À propos d'une observation marocaine. *Bull Soc Pathol Exot* 92(1):20–22, 1999.

Amarante, A.F., M.A. Barbosa, T.C. Oliveira-Sequeira, S. Fernandes. Epidemiology of sheep myiases in São Paulo State, Brazil. *Trop Anim Health Prod* 24(1):36–39, 1992.

Barriga, O.O. *Veterinary Parasitology for Practitioners*, 2nd ed. Edina: Burgess International Group; 1997.

Baird, J.K., C.R. Baird, C.W. Sabrosky. North American cuterebrid myiasis. Report of seventeen new infections of human beings and review of disease. *J Am Acad Dermatol* 21 (4 Pt 1):763–772, 1989.

Chodosh, J., J. Clarridge. Ophthalmomyiasis: A review with special reference to *Cochliomyia hominivorax*. *Clin Infect Dis* 14(2):444–449, 1992.

Ciftcioglu, N., K. Altintas, M. Haberal. A case of human orotracheal myiasis caused by *Wohlfahrtia magnifica*. *Parasitol Res* 83(1):34–36, 1997.

Daniel, M., H. Sramova, E. Zalabska. *Lucilia sericata* (Diptera: Calliphoridae) causing hospital-acquired myiasis of a traumatic wound. *J Hosp Infect* 28(2):149–152, 1994.

Dar, M.S., M.B. Amer, F.K. Dar, V. Papazotos. Ophthalmomyiasis caused by sheep nasal bot, *Oestrus ovis* (Oestridae) larvae, in Benghazi area of eastern Libya. *Trans R Soc Trop Med Hyg* 74(3):303–306, 1980.

Delir, S., F. Handjani, M. Emad, S. Ardehali. Vulvar myiasis due to *Wohlfahrtia magnifica*. *Clin Exp Dermatol* 24(4):279–280, 1999.

Doby, J.M., J. Deunff. Considérations sur la fréquence respective des espèces d'hypodermes (Insecta Diptera Oestroidea) à l'origine des cas humains d'hypodermose en France. *Ann Parasitol Hum Comp* 57(5):497–505, 1982.

Dorchies, P. Physiopathologie comparée de la myiase à *Oestrus ovis* (Linne 1761) chez l'homme et chez les animaux. *Bull Acad Natl Med* 181:673–683, 1997.

Fleischmann, W., M. Russ, D. Moch, C. Marquardt. Biochirurgie-Sind Fliegenmaden wirklich die besseren Chirurgen? *Chirurg* 70(11):1340–1346, 1999.

Glass, E.N., A.M. Cornetta, A. deLahunta, S.A. Center, M. Kent. Clinical and clinicopathologic features in 11 cats with *Cuterebra larvae* myiasis of the central nervous system. *J Vet Intern Med* 12(5):365–368, 1998.

Gupta, S.C., S. Kumar, A. Srivastava. Urethral myasis. *Trop Geogr Med* 35:73–74, 1983.

Husain, A., S. Husain, G.N. Malaviya, R.R. Bahadur. Myiasis in leprosy. *Acta Leprol* 8(3):137–141, 1993.

Iori, A., B. Zechini, L. Cordier, E. Luongo, G. Pontuale, S. Persichino. A case of myiasis in man due to *Wohlfahrtia magnifica* (Schiner) recorded near Rome. *Parassitologia* 41(4):583–585, 1999.

Jelinek, T., H.D. Nothdurft, N. Rieder, T. Loscher. Cutaneous myiasis: Review of 13 cases in travelers returning from tropical countries. *Int J Dermatol* 34(9):624–626, 1995.

Kalelioglu, M., G. Akturk, F. Akturk, *et al*. Intracerebral myiasis from *Hypoderma bovis* larva in a child. Case report. *J Neurosurg* 71(6):929–931, 1989.

Krafsur, E.S., D.A. Lindquist. Did the sterile insect technique or weather eradicate screwworms (Diptera: Calliphoridae) from Libya? *J Med Entomol* 33(6):877–887, 1996.

Lukin, L.G. Human cutaneous myiasis in Brisbane: A prospective study. *Med J Aust* 150(5):237–240, 1989.

Mateos, M., A. León, P. González Herranz, J. Burgos, J.A. López Mondejar, F. Baquero. Infestación por *Lucilia sericata* de los orificios cutáneos de osteotaxo en alargamiento de tibias: a propósito de un caso. *Enferm Infecc Microbiol Clin* 8(6):365–367, 1990.

Merino, F.J., A. Campos, T. Nebreda, C. Canovas, F. Cuezva. Miasis cutánea por *Sarcophaga* sp. *Enferm Infecc Microbiol Clin* 18(1):19–21, 2000.

Nacapunchai, D., C. Lamon, N. Sukprasert. A first record from Thailand of human external ophthalmomyiasis due to *Oestrus ovis*. *Southeast Asian J Trop Med Public Health* 29(1):133–136, 1998.

Navajas, A., I. Cardenal, M.A. Pinan, A. Ortiz, I. Astigarraga, A. Fdez-Teijeiro. Hypereosinophilia due to myiasis. *Acta Haematol* 99(1):27–30, 1998.

Omar, M.S., R.E. Abdalla. Cutaneous myiasis caused by tumbu fly larvae, *Cordylobia anthropophaga* in southwestern Saudi Arabia. *Trop Med Parasitol* 43(2):128–129, 1992.

Pampiglione, S., S. Giannetto, A. Virga. Persistence of human myiasis by *Oestrus ovis* L. (Diptera: Oestridae) among shepherds of the Etnean area (Sicily) for over 150 years. *Parassitologia* 39(4):415–418, 1997.

Powers, N.R., M.L. Yorgensen, P.D. Rumm, W. Souffront. Myiasis in humans: An overview and a report of two cases in the Republic of Panama. *Mil Med* 161(8):495–497, 1996.

Rastegaev, IuM. [Myiasis in man caused by larvae of the horse botfly, *Rhinoestrus purpureus* Br.]. *Med Parazitol (Mosk)* 49(5):86–88, 1980.

Reichard, R. Case studies of emergency management of screwworm. *Rev Sci Tech* 18:145–163, 1999.

Reunala, T., L.J. Laine, O. Saksela, T. Pitkanen, K. Lounatmaa. Furuncular myiasis. *Acta Derm Venereol* 70(2):167–170, 1990.

Rodríguez Diego, J.G., T. Blandino, M. Alonso, E. Mendoza, G. Seoane, N. Fregel.

[Presence in Cuba of screw worms (*Cochliomyia hominivorax*) in the livestock]. *Rev Elev Med Vet Pay Trop* 49:223–225, 1996.

Royce, L.A., P.A. Rossignol, M.L. Kubitz, F.R. Burton. Recovery of a second instar *Gasterophilus larva* in a human infant: A case report. *Am J Trop Med Hyg* 60(3):403–404, 1999.

Sachdev, M.S., H. Kumar, S. Roop, A.K. Jain, R. Arora, V.K. Dada. Destructive ocular myiasis in a noncompromised host. *Indian J Ophthalmol* 38(4):184–186, 1990.

Sampson, C.E., J. MaGuire, E. Eriksson. Botfly myiasis: Case report and brief review. *Ann Plast Surg* 46(2):150–152, 2001.

Soulsby, E.J.L. *Helminths, Arthropods and Protozoa of Domesticated Animals*, 7th ed. Philadelphia: Lea & Febiger; 1982.

Starr, J., J.H. Pruett, J.W. Yunginger, G.J. Gleich. Myiasis due to *Hypoderma lineatum* infection mimicking the hypereosinophilic syndrome. *Mayo Clin Proc* 75(7):755–759, 2000.

Sutherst, R.W., J.P. Spradbery, G.F. Maywald. The potential geographical distribution of the Old World screw-worm fly, *Chrysomya bezziana*. *Med Vet Entomol* 3(3):273–280, 1989.

Taylor, D.B., A.L. Szalanski, R.D. Peterson II. Identification of screwworm species by polymerase chain reaction-restriction fragment length polymorphism. *Med Vet Entomol* 10(1):63–70, 1996.

Ugwu, B.T., P.O. Nwadiaro. *Cordylobia anthropophaga* mastitis mimicking breast cancer: Case report. *East Afr Med J* 76(2):115–116, 1999.

Vincent, S., J.M. Vian, M.P. Carlotti. Partial sequencing of the cytochrome oxydase b subunit gene I: A tool for the identification of European species of blow flies for postmortem interval estimation. *J Forensic Sci* 45(4):820–823, 2000.

Zayed, A.A. Studies on *Rhinoestrus purpureus* (Diptera: Oestridae) larvae infesting donkeys (*Equus asinus*) in Egypt. III. Pupal duration under controlled conditions. *Vet Parasitol* 44(3–4):285–290, 1992.

PENTASTOMIASES

ICD-10 B88.8 Other specified infestations

Synonyms: Tongue worm infection, porocephalosis, porocephaliasis.

Etiology: There are two genera of pentastomids that are of medical interest: *Linguatula* and *Armillifer*, both of the family Porocephalidae. On rare occasions, *Porocephalus* (a snake parasite, with rodents as intermediate hosts), *Leiperia* (a crocodile parasite, with fish as intermediate hosts), and *Raillietiella* (a lizard parasite, with cockroaches as intermediate hosts) have been mentioned as human parasites.

Owing to the morphological and biological peculiarities of the pentastomids, their taxonomy and phylogenetic status are not yet well defined. On the basis of ultrastructural, embryologic, and genetic studies, they can be considered a class related to the arthropods (Self, 1982). Interestingly, almost all the adult parasites infest a host higher on the phylogenetic scale than the hosts of the larval forms, which suggests that the parasite evolved along with the host. The fact that the reverse is true in the case of certain pentastomids is difficult to explain, however.

In their adult stage, pentastomids are commonly parasites of the respiratory system of reptiles or carnivores, and in their larval stages, of herbivores. However, although their specific hosts seem to be limited, infections have been found in many animals. Except for a few epidemiological studies, human infection by pentastomids is infrequent: only eight cases had been reported in the United States up to 1991 (Guardia *et al.*, 1991), and nine cases had been reported worldwide from 1989 to mid-2001.

1. Infection due to *Linguatula serrata*

Synonyms: Linguatuliasis, linguatulosis.

Etiology: *Linguatula serrata* is a linguiform parasite with discreet transverse segmentation. The adult female measures about 10 cm long, and the male barely 2 cm. In its adult form, *L. serrata* lodges in the nasal passages, frontal sinuses, and tympanic cavity of dogs, other canids, and felids, where it ingests mucus and blood. Few cases of adult specimens have been found in man.

The development cycle of the parasite requires herbivorous intermediate hosts, mainly sheep, goats, and lagomorphs. Bovines, deer, equines, swine, and various other mammals can also serve as intermediate hosts. Man is an accidental and aberrant intermediate host. *Linguatula* lays its eggs in the upper respiratory passages of the host, and they are then expelled into the environment by sneezing or splitting, or if swallowed, with the feces. The eggs ingested by the intermediate host with food or water release the first-stage larvae in the intestine; they possess four clawed feet and an apparatus that enables them to perforate the intestinal wall. The larvae migrate through the blood to the internal organs and encyst in the lymph glands, the liver, spleen, lungs, and other organs, where they form small pentastomid nodules that are discovered during the veterinary inspection of meat. Between 250 and 300 days after infection and after some 12 molts within the cyst, the larva reaches the nymph, or infective stage. It is about 5 mm and resembles the adult parasite. The nymph can break the cystic envelope, migrate through the peritoneal cavity, and penetrate different tissues. If a carnivore consumes the tissues or organs of an infected intermediate host, the infective nymph migrates through the stomach and esophagus to the nasopharynx, where after several molts it reaches maturity and begins oviposition.

Geographic Distribution and Occurrence: *L. serrata* is widely distributed throughout the world, but human infection is infrequent. Most cases have been reported in several countries of North Africa, Europe, and the Middle East. In the Americas, human linguatuliasis has been diagnosed in Brazil, Canada, Chile, Colombia, Cuba, Panama, and the US. From 1989 to mid-2001, only one ocular case, in Ecuador, was reported worldwide (Lazo *et al.*, 1999).

The infection rate in dogs is very high in some areas. *L. serrata* was found in 43.3% of stray dogs in Beirut, Lebanon, in 38% in parts of India, and in a high percentage in Mexico City. The highest rates are seen in areas where dogs are fed raw viscera from sheep and goats. Infected dogs have been found in the Midwest and in Georgia, US, but the prevalence rate obtained by coprologic examination was very low (Ehrenford and Newberne, 1981). Data on the frequency of nymphal infection in domestic herbivores are not available. In Lebanon, 4 of 10 goat livers acquired in randomly selected butcher shops had larvae in the hepatic lymph nodes, and 2 of 10 sheep livers were parasitized. In the US, the principal intermediate hosts seem to be wild rabbits, which have been found infected in several southern and southeastern states (Gardner *et al.*, 1984). A study conducted in eight southeastern states found that 2% of 260 *Sylvilagus floridanus* rabbits had nymphs of *L. serrata*, but the infections were mild (Andrews and Davidson, 1980).

The Disease in Man: Man can become infected by ingesting either eggs or nymphs. When the infection occurs from the ingestion of eggs, the larvae become encapsulated in various organs, where they can survive up to two years. When the larvae die, they are absorbed or the cyst can calcify. The larvae locate mainly in the liver, either below Glisson's capsule or in the parenchyma and, to a lesser extent, in the mesentery and intestinal wall. The encysted nymphs do not produce clinical symptoms, and the infection is almost always discovered during surgery, radiological examination, or autopsy. Clinical cases of prostatitis, ocular infection (anterior chamber of the eye), and acute abdomen have been described; their origin is a parasitized, inflamed lymph node adhering to the intestinal wall. The "halzoun" and "marrara" syndromes (infection of the human nasopharynx) are attributed to infection caused by the nymph of *L. serrata* ingested with the raw or undercooked liver or lymph glands of infested goats and sheep. Halzoun occurs in Greece, Lebanon, and Turkey, and marrara in Sudan. The symptoms appear a few minutes to a half-hour after the infective food is eaten. The variation in the incubation period probably depends on the place where the nymphs are released from their cysts, since the ones that are swallowed require more time to migrate to the tonsils and nasopharyngeal mucosa than the ones that become free in the mouth. The most prominent symptoms are throat irritation and pain. Sometimes there is congestion and intense edema of the region, which may extend to the larynx, eustachian tube, conjunctiva, nose, and lips. Lacrimation and nasal discharge are common. At times, there is also dyspnea, dysphagia, vomiting, headaches, photophobia, and exophthalmia. The most serious symptomatology is believed to occur in persons sensitized by visceral infections with *L. serrata*. The course of the disease is rapid and benign. About half of the patients recover in less than one day; in others the illness may last one to two weeks.

The Disease in Animals: The adult parasite causes a mucopurulent nasal catarrh, with sneezing, copious nasal discharge, and sometimes epistaxis in dogs. However, in mild infections no lesion is found in the nasal conchae. Larval infection in domestic herbivores and omnivores (intermediate hosts) is asymptomatic. Only heavy parasite burdens can damage the affected organs.

Source of Infection and Mode of Transmission: The natural reservoirs are wild and domestic canids and, rarely, felids. Carnivores acquire the infection by ingesting viscera and tissues of infected intermediate hosts. In endemic areas, the cycles between dogs and goats and between dogs and sheep are of special interest. Hunting dogs become infected when they catch infected lagomorphs. In the wild cycle, the infection circulates between wild herbivores and their carnivore predators. Herbivores become infected by ingesting pasture contaminated with feces or nasal secretions of the canids.

Man acquires the visceral form by consuming vegetables or water contaminated with parasite eggs shed with the fecal matter, saliva, or nasal discharge of dogs or other definitive hosts. Man contracts halzoun or marrara by consuming raw liver or lymph nodes from sheep, goats, or other infected domestic herbivores.

Diagnosis: The visceral form (small pentastomid nodules) caused by nymphs is rarely diagnosed in living persons or domestic animals, except during surgery. X-rays showing calcified cysts may arouse suspicion of the infection's presence. Specific diagnosis is effected by identification of the nymph in a biopsy specimen. Histopathological examination reveals a granulomatous reaction with multiple eosinophilic abscesses, at the center of which degenerated nymphs are found. In very old cases, there may not be pathological findings around the calcified cysts. In cases of halzoun or marrara, the nymph should be obtained for identification. In dogs with suspicious nasal catarrh, diagnosis can be confirmed by detecting eggs in the nasal secretion or feces.

Control: Visceral infection from ingestion of the eggs can be prevented by guarding against contamination of untreated water or raw food with carnivore depositions and washing hands carefully before eating. Halzoun and marrara or nasal infection with the adult parasite can be prevented by not consuming raw or undercooked viscera. Likewise, dogs must not be fed the raw viscera of goats, sheep, or other herbivores.

2. Infection due to *Armillifer* spp.

Etiology: *Armillifer armillatus* is the agent of this infection. Human infection by *A. moniliformis* (three cases in China, the Philippines, and the Indonesian island of Java) and by *A. grandis* has been reported rarely. In 1996, a local Chinese journal described the first human case of infection with larvae of *A. agkistrodontis*. These pentastomids have a cylindrical body and well defined segmentation. In the adult stage, they live in the respiratory tract of snakes. The pre-adult stages are found in rodents, livestock, and many other animals, including man.

The life cycle of *Armillifer* is similar to that of *Linguatula*, but the definitive hosts are snakes and the intermediate hosts are rodents and other wild mammals. The female of *Armillifer* deposits eggs in the respiratory cavities of snakes, and the eggs are expectorated or swallowed and then eliminated with the feces. In the cases that are known, the life cycle of the other species is similar (for example, *Porocephalus crotali* in the rattlesnake).

Geographic Distribution and Occurrence: *A. armillatus* and *A. grandis* are African species; *A. moniliformis* is found in Asia, and *A. agkistrodontis* has been described in China. Armilliferiasis occurs mainly in West Africa (Nigeria, Democratic Republic of Congo) and South and Southeast Asia; it seems to be infrequent in eastern and southern Africa, and no cases have been diagnosed in the Americas. Encysted larvae were found in 22.5% of adults autopsied in a hospital in Kinshasa, Democratic Republic of Congo, in 8% of the autopsies in Cameroon, and in 1.4% of the radiographs taken in a university hospital in Ibadan, Nigeria. In addition, autopsies found a 45.4% infection rate in Senoi natives in Malaysia. The most frequent localizations are the liver and lungs. Between 1989 and mid-2001, eight cases were described in the world: one in Benin during a diagnostic laparoscopy, one fatal case in France, three cases of abdominal calcification and one fatal case in Nigeria, one case in the autopsy of a Nigerian in Canada, and one case of *A. agkistrodontis* in China. The three cases of calcification in Nigeria were found during radiographic examination of 214 patients, thus revealing a prevalence of 1.4% in this population (Nzeh *et al.*, 1996).

The Disease in Man: Man is infected only with the larval forms; no cases of infection caused by the adult are known. The infection is similar to the visceral form of linguatuliasis and generally asymptomatic. The infected person usually harbors few nymphs (from 1 to 12). Severe infections can give rise to serious illness, especially when the larvae lodge in vital organs where they can produce multifocal abscesses, tumors, or obstruction of ducts. In the case in China, high fever, abdominal pain, diarrhea, moderate anemia, eosinophilia, hepatosplenomegaly, and polyps in the colon were observed. In the ocular case, the patient complained of pain, conjunctivitis, and vision problems. The autopsy of the Nigerian in Canada, in which death was due to a longstanding infection, found nodules in the liver, lungs, pleura, and peritoneum, but there was no inflammatory or degenerative reaction around the nodules. In the case of an 18-year-old woman in Nigeria, the patient suffered from fever, dizziness, weakness, jaundice, hypotension, and a confused mental state. She died shortly after being admitted, and the autopsy revealed disseminated infection encompassing the thoracic and abdominal serous membranes and internal organs (Obafunwa *et al.*, 1989). The diagnostic laparoscopy of a woman from Benin who had abdominal pain for 10 years found hundreds of calcified masses 1 to 2 cm in diameter in the abdominal cavity. Microscopy of the nodules revealed questionable remains of parasites, but the X-ray showed crescent- or horseshoe-shaped calcifications that were attributed to *Armillifer* (Mulder, 1989).

The Disease in Animals: Nonhuman primates are also accidental hosts of the infection. The larvae of *Armillifer* spp. are found mainly in Old World primates and less commonly in those of the Americas. The infection is usually asymptomatic.

Source of Infection and Mode of Transmission: The reservoirs and definitive hosts of *Armillifer* spp. are snakes, probably including all members of the families Boidae and Viperidae (Self, 1982). Snakes become infected when they ingest wild mammals infected with the nymph.

Man contracts the infection by consuming water or vegetables contaminated with eggs eliminated in the feces or saliva of infected snakes, by consuming raw or undercooked snake meat, or by placing hands to the mouth after handling contaminated snake meat. The other intermediate hosts also become infected by ingesting the parasite eggs. *Armillifer* eggs are very resistant to environmental factors.

Diagnosis: Some cases can be diagnosed by radiographic examination, which reveals the calcified, half-moon-shaped larvae. In the overwhelming majority of cases, however, the encapsulated nymphs of the pentastomids are found during autopsies or laparotomies performed for other reasons. Jones and Riley (1991) identified a protein of *Porocephalus crotali* that combined with rat immune serum in the Western blot test; an enzyme-linked immunosorbent assay can thus presumably be designed for the diagnosis of pentastomiasis.

Control: Preventive measures for humans consist of observing the rules of food hygiene: not consuming suspect water or raw vegetables, and washing the hands after handling suspect meat and before eating.

Bibliography

Andrews, C.L., W.R. Davidson. Endoparasites of selected populations of cottontail rabbits *(Sylvilagus floridanus)* in the southeastern United States. *J Wildl Dis* 16(3):395–401, 1980.

Ehrenford, F.A., J.W. Newberne. An aid to clinical diagnosis of tongue worms *(Linguatula serrata)* in dogs. *Lab Anim Sci* 31(1):74–76, 1981.

Gardiner, C.H., J.W. Dyke, S.F. Shirley. Hepatic granuloma due to a nymph of *Linguatula serrata* in a woman from Michigan: A case report and review of the literature. *Am J Trop Med Hyg* 33(1):187–189, 1984.

Guardia, S.N., H. Sepp, T. Scholten, I. Morava-Protzner. Pentastomiasis in Canada. *Arch Pathol Lab Med* 115(5):515–517, 1991.

Jones, D.A., J. Riley. An ELISA for the detection of pentastomid infections in the rat. *Parasitology* 103(Pt 3):331–337, 1991.

Lazo, R.F., E. Hidalgo, J.E. Lazo, *et al.* Ocular linguatuliasis in Ecuador: Case report and morphometric study of the larva of *Linguatula serrata. Am J Trop Med Hyg* 60(3):405–409, 1999.

Mulder, K. Porocephalosis. *Dtsch Med Wochenschr* 114(49):1921–1923, 1989.

Nzeh, D.A., J.K. Akinlemibola, G.C. Nzeh. Incidence of *Armillifer armillatus* (pentastome) calcification in the abdomen. *Cent Afr J Med* 42(1):29–31, 1996.

Obafunwa, J.O., A. Busuttil, E.J. Nwana. Sudden death due to disseminated porocephalosis—a case history. *Int J Legal Med* 105(1):43–46, 1992.

Self, J.T. Pentastomiasis. *In:* Hillyer, G.V., C.E. Hopla, section ed. Section C, Vol. 3: *CRC Handbook Series in Zoonoses.* Boca Raton: CRC Press; 1982.

TICK INFESTATIONS

ICD-10 B88.8 Other specified infestations

Etiology: The agents of these infestations are various species of the genera *Argas, Amblyomma, Boophilus, Dermacentor, Haemaphysalis, Hyalomma, Ixodes, Ornithodoros,* and *Rhipicephalus.* Man is not affected by specific ticks, but can occasionally be infested by ticks of other vertebrates that transmit various infections (Table 4). Ticks are divided into two groups: the family Argasidae, comprised of soft ticks whose bodies are covered by a coriaceous tegument, with the mouthparts located on the ventral surface, and the family Ixodidae, comprised of ticks which have an enlargement of the shield-shaped cuticle on their backs, and mouthparts on the anterior end. That shield covers the entire back in the males, but just the anterior half of the back in females, to permit their bodies to engorge while feeding.

The only soft ticks that are important in human medicine are those of the genus

TABLE 4. Ticks that infect man, and organisms and infections they transmit.

Tick	Transmission area	Organism transmitted
Amblyomma americanum	Southern US and Mexico	*Francisella tularensis*
		Rickettsia rickettsii
		Ehrlichia spp.
Amblyomma cajennense	Texas (US) to tropical South America	*Rickettsia rickettsii*
Amblyomma hebraeum	South Africa	*Rickettsia conorii*
Amblyomma triguttatum	Australia	*Coxiella burnetii*
Amblyomma variegatum	Caribbean	*Rickettsia africae*
Boophilus decoloratus	South Africa and tropical Africa	*Rickettsia conorii*
		Bunyaviruses of the tick-borne hemorrhagic fevers
Dermacentor spp.	Asia	*Rickettsia sibirica*
Dermacentor andersoni	Western Canada and US	*Francisella tularensis*
		Rickettsia rickettsii
Dermacentor marginatus	Siberia	Flaviviruses of the tick-borne arboviral encephalitides[a]
Dermacentor reticulatus	Siberia	Flaviviruses of the tick-borne arboviral encephalitides[a]
Dermacentor variabilis	Western Canada, US, and Mexico	*Francisella tularensis*
		Rickettsia rickettsii
Haemaphysalis spp.	Asia	*Rickettsia sibirica*
Haemaphysalis bispinosis	Southern China	*Borrelia burgdorferi*
Haemaphysalis leachi	South Africa	*Rickettsia conorii*
Haemaphysalis spinigera	India	Flaviviruses of the tick-borne arboviral encephalitides[a]
Hyalomma aegyptium	South Africa	*Rickettsia conorii*
Hyalomma anatolicum	Eurasia and South Africa	Bunyaviruses of the tick-borne hemorrhagic fevers
Hyalomma excavatum	Somalia	Bunyaviruses of the tick-borne hemorrhagic fevers
Hyalomma impeltatum	Somalia	Bunyaviruses of the tick-borne hemorrhagic fevers
Hyalomma marginatum	Eurasia and South Africa	Bunyaviruses of the tick-borne hemorrhagic fevers
Ixodes cookei	Eastern Canada and US	Flaviviruses of the tick-borne arboviral encephalitides

TABLE 4. Continued.

Tick	Transmission area	Organism transmitted
Ixodes granulatus	Southern China	*Borrelia burgdorferi*
Ixodes holocyclus	Australia	*Rickettsia australis*
Ixodes ovatus	Japan	Virus of tick-borne Asian encephalitis
Ixodes pacificus	Western US	*Borrelia burgdorferi*
Ixodes persulcatus	Asia, northern China, eastern Russian Federation	*Borrelia burgdorferi* *Ehrlichia* of the *Phagocytophila* group Flaviviruses of the tick-borne arboviral encephalitides
Ixodes ricinus	Europe	*Babesia divergens* *Borrelia burgdorferi* *Ehrlichia* of the *Phagocytophila* group Flaviviruses of the tick-borne arboviral encephalitides
Ixodes scapularis (I. dammini)	Central and eastern US	*Babesia microti* *Borrelia burgdorferi* *Ehrlichia* spp.[a]
Ornithodoros hermsi	US	*Borrelia recurrentis*
Ornithodoros hispanica	Africa	*Borrelia recurrentis*
Ornithodoros moubata	Africa	*Borrelia recurrentis*
Ornithodoros rudis	Latin America	*Borrelia recurrentis*
Ornithodoros talaje	Latin America	*Borrelia recurrentis*
Ornithodoros tholozani	Middle East	*Borrelia recurrentis*
Ornithodoros turicata	US	*Borrelia recurrentis*
Rhipicephalus appendiculatus	South Africa	*Rickettsia conorii*
Rhipicephalus sanguineus	Mediterranean and South Africa	*Ehrlichia* spp. *Rickettsia conorii*

[a] Confirmation needed.

Ornithodoros, which transmit the relapsing fevers in man caused by strains of *Borrelia recurrentis*, and several species of *Argas*, in particular those of chickens, pigeons, and other birds that attack man when they cannot find their natural host. The species of *Ornithodoros* that infest man live hidden in the ground, in tools and equipment, and in the cracks of shack or cabin walls, and emerge at night to suck blood from people or chickens that take shelter there. The females measure 7–8 mm in length before feeding and up to 11 mm immediately thereafter; they produce groups of 20 to 100 eggs on alternate days, for a total of 500 to 2,000 in a lifetime. After approximately eight days at 30°C, the eggs hatch and hexapodal larvae, which do not feed, emerge and molt into nymphs in four days. The nymphs that go through four stages molt into adult males; those that go through five stages molt into adult females. Each nymph has one blood meal lasting 20–25 minutes. Adult specimens emerge about four months after oviposition. The female mates and produces eggs 10 to 15 days after each blood meal, and can mate up to 40 times before dying. Also, more than half of the females can survive between 9 and 56 months without feeding. The cycle of *Argas* is similar to that of *Ornithodoros*, but the larvae feed by day as well as by night and can remain attached to the host's skin, sucking blood, for several days.

Among the hard ticks, the species of the genera *Amblyomma*, *Boophilus*, *Dermacentor*, *Haemaphysalis*, *Hyalomma*, *Ixodes,* and *Rhipicephalus* are important in human medicine. The life cycle of all these ticks is similar, with small variations among the genera. The female produces several thousand eggs at a time for a few days, and then dies. Hexapodal larvae emerge from the eggs; they measure about 1 mm in length, feed on blood for a few days, and molt into nymphs a few days thereafter. Similarly, the nymphs feed on blood and molt into adults. The adults mate, the female sucks blood in amounts that can exceed 10 times her body weight for several days—an engorged hard tick is the size of a pea—and falls to the ground, seeks out a protected place, and begins to produce eggs. Hard one-host ticks remain with a host from the larval stage until adulthood; two-host ticks remain with one host during the larval and nymph stages, but molt on the ground and the adults have to seek out another host; three-host ticks molt on the ground and need a different host in each stage—larva, nymph, and adult. These differences are important in the spread of disease and the design of tick control plans.

Geographic Distribution and Occurrence: The transmission areas of tick-borne infections are shown in Table 4. The distribution of the ticks themselves is diverse; those of the genus *Amblyomma* are mainly parasites of small and large mammals distributed throughout the tropical and subtropical areas of the Americas and sub-Saharan Africa. Ticks of the genus *Boophilus* are parasites of cattle, and, exceptionally, of other herbivores, and are distributed in tropical to temperate zones throughout the world. Human infection is exceptional. Ticks of the genus *Dermacentor* are parasites of rodents and large mammals ranging from the tropical zone of Latin America to Canada. Ticks of the genus *Haemaphysalis* are parasites of small mammals and birds and are found throughout the world. Those of the genus *Hyalomma* are mainly parasites of domestic animals found in the Old World below the 45th parallel North. Ticks of the genus *Ixodes* are parasites of birds as well as large and small mammals and are distributed worldwide. *Rhipicephalus* are ticks of a variety of African and Eurasian animals; only *Rhipicephalus sanguineus* is distributed worldwide.

Humans can be infested by 12 species of Argasidae (*Argas* and *Ornithodoros*) and 22 species of Ixodidae (4 of the genus *Amblyomma*, 7 of *Dermacentor*, 3 of *Haemaphysalis*, 2 of *Hyalomma,* and 6 of *Ixodes*) (Estrada-Pena and Jongejan, 1999). In the US, 44 species of ticks have been found on humans: 11 species of soft ticks and 33 of hard ticks. But four of the former were acquired outside the country and are not species native to the US. The most common were *Amblyomma americanum* in the south and near the Atlantic Ocean; *Dermacentor variabilis* and *Ixodes scapularis* in the east; *Dermacentor andersoni* in the west; *Ixodes pacificus* near the Pacific; and *Ornithodoros* spp. mainly in the west (Merten and Durden, 2000). North Carolina reported human infestations with *Otobius megnini*, *Amblyomma maculatum*, *Haemaphysalis leporispalustris*, *Ixodes cookei*, *Ixodes dentatus*, and *R. sanguineus*. *O. megnini* was the first specimen of this species found in North Carolina in over 50 years (Harrison *et al.*, 1997).

Since tick infestations in man are occasional, their frequency is difficult to assess. In one locality in Italy, during 1995 and 1996, 240 infested individuals were found, with an average of 1.3 ticks per person; 89% were infested with *Ixodes ricinus* in all stages; 10% with *R. sanguineus* nymphs and adults; and 1% with *Dermacentor marginatus* adults. Eleven percent of the cases occurred in children, 26% in students, 22% in workers, and 24% in retired persons. During the period studied, the prevalence of bites was 5 per 1,000 residents (Manfredi *et al.*, 1999). A report from a medical school in the state of Georgia, US, indicates that 521 infestations were recorded in two and a half years, with an average of 1.3 ticks per person (Felz and Durden, 1999). In Chile, 2.2% of 1,384 patients referred to a university clinic for "spider bites" between 1955 and 1995 really had tick bites.

The Disease in Man: Ticks cause damage directly by biting and by sucking blood, since they cause allergic reactions by injecting toxins and transmit infections. It has also been found that ticks cause a depressed immune response (Barriga, 1999), but the importance of that is probably minimal. It may be that the direct damage ticks cause is slight in human beings because the majority of infestations are due to a single arthropod and the patient does not notice it. The case of *Amblyomma testudinarium* of Japan is noteworthy, since it caused infestations with more than 100 larvae (Nakamura-Uchiyama *et al.*, 2000). The mouthparts that remain in the wound when the tick is removed can cause a granuloma that looks like a pustule and lasts for several weeks. Despite the fact that *O. megnini*, the ear tick of many animals, is exceptional in man, cases of otocariasis in man are described with some frequency (Indudharan *et al.*, 1999).

Ticks are generally not included among the arthropods that cause allergies; however, there are reports of severe allergic reactions. For example, symptoms have been reported ranging from erythematous reactions to ulcerative lesions caused by *Argas reflexus* (pigeon tick) (Veraldi *et al.*, 1998), very extensive urticarias, caused particularly by *Argas* (Basset-Stheme *et al.*, 1999), cases of anaphylaxia caused by the genera *Argas* and *Ixodes* (Lavaud *et al.*, 1999), and even cases of anaphylactic shock caused by *I. ricinus* (Moneret-Vautrin *et al.*, 1998).

A paralysis caused by the female of certain ticks feeding on their hosts has been described in both animals and humans; approximately 20 species have been identified: *D. andersoni* and *D. variabilis* in Canada and the US; *Haemaphysalis, Hyalomma,* and *Ixodes* in Europe; *Ixodes* and *Rhipicephalus* in South Africa; *Ixodes holocyclus* in Australia; and *Argas persicus* in chickens in many countries (Barriga, 1997). While it is suspected that the paralysis is due to a toxin, it has been identified only in the case of the Australian tick *I. holocyclus*. Grattan-Smith *et al.* (1997) described six cases of paralysis caused by ticks in Australian children. The patients experienced an ascending symmetrical flaccid paralysis that causes respiratory paralysis after about a week; the illness ends when the arthropod is removed, but recovery is slow. In the state of Washington, US, a review was conducted of the 33 cases (with two deaths) reported between 1946 and 1996 (Dworkin *et al.*, 1999).

Transmission of infection is the most serious concern in connection with tick infestation of humans. Walker (1998) conducted a review of the problem in the US, and Benenson (1995) conducted a worldwide review. Table 4 presents a summary of the state of knowledge up to the year 2000.

The Disease in Animals: The disease in animals has the same four pathogenic components as the disease in man. Since the number of ticks that attack a single animal can be very high, inflammation, pain, and pruritis are intense, due either to the trauma or hypersensitivity, and distract the cattle from feeding, in addition to causing weight loss. Also, the wounds caused by the ticks can ruin the skins for industrial use and attract fly attacks that result in myiasis. The sucking of blood can be significant when the infestation is intense and can also promote weight loss, since the cattle have to expend energy to replace the blood loss. The combined effect of these factors is often called "tick worry." Paralysis caused by ticks is no longer a widespread problem in cattle, as it was 70 years ago, but cases are still reported regularly in the scientific publications. With respect to the transmission of disease, ticks play a role as important for animals as mosquitoes play for humans. Some of the most severe cattle diseases are tick-borne, such as babesiosis (see chapter on Babesiosis), theileriosis, cowdriosis (hydropericardium), and anaplasmosis (Uilenberg, 1997).

Source of Infestation: The source of infestation is the environment contaminated with ticks; in the case of hard ticks, the vegetation where the hungry larvae are found in large numbers; in the case of soft ticks, the dwellings with cracks where they can find shelter during the day. While infested animals are the source of contamination of the environment, they are rarely a direct source of infection for man or other animals.

Diagnosis: Diagnosis is made by removing and studying the tick. Studying them should not be difficult because even the tick larvae measure more than 1 mm, and they are red or dark after feeding. However, the tick is often located on parts of the body where the infested person cannot see it, including behind the ears, where even the doctor can miss it if he or she is not specifically looking for it. When removing a tick, it is important to extract the mouthparts from the skin to prevent the formation of granulomas; to ensure this, the body must be pulled continuously for one minute, without excessive force, in a direction perpendicular to the patient's skin, until the grip is loosened. It is advisable to remove the tick with tweezers or a plastic sheet to avoid contact with its blood if it should explode, since the fluid may contain pathogenic organisms. Taxonomic identification is rarely necessary but, if it is desired, the specimens should be packaged in 70% alcohol and sent to the Department of Agriculture or university veterinary services.

Control: Control of animal ticks is based essentially on the periodic application of acaricides to animals at risk for infestation. An inevitable consequence of this method is the development of strains of ticks resistant to the acaricide. This situation is common in cattle-raising countries with high rates of tick infestation, such as Brazil and South Africa. Modification of the environment to make it unsuitable for the proliferation of ticks is complicated, and not enough is known about their ecology to ensure success. A large number of biological control experiments have been carried out employing the natural enemies of ticks (Samish and Rehacek, 1999), but practical solutions have not been found. Many experiments have also been conducted in an attempt to develop breeds of cattle with a natural resistance to these arthropods, but, despite encouraging results, a meaningful solution has not been found. In an attempt to increase the host's resistance, Australian investigators developed a vaccine against the *Boophilus microplus* tick; this inhibits by about 75% the fertility of the ticks that feed on vaccinated animals. However, in the short term, the ticks continue to bite and transmit infections; over the long term, that reduction in fertility could be insufficient to decrease the proliferation of arthropods in the pasturelands. The European Union supports a project for the integrated control of ticks and tick-borne disease, with the objective of increasing livestock productivity through the control of ticks, vaccination, and the comprehensive diagnosis of the diseases (Jongejan, 1999). Also, techniques involving remote sensors and geographic information systems are starting to be used to help control these pests (Thomson and Connor, 2000).

From the standpoint of human infestations, attempts are rarely made to eliminate ticks from an entire area—although it could be tried in the endemic area for Lyme disease in the US. Rather, efforts are directed at protecting hunters and tourists who enter areas populated with ticks. For this, it is sufficient to wear clothing that covers the body completely, including high boots with pants legs closed around the boot tops. The use of repellents is also recommended. DEET (N, N-diethyl-m-toluamide) is an excellent insect repellent, although less effective against ticks than permethrin. The concomitant use of both is particularly effective (Mafong and Kaplan, 1997). The US Army recommends this combination for soldiers on maneuvers.

Bibliography

Barriga, O.O. Evidence and mechanisms of immunosuppression in tick infestations. *Genet Anal* 15:139–142, 1999.

Barriga, O.O. *Veterinary Parasitology for Practitioners*, 2nd ed. Edina: Burgess International Group; 1997.

Basset-Stheme, D., P. Couturier, J. Sainte-Laudy. Urticaire géante par piqure d'*Argas reflexus*: à propos d'un cas. *Allerg Immunol (Paris)* 31:61–62, 1999.

Benenson, A.S., ed. *Control of Communicable Diseases in Man*, 16th ed. An official report of the American Public Health Association. Washington, D.C.: American Public Health Association; 1995.

Blankenship, M.L. Mite dermatitis other than scabies. *Dermatol Clin* 8:265–275, 1990.

Dworkin, M.S., P.C. Shoemaker, D.E. Anderson. Tick paralysis: 33 human cases in Washington State, 1946–1996. *Clin Infect Dis* 29:1435–1439, 1999.

Engel, P.M., J. Welzel, M. Maass, U. Schramm, H.H. Wolff. Tropical rat mite dermatitis: Case report and review. *Clin Infect Dis* 27:1465–1469, 1998.

Estrada-Pena, A., F. Jongejan. Ticks feeding on humans: A review of records on human-biting Ixodoidea with special reference to pathogen transmission. *Exp Appl Acarol* 23:685–715, 1999.

Felz, M.W., L.A. Durden. Attachment sites of four tick species (Acari: Ixodidae) parasitizing humans in Georgia and South Carolina. *J Med Entomol* 36:361–364, 1999.

Flynn, R.J. *Parasites of Laboratory Animals*. Ames: Iowa State University Press; 1973.

Grattan-Smith, P.J., J.G. Morris, H.M. Johnston, *et al.* Clinical and neurophysiological features of tick paralysis. *Brain* 120(Pt 11):1975–1987, 1997.

Harrison, B.A., B.R. Engber, C.S. Apperson. Ticks (Acari: Ixodida) uncommonly found biting humans in North Carolina. *J Vector Ecol* 22:6–12, 1997.

Indudharan, R., M. Ahamad, T.M. Ho, R. Salim, Y.N. Htun. Human otoacariasis. *Ann Trop Med Parasitol* 93:163–167, 1999.

Jongejan, F. Integrated control of ticks and tick-borne diseases. *Parassitologia* 41(Suppl 1):57–58, 1999.

Lavaud, F., F. Bouchet, P.M. Mertes, S. Kochman. Allergie aux piqures d'insectes hematophages: manifestations cliniques. *Allerg Immunol (Paris)* 31:311–316, 1999.

Manfredi, M.T., V. Dini, S. Piacenza, C. Genchi. Tick species parasitizing people in an area endemic for tick-borne diseases in north-western Italy. *Parassitologia* 41:555–560, 1999.

Mafong, E.A., L.A. Kaplan. Insect repellents. What really works? *Postgrad Med* 102:63, 68–69, 74, 1997.

McKeever, P.J., S.K. Allen. Dermatitis associated with *Cheyletiella* infestation in cats. *J Am Vet Med Assoc* 147:718–720, 1979.

Merten, H.A., L.A. Durden. A state-by-state survey of ticks recorded from humans in the United States. *J Vector Ecol* 25:102–113, 2000.

Miller, W.H. *Cheyletiella* infestation. *In:* Parish, L.C., W.B. Nutting, R.M. Schwartzman, eds. *Cutaneous Infestations of Man and Animal.* New York: Praeger; 1983.

Moneret-Vautrin, D.A., E. Beaudouin, G. Kanny, L. Guerin, J.F. Roche. Anaphylactic shock caused by ticks (*Ixodes ricinus*). *J Allergy Clin Immunol* 101(1 Pt 1):144–145, 1998.

Nakamura-Uchiyama, F., Y. Komuro, A. Yoshii, Y. Nawa. *Amblyomma testudinarium* tick bite: One case of engorged adult and a case of extraordinary number of larval tick infestation. *J Dermatol* 27:774–777, 2000.

Paradis, M. Mite dermatitis caused by *Cheyletiella blakei. J Am Acad Dermatol* 38(6 Pt 1):1014–1015, 1998.

Pecheur, M., H. Wissocq. Un cas de gale due à *Cheyletiella parasitovorax* chez un chat. *Ann Med Vet* 125:191–192, 1981.

Samish, M., J. Rehacek. Pathogens and predators of ticks and their potential in biological control. *Annu Rev Entomol* 44:159–182, 1999.

Thomson, M.C., S.J. Connor. Environmental information systems for the control of arthropod vectors of disease. *Med Vet Entomol* 14:227–244, 2000.

Uilenberg, G. General review of tick-borne diseases of sheep and goats world-wide. *Parassitologia* 39:161–165, 1997.

Veraldi, S., M. Barbareschi, R. Zerboni, G. Scarabelli. Skin manifestations caused by pigeon ticks (*Argas reflexus*). *Cutis* 61:38–40, 1998.

Walker, D.H. Tick-borne infectious diseases in the United States. *Annu Rev Public Health* 19:237–269, 1998.

TUNGIASIS

ICD-10 B88.1 Tungiasis [sandflea infestation]

Synonyms: Chigoe, jigger flea, burrowing flea, sand flea, dermatophiliasis.

Etiology: The agent of this infestation is *Tunga (Sarcopsylla) penetrans*, a small flea. The ovigerous female is an obligate parasite of warm-blooded animals, including swine, man, nonhuman primates, and dogs. It is easy to identify because it is small (about 1 mm long), it does not have pronotal or genal combs, and it has an angular head.

The fertilized female becomes encrusted in the skin of the host, where she feeds continuously. Her abdominal segments gradually enlarge over a period of about two weeks until she reaches the size of a pea (approximately 5 mm in diameter). As she increases in size, the host epidermis surrounds and encloses her in an excrescence similar to a wart that encloses inflammatory cells. This formation usually ulcerates and can develop secondary infections. Meanwhile, the female expels her eggs through an orifice on top of the excrescence. If the eggs fall on sandy soil, the larvae are born in three or four days. These larvae molt twice within 10 to 14 days and are transformed into pupae that bury themselves in the soil for another 10 to 14 days. At the end of the pupal stage, the adult fleas emerge. The female lays about 200 eggs and then dies. Both the young males and females feed on the blood of animals. After mating, the male dies and the female penetrates the skin of an animal and reinitiates the cycle with oviposition.

Geographic Distribution and Occurrence: *T. penetrans* is believed to be native to the tropical and subtropical regions of Central America, the Caribbean, and South America. It was first reported in the American tropics in 1526 and in Africa in 1732. It was probably carried from America to Africa in the seventeenth century and reintroduced in 1872 by a British ship that arrived from South America and unloaded its sand ballast on the beaches of Angola. Whether by this means or because some members of the crew were infested with *T. penetrans*, the flea was introduced into Angola. From there it spread through the entire western coast of Africa and ultimately reached eastern Africa and Madagascar. Outside Africa and the Americas, *T. penetrans* is present in western India and Pakistan, where it was probably introduced by workers returning home from Africa (Connor, 1976).

Thus, infestations occur in Central and South America, the Caribbean, tropical Africa, India, and Pakistan (Lowry *et al.*, 1996). To cite examples from studies carried out near the end of the twentieth century, infestations were reported in 11 (25%) of 44 children examined in the Republic of the Congo (Obengui, 1989); 49 (22.5%) of 280 in Nigeria (Nte and Eke, 1995); 32 (31.4%) of 102 in the West Indies (Chadee, 1994); and, in a subsequent report, 267 (20.4%) of 1,307 in the West Indies (Chadee, 1998). By contrast, in the rest of the world the infestation is so rare that individual cases are worthy of publication. Between 1989 and mid-2001, 1 case each was reported in Australia, Brazil, Chile, Denmark, France, Germany, New Zealand, and Switzerland; 2 cases were reported in Great Britain, 2 in Israel, 5 in Italy, 4 in Mexico, 2 in the Netherlands, and 6 in the US (in addition to 14 reported previously) (Sanusi *et al.*, 1989). In addition, Caumes *et al.* (1995) found 16 cases in French nationals who had traveled abroad, and Matías (1989) reported an epidemic of unknown magnitude in Rio Grande do Sul, Brazil. In all these cases except Brazil and Mexico, the infestation was contracted outside the country. In Mexico, the last cases of human tungiasis prior to those mentioned above were reported in 1948; authors believe that those 4 new cases are an indication that the parasite is reappearing in that country.

In some regions of Africa, human *T. penetrans* infestation can reach very high prevalence rates. In a village in the state of Lagos, Nigeria, 41.5% of 373 children 6 to 14 years old were found to be harboring the fleas between their toes. Prevalence declines with age, probably because the skin is thicker and also because footwear is used more often (Ade-Serrano and Ejezie, 1981).

Little information is available about the frequency of infestation in animals. Outbreaks have been described in Tanzania and the Democratic Republic of Congo among swine (Cooper, 1967; Verhulst, 1976), and in French Guiana, among dogs (Rietschel, 1989).

The Disease in Man and Animals: The flea usually penetrates the human epidermis on the sole of the foot, the toes, under the edge of the toenails, and in the interdigital spaces, but it can lodge in any exposed part of the body. Upon penetration, the insect produces a mild but persistent pruritus and later, as it increases in size, a chronic proliferating inflammation that completely surrounds the site, except for a small orifice on the top. Ulceration and secondary infections are common. When the flea finally lays its eggs, its body collapses and is expelled by tissue reaction, usually in the form of a draining abscess, leaving behind a crateriform ulceration. At first, the lesion looks like a black spot on a taut area of skin, but later it assumes the appearance of a wart, then an ulcer, and finally it turns into a small oozing abscess. The lesions originated by *Tunga* sp. offer favorable conditions for secondary infections. A study conducted in the West Indies found 7 different bacteria (*Streptococcus pyogenes*, non-group A beta-hemolytic *Streptococcus*, *Klebsiella aerogenes*, *Enterobacter agglomerans*, *Staphylococcus aureus*, *Escherichia coli*, and *Bacillus* sp.) in infections associated with *Tunga* lesions (Chadee, 1998). In Senegal, 11 cases of tetanus infection were found in 44 cases of tungiasis (Obengui, 1989).

In Nigeria, the most common symptoms seen in 49 children with tungiasis were pruritus and ulceration. In all cases, the infestation was in the feet, but no case had been considered serious enough to take the child to a clinic (Nte and Eke, 1995). The pain is particularly intense when the flea penetrates under a nail. Usually only one or two lesions are found on a single individual, but sometimes there can be hundreds. In a series of 102 patients, the highest prevalence of infestation was found in the groups 5 to 9 years of age, 10 to 14, and over 55, with averages of 9, 5–6, and 12 fleas per person, respectively (Chafee, 1994).

In the outbreak among swine in Tanzania, infestations were observed on the scrotum, feet, snout, and teats, but they had not caused any marked inflammation, pruritus, or pain (Cooper, 1967). The outbreak in the Democratic Republic of Congo was characterized especially by agalactia in the sows and consequent death of the suckling pigs, which could not feed because the intense concentration of *T. penetrans* in the maternal nipples compressed or obstructed the lactiferous ducts (Verhulst, 1976).

Source of Infestation and Mode of Transmission: *T. penetrans* is found primarily in dry, sandy places, inside and around precarious human dwellings, and in pigsties, stables, and hen houses. Humans contract tungiasis by walking barefoot in soil containing fleas that originated from infested dogs or swine. Dogs, and sometimes swine, can carry the infestation inside huts with earthen floors. Conversely, man can introduce the flea into the animal environment.

Diagnosis: In areas where *T. penetrans* is common, diagnosis can be based on the finding of the characteristic lesions. Specific diagnosis can be made by extracting the flea from the skin and examining it microscopically.

Control: The application of pesticides (insecticides, development regulators, hormonal analogs, etc.) in contaminated environments can eliminate the source of infestation. The application of pesticides on infested animals can eliminate the source of the infestation. Flea control has been greatly facilitated by the development of new insecticides and chitin formation inhibitors, which are now being used systemically in domestic animals. Humans can protect themselves individually by wearing shoes. However, this simple preventive measure is difficult to apply because of the low economic level of the population and the tropical climate in affected regions. Indeed, it has been recommended for the control of the ancylostomiases for more than 70 years, so far with very little effect.

Tungiasis by itself is a mild condition; the risk lies in secondary infections. For that reason, the flea should be extracted and the wound should be treated with disinfectants and kept clean until a scar forms.

Bibliography

Ade-Serrano, M.A., G.C. Ejezie. The prevalence of tungiasis in Oto-Ijanikin village, Badagry, Lagos State. Nigeria. *Ann Trop Med Parasitol* 75(4):471–472, 1981.

Caumes, E., J. Carriere, G. Guermonprez, F. Bricaire, M. Danis, M. Gentilini. Dermatoses associated with travel to tropical countries: A prospective study of the diagnosis and management of 269 patients presenting to a tropical disease unit. *Clin Infect Dis* 20(3):542–548, 1995.

Chadee, D.D. Distribution patterns of *Tunga penetrans* within a community in Trinidad, West Indies. *J Trop Med Hyg* 97(3):167–170, 1994.

Chadee, D.D. Tungiasis among five communities in south-western Trinidad, West Indies. *Ann Trop Med Parasitol* 92(1):107–113, 1998.

Connor, D.H. Tungiasis. *In*: Binford, C.H., D.H. Connor, eds. Vol. 2: *Pathology of Tropical and Extraordinary Diseases.* Washington, D.C.: Armed Forces Institute of Pathology; 1976.

Cooper, J.E. An outbreak of *Tunga penetrans* in a pig herd. *Vet Rec* 80(11):365–366, 1967.

Lowry, M.A., J.L. Ownbey, P.L. McEvoy. A case of tungiasis. *Mil Med* 161(2):128–129, 1996.

Matias, R.S. Epidemia de tungiase no Rio Grande do Sul. *Rev Soc Bras Med Trop* 22(3):137–142, 1989.

Nte, A.R., F.U. Eke. Jigger infestation in children in a rural area of Rivers State of Nigeria. *West Afr J Med* 14(1):56–58, 1995.

Obengui. La tungose et le tetanos au C.H.U. de Brazzaville. *Dakar Med* 34(1):44–48, 1989.

Rietschel, W. Beobachtungen zum Sandfloh (*Tunga penetrans*) bei Mensch und Hund in Franzosisch Guayana. *Tierarztl Prax* 17(2):189–193, 1989.

Sanusi, I.D., E.B. Brown, T.G. Shepard, W.D. Grafton. Tungiasis: Report of one case and review of the 14 reported cases in the United States. *J Am Acad Dermatol* 20(5 Pt 2):941–944, 1989.

Verhulst, A. *Tunga penetrans (Sarcopsylla penetrans)* as a cause of agalactia in sows in the Republic of Zaire. *Vet Rec* 98(19):384, 1976.

ZOONOTIC SCABIES

ICD-10 B86 Scabies

Synonyms: Scabiosis, mange, sarcoptic acariasis, sarcoptic itch, seven-year itch.

Etiology: The agent of human scabies is *Sarcoptes scabiei* var. *hominis*, an oval mite. The female measures up to 450 μm by 350 μm and the male, up to 240 μm by 200 μm. This species has varieties that infest some 40 species of mammals, from primates to marsupials (Elgart, 1990). By and large, each variety is strongly host-specific, although some can infest other species and cause temporary illness. Since the varieties on the different hosts are morphologically indistinguishable, until recently their identification was based solely on empirical testing. However, Lee and Cho (1995) proposed that *Sarcoptes* in humans and swine belonged to different varieties but that the dog mite was a different species. Serological (Arlian *et al.*, 1996) and genetic (Walton *et al.*, 1999) differences that have been found, at least in some varieties, could provide more solid grounds for differentiating them.

Other mites that cause zoonotic scabies in man are *Notoedres cati* (also of the Sarcoptidae family), which produces head scabies in cats, and *Cheyletiella*, the dog, cat, and rabbit mite (see the chapter on Dermatitis Caused by Mites of Animal Origin). In contrast, *Otodectes cynotis* (family Psoroptidae), which causes dog ear scabies, does not seem to affect man (Park *et al.*, 1996).

The mites of sarcoptic scabies lodge in furrows that they excavate in the epidermis of the host and lay their eggs there. The six-legged larvae emerge from the eggs after two days and dig lateral tunnels to migrate to the surface; there they hide under the epidermic scales or in hair follicles. Two to three days later, the larvae give rise to eight-legged, first-stage nymphs, or protonymphs, which transform into tritonymphs; lastly, they reach the adult stage. The adults mate on the surface, and the females begin building tunnels (from 0.5 to 5 mm a day), where they lay their eggs. The entire life cycle can take 10 to 14 days.

The life cycle of *Notoedres* is similar to that of *Sarcoptes*, although a bit slower; the cycle from egg to adult usually takes about 17 days. Unlike *Sarcoptes*, the larvae and nymphs of *Notoedres* move about freely on the skin of the host. Notoedric scabies affects the head of cats and occasionally causes temporary dermatitis in humans.

Sarcoptic scabies affects humans and a large number of domestic and wild animals. Specific names used to be assigned to the mites of each animal species, such as *S. scabiei* for the human parasite, *S. equi* for the horse parasite, and *S. ovis* for the sheep parasite. Now only one species—*S. scabiei*—is recognized, and the mite of each animal species is regarded as a subspecies.

Geographic Distribution and Occurrence: *Sarcoptes* is distributed worldwide. Human scabies is prevalent primarily among socioeconomic classes whose members are poor and often, malnourished, and who have inadequate hygiene; overcrowding promotes the spread of the mite and poor hygiene is conducive to its persistence. However, in the US and Europe, there has been a wave of human infestations unrelated to socioeconomic status, hygiene level, age, sex, or race. Epidemiologists have observed that epidemics of human scabies occur every 30 years and have speculated that a considerable portion of the human population is protected by a certain level of immunity during periods between epidemics.

All animals raised by man for food or transportation are susceptible to *S. scabiei*. Among pets and laboratory animals, the mite is found in dogs, rabbits, hamsters, and some nonhuman primates. The infestation is also seen in zoo animals.

Man is affected by sarcoptic scabies of dogs, cattle, goats, swine, and horses, by notoedric scabies of cats, and by cheyletiellosis of dogs, cats, and rabbits (Beck, 1996; Mitra *et al.*, 1993; Parish and Schwartzmann, 1993). Skerratt and Beveridge (1999) reported that man can also acquire the scabies of the Australian wombat. For further information on *Cheyletiella* spp., see the chapter on Dermatitis Caused by Mites of Animal Origin.

Sarcoptes of goats seems not to be very host-specific, inasmuch as there was a report of one epidemic in goats that then spread to cattle, sheep, and dogs, and eventually affected 42 persons. Nineteen goats and one cow died, but the infestation was self-limiting in some human cases (Mitra *et al.*, 1993). The sarcoptic scabies of swine also seems to be transmitted easily to man. Of 48 individuals working with swine infested by *Sarcoptes* in India, 30 (65%) had signs of scabies, and mites were recovered on 20 persons (67%) (Chakrabarti, 1990). Dog scabies is also often transferred to man. In most cases, the symptoms in humans disappear when the animals are treated and contagion ceases to be constant (Fontaine, 2000). Owing to the difficulty of identifying the origin of the mites, the frequency of zoonotic scabies in man is not known. Nevertheless, Normaznah *et al.* (1996) found that 25% of 312 aborigines in Malaysia had antibodies to *S. scabiei* var. *canis*. Arlian *et al.* (1996) found that *Sarcoptes* of man, dogs, and swine had both common and exclusive antibodies. Consequently, it may be possible to differentiate them by serology.

The Disease in Man: The disease caused by the homologous (human) variety of *S. scabiei* is characterized by tunnels in the corneous layer of the skin that are between a few millimeters and 2 cm long. The furrows are very thin and sinuous and are difficult to observe without the aid of a magnifying glass; they are generally not very abundant and are situated primarily in the interdigital spaces, back of the hand, elbows, axillae, torso, inguinal region, chest, penis, and navel. Fiminani *et al.* (1997) conducted a detailed morphological study of dermal pathology caused by *Sarcoptes*.

The most prominent symptom is itching, which is especially intense at night, forcing patients to scratch themselves. Such scratching can cause lesions, new foci of scabies and, often, purulent secondary infections. Irritation and pruritis are manifested one or two weeks after infestation and are due primarily to a type I allergic reaction. Scabies can persist for a long time if not treated; in fact, homologous human scabies is unlikely to heal by itself.

It is believed that animal mites do not generally excavate tunnels in human skin and that the infestation is more superficial. This does not, however, explain the sometimes intense itching that zoonotic infestations cause. A researcher who experimentally infested herself with canine *Sarcoptes* was able to confirm by histopathologic examination the existence of mite tunnels in her skin (Kummel, cited in Schwartzmann, 1983). The lesion can vary from a pruriginous papular eruption, which is the most common form, to an intense allergic sensitization with the appearance of vesicles. Excoriations from scratching are also frequent. The location of lesions in 22 patients infested by *S. scabiei* var. *canis* corresponded to the places most exposed to infested dogs, such as forearms, hands, torso, and thighs (Smith and Claypole, 1967). In 35 patients who were in contact with water buffaloes infested with *S. scabiei* var. *bubalis*, the lesions were distributed on the face, fingers, hands, thighs, and legs (Chakrabarti *et al.*, 1981). In 30 persons infested with swine *Sarcoptes*, the lesions occurred on hands and legs (Chakrabarti, 1990). Zoonotic scabies is unlikely to affect the interdigital folds and external genital organs, which are often affected by homologous scabies. In addition, zoonotic scabies heals by itself and does not last more than one to three weeks. Spontaneous healing is attributed to the fact that the parasites do not multiply or only reproduce for a short time on the heterologous host. An infestation that lasts longer is usually due to ongoing exposure and permanent superinfestation. Treatment of the animal species originating the scabies is usually sufficient to eliminate human zoonotic scabies without treatment in a couple of weeks.

The Disease in Animals: Sarcoptic scabies in animals generally starts on the head and on areas of the body with delicate skin (Davis and Moon, 1990). In equines, the lesions are observed on the head and neck; in dogs, on the ear flaps, snout, and elbows. As with the human parasites, the animal mites produce an allergic sensitization with intense itching and the formation of papules and vesicles. Vigorous scratching by the affected animals causes the vesicles to open and become covered with scales and then scabby plaques, which often ooze a serous liquid. Over time, there is a proliferation of the connective tissue and hyperkeratinization, causing the skin to thicken and form creases. Hair loss in the affected areas as a result of scratching is also frequent. Scabies limited to a small area does not particularly affect an animal's health, but when it spreads to large areas of the body it can have an adverse impact and even cause death.

Source of Infestation and Mode of Transmission: *Sarcoptes* is transmitted mainly by recently inseminated females before they begin to build their tunnels. *Notoedres*, in contrast, is transmitted by larvae or nymphs. In both cases, the skin of the susceptible individual must be in close contact with the skin of the infested individual. In the case of interhuman transmission of *Sarcoptes*, the mite has been found on fomites, and thus contagion through contaminated objects seems possible. Since the parasite can survive for several days off an animal's body on clothing, towels, bedclothes, animal bedding, harnesses, and horse blankets, these objects can serve as sources of infestation.

Each animal species is a reservoir of the mite that attacks its own kind, but cross-transmission between species occasionally occurs. Human scabies is transmitted primarily from person to person, but several animals, such as horses, dogs, cattle, bubalids, sheep, goats, swine, camels, and zoo animals, can occasionally transmit it to man. One of the most common sources of zoonotic scabies is the dog. Infestation by *S. scabiei* var. *canis* occurs through close contact with scabietic dogs and can appear in several members of the family at the same time. It has been estimated that almost 1% of the dogs in the UK have scabies; a study of 65 persons who had been in contact with 28 scabietic dogs confirmed the presence of scabietic lesions in 34 of them. In the US Army dermatology clinic at Fort Benning, Georgia, 20 cases of scabies acquired from dogs were observed in the course of one year (Smith and Claypole, 1967). The University of Pennsylvania found that around 33% of dogs with scabies caused infestations in members of their owners' families (Schwartzmann, 1983). The School of Veterinary Medicine of São Paulo, Brazil tracked human infestation among 143 individuals who were exposed to 27 dogs with sarcoptic scabies; cutaneous lesions compatible with scabiosis were found in 58 (40.6%) of them (Larsson, 1978). When scabies was still common in domestic animals in the Netherlands, around 25% of the veterinarians in rural areas were infested with *Sarcoptes* of zoonotic origin. Scabies of animal origin is also observed in rural inhabitants. Transmission of sarcoptic scabies (*S. scabiei* var. *bubalis*) from water buffaloes to man was described in India. Of 52 persons who had been in contact with scabietic buffaloes, 35 (67.3%) had symptoms of scabies, and the presence of the mite was confirmed in 22 (42.3%). All of the persons who contracted the infestation (people in charge of handling and milking the buffaloes) had intense pruritus a few hours after initial contact with the affected animals (Chakrabarti *et al.*, 1981).

Zoonotic scabies is not an important public health problem because it resolves spontaneously and is not transmitted between humans.

Diagnosis: The presence of sarcoptic scabies is suspected because of intense pruritus and typically located lesions. For the specific diagnosis of homologous infestations in man and animals, the recommendation is to cover the papules and a scalpel blade with a thin layer of mineral oil so that the mites and skin scales stick to it, scrape five to seven times until a small amount of blood is drawn, and examine the scrapings under a microscope to detect the presence of mites. A solution of 10% to 15% sodium or potassium hydroxide can be added to the microscope slide, which can then be heated slightly for 5 minutes to clarify the cornified cells that hinder observation. Since this procedure is painful for patients, in human cases the recommendation is to try and remove the mite from the furrows with a needle. However, the sensitivity of this method is so low that it is almost not worth attempting. Direct examination of the skin with an epifluorescent microscope is also recommended, since this method is quick, painless, and sensitive to the diagnosis of scabies (Argenziano *et al.*, 1997).

Zoonotic scabies in humans is more difficult to diagnose because the mites are much less numerous and most seem to move about on the skin. Transparent cellophane tape can be applied to the skin and then examined under a microscope in the hope that a mite has been picked up, but this is not very effective because there is no precise method of determining where the mites are.

Control: In order to prevent human scabies of zoonotic origin, infestation of animals must be prevented or contact with animals suspected of being infested must be avoided. It is easier and more effective to treat pets with acaricides in order to eradicate the infestation. When there is professional contact with animals that may be infested (handling of swine, goats, etc.), gloves and high boots of a material that mites cannot penetrate should be used.

Bibliography

Argenziano, G., G. Fabbrocini, M. Delfino. Epiluminescence microscopy. A new approach to *in vivo* detection of *Sarcoptes scabiei*. *Arch Dermatol* 133(6):751–753, 1997.

Arlian, L.G., M.S. Morgan, J.J. Arends. Immunologic cross-reactivity among various strains of *Sarcoptes scabiei*. *J Parasitol* 82(1):66–72, 1996.

Beck, W. [Animal mite-induced epizoonoses and their significance in dermatology]. *Hautarzt* 47(10):744–748, 1996.

Chakrabarti, A. Some epidemiological aspects of animal scabies in human population. *Int J Zoonoses* 12(1):39–52, 1985.

Chakrabarti, A. Pig handler's itch. *Int J Dermatol* 29(3):205–206, 1990.

Chakrabarti, A., A. Chatterjee, K. Chakrabarti, D.N. Sengupta. Human scabies from contact with water buffaloes infested with *Sarcoptes scabiei* var. *bubalis*. *Ann Trop Med Parasitol* 75(3):353–357, 1981.

Davis, D.P., R.D. Moon. Dynamics of swine mange: A critical review of the literature. *J Med Entomol* 27(5):727–737, 1990.

Elgart, M.L. Scabies. *Dermatol Clin* 8(2):253–263, 1990.

Fimiani, M., C. Mazzatenta, C. Alessandrini, E. Paccagnini, L. Andreassi. The behaviour of *Sarcoptes scabiei* var. *hominis* in human skin: An ultrastructural study. *J Submicrosc Cytol Pathol* 29(1):105–113, 1997.

Fontaine, J. Zoonoses et dermatoses: le point de vue du veterinaire. *Rev Med Brux* 21(4):A247–250, 2000.

Larsson, M.H. Evidências epidemiológicas da ocorrência de escabiose em humanos, causada pelo *Sarcoptes scabiei* (Degeer, 1778) var. *canis* (Botirguignon, 1853). *Rev Saude Publica* 12(3):333–339, 1978.

Lee, W.K., B.K. Cho. [Taxonomical approach to scabies mites of human and animals and their prevalence in Korea]. *Korean J Parasitol* 33(2):85–94, 1995.

Mitra, M., S.K. Mahanta, S. Sen, C. Ghosh, A.K. Hati. *Sarcoptes scabiei* in animals spreading to man. *Trop Geogr Med* 45(3):142–143, 1993.

Normaznah, Y., K. Saniah, M. Nazma, J.W. Mak, M. Krishnasamy, S.L. Hakin. Seroprevalence of *Sarcoptes scabiei* var. *canis* antibodies among aborigines in peninsular Malaysia. *Southeast Asian J Trop Med Public Health* 27(1):53–56, 1996.

Parish, L.C., R.M. Schwartzman. Zoonoses of dermatological interest. *Semin Dermatol* 12(1):57–64, 1993.

Park, G.S., J.S. Park, B.K. Cho, W.K. Lee, J.H. Cho. [Mite infestation rate of pet dogs with ear dermatoses]. *Korean J Parasitol* 34(2):143–150, 1996.

Skerratt, L.F., I. Beveridge. Human scabies of wombat origin. *Aust Vet J* 77(9):607, 1999.

Schwartzman, R.M. Scabies in animals. *In*: Parish, L.C., W.B. Nutting, R.M. Schwartzman, eds. *Cutaneous Infestations of Man and Animal*. New York: Praeger; 1983.

Smith, E.B., T.F. Claypoole. Canine scabies in dogs and in humans. *JAMA* 199(2):59–64, 1967.

Walton, S.F., J.L. Choy, A. Bonson, *et al.* Genetically distinct dog-derived and human-derived *Sarcoptes scabiei* in scabies-endemic communities in northern Australia. *Am J Trop Med Hyg* 61(4):542–547, 1999.

INDEX

NOTES

NOTES

NOTES

NOTES

NOTES